# Clinical Anesthesiology

# Clinical Anesthesiology

Edited by Pam Kellner

hayle medical
New York

Hayle Medical,
750 Third Avenue, 9th Floor,
New York, NY 10017, USA

Visit us on the World Wide Web at:
www.haylemedical.com



ISBN: 978-1-63241-526-4



**Cataloging-in-Publication Data**

Clinical anesthesiology / edited by Pam Kellner.
p. cm.
Includes bibliographical references and index.
ISBN 978-1-63241-526-4
1. Anesthesiology. I. Kellner, Pam.

RD81 .C55 2018
617.96--dc23

# Table of Contents

# Preface

This book has been an outcome of determined endeavour from a group of educationists in the field. The primary objective was to involve a broad spectrum of professionals from diverse cultural background involved in the field for developing new researches. The book not only targets students but also scholars pursuing higher research for further enhancement of the theoretical and practical applications of the subject.

Clinical anesthesiology focuses on the use of anesthesia for medical purposes. It places a person in a temporary state of unconsciousness. Anesthesia is categorized into regional anesthesia or general anesthesia. Regional anesthesia is mainly used in cases in which only a particular region of the body needs to be numbed such as in childbirth. This book presents the complex subject of anesthesiology in the most comprehensible and easy to understand language. It strives to provide a fair idea about this discipline and to help develop a better understanding of the latest advances within this field. The readers would gain knowledge that would broaden their perspective about the subject matter.

It was an honour to edit such a profound book and also a challenging task to compile and examine all the relevant data for accuracy and originality. I wish to acknowledge the efforts of the contributors for submitting such brilliant and diverse chapters in the field and for endlessly working for the completion of the book. Last, but not the least; I thank my family for being a constant source of support in all my research endeavours.

**Editor**

1

# Posterior Cingulate Cortex-Related Co-Activation Patterns: A Resting State fMRI Study in Propofol-Induced Loss of Consciousness

**Enrico Amico[1,2]*, Francisco Gomez[1], Carol Di Perri[7], Audrey Vanhaudenhuyse[1,6], Damien Lesenfants[1], Pierre Boveroux[1,4], Vincent Bonhomme[1,4,5], Jean-François Brichant[4], Daniele Marinazzo[2], Steven Laureys[1,3]**

**1** Coma Science Group, Cyclotron Research Centre, University of Liège, Liège, Belgium, **2** Faculty of Psychology and Educational Sciences, Department of Data Analysis, Ghent University, Ghent, Belgium, **3** Department of Neurology, University of Liège, Liège, Belgium, **4** Department of Anesthesia and Intensive Care Medicine, CHU Sart Tilman Hospital, University of Liège, Liège, Belgium, **5** Department of Anesthesia and Intensive Care Medicine, CHR Citadelle, University of Liège, Liège, Belgium, **6** Department of Algology and Palliative Care, CHU Sart Tilman Hospital, University of Liège, Liège, Belgium, **7** Department of Neuroradiology, National Neurological Institute C. Mondino, Pavia, Italy

## Abstract

***Background:*** Recent studies have been shown that functional connectivity of cerebral areas is not a static phenomenon, but exhibits spontaneous fluctuations over time. There is evidence that fluctuating connectivity is an intrinsic phenomenon of brain dynamics that persists during anesthesia. Lately, point process analysis applied on functional data has revealed that much of the information regarding brain connectivity is contained in a fraction of critical time points of a resting state dataset. In the present study we want to extend this methodology for the investigation of resting state fMRI spatial pattern changes during propofol-induced modulation of consciousness, with the aim of extracting new insights on brain networks consciousness-dependent fluctuations.

***Methods:*** Resting-state fMRI volumes on 18 healthy subjects were acquired in four clinical states during propofol injection: wakefulness, sedation, unconsciousness, and recovery. The dataset was reduced to a spatio-temporal point process by selecting time points in the Posterior Cingulate Cortex (PCC) at which the signal is higher than a given threshold (i.e., BOLD intensity above 1 standard deviation). Spatial clustering on the PCC time frames extracted was then performed (number of clusters = 8), to obtain 8 different PCC co-activation patterns (CAPs) for each level of consciousness.

***Results:*** The current analysis shows that the core of the PCC-CAPs throughout consciousness modulation seems to be preserved. Nonetheless, this methodology enables to differentiate region-specific propofol-induced reductions in PCC-CAPs, some of them already present in the functional connectivity literature (e.g., disconnections of the prefrontal cortex, thalamus, auditory cortex), some others new (e.g., reduced co-activation in motor cortex and visual area).

***Conclusion:*** In conclusion, our results indicate that the employed methodology can help in improving and refining the characterization of local functional changes in the brain associated to propofol-induced modulation of consciousness.

**Editor:** Yong He, Beijing Normal University, Beijing, China

**Funding:** This research was supported by the Belgian Funds for Scientific Research (FRS), European Commission (DECODER), Belgian Science Policy (CEREBNET), McDonnell Foundation, European Space Agency, Wallonia-Brussels Federation Concerted Research Action Mind Science Foundation, University of Liège. The funders had no role in study design, data collection and analysis, decision to publish, or preparation of the manuscript.

* Email: eamico@ulg.ac.be

## Introduction

Functional magnetic resonance imaging (fMRI) technique has been widely used in the investigation of brain connectivity patterns at rest [1,2]. Blood-oxygen-level dependent (BOLD) signal activity at rest is organized in correlated spatial patterns, which are called "resting state networks" (i.e. RSNs). These networks have been increasingly investigated and their modulation or disruption has been associated to several pathophysiological conditions [3,4], together with the importance of these RSNs to provide information about brain dynamic organization, as a complement to structural information.

In particular, in altered states of consciousness it's important to see which functional connections remain unaltered and which ones are modified or disrupted [5,6]. In this regards, functional connectivity studies of RSNs in induced sedation through anesthesia, have shown widespread changes in fronto-parietal networks, compared with the relative preservation of sensory networks, suggesting a major role of higher-order frontoparietal associative network activity in the loss of consciousness phenom-

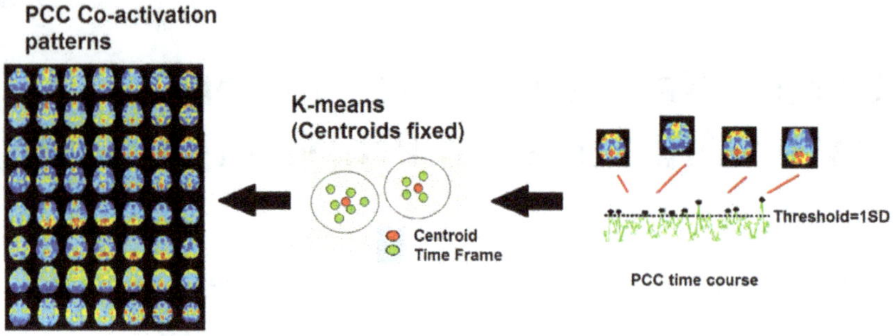


**Figure 1. Co-activation patterns (CAPs).** The approach is similar to the ones proposed in [16] and [15]. After the extraction of a seed region, in this case Posterior Cingulate Cortex (PCC), a threshold equal to 1 standard deviation(SD) was applied, as to consider only the time points corresponding to peaks in the BOLD signal; next, the spatial maps (namely, time frames), associated with these time points are collected and clusterized using k-means, with a number of clusters fixed to 8. The centroids were kept fixed as well, to allow cluster comparison between the different clinical conditions. The within-cluster time frames were then averaged to obtain 8 spatial PCC-related co-activation patterns. Finally, the computation was iterated over the 4 different states of consciousness (wakefulness, sedation, unconsciousness, recovery), obtaining 8 PCC-related co-activation patterns for each state.

ena [7,8]. Moreover, functional impairment of highly connected frontoparietal areas seems to have greater repercussions on global brain function than on less centrally connected sensorimotor areas [9,10].

Additionally, recent studies have been shown that functional connectivity of cerebral areas is not a static phenomenon, but exhibits spontaneous fluctuations over time [11–13]. Previously, fluctuations of functional connectivity have been thought to reflect changing levels of vigilance, task switching or conscious processing. There is evidence that fluctuating connectivity is an intrinsic phenomenon of brain dynamics that persists even during anesthesia [11]. Fluctuations of functional connectivity within an attention network in macaques have been demonstrated and interpreted as mechanistically important network information [14]. Still, the relationship between changes of consciousness and network dynamics is not understood yet.

Lately, a new approach in exploring functional brain connectivity, using point process analysis, has been proposed by Tagliazucchi et al. [15]. The main idea in this work is that important features of brain functional connectivity at rest can be obtained from BOLD fluctuations, isolating the periods in which the signal crosses some amplitude threshold. In this way the study of the dynamics of a continuous BOLD time series is reduced to the exploration of a discretized one (a point process), defined by time and location of BOLD signal threshold crossings. Through point process analysis, Tagliazucchi and colleagues showed that much of the information regarding a specific RSN is actually contained in a fraction of critical time points (i.e. BOLD signal peaks) of a resting state dataset. This idea has next been adopted by Liu et al. [16], in a study showing that seed-based RSNs extracted from fMRI BOLD signal are averages of multiple distinct spatial co-activations patterns (CAPs) at different time points, and that the analysis of these patterns might provide more fine-grained information on brain functional network organization.

In the present study we want to extend and apply this methodology for the investigation of fMRI resting state spatial pattern changes during propofol-induced modulation of consciousness, with the central aim of extracting new information regarding brain networks consciousness-dependent fluctuations.

## Materials and Methods

### Ethics Statement

The study was approved by the Ethics Committee of the Medical School of the University of Liège (University Hospital, Liège, Belgium). The subjects provided written informed consent to participate in the study.

### Clinical Protocol

The present work is a reanalysis of previous published data [7,8]. Eighteen healthy right-handed volunteers participated in the study. Subjects fasted for at least 6 h from solids and 2 h from liquids before sedation. During the study and the recovery period, electrocardiogram, blood pressure, pulse oxymetry (SpO2), and breathing frequency were continuously monitored (Magnitude 3150M; Invivo Research, Inc., Orlando,FL). Propofol was infused through an intravenous catheter placed into a vein of the right hand or forearm. An arterial catheter was placed into the left radial artery. Throughout the study, the subjects breathed spontaneously, and additional oxygen (5 l/min) was given through a loosely fitting plastic facemask. The level of consciousness was evaluated clinically throughout the study with the scale used by Ramsay et al. [17].

The subject was asked to strongly squeeze the hand of the investigator. She/he was considered fully awake or to have recovered consciousness if the response to verbal command (squeeze my hand) was clear and strong (Ramsay 2), in sedation if the response to verbal command was clear but slow (Ramsay 3), and in unconsciousness if there was no response to verbal command (Ramsay 5–6). For each consciousness level assessment, Ramsay scale verbal commands were repeated twice. Functional MRI acquisitions consisted of resting-state functional MRI volumes repeated in four clinical states: normal wakefulness (Ramsay 2), sedation (Ramsay 3), unconsciousness (Ramsay 5), and recovery of consciousness (Ramsay 2). The typical scan duration was half an hour in each condition. The number of scans per session (197 functional volumes) was matched in each subject to obtain a similar number of scans in all four clinical states. Functional images were acquired on a 3 Tesla Siemens Allegra scanner (Siemens AG, Munich, Germany; Echo Planar Imaging sequence using 32 slices; repetition time = 2460 ms, echo time = 40 ms, field of view = 220 mm, voxel size = $3.45\times3.45\times3$ mm$^3$, and matrix size = $64\times64\times32$).

**Table 1.** Stereotactic coordinates of peak voxels in clusters of PCC-CAPs showing a linear correlation with propofol-induced changes in consciousness.

| CAP 1 | x | y | z | Z-value | FDR-p |
|---|---|---|---|---|---|
| Right Superior Frontal Gyrus | 18 | 42 | 48 | 5.41 | 0.002 |
| Left Superior Medial Frontal Gyrus | −9 | 60 | 30 | 5.12 | 0.002 |
| Left Mid Orbital Gyrus | 0 | 57 | −9 | 4.65 | 0.004 |
| Right Superior Medial Frontal Gyrus | 9 | 57 | 36 | 4.06 | 0.016 |
| **CAP 2** | **x** | **y** | **z** | **Z-value** | **FDR-p** |
| Left Superior Medial Frontal Gyrus | −3 | 60 | 9 | 6.55 | <0.001 |
| Left Superior Frontal Gyrus | −15 | 60 | 24 | 6.55 | <0.001 |
| Right Precuneus | 3 | −54 | 36 | 5.54 | <0.001 |
| Left Middle Cingulate Cortex | 0 | −36 | 39 | 3.09 | 0.011 |
| Right ParaHippocampal Gyrus | 24 | −21 | −18 | 4.47 | <0.001 |
| Right Angular Gyrus | 60 | −63 | 33 | 3.97 | <0.001 |
| Left Middle Temporal Gyrus | −63 | −15 | −24 | 3.38 | 0.005 |
| **CAP 3** | **x** | **y** | **z** | **Z-value** | **FDR-p** |
| Left Anterior Cingulate Cortex | 0 | 39 | 15 | 5.23 | 0.003 |
| Thalamus | 0 | −12 | 0 | 4.48 | 0.012 |
| **CAP 5** | **x** | **y** | **z** | **Z-value** | **FDR-p** |
| Right Superior Medial Frontal Gyrus | 3 | 57 | 12 | 6.55 | <0.001 |
| Left Superior Medial Frontal Gyrus | 0 | 57 | 3 | 6.55 | <0.001 |
| Left Precentral Gyrus | −39 | −18 | 60 | 5.47 | <0.001 |
| Right Cerebellum | 27 | −33 | −33 | 5.053 | <0.001 |
| Hippocampus | 15 | −33 | −9 | 3.47 | 0.011 |
| Right Precuneus | 3 | −57 | 21 | 4.83 | <0.001 |
| Left Middle Temporal Gyrus | −66 | −15 | −21 | 4.75 | <0.001 |
| Right Inferior Occipital Gyrus | 48 | −81 | −6 | 4.03 | 0.002 |
| Left Superior Frontal Gyrus | −21 | 30 | 48 | 4.51 | <0.001 |
| Right Postcentral Gyrus | 57 | −15 | 48 | 4.28 | <0.001 |
| Right Precentral Gyrus | 48 | −15 | 60 | 3.64 | 0.006 |
| Left Precuneus | −9 | −45 | 39 | 3.61 | 0.007 |
| **CAP 6** | **x** | **y** | **z** | **Z-value** | **FDR-p** |
| Left Middle Frontal Gyrus | −24 | 30 | 54 | 7.52 | <0.001 |
| Right Superior Frontal Gyrus | 27 | 27 | 54 | 7.11 | <0.001 |
| Right Middle Frontal Gyrus | 45 | 18 | 48 | 5.68 | <0.001 |
| Right Precuneus | 9 | −54 | 15 | 6.12 | <0.001 |
| Left Hippocampus | −15 | −33 | −6 | 5.09 | <0.001 |
| Left Middle Temporal Gyrus | −57 | −18 | −24 | 5.55 | <0.001 |
| Right Fusiform Gyrus | 30 | −27 | −21 | 4.71 | <0.001 |
| Right ParaHippocampal Gyrus | 30 | −36 | −9 | 3.69 | 0.005 |
| **CAP 7** | **x** | **y** | **z** | **Z-value** | **FDR-p** |
| Left Thalamus | 6 | −12 | 9 | 5,48 | <0.001 |
| Right Thalamus | 6 | −12 | 0 | 5,48 | <0.001 |
| Left Anterior Cingulate Cortex | 0 | 48 | 9 | 5,25 | <0.001 |
| Left Precuneus | −15 | −60 | 21 | 4,67 | 0,001 |
| Right Precuneus | 12 | −51 | 15 | 4,43 | 0,002 |
| Right Calcarine Gyrus | 12 | −60 | 15 | 4,37 | 0,002 |
| Right Middle Frontal Gyrus | 33 | 30 | 45 | 4,19 | 0,003 |
| Right Superior Frontal Gyrus | 24 | 33 | 54 | 3,61 | 0,012 |
| Right Inferior Temporal Gyrus | 54 | 3 | −39 | 3,93 | 0,006 |

**Table 1.** Cont.

| CAP 7 | x | y | z | Z-value | FDR-p |
|---|---|---|---|---|---|
| Left Middle Cingulate Cortex | 0 | −33 | 48 | 3,86 | 0,007 |
| Hippocampus | −24 | −9 | −21 | 3,84 | 0,007 |
| Right Inferior Frontal Gyrus | 48 | 39 | 15 | 3,74 | 0,009 |
| Right Inferior Parietal Lobule | 51 | −51 | 57 | 3,47 | 0,016 |
| **CAP 8** | **x** | **y** | **z** | **Z-value** | **FDR-p** |
| Left Postcentral Gyrus | −54 | −18 | 54 | 6,58 | <0.001 |
| Right Postcentral Gyrus | 63 | −12 | 42 | 4,86 | 0,001 |
| Right Precentral Gyrus | 48 | −6 | 60 | 3,91 | 0,011 |
| Right Middle Temporal Gyrus | 60 | −12 | −24 | 4,76 | 0,002 |
| Left Superior Medial Frontal Gyrus | 0 | 57 | 6 | 3,82 | 0,013 |
| Left Anterior Cingulate Cortex | −12 | 45 | 0 | 3,65 | 0,018 |
| Left Middle Temporal Gyrus | −57 | −6 | −18 | 4,43 | 0,005 |
| Left Rolandic Operculum | −39 | 0 | 15 | 4,32 | 0,005 |
| Left Insula Lobe | −42 | −9 | 3 | 3,84 | 0,012 |
| Right Rolandic Operculum | 48 | −12 | 21 | 4,15 | 0,007 |
| Left Amygdala | −27 | −3 | −24 | 3,95 | 0,011 |
| Right Hippocampus | 30 | −3 | −24 | 3,95 | 0,011 |

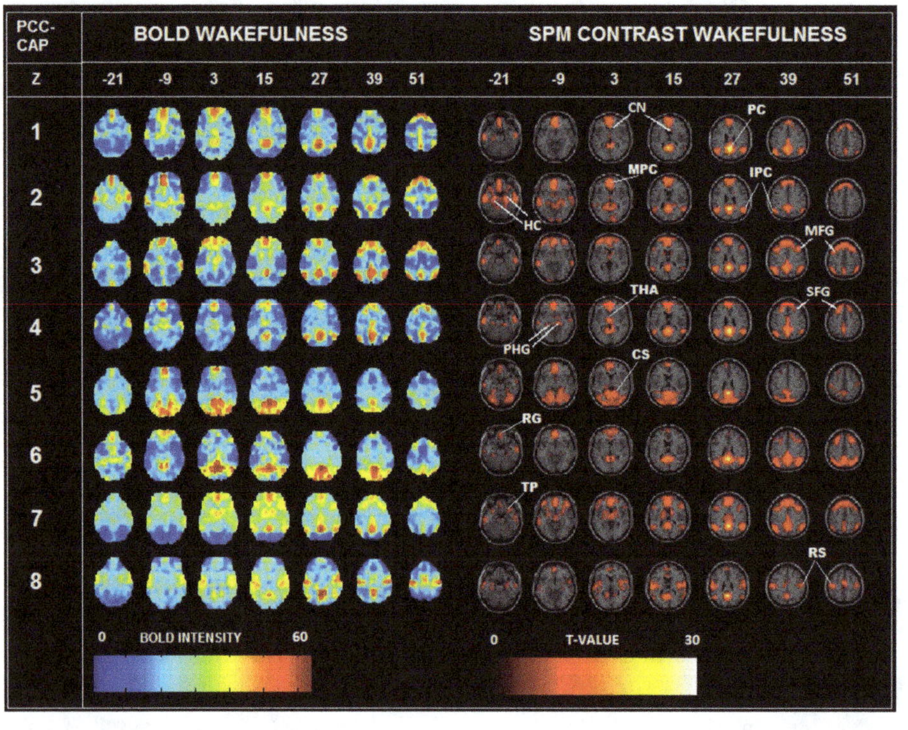


**Figure 2. PCC-CAPs in wakefulness.** Left: PCC co-activation patterns in wakefulness (colormap normalized by BOLD intensity), current dataset (18 subjects). Note the similarity of these patterns with the ones showed in Fig. 2 of [16]. Right: t-test on the same CAPs in the awake state showing statistically significant PCC co-activations. The seven slices shown in the maps are at Z = −21, −9, 3, 15, 27, 39, 51, respectively. The activation of precuneus (PC) appears in all 8 CAPs (see Z = 27); superior frontal gyrus (SFG) is co-activated in CAPs 1, 2, 3, 4, 6, 7 (Z = 39 and 51); the mesial prefrontal cortex (MPC) in CAPs 1, 2, 3, 4, 5, 6, 7 (Z = 3); rectus gyrus (RG) in CAPs 1, 2, 3,4, 5, 6, 7 (Z = −21); thalamus(THA) in CAPs 4 and 7 (Z = 3); caudate nucleus (CN) in CAPs 1, 3, 7 (Z = 15); temporal pole (TP) in all CAPs (slice Z = −21); hippocampus(HC) in CAPs 2, 4, 6, 8 (Z = −21); parahippocampus gyrus(PHG) in CAPs 2 and 4 (Z = −9); intraparietal cortex(IPC) all CAPs (Z = 27); medial frontal gyrus(MFG) in CAPs 3, 6, 7 (Z = 39); cuneus(CS) in CAPs 4 and 5 (Z = 3); rolandic stripe(RS) in CAPs 5 and 8 (Z = 51). Note how all these region-specific PCC co-activations survive to the t-test (e.g. HC for CAPs 2, 4, 6, 8; MFG for CAPs 3, 6, 7; PHG for CAPs 2, 4 etc.)

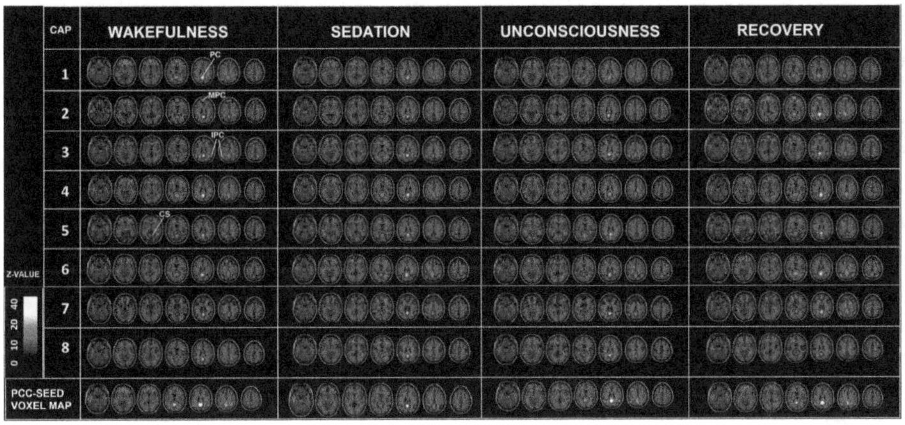


**Figure 3. CAPs at different levels of consciousness.** Co-activation patterns (t-contrast) in wakefulness (left), sedation (middle-left), unconsciousness (middle-right), recovery (right), corrected at FDR $p<0.05$. Lower panel shows PCC seed-voxel correlation maps for each state. The seven slices shown in the maps are at Z = −21, −9, 3, 15, 27, 39, 51, respectively. Spatial patterns in wakefulness and recovery do not significantly differ from each other. Precuneal (PC) activations are preserved in all CAPs in all conditions (Z = 27 and Z = 39); mesial prefrontal (MPC) cortical activity is preserved in CAPs 1, 2, 3, 4 and 7 during wakefulness, sedation and recovery (Z = 27); intraparietal cortex (IPC) activation is preserved in CAPs 1, 2, 3, 4, 6 and 7 in all conditions (Z = 39); cuneus(CS) in CAPs 4 and 5 in all conditions (Z = 3). Note that PCC-CAPs add spatial region-specific information to the network characterization across the different stages of consciousness, when compared to the equivalent PCC seed-based contrast (last row), which exhibit a prominent drop of frontal activation during sedation and unconsciousness.

## fMRI preprocessing

The fMRI data were preprocessed using Statistical Parametric Software (SPM8), performing the typical preprocessing steps of functional connectivity analysis. These steps included motion correction, spatial smoothing (FWHM = 8 mm), temporal filtering with a bandpass filter (0.005 to 0.1 Hz), and the removal of linear and quadratic temporal trends. In addition, the brain-averaged signal, the time series of regions of interest in the white matter and cerebrospinal fluid, and six affine motion parameters were regressed out from the dataset. The fMRI data of each subject was first spatially coregistered to high-resolution anatomical images and then to the 152-brain Montreal Neurological Institute (MNI) space. It has recently been shown that even after standard motion correction, residual head movements can still inflate connectivity measures [18]. In order to evaluate the extent of these residual motion artifact in CAPs, for each subject and for each state of consciousness, we computed the two indices proposed by [18], i.e. Framewise Displacement (FD) and DVARS: D referring to temporal derivative of timecourses, VARS referring to root mean square (RMS) variance over voxels. FD is a scalar quantity that expresses instantaneous head motion, while DVARS is a measure of how much the intensity of a brain image changes in comparison to the previous timepoint [18]. Secondly, we defined as motion corrupted the frames in which FD and DVARS values were both above 0.5 mm for FD and 0.5% Bold for DVARS, as suggested in the same paper. Next, for each state of consciousness, we checked if there were corrupted time frames in our PCC-CAPs, and the percentage of these frames over the whole sample (see also Figure S4). We noticed that the percentage of corrupted time frames in wakefulness was 5% of the total number of frames collected; in sedation 3%; in unconsciousness 8%; in recovery 1%. However, there was no significant difference between CAPs calculated with or without artifact removal. Additionally, the preprocessed fMRI data were resampled to $3\times3\times3$ mm$^3$ in the MNI space, and the signal of each voxel was demeaned and normalized by its temporal standard deviation (SD).

## Co-activation patterns construction

After preprocessing, the dataset was reduced to a spatio-temporal point process [15] by selecting time points in the seed region at which the signal is higher than a given threshold. In this work we used a $6\times6\times6$ mm$^3$ cube centered at the posterior cingulate cortex (i.e. PCC, [0, 53, 26] in MNI coordinates, identical to Liu et al. [16]). We chose PCC as seed to study default mode network (DMN) variability during consciousness modulation, since PCC is widely known as a central node in the DMN [19,20]. CAPs construction can then be summarized in three steps (Fig. 1):

1. First, we collected all the points in the normalized PCC time course where the BOLD signal was above threshold. In our study we fixed the threshold at 1 SD, roughly the 15% of the whole dataset. This percentage did not significantly vary across the four levels of consciousness. For each of these points in the PCC, and for each of the 4 levels of consciousness, we collected the relative spatial maps (Fig. 1). These spatial maps, or time frames [16], represent whole-brain patterns of functional activations correlated to PCC BOLD peaks, previously extracted using this thresholding approach.
2. In order to achieve a spatio-temporal mapping of correlated activity we clustered all the time frames which were significantly co-activated with PCC, in the same way as described in [16]. The sorting of the time frames was performed by K-means clustering, a machine learning classification method able to group unlabeled data into clusters. Once that the desired number of clusters has been fixed, K-means iteratively optimizes the position of the centers in order to minimize the total variance within each cluster [21]. We performed K-means (number of clusters fixed at 8) over all the spatial maps collected to classify the time frames based on their spatial similarity, and then averaging them within-cluster to extract 8 different spatial PCC-related co-activation patterns (i.e. CAPs [16]). Here, since we also aimed to compare different PCC-CAPs between different conditions (i.e. 4 different levels of consciousness), we added an extra step. With the purpose of

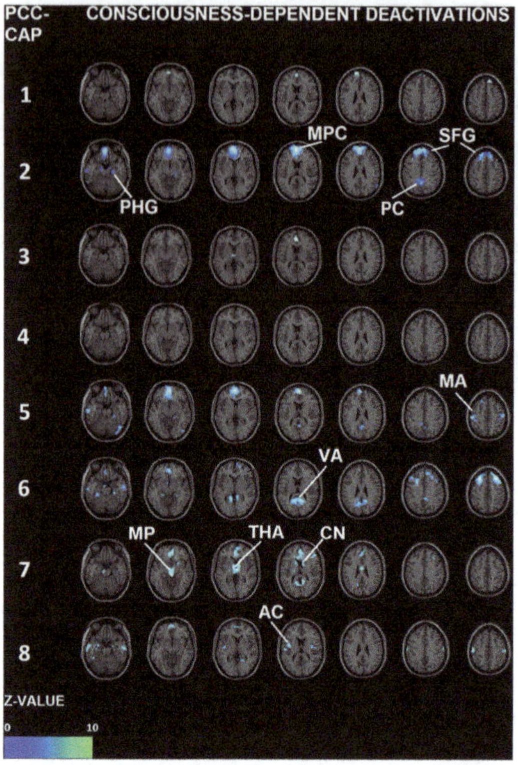


**Figure 4. Decreases in CAPs.** This figure shows the local decreases in co-activation from wakefulness to unconsciousness, using the same t-contrast as in [7]. All the images report contrast which are significant at $p<0.05$, FDR corrected. The seven slices shown in the maps are at Z = −21, −9, 3, 15, 27, 39, 51, respectively. CAPs consciousness-dependent deactivations appear in mesial prefrontal cortex (MPC), CAPs 1, 2, 5 (see Z = 15); superior fontal gyrus (SFG) in CAP 2 (Z = 39 and 51); thalamus (THA) in CAPs 3 and 7 (Z = 3); mesencephalon (MP) in CAP 7 (Z = −9); motor area (MA) in CAP 5 and CAP 8 (Z = 51); parahippocampal gyrus (PHG) in CAPs 2, 5, 6 (Z = −21); caudate nucleus (CN) in CAP 7 (Z = 15); visual area (VA) in CAP 6 (Z = 15); auditory cortex (AC) in CAP 8 (Z = 15) and precuneus (PC) in CAP 2 (Z = 39). For details see also Fig. 5 and Table 1.

obtaining a robust benchmark baseline against which to track modifications related to level of consciousness, we first ran k-means clustering over the PCC time frames collected on an independent dataset from the 1000 Functional Connectome Project (FCP, *www.nitrc.org/projects/fcon_1000/*), which includes wakefulness resting-state functional magnetic resonance imaging (fMRI) collected at multiple sites (247 subjects), as used by Liu and colleagues [16].

3. The eight PCC-CAPs centroids obtained from the clustering of the 1000 Functional Connectome Project dataset (FCP, *www.nitrc.org/projects/fcon_1000/*) were then kept fixed, and spatial clustering on the PCC time frames extracted from our propofol dataset, for each condition (i.e. wakefulness, sedation, unconsciousness, recovery), was then performed around these centroids, averaging the within-cluster spatial maps to obtain 8 different PCC-CAPs for each level of consciousness. The clustering with centroid fixed allowed us to compare PCC-CAPs between states (i.e. CAP1 in wakefulness with CAP1 in sedation, etc.), and to follow thus the fluctuation of each PCC-CAP over the course of consciousness modulation.

## Statistical analysis

All statistical analyses were carried out using SPM8. For each CAP, individual time frames were entered in a second-level analysis, corresponding to a random effects model in which subjects are considered random variables. These second-level analyses consisted of analyses of variance (repeated measures analysis of variance) with the four clinical conditions as factors: normal wakefulness, sedation, unconsciousness, and recovery of consciousness. The error covariance was not assumed to be independent between regressors, and a correction for non-sphericity was applied. We used one-sided T contrasts, as implemented in Statistical Parametric Mapping software, to test for significant effects in all our analyses. After model estimation, a first T contrast searched for areas co-activated with the PCC during normal wakefulness, sedation, unconsciousness and recovery. Afterwards, in a second analysis a linear one-tailed T contrast was computed for each CAP, searching for a linear relationship between PCC co-activation patterns and the level of consciousness of the subjects across the four conditions (i.e., normal wakefulness, sedation, unconsciousness, and recovery of consciousness, SPM contrast [1.5 −0.5 −1.5 0.5], as previously described in [7]).

It should here be noted that during the recovery of consciousness subjects showed residual plasma propofol levels and lower reaction times scores (table 1 in [7]). Therefore we fixed different SPM contrast values for wakefulness (1.5) and recovery (0.5).

Results were considered significant at $p<0.05$, corrected for multiple comparisons with False Discovery Rate (FDR [22]), as in [7].

## Results

We studied PCC-CAPs in our 18 subjects fMRI resting state dataset, for all the 4 different states of consciousness acquired, i.e. normal wakefulness, sedation, unconsciousness, recovery (see **Material and Methods** section for details). Fig. 2 shows the CAPs obtained in our study, before and after t-contrast on the significant co-activations. These spatial patterns are well reproduced in our smaller cohort (compared to the one obtained from the 1000 Functional Connectome Project dataset, depicted in Fig. 2 of [16]), and they also appear to be statistically significant(see Legend Fig. 2 for details).

Fig. 3 illustrates significant PCC co-activations in wakefulness, sedation, unconsciousness and recovery. The coarse core of the patterns throughout the consciousness modulation seem to be preserved (see Legend Fig. 3 for details). The comparison with the common seed-voxel analysis (bottom) helps to understand the advantage of this methodology, that is the ability to differentiate spatially the activation, adding fine grained information [16].

Preserved CAPs aside, some regions are no longer co-activated with the PCC in states of propofol-reduced consciousness. As to better quantify this phenomenon we decided to use a contrast that correlates with levels of consciousness. Fig. 4 illustrates the regions in each PCC-CAP where activity follows consciousness modulation. Interestingly, results show several region specific drops in CAPs activation that we are able to differentiate thanks to the employed methodology, some of them already shown in literature, some others not. In Fig. 4, CAP 1, 2 5 and 7 show drop in the prefrontal cortex, CAP 3 and 7 isolates the thalamic drop, the auditory and motor cortex decreases come up in CAP 8 and 5, drop of the visual area in CAP 6 (see also Fig. 5 and Table 1 for details).

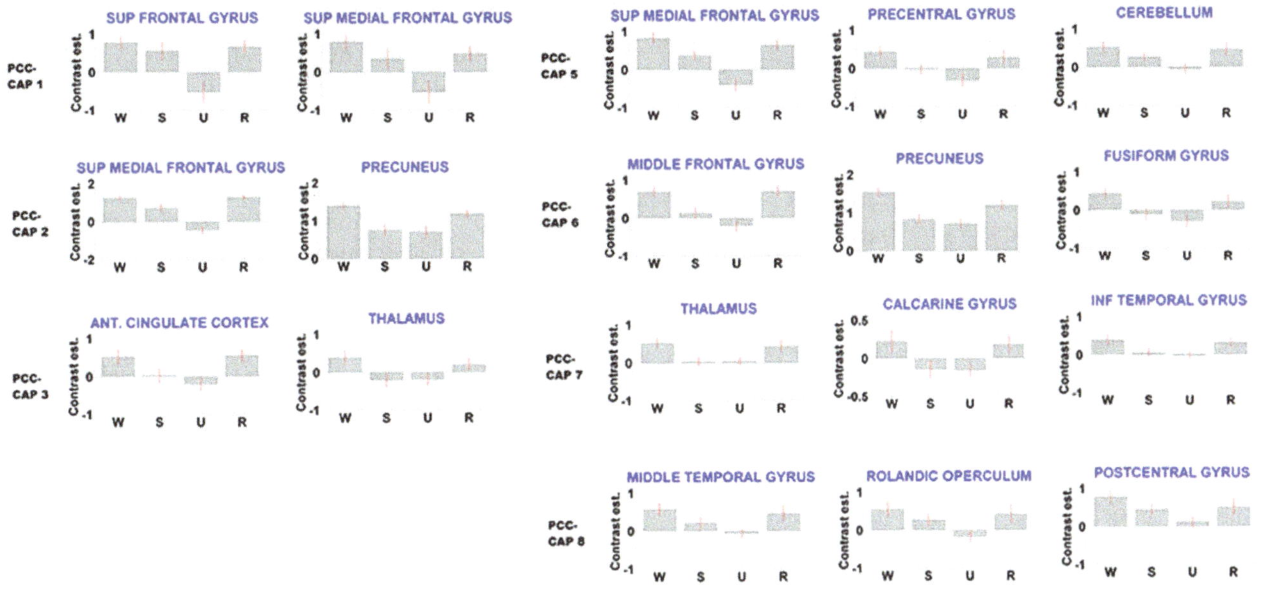


**Figure 5. Region specific consciousness modulation in CAPs.** Parameters estimates for the t-contrast employed, identical as in [7], for some indicative regions where PCC-related activation correlates with propofol-induced changes in consciousness. (mean ± SE; x axis labels: W = wakefulness; S = sedation; U = unconsciousness; R = recovery). Note how PCC co-activation in these regions significantly follows consciousness modulation (see also Table 1).

## Discussion

With the aim to investigate changes in global and local brain activity, in this study we assessed propofol-induced changes in PCC co-activation functional patterns, during wakefulness, sedation, unconsciousness, and wakefulness recovery. Our results contribute to a growing literature addressing the changes in functional connectivity accompanying the loss of consciousness [23–26]. The approach proposed, based on the clustering of instantaneous PCC-related spatial maps, helps in the refinement and the differentiation in the spatial modulation of the default mode network when switching from wakefulness to unconsciousness.

Two key aspects of the methodology proposed in [16], and extended here, are worth discussing. One is the choice of the threshold, that is a crucial step for the construction of a spatio-temporal point process from BOLD time series. We decided to fix our threshold at 1 SD, as in [15], rather than address the threshold in terms of time frame similarity with the seed-based correlation map (see Fig. 1B in [16]). The hypothesis behind this choice is that BOLD signal point processing can help in the spatial characterization of functional connectivity patterns, better than standard correlation analysis (see also Figure S2 and S3). This data-driven evidence is independent of the assumption that BOLD signal peaks may or may not reflect cortical activations [15,27]. In this study we simply focused on spatial clustering of point processed BOLD time series, which allowed us to better characterize functional spatial interaction with the PCC during modulation of consciousness. On the other hand, the employed point process methodology is not purely dominated by hemodynamics. Indeed, co-activations patterns obtained after deconvolving the hemodynamic response function (HRF) at rest as in [27], are not qualitatively different from the ones presented in Fig. 2 (see also Figure S1).

Furthermore, the results from our PCC coactivation patterns seem in line with the ones obtained by Liu [16], in a different cohort and with a different choice of the threshold. This comes out on the side of point process methodology and of the importance of these BOLD signal peaks in spatial differentiation of network co-activations. Also, the use of clustering with centroid fixed, that is new with respect to the approach proposed in [16], can be an useful benchmark for statistical comparison of functional changing patterns between conditions (conscious states in this case, but it could also be used in pathological conditions, etc.).

A primary result is that the core of PCC-CAPs is preserved in anesthesia (Fig. 3). This is in line with other studies [7,14], where, using standard seed-based functional connectivity, the preservation of a core network of correlated regions independent on the level of consciousness was confirmed. The origin of these functional networks could be related to the fixed structural connection present in the awake brain, albeit anesthetized. This partial preservation of functional connectivity in the absence of consciousness has been suggested to possibly reflect preserved anatomical connections dissociated from higher cognitive functions [28].

Also, this approach adds new information on region specific drops in connectivity between the seeds in the DMN area and whole brain connectivity, correlating with levels of consciousness (Fig. 4 and Fig. 5): prefrontal drops (CAP 1, 2, 5, 7) are in line with previous findings in the field, showing widespread changes in prefrontal connectivity [7,9,10]: at the cortical level, hypnotic anesthetic agents have traditionally been considered to decrease activity in a widespread bilateral frontoparietal network. The primary action of hypnotic anesthetic agents would be to functionally disconnect different parts of the cortex, which would probably impair the ability to integrate information [8,23,29]. A recent electroencephalography study similarly suggests the presence of some anterior-posterior functional uncoupling in the brain, during anesthesia-induced loss of consciousness [30].

The disconnection of the thalamic area, already noted in [31,32], is highlighted in CAP 3 and 7. Using positron emission tomography, thalamic metabolism has been shown to decrease significantly during anesthesia-induced unconsciousness [24]. Furthermore, a model has been suggested in which the thalamus orchestrates the commonly observed increased and coherent alpha frequency activity in the frontal cortex during propofol-induced unconsciousness. This steady thalamic alpha rhythm could impede conduction and thus responsiveness to external stimuli [33].

Decrease of activation in the visual area (CAP 6) during anesthesia has previously been studied in monkeys [34,35], where it has been shown how local and global processing in the visual area might depend gradually on the depth of anesthesia. It may also critically depend on information integration mechanisms that function properly only in the awake and perceiving animal [34]. Here, this disconnection is shown in fMRI resting state on humans: thus, this approach seem to enlighten instantaneous spatial connectivity changes between DMN and other external areas, unlikely to be seen with other commonly used correlation analysis (e.g. seed-based functional connectivity).

Similarly, the PCC-related primary motor disconnection is pointed out here (CAP 5 and 8) on fMRI resting state data. These results are in line with previous transcranial magnetic stimulation (TMS) and electroencephalographic (EEG) studies, that indicate intracortical inhibition of central motor circuitry during incremental suppression by a potentiator of GABA agonist (propofol) in a dose-dependent manner [36,37]. The decrease in auditory cortex PCC-coactivation (CAP8) is in agreement with previous findings, in animals [38] and humans [39]. Our finding of decreased auditory cortex co-activation could be related to the hypothesis that propofol bilaterally attenuates the auditory-induced BOLD signal activation of the auditory cortex in a dose-dependent manner [40]. However, it should be noted that activation studies and resting state acquisitions offer different assessments of the underlying neurophysiological activity, in response to external stimulation or during resting conditions, respectively.

A limitation to this approach is the choice of the seed, that needs to be based on a strong priori hypothesis: whole brain connectivity analysis can improve research in this direction. Finally, since it has recently been shown that EEG directional connectivity shows characteristic changes during propofol-induced unconsciousness [41], the nature of BOLD peaks and their correlation with cortical activity needs to be explored using combined fMRI-EEG recordings.

In conclusion, our result show that functional changes in the brain associated to propofol-induced modulation of consciousness can be efficiently revealed by tracking the patterns of co-activation in the Posterior Cingulate Cortex, an area with a central role in the dynamical connectivity at rest. This methodology, based on point process analysis, can help in refining the characterization of local functional disconnections following the partial or total loss of consciousness.

## Supporting Information

**Figure S1 CAPs from BOLD and deconvolved BOLD signal.** To avoid the possibility that the PCC-coactivation patterns were only due to different hemodynamic response functions in the different areas of the brain, we applied the approach proposed in Wu et al. [27], where point process is used to deconvolve the HRF at rest from the BOLD signal. As shown above, the CAPs obtained from the BOLD signal reported in the manuscript are confirmed when obtained from the deconvolved BOLD, suggesting a connection between spatial functional co-activations and neuronal brain response.

**Figure S2 CAPs from negative BOLD peaks.** CAPs obtained using positive threshold crossing (left) and negative threshold crossing (right), during wake resting state (CAPs colormap in absolute Z-value, to make patterns comparable). After the clustering, the specificity of the spatial patterns obtained using positive peaks in BOLD is not reproducible using negative peaks; positive BOLD peaks allow to reconstruct a richer variety of patterns.

**Figure S3 Sliding window correlation vs CAPs.** PCC co-activation patterns in wakefulness (left) compared to the 8 patterns obtained after spatial clustering of the N PCC-correlation maps computed using sliding window correlation, with window size varying from 5 time points (i.e. 12 s window, TR = 2.46 s) to 20 time points (i.e. 50 s window). Note that the region-specific patterns obtained with point process on the BOLD peaks are not recovered by using sliding window correlation. This approach seems to add more refined information in the spatial differentiation of functional networks.

**Figure S4 Motion correction in CAPs.** Example of the procedure discussed in **Materials and Methods**, for one subject, for each level of consciousness (i.e. wakefulness, sedation, unconsciousness, recovery). In order to evaluate the extent of these residual motion artifact in CAPs, for each subject and for each state of consciousness, we computed the two indices proposed by [18], i.e. Framewise Displacement (FD) and DVARS. FD is a scalar quantity that expresses instantaneous head motion, while DVARS is a measure of how much the intensity of a brain image changes in comparison to the previous time point [18]. Secondly, we defined as motion corrupted the frames (ArtFrames in the figure) in which FD and DVARS values were both above 0.5 mm for FD and 0.5.

## Author Contributions

Conceived and designed the experiments: DM SL EA. Performed the experiments: AV DL PB JB VB CD. Analyzed the data: EA FG. Wrote the paper: EA DM SL.

## References

1. Greicius MD, Krasnow B, Reiss AL, Menon V (2003) Functional connectivity in the resting brain: a network analysis of the default mode hypothesis. Proceedings of the National Academy of Sciences 100: 253–258.
2. Fox MD, Snyder AZ, Vincent JL, Corbetta M, Van Essen DC, et al. (2005) The human brain is intrinsically organized into dynamic, anticorrelated functional networks. Proceedings of the National Academy of Sciences of the United States of America 102: 9673–9678.
3. Fox MD, Raichle ME (2007) Spontaneous uctuations in brain activity observed with functional magnetic resonance imaging. Nature Reviews Neuroscience 8: 700–711.
4. Fox MD, Greicius M (2010) Clinical applications of resting state functional connectivity. Frontiers in systems neuroscience 4: 19–24.
5. Boly M, Tshibanda L, Vanhaudenhuyse A, Noirhomme Q, Schnakers C, et al. (2009) Functional connectivity in the default network during resting state is preserved in a vegetative but not in a brain dead patient. Human brain mapping 30: 2393–2400.
6. Vanhaudenhuyse A, Noirhomme Q, Tshibanda LJF, Bruno MA, Boveroux P, et al. (2010) Default network connectivity reects the level of consciousness in non-communicative brain-damaged patients. Brain 133: 161–171.
7. Boveroux P, Vanhaudenhuyse A, Bruno MA, Noirhomme Q, Lauwick S, et al. (2010) Breakdown of within-and between-network resting state functional

magnetic resonance imaging connectivity during propofol-induced loss of consciousness. Anesthesiology 113: 1038–1053.
8. Schrouff J, Perlbarg V, Boly M, Marrelec G, Boveroux P, et al. (2011) Brain functional integration decreases during propofol-induced loss of consciousness. Neuroimage 57: 198–205.
9. Martuzzi R, Ramani R, Qiu M, Rajeevan N, Constable RT (2010) Functional connectivity and alterations in baseline brain state in humans. NeuroImage 49: 823–834.
10. Deshpande G, Kerssens C, Sebel PS, Hu X (2010) Altered local coherence in the default mode network due to sevourane anesthesia. Brain research 1318: 110–121.
11. Hutchison RM, Womelsdorf T, Allen EA, Bandettini PA, Calhoun VD, et al. (2013) Dynamic functional connectivity: Promises, issues, and interpretations. NeuroImage 80: 360–368.
12. Allen EA, Damaraju E, Plis SM, Erhardt EB, Eichele T, et al. (2012) Tracking whole-brain connectivity dynamics in the resting state. Cerebral Cortex : bhs352.
13. Chang C, Glover GH (2010) Time–frequency dynamics of resting-state brain connectivity measured with fmri. Neuroimage 50: 81–98.
14. Hutchison RM, Womelsdorf T, Gati JS, Everling S, Menon RS (2012) Resting-state networks show dynamic functional connectivity in awake humans and anesthetized macaques. Human brain mapping 34: 2154–2177.
15. Tagliazucchi E, Balenzuela P, Fraiman D, Chialvo DR (2012) Criticality in large-scale brain fmridynamics unveiled by a novel point process analysis. Frontiers in Physiology 3: 15–25.
16. Liu X, Duyn JH (2013) Time-varying functional network information extracted from brief instances of spontaneous brain activity. Proceedings of the National Academy of Sciences 110: 4392–4397.
17. MacLaren R, Plamondon JM, Ramsay KB, Rocker GM, Patrick WD, et al. (2000) A prospective evaluation of empiric versus protocol-based sedation and analgesia. Pharmacotherapy: The Journal of Human Pharmacology and Drug Therapy 20: 662–672.
18. Power JD, Barnes KA, Snyder AZ, Schlaggar BL, Petersen SE (2012) Spurious but systematic correlations in functional connectivity mri networks arise from subject motion. Neuroimage 59: 2142–2154.
19. Fransson P, Marrelec G (2008) The precuneus/posterior cingulate cortex plays a pivotal role in the default mode network: Evidence from a partial correlation network analysis. Neuroimage 42: 1178–1184.
20. Leech R, Kamourieh S, Beckmann CF, Sharp DJ (2011) Fractionating the default mode network: distinct contributions of the ventral and dorsal posterior cingulate cortex to cognitive control. The Journal of Neuroscience 31: 3217–3224.
21. Hastie T, Tibshirani R, Friedman J, Hastie T, Friedman J, et al. (2009) The elements of statistical learning, volume 2. Springer.
22. Genovese CR, Lazar NA, Nichols T (2002) Thresholding of statistical maps in functional neuroimaging using the false discovery rate. Neuroimage 15: 870–878.
23. Alkire MT, Hudetz AG, Tononi G (2008) Consciousness and anesthesia. Science 322: 876–880.
24. Fiset P, Paus T, Daloze T, Plourde G, Meuret P, et al. (1999) Brain mechanisms of propofolinduced loss of consciousness in humans: a positron emission tomographic study. The Journal of neuroscience 19: 5506–5513.
25. Boveroux P, Bonhomme V, Boly M, Vanhaudenhuyse A, Maquet P, et al. (2008) Brain function in physiologically, pharmacologically, and pathologically altered states of consciousness. International anesthesiology clinics 46: 131–146.
26. Sanders RD, Tononi G, Laureys S, Sleigh J (2012) Unresponsiveness≠unconsciousness. Anesthesiology 116: 946.
27. Wu GR, Liao W, Stramaglia S, Ding JR, Chen H, et al. (2013) A blind deconvolution approach to recover effective connectivity brain networks from resting state fmri data. Medical image analysis 17: 365–374.
28. Peigneux P, Orban P, Balteau E, Degueldre C, Luxen A, et al. (2006) Offline persistence of memoryrelated cerebral activity during active wakefulness. PLoS biology 4: e100.
29. Lee U, Mashour GA, Kim S, Noh GJ, Choi BM (2009) Propofol induction reduces the capacity for neural information integration: implications for the mechanism of consciousness and general anesthesia. Consciousness and cognition 18: 56–64.
30. John ER, Prichep LS (2005) The anesthetic cascade: a theory of how anesthesia suppresses consciousness. Anesthesiology 102: 447–471.
31. Ying SW, Goldstein PA (2005) Propofol-block of sk channels in reticular thalamic neurons enhances gabaergic inhibition in relay neurons. Journal of neurophysiology 93: 1935–1948.
32. Guldenmund P, Demertzi A, Boveroux P, Boly M, Vanhaudenhuyse A, et al. (2013) Thalamus, brainstem and salience network connectivity changes during propofol-induced sedation and unconsciousness. Brain connectivity 3: 273–285.
33. Vijayan S, Ching S, Purdon PL, Brown EN, Kopell NJ (2013) Thalamocortical mechanisms for the anteriorization of alpha rhythms during propofol-induced unconsciousness. The Journal of Neuroscience 33: 11070–11075.
34. Lamme VA, Zipser K, Spekreijse H (1998) Figure-ground activity in primary visual cortex is suppressed by anesthesia. Proceedings of the National Academy of Sciences 95: 3263–3268.
35. Tenenbein PK, Lam AM, Klein M, Lee L (2006) Effects of sevourane and propofol on ash visual evoked potentials. Journal of Neurosurgical Anesthesiology 18: 310.
36. Ziemann U, Lönnecker S, Steinhoff B, Paulus W (1996) Effects of antiepileptic drugs on motor cortex excitability in humans: a transcranial magnetic stimulation study. Annals of neurology 40: 367–378.
37. Kalkman CJ, Drummond JC, Ribberink AA, Patel PM, Sano T, et al. (1992) Effects of propofol, etomidate, midazolam, and fentanyl on motor evoked responses to transcranial electrical or magnetic stimulation in humans. Anesthesiology 76: 502–509.
38. Gaese BH, Ostwald J (2001) Anesthesia changes frequency tuning of neurons in the rat primary auditory cortex. Journal of neurophysiology 86: 1062–1066.
39. Plourde G, Belin P, Chartrand D, Fiset P, Backman SB, et al. (2006) Cortical processing of complex auditory stimuli during alterations of consciousness with the general anesthetic propofol. Anesthesiology 104: 448–457.
40. Dueck M, Petzke F, Gerbershagen H, Paul M, Hesselmann V, et al. (2005) Propofol attenuates responses of the auditory cortex to acoustic stimulation in a dose-dependent manner: A fmri study. Acta anaesthesiologica scandinavica 49: 784–791.
41. Untergehrer G, Jordan D, Kochs EF, Ilg R, Schneider G (2014) Fronto-parietal connectivity is a non-static phenomenon with characteristic changes during unconsciousness. PloS one 9: e87498.

# 2

# Portable Optical Epidural Needle-A CMOS-Based System Solution and Its Circuit Design

**Cihun-Siyong Alex Gong[2,3], Shih-Pin Lin[1], M. Susan Mandell[4], Mei-Yung Tsou[1], Yin Chang[5], Chien-Kun Ting[1]***

**1** Department of Anesthesiology, Taipei Veterans General Hospital and National Yang-Ming University, Taipei, Taiwan, **2** Department of Electrical Engineering, School of Electrical and Computer Engineering, College of Engineering, Chang Gung University, Taoyuan, Taiwan, **3** Portable Energy System Group, Green Technology Research Center, College of Engineering, Chang Gung University, Taoyuan, Taiwan, **4** Department of Anesthesiology, University of Colorado Health Sciences Center, Aurora, Colorado, United States of America, **5** Institute of Biomedical Engineering, National Yang-Ming University, Taipei, Taiwan

## Abstract

Epidural anesthesia is a common anesthesia method yet up to 10% of procedures fail to provide adequate analgesia. This is usually due to misinterpreting the tactile information derived from the advancing needle through the complex tissue planes. Incorrect placement also can cause dural puncture and neural injury. We developed an optic system capable of reliably identifying tissue planes surrounding the epidural space. However the new technology was too large and cumbersome for practical clinical use. We present a miniaturized version of our optic system using chip technology (first generation CMOS-based system) for logic functions. The new system was connected to an alarm that was triggered once the optic properties of the epidural were identified. The aims of this study were to test our miniaturized system in a porcine model and describe the technology to build this new clinical tool. Our system was tested in a porcine model and identified the epidural space in the lumbar, low and high thoracic regions of the spine. The new technology identified the epidural space in all but 1 of 46 attempts. Experimental results from our fabricated integrated circuit and animal study show the new tool has future clinical potential.

**Editor:** Giovanni Landoni, San Raffaele Scientific Institute, Italy

**Funding:** This study was supported by the following: 1. National Science Council (NSC), Taiwan, grant numbers NSC 102-2218-E-182-003- and 100-2221-E-075-003-MY3. This funder supported the study design. 2. Chang Gung University , grant numbers UERPD2D0051 and UERPD2D0011 . This funder supported the data collection, analysis, and preparation of the manuscript. 3. Ministry of Science and Technology, Taiwan, grant number MOST 103-2221-E-182-070. This funder played a role in supporting the study implementation. 4. Taipei Veterans General Hospital (supporting animal studies), grant number 103DHA0100493.

* Email: ckting@vghtpe.gov.tw

## Introduction

Epidural analgesia is a common but technically challenging method for providing pain relief [1,2]. Care providers use anatomic landmarks and tactile information to locate a space that is only 2–7 mm in diameter [2]. The space is detected as a loss of resistance to pressure exerted on a syringe barrel coupled to a needle that travels through the patient's tissue planes [2]. This requires the provider to sense differences between ligament tissue tone and the epidural space while blindly advancing a fluid or air filled syringe. Anatomic variation between patients and the experience of the provider play a large role in how well an epidural works [3,4]. Inability to correctly locate the epidural space is one of the common reasons for the 5–10% failure rate reported in the literature [5]. It can also lead to complications including dural puncture with resulting post-dural puncture headache or spinal nerve injury.

We previously reported successful identification of the epidural space in real time using a novel system developed in our laboratory [6,7]. We tested if optical probes mounted inside a standard Tuohy needle could identify the epidural space in a porcine model. Our optical system performed well. Dual wavelength optical impulses (650 and 532 nm) reliably identified the ligamentum flavum. Because the ligamentum flavum is the entry point to the epidural space (farthest tissue plane from the cerebrospinal fluid), the approach improves the safety of the instrument. The fidelity of the optical signals was sufficient to implement an intelligent recognition system for needle placement [8]. The primary limitation of our optical model was the large cumbersome setup with a long electrical connection coming out of the needle and connection to a computer.

Our laboratory therefore used novel technology to develop a more compact and mobile optical guided probe for practical clinical use. We used a complementary metal oxide semiconductor (CMOS) to construct a miniature optical probe. The CMOS is a type of digital circuitry in chip technology. It allows for a high density of logic functions and is therefore more compact than other forms of integrated technology. The immunity to noise and low static power consumption makes this an ideal technology to use for optic guided epidural needle insertion.

We questioned if the smaller probe performed as well as our previous fiberoptic-guided needle. The probe was therefore tested in the same *invivo* porcine model used in our original study. We aimed to determine if the optic signals from CMOS technology could reliably identify the tissue planes during needle passage into the epidural space. The electronic circuitry of our novel probe construction is described.

## Methods

### Porcine model

Our study was approved by the Institutional Animal Care and Use Committee of Taipei Veterans General Hospital. We conducted invivo studies in four Duroc and Landrance pigs each weighing approximately 25 kg. General anesthesia was induced with intramuscular injection of Tiletamine-zolazepam (5 mg/kg) and maintained with isoflurane (1.5–2%) through an endotracheal tube during the whole course of study. Animals were then placed in the left lateral position for epidural needle insertion. Vital signs were continuously monitored during the procedure.

A standard 17 G Tuohy needle with newly designed miniature optical stylet were inserted into the lumbar and then low and high thoracic segments of the porcine vertebral column. The needle was advanced until the alarm sounded because the signal indicated entry into the epidural space. Approximately 10–12 punctures at different spinal levels were performed in each pig. Electronic signals from the 650 nm wavelength were retrieved for analysis. To test the accuracy of our system, the stylet was removed when optic properties indicated the needle tip was in the epidural space. A catheter was then inserted and placement confirmed using ultrasonography (Vivid e, GE healthcare, London, United Kingdom). Radiography following injection of the catheter with contrast medium was then done as a second confirmation that the needle entered the epidural space.

### Statistical Analysis

Parametrical data are presented as the mean±SD. Linear mixed model analysis did not identify any variation in the optical signal at different levels along the vertebral column in our previous study [7]. The optical characteristics of the tissue were consistent regardless of axial position on the spine, a naïve pooled technique was used to put all data together from different spine level for analysis statistically. A paired $t$ test was used to compare the signal amplitude of 650 nm between the epidural space and the ligamentum flavum. The results were considered to be statistically significant for $P$ values less than 0.05. A receiver operating characteristic curve (ROC) was used to determine the optimal cutoff values for signal amplitudes of 650 nm to differentiate the epidural space from the ligamentum flavum. Area under the ROC curve with its 95% CIs was also calculated to evaluate the predictive validity of 650 nm All statistical analyses were performed with SPSS software (v.17; SPSS Inc., Chicago, IL).

### Optical Needle

The optic system has been previously described [6,7]. In brief, a fiberoptic bundle was inserted into a hollow stylet of a standard 17 G Tuohy needle (Arrow, Teleflex Incorporated, Limerick PA). The fibers were sealed into a single bundle, manually beveled to fit the shape of the Tuohy needle tip and inserted into a hollow stylet. Our previous studies used two wavelengths (532 and 650 nm) to test the optic system. The 532-nm wavelength did not perform as well as the 650 nm wavelength in our previous invivo study [6,7]. We therefore only used 650 nm wavelength in this study to determine how new CMOS-chip technology influenced signal recovery. An Avalanche photodiode (S5345 Hamamatsu Photonics, KK Shizuoka, Pref Japan) converted the optic to an electrical signal. The signal was amplified so it could be read by the operator. In our new system, an optical impulse triggered alarm was added to inform the user when the epidural space was detected. The threshold of the alarm was set using the reflection signals of ligamentum flavum and epidural space from our previous study results.

### The CMOS chip

We modified our previously described fiberoptic epidural stylet in order to produce a compact instrument more suitable for mobile clinical use. The instrument was composed of a fiberoptic light source that is translated into a visual signal and linked to an alarm indicating location of the target tissue. The components of our epidural needle were integrated into a single chip using solid-state electronics. The conceptual drawing of this work is shown in Fig. 1. We therefore used an application-specific device (Fig. 2). In this system, a chip with different sub-circuits performed the same signal processing as our previous off-the-shelf discrete components.

**Overview of the System.** Advanced Semi Conductor Development (ASD) was used to miniaturize the optic system. This is a highly integrated semiconductor using distinct building blocks. In our system, the off-ASD laser diode (LD) used for the Light Emitter was driven by the LD Modulator block (Fig. 2). The Clock Generator Block modulated signals required by the enabled LD Modulator. The LD Power Controller dominated the average optical output power of the LD through a feedback loop formed by the LD. The loop consisted of the photodiode (PD) used for sensing the light emitted from the LD, the LD Modulator block, and the LD Power Controller.

The Light Detectors shown in Fig. 1 received the tissue-reflected signals for post processing. There were two stages in signal readout: the signal was first amplified through a photomultiplier tube (PMT) and then processed through a transimpedance amplifier (TIA). Of the three options for PMT readout; the "gated integrator", the "continuous current", and the "photo counting", we chose the gated integrator for our laser application because the arrival times of the periodic PMT output current pulses were known.

The output of the TIA was linked to a clock signal through a blend circuit to generate a driving signal (buzzer) for an alarm. The audio alarm was added to alert the clinician that the target point (epidural space) was reached. The target point was identified when signals from the ligamentum-flavum-reflected light was lost. The system was battery-powered and its supply regulated by the Power Management Circuit block. The standard operation procedure of the implemented epidural space (ES) identification prototype is illustrated with Fig. 3.

## Results

There were a total of 46 punctures recorded in 4 pigs. The epidural space was identified using the optical impulses. Ultrasound and contrast studies showed the epidural catheter was correctly placed in 45 attempts, indicating a 97.82% success rate (Table 1).

Fig. 4 illustrates a total of 46 needle insertions that were performed in the four pigs. The averaged magnitude of the reflective signals at the epidural space was 3.516+/0.093 at 650 nm, and at the ligamentum, it was 3.743+/0.117. A paired $t$ test showed significant differences between the averaged magnitudes for the light reflected from the ligamentum flavum and the epidural space in the 650 nm wavelengths ($P<0.001$). ROC analysis verified the difference in optical properties between the ligamentum flavum and epidural space at wavelengths of 650 nm

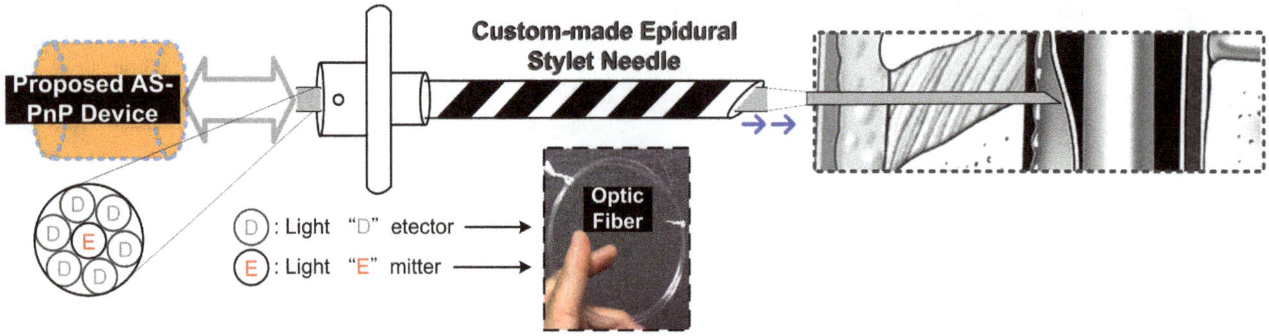


**Figure 1. Conceptual drawing of the optic system.**

based on the sensitivity and specificity [9,10]. Fig. 5 shows the ROC curve of the test. The test showed good discrimination between the epidural space and ligamentum flavum (Table 2). The area under curve for 650 nm was 0.927 (95% CI 0.874–0.980).

## Discussion

Our studies showed that optical analysis of tissue planes can be successfully miniaturized for use in clinical medicine using chip technology. The miniaturized system replicates the findings obtained from our previous optic analysis. This suggests that new chip technology can facilitate a number of logical functions needed for optical resolution of tissue planes that previously required large and bulky equipment. The miniature version of our optical device is compact and portable and is therefore more suitable for clinical use.

In our previous study, we showed that reflective light could be used to guide epidural placement [6,7]. There were more successful epidural placements using the optical system compared to experienced operators [11,12]. The reliable reflective optical impulses from the ligamentum flavum and epidural space provide more consistent information for guiding needle placement compared to tactile techniques. Only one person is required for optic guided needle placement. However, the equipment needed for optical placement was large and not easily portable. These are important design limitations. Therefore, we designed a small and portable version of our optical device by the selective use of chip technology.

There are two common problems leading to failed epidural placement. First is identification of an accurate trajectory leading from the skin to the ligamentum flavum. Second is placement of the needle tip into epidural space without passing through the dura mata. Our device was built to identify the epidural space and prevent accidental dural punctures. It does not identify needle trajectory for guiding purpose. However, surface 2D ultrasound can be used to estimate an accurate trajectory from the skin to epidural space [13].

We tested the reliability of our new optical system using our older system as a standard for performance. Our previous model identified the epidural space in all passages of the optical needle [6,7]. The average magnitude of the reflective signals at the epidural space was similar between our previous system

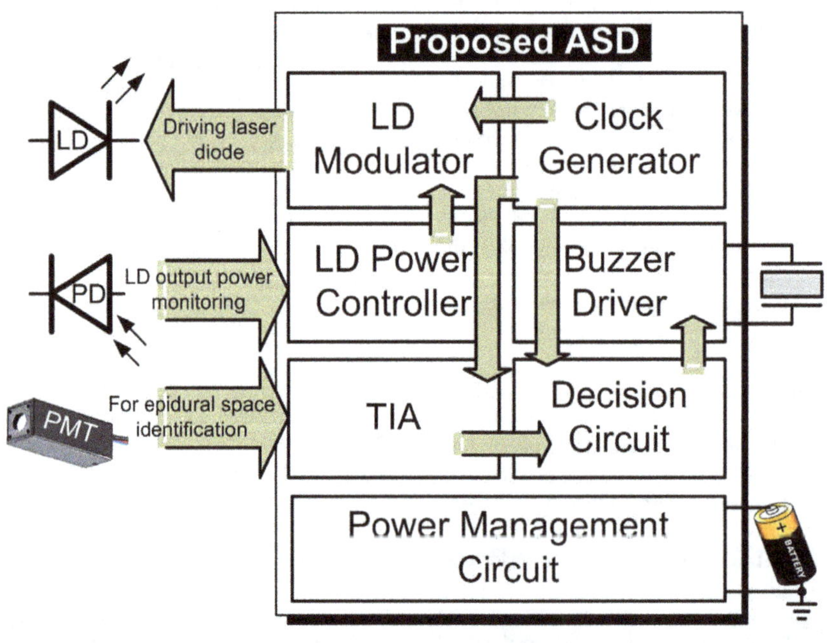


**Figure 2. Proposed application-specific device for the optical needle placement.**

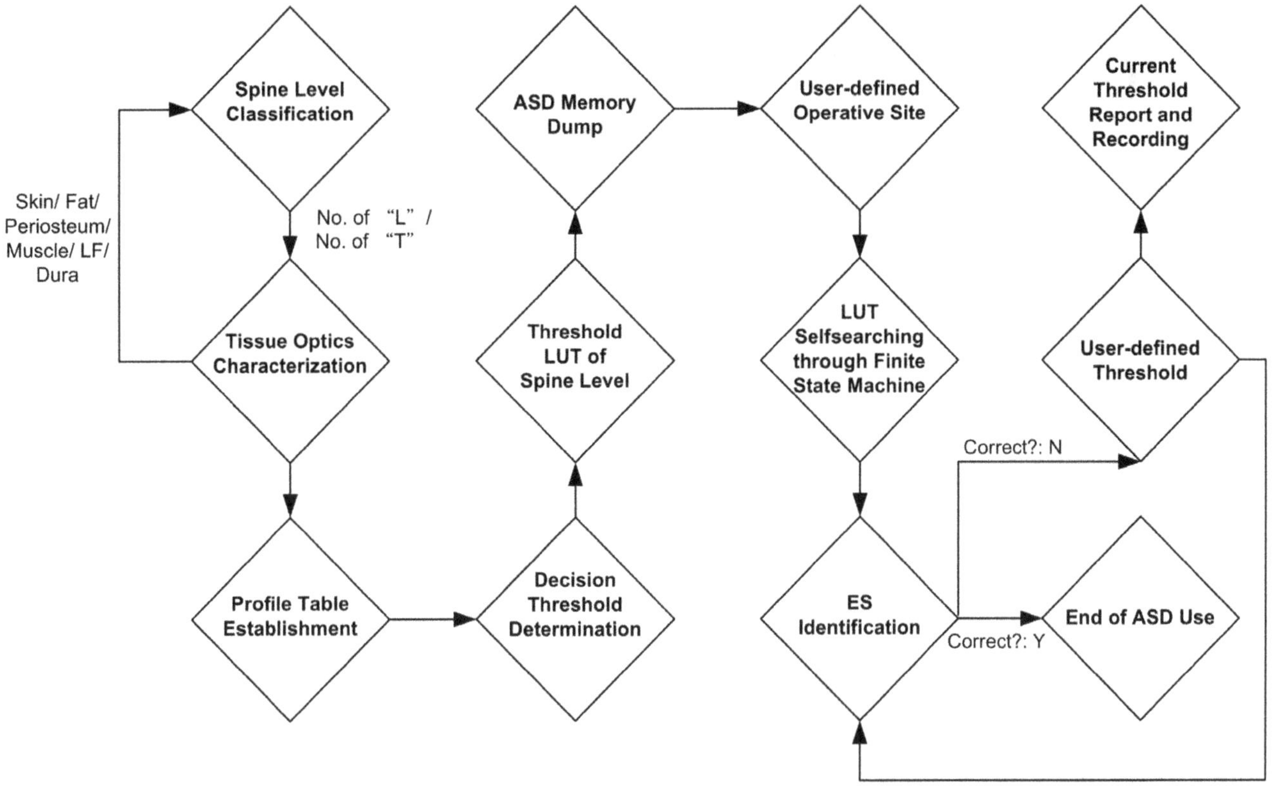


**Figure 3. Standard operation procedure of proposed assistive system.**

(3.565±0.194) and our new device (3.516+/0.093). A similar concordance was noted for the reflective signals at the ligamentum flavum (3.842±0.191) in our previous and new system (3.743+/0.117). Similar to our previous system, there were no significant differences in the optical characteristics of tissues at different levels of the spinal column [7]. Thus, there is no need to adjust the optical settings at different levels of epidural insertion.

The difference between the average magnitudes for the reflected light of the epidural space and ligamentum flavum was significant for our new miniaturized and original devices. This indicates that

**Table 1.** Results of Animal Study.

| Pig # | 1 | 2 | 3 | 4 |
|---|---|---|---|---|
| **Spine level** | | | | |
| **L4-5** | O | O | | O |
| **L3-4** | O | | O | O |
| **L2-3** | O | O | | O |
| **L1-2** | O | O | O | O |
| **T14-L1** | | O | O | |
| **T13-14** | O | O | O | O |
| **T12-13** | O | O | O | O |
| **T11-12** | O | | X | O |
| **T10-11** | O | O | O | O |
| **T9-10** | | O | O | O |
| **T8-9** | O | O | O | O |
| **T7-8** | O | O | | O |
| **T6-7** | O | O | O | O |
| **T5-6** | | O | O | O |

O: Successful, X: Fail.

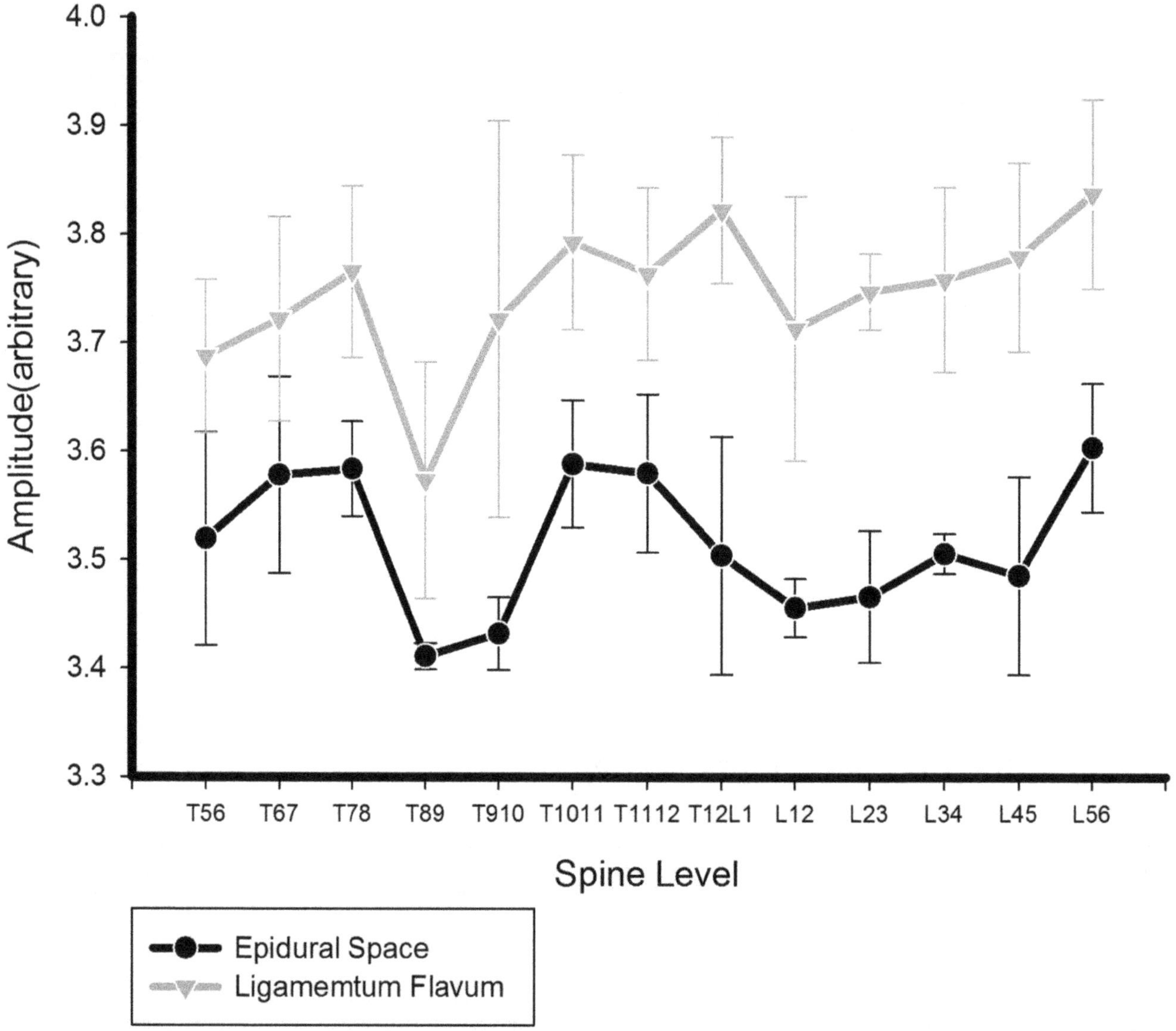


**Figure 4. The reflective amplitude at different spinal levels in the porcine model (mean+/SD).**

the optic signals can discriminate between the two anatomic structures without overlap. The ROC analysis verified the differences in optical properties between the two anatomic structures. The distinct differences in reflective optical patterns of the epidural space and ligamentum flavum may account for the higher degree of accuracy when placing the epidural needle compared to the average 10% failure rate using conventional tactile techniques [5,14].

One of the possible errors in epidural placement can occur during interpretation of the optical signals. We have previously shown that reflective light impulses can be analyzed using discriminate analysis to identify the epidural space [8]. The data were tested using linear discriminate analysis to "decide" if the needle had entered the epidural space. However the discriminate analysis only had 80% sensitivity and specificity.

We therefore used a clock signal linked to a buzzer in our new system to alert the operator that the needle was within the epidural space. We linked the output of the transimpedance amplifier to a clock signal through a blend circuit to drive a signal to alert the operator that the signals from the ligamentum flavum-reflected light was lost. Using this technique there was only one failed attempt. We reason the failure is due to limitations in the standard operation procedure of the assistive system. The system alarmed when the needle tip passed into a pseudo-space before the ligamentum flavum. The pseudo-space has the same fiberoptic qualities as the epidural space. However, ligamentum flavum signals were not observed prior to entry. This indicates that a new assistive design is required to incorporate more complex information that sequentially identifies the ligamentum flavum and epidural space (loss of signal).

The decision threshold plays a key role in successful identification. The determination of threshold involves a choice of statistical methods. Currently, a small sample size is the primary problem to make this determination. We are currently working on ways to improve the performance of our standard operation procedure. The system requires a decision maker that simultaneously learns from large amount of unlabeled data, together with labeled data, and sets a reliable threshold. We are examining different ways to achieve this. The accuracy of the optical system should also be modified. Semiconductor technology suffers process

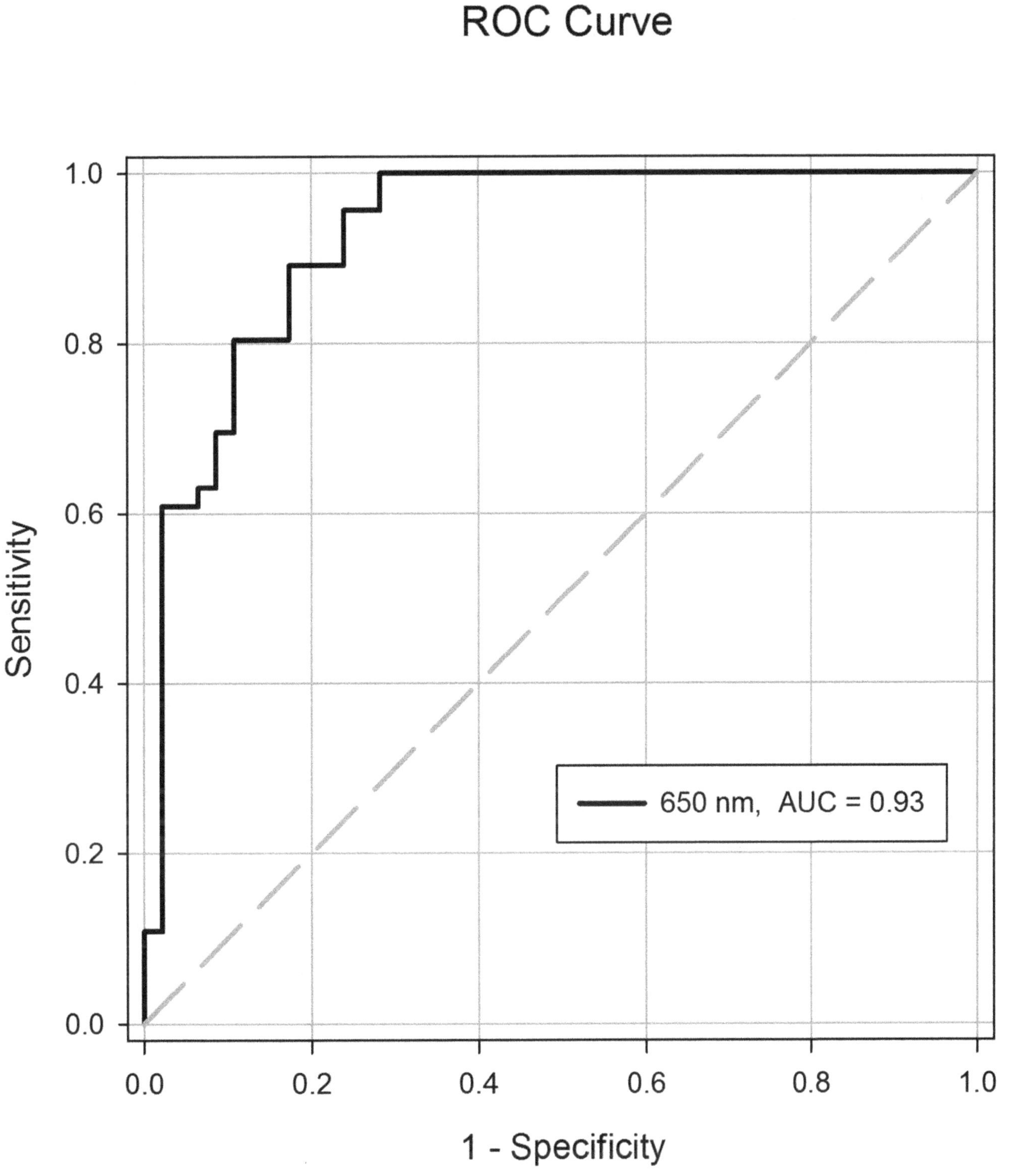


**Figure 5. The receiver operating characteristic (ROC) cure of observations from epidural puncture in the porcine model.** The area under curve for 650 nm is 0.93.

variations which result in device imperfection. This affects the accuracy of light reception and degrades signal conditioning performance. The next-generation design will focus on adding a better on-system automatic calibrator to adjust itself after startup.

Our device is simple, sensitive and portable. Further, the data provides recordable information for review and quality improvement. Direct observation of the reflected light using an oscilloscope may also facilitate training because both the student and instructor can observe the same information simultaneously. One of the

**Table 2.** Receiver Operating Characteristic Curve Analysis.

| | Mean | SD | SEM | 95%CI | P-value |
|---|---|---|---|---|---|
| LF | 3.743 | 0.117 | 0.017 | | |
| ES | 3.516 | 0.093 | 0.014 | | |
| AUC | 0.927 | | 0.027 | 0.874–0.980 | <0.001 |

LF: Ligamentum flavum; ES: Epidural Space; AUC: Area under curve; CI confidence interval.

limitations of our technique observed in our previous study was that the amplitude of the reflective light was influenced by the direction of the needle bevel. However, this influence became minimal with greater use of the optic guided needle indicating that there was a learning curve required for efficient use [6–8].

The findings of our study are derived from an animal model and we did not test our devise in a human population. We anticipate the optical characteristics of human epidural space are similar. The tissue composition and anatomic order of tissue planes are identical. We were able to compensate for anatomic differences based on size of the study animal. The distance from the ligamentum flavum to the dura was 2 to 4 mm in the lumbar and thoracic of piglet. It varied with size and weight of piglet. These variations did not affect the outcome of our study. In conclusion, our optical epidural needle is a reliable method. The device can decrease failed epidural catheters. By taking the advantage of CMOS widely used in many advanced and miniaturized medical applications [15], our new ASD is compact and portable.

## Addendum (System Specifications and Rationale)

In this section, we describe the system in detail, outlining our rationale for circuit design.

**Control of optical power (Fig. S1).** We controlled average optical power to prevent instrument damage by comparing gate voltage of the transistor MP7 (the produced current ipd from the incident light of the PD), against the reference voltage Vref1. The resistor R1 and capacitor C1 are frequency compensation components used to assure stability of the LD Power Controller.

**LD modulator schematics (Fig. S2).** Minimal threshold current, *ith* was needed to properly drive the LD [16]. We chose a transistor with off-chip bias tuning instead of an on-chip constant bias for better temperature coefficient compensation. The feedback power control current was generated by the MN5-R2 path through a unity-gain buffer formed by the two transistors MN3 and MN4. The source-coupled circuit constructed by the MN6, MN7, and MN8 supplied the total current producing maximal optical power modulation. Vref2 drove the MN7 to provide half the current. To prevent "ripple (residual variation on the Vmod provider/Clock Generator) we designed an active power regulator shown in Fig. S3. This prevented large transient current that exceeds the limit of the emitted optical LD optical power.

**Power Management Circuit.** The supply regulator (Power Management Circuit in Fig. 2) had three sub-building blocks (Fig. S3): 1. the battery-powered Voltage Reference with supply-independent reference current through the generated biaε V ref and whose zero current mirroring condition could be broken by its Startup circuit; 2. the amplifier formed a negative feedback loop so low-ripple supply generation could be imposed by comparison with the Vref to control the power transistor Mp; 3. the feedback voltage divider network consisting of the passive components (Rc, Cc. etc.) used for on-the-fly generation of the Vfb associated with the ripple on the Vdd.

**Clock Generator (Fig. S4).** We used output CLK-out to generate clock signals in demand for our ASD. The Vmod was obtained by processing the CLK-out in a low-pass filter followed by an AC-coupled circuit with its output biased at the Vdd. The low-pass filtering circuit assured an ASD safety window so the rising and the falling edges of the Vmod would be within the range protecting the LD from over light power. We noted the low-level supply Vdd2 offered a low-frequency generation with low-power consumption and was not an "unregulated" energy source. The power supply stabilization allowed the LD Modulator to drive the LD without damage.

The ring oscillator of the Clock Generator is shown in Fig. S4. The loop formed by the current-starved inverters and NAND circuit were sized to satisfy the Barkhausen criterion to start oscillation with an expected frequency at power-up. The sw from the combination of power-on-reset signal and special-purpose control signal activated/deactivated the Clock Generator. Transistors MP8–MP10 and MN9–MN11 were used as a low-power Schmitt trigger [17]. The signal comparison with hysteresis could reject its on-input noise to achieve pulse shaping. The circuit of the MP11–MP12 and MN12–MN13 functioned as level converters to other building blocks.

**TIA and the Decision Circuit building blocks (Fig. S5).** The output signal of the PMT was fed into a clocked integrator where the input is synchronous sampled by the CMOS switch (gated by CLK-out). The amplified signal representing the reflected light from the tissue was integrated and unity-gain buffered in time to be processed. Once the acceptable level of the charge accumulated on the C1, it was sampled and subtracted from the previously sample through the controlling of the t1 and t2. The resulting value was compared with the Threshold, which can be set by the user to better identify the target. All the clock signals shown in the timing diagram of Fig. S5 were generated by the on-chip Timer. The operational amplifiers (Fig. S5) were placed with the same structures as shown in Fig. S3(c) with the exception of transistor sizing and offset nulling technique.

Offset Nulling was used to calibrate each of the amplifiers involved to minimize the process-and-fabrication-induced mismatch between the differential pairs. This is standard practice in modern semiconductor design [18]. This improves decision making. Circuit detail of the offset nulling technique is shown in Fig. S6(a). The transistors separately controlled by the Offset Nulling and biased at the Bias_aux function as an auxiliary pair whose source terminals the $Aux_{left}$ and $Aux_{right}$ were connected with the counterparts of the amplifier input pair in parallel, respectively. Fig. S6(b) shows the circuit driving the buzzer (the Buzzer Driver) for target identification. Once the epidural space was identified the Decision Output was kept constant until the system was manually reset. The AND gate involved was able to control its output slew rate (current-starved design similar to the counterparts shown in Fig. S4) so that it did not cause ill effect in the buzz sound.

The ASD was realized in a 0.35-μm CMOS process. The fabricated chip for epidural space identification was tested using PCBs (Printed Circuit Boards), as shown in Fig. S7. The required test currents used to emulate the currents associated with the emitted light and the reflected counterpart were generated by a potentiostat/galvanostat, supplied with the EC-Lab, which supports programmable μA-level current generation. For practical use, it was powered by an energy source with three serially connected small-size 2.5-V end-point-voltage batteries to provide two unregulated power supplies: Vbat = 7.5 V and Vdd1 = 5 V. The regulated counterparts Vdd = 5 V and Vdd2 = 2.5 V were generated by the on-chip active regulator. The proposed ASD system consumes an average current of 65 mA in total, with approximately 60% in the LD-associated devices and circuits. The Buzzer Driver dominated the rest of the power consumption. An 1-KHz clock was generated from its building block with sub-microwatt average power dissipation. The system emitted an average light power of 3 mW to the targets and received reflected feedback of 4.5 μA in the PMT output at the ligamentum flavum and 0.7 μA at the epidural space. The effective bandwidth (−3 dB) of the TIA was set as 9 KHz to keep errors below 3% for an internal CLK out rising/falling time of approximately 40 us. An oscilloscope trace showing buffered output of the input of the Buzzer Driver can be seen from Fig. S8, which clearly demonstrates that the proposed design could ring an alarm when the epidural space was identified. An important factor indicating the ASD performance is the loop transient response versus power supply variation. The regulator was designed to prevent the ripple onto its output when a predetermined maximum output load of 80 mA was connected. The experimental regulator output performance is shown in Fig. S9 where an average of 250-mV peak-to-peak Vdd voltage variation was measured for the ASD.

## Supporting Information

**Figure S1 Circuit Schematic of the LD Power Controller.**

**Figure S2 Circuit Schematic of the LD modulator.**

**Figure S3 Schematic of the Power Management Circuit.**

**Figure S4 Design of the Clock Generator.**

**Figure S5 The proposed TIA and analog part of the Decision Circuit.**

**Figure S6** (a) The offset nulling technique. (b) The Buzzer Driver circuit.

**Figure S7 Measurement setup of the fabricated ASD chip.**

**Figure S8 Measured buffered output of the Buzzer Driver input in an epidural space identification test.**

**Figure S9 Measured regulator output performance of our ASD.**

## Author Contributions

Conceived and designed the experiments: CSAG CKT. Performed the experiments: CSAG CKT. Analyzed the data: SPL. Contributed reagents/materials/analysis tools: MYT YC. Contributed to the writing of the manuscript: CSAG CKT MSM.

## References


1. Konrad C, Schupfer G, Wietlisbach M, Gerber H (1998) Learning manual skills in anesthesiology: Is there a recommended number of cases for anesthetic procedures? Anesth Analg 86(3): 635–9.
2. Scott DB (1997) Identification of the epidural space: loss of resistance to air or saline? Reg Anesth 22(1): 1–2.
3. Curatolo M, Orlando A, Zbinden AM, Scaramozzino P, Venuti FS (1995) A multifactorial analysis to explain inadequate surgical analgesia after extradural block. Br J Anaesth 75(3): 274–81.
4. Hood DD, Dewan DM (1993) Anesthetic and obstetric outcome in morbidly obese parturients. Anesthesiology 79(6): 1210–8.
5. Rigg JR, Jamrozik K, Myles PS, Silbert BS, Peyton PJ, et al. (2002) Epidural anaesthesia and analgesia and outcome of major surgery: a randomised trial. Lancet 359(9314): 1276–82.
6. Ting CK, Chang Y (2010) Technique of fiber optics used to localize epidural space in piglets. Opt Express 24; 18(11): 11138–47.
7. Ting CK, Tsou MY, Chen PT, Chang KY, Mandell MS, et al. (2010) A new technique to assist epidural needle placement: fiberoptic-guided insertion using two wavelengths. Anesthesiology 112(5): 1128–35.
8. Lin SP, Mandell MS, Chang Y, Chen PT, Tsou MY, et al. (2012) Discriminant analysis for anaesthetic decision-making: an intelligent recognition system for epidural needle insertion. Br J Anaesth 108(2): 302–7.
9. Lasko TA, Bhagwat JG, Zou KH, Ohno-Machado L (2005) The use of receiver operating characteristic curves in biomedical informatics. J Biomed Inform 38(5): 404–15.
10. Pepe MS (2003) The statistical evaluation of medical tests for classification and prediction. Oxford: Oxford University Press. 318 p.
11. Desjardins AE, Hendriks BH, van der Voort M, Nachabe R, Bierhoff W, et al. (2011) Epidural needle with embedded optical fibers for spectroscopic differentiation of tissue: ex vivo feasibility study. Biomedical Optics Express 2(6): 1452–61.
12. Rathmell JP, Desjardins AE, van der Voort M, Hendriks BH, Nachabe R, et al. (2010) Identification of the epidural space with optical spectroscopy: an in vivo swine study. Anesthesiology 113(6): 1406–18.
13. Karmakar MK, Li X, Ho AM, Kwok WH, Chui PT (2009) Real-time ultrasound-guided paramedian epidural access: evaluation of a novel in-plane technique. Br J Anaesth 102(6): 845–54.
14. McLeod A, Roche A, Fennelly M (2005) Case series: Ultrasonography may assist epidural insertion in scoliosis patients. Can J Anaesth 52(7): 717–20.
15. Khan TH, Shrestha R, Wahid KA (2014) A Modular and Programmable Development Platform for Capsule Endoscopy System. J. Medical Systems 38: 57.
16. Zivojinovic P, Lescure M, Tap-Béteille H (2001) Design and stability analysis of a CMOS feedback laser driver. IEEE Transactions on Instrumentation and Measurement 53(1): 102–8.
17. Al-Sarawi SF (2002) Low power Schmitt trigger circuit. Electron Lett 38(18): 1009–10.
18. Weste HE, Harris DM (2010) CMOS VLSI Design: A Circuits and Systems Perspective. Addison-Wesley, NY, USA, 4th edition. 864 p.

3

# Implementation of the Surgical Safety Checklist in Switzerland and Perceptions of Its Benefits: Cross-Sectional Survey

**Stéphane Cullati[1*], Marc-Joseph Licker[2], Patricia Francis[1], Adriana Degiorgi[3], Paula Bezzola[4], Delphine S. Courvoisier[5], Pierre Chopard[1]**

**1** Quality of care service, University Hospitals of Geneva, Geneva, Switzerland, **2** Division of anesthesiology, University Hospitals of Geneva, Geneva, Switzerland, **3** Quality of care unit, Ente Ospedaliero Cantonale, Lugano, Switzerland, **4** Patient Safety Foundation Switzerland, Zürich, Switzerland, **5** Division of clinical epidemiology, University Hospitals of Geneva, Geneva, Switzerland

## Abstract

***Objectives:*** To examine the implementation of the Surgical Safety Checklist (SSC) among surgeons and anaesthetists working in Swiss hospitals and clinics and their perceptions of the SSC.

***Methods:*** Cross-sectional survey at the 97th Annual Meeting of the Swiss Society of Surgery, Switzerland, 2010. Opinions of the SSC were assessed with a 6-item questionnaire.

***Results:*** 152 respondents answered the questionnaire (participation rate 35.1%). 64.7% respondents acknowledged having a checklist in their hospital or their clinic. Median implementation year was 2009. More than 8 out of 10 respondents reported their team applied the Sign In and the Time Out very often or quasi systematically, whereas almost half of respondents acknowledged the Sign Out was applied never or rarely. The majority of respondents agreed that the checklist improves safety and team communication, and helps to develop a safety culture. However, they were less supportive about the opinion that the checklist facilitates teamwork and eliminates social hierarchy between caregivers.

***Conclusions:*** This survey indicates that the SSC has been largely implemented in many Swiss hospitals and clinics. Both surgeons and anaesthetists perceived the SSC as a valuable tool in improving intraoperative patient safety and communication among health care professionals, with lesser importance in facilitating teamwork (and eliminating hierarchical categories).

**Editor:** David Warburton, University of Southern California, United States of America

**Funding:** The authors have no support or funding to report.

**Competing Interests:** The authors have declared that no competing interests exist.

* Email: stephane.cullati@hcuge.ch

These authors contributed equally to this work.

## Introduction

In Switzerland, over 1 million operations are carried out annually and major complications are expected to occur in 3 to 20% of patients with a mortality rate between 0.8 and 1.5% [1]. Although surgical procedures are performed to save lives and to improve patient's quality of life, unsafe practice and medical errors have also been incriminated in causing serious complications. Such preventable complications have been estimated to increase the total hospital cost by an average 10% [2].

With the increasing burden of patients' comorbidities [3–6], the complexity of the surgical operation and application of advanced technologies, the achievement and maintenance of clinical excellence has become increasingly challenging. Many lessons have been learned from the aviation industry where checklists and training in crew resource management have largely contributed to decrease the incidence of accidents and strengthen safety culture [7–9].

In 2007, the World Health Organization (WHO) initiated the Safer Surgery Saves Lives project [10], in which standards for the safe delivery of surgical care and a 19-item Surgical Safety Checklist (SSC) were developed [11]. This SSC encompasses the three phases of any operation that mirror the take-off cruise and landing phases of the aviation-industry. Before anaesthesia induction ("sign in"), the team confirms patient identity, surgical site, anaesthetic concerns, allergies and estimated surgical blood losses. Before skin incision ("time out"), the entire team is introduced, the anticipated critical events are reviewed, sterility and antibiotic administration is confirmed, and, imaging and other diagnostic elements are displayed if appropriate. Before the patient leaves the operating room (OR) ("sign out"), the swab count is confirmed, procedure name and handling of specific tissue/fluid specimen is confirmed and, equipment, postoperative treatment and patient destination are addressed. This SSC was trialled in eight different countries, representing a wide spectrum of health care systems and environments. Using a pre-post-design and including more than 8'000 patients, the implementation of the SSC resulted in a 30% reduction in operative mortality and major complications, in both high and low income countries [12]. A meta-analysis confirmed the effectiveness of the SSC for mortality (relative risk (RR) 0.57, 95% confidence interval (CI): 0.42–0.76) and complications (RR 0.63, 95% CI 0.58–0.67) [13], however the risk of bias remains elevated considering the large number of low quality studies, as noted in two systematic reviews [13,14].

Acknowledging the positive impact the SSC could have on patient safety, the UK National Patient Safety Agency issued an alert stating that the SSC (in its modified version) should be completed for every surgical patient from February 2010 onwards [15]. Likewise, national health regulatory authorities in France [16] and Ireland [17] endorsed the mandatory use of SSC for all patients undergoing surgery. In other Western countries, professional health organisations for surgical care have recommended the routine utilization of SSC [18]. In Switzerland, the Patient Safety Foundation has dealt with safety issues and quality of care since 2003 and a recent survey among directors of surgery departments reported that the SSC was used in 74% of hospitals [19]. However, despite an "official" adhesion to SSC of the majority of perioperative health care professionals [20–23], there are many barriers hindering the success of its implementation [24] and the promotion of a true safety culture [20,22,23,25–30]. A recent survey among Swiss surgical healthcare professionals showed moderate satisfaction with the SSC [31]. This mixed picture suggests that the implementation of the checklist is facing not only barriers from healthcare organizations but also barriers related to the perception of the benefit of the SSC. We know little about perceptions of the SSC among Swiss surgeons and anaesthetists.

The objective of this study was twofold: to report on the initial implementation of SSC among Swiss hospitals and to describe personal opinions of surgeons and anaesthetists towards the SSC.

## Methods

### Setting and design

The study was initiated in 2010 by a multidisciplinary team including anaesthetists, surgeons, a psychologist, a sociologist and clinical quality officers from the University Hospital of Geneva, in collaboration with the Swiss Patient Safety Foundation in Zurich. A comprehensive questionnaire was developed to address various aspects of the SSC: its implementation in the respondent's hospital/clinic, self-reported compliance and general perceptions of the SSC. The questionnaire was designed to provide a comprehensive view of the application and the attitude towards the SSC among practicing Swiss surgeons and anaesthetists. The questionnaire was translated in German, French and Italian. Each translation was conducted by two native translators and pre-tested.

The questionnaire was distributed to all participants of the joint meeting of the Swiss Society of Surgery and the Swiss Society of Anaesthesia and Reanimation that was held during the 97th Annual Meeting of the Swiss Society of Surgery in Interlaken in June 2010 (26th–28th). The purpose of the cross-sectional survey was addressed in an explanatory letter and presented by the chairman of the plenary lecture. Questionnaires were distributed by bilingual medical students, along with a Swiss chocolate to attendees agreeing to participate. No consent was asked to an Institutional Review Board because the survey was administered during a congress and no identifying information was asked to respondents.

### Variables of interest (outcome)

**Implementation of the SSC.** The implementation of the SSC was addressed by asking participants whether the SSC was applied in their institutions (yes, no, don't know, I don't know this surgical safety checklist), whether they received support from their administrative and clinical managing authorities (no, little, medium, strong, or very strong support) and whether different sections – Sign In, Time out, Sing Out, Others – were included in their SSC (yes, no),

**Perceived compliance to the SSC.** The SSC's use was addressed with the following question: "please indicate if these checklist sections are applied either never (0%), rarely (1–29%), partially (30–59%), very often (60–90%), or quasi systematically (> 90%) within your surgical/anaesthetic team (i.e., the one with which you operate most often)". Space was also allocated for free commentary.

**Perception of the SSC.** Based on the literature assessing the perception of the checklist, a list of 8 questions was built to assess the general perceptions of the SSC. Respondents had to report their agreement with each item on a scale ranging from 1 (don't agree at all) to 5 (fully agree) with an additional "No opinion" option.

### Descriptive variables

The first question addressed the sector of employment (public or private) where the SSC was implemented. Sociodemographic and professional characteristics of the participants included sex, age (year of birth), profession (surgeon, anaesthetist), postgraduate training abroad ("After completing your specialist training, have you followed part of your postgraduate training in another country"? yes vs. no), type of employment (private or public sector; University or non-University hospital), workload (number of interventions performed each year) and clinical experience (number of years of clinical practice in the specialty).

### Statistical analysis

Given the exploratory nature of this cross-sectional survey, no power calculation was conducted. Characteristics are presented as frequencies, means, standard deviations and medians as appropriate. To describe physician's attitude and perception regarding the SCC, the 5-point Likert scale was collapsed into a 3-point scale (positive, neutral, negative). We examined sub-groups differences with t-test if the outcome was continuous and with Chi-square test if the outcome was ordinal or dichotomous. In case of small sample size in sub-groups, we used the Fischer exact test. When a continuous outcome was not normally distributed, we used the Wilcoxon-Mann-Whitney test. The level of significance was set at $p<0.05$ and all tests were two-sided. All statistical analyses were completed using the SPSS software (version 18; SPSS Inc, Chicago, IL).

## Results

### Participants

Out of 433 questionnaires distributed at the meeting, 152 were returned (response rate 35.1%). As described in Table 1, the majority of respondents were men (62.6%), German speaking (84.2%), surgeons (61.6%) and employed in a public hospital (78.4%) with a median of 500 surgical procedures being performed annually. Their mean age was 44.5 years and, on average, they had been in practice for 16 years.

**Table 1.** Characteristics of participating physicians (N = 152).

| | N (%)[a] |
|---|---|
| Sex (N = 139) | |
| Men | 87 (62.6) |
| Age [year] (N = 135) | |
| Mean age (SD) | 44.5 (11.1) |
| Range | 20–79 |
| *by age classes:* | |
| 20–37 | 48 (35.6) |
| 38–50 | 45 (33.3) |
| 51 and older | 42 (31.1) |
| Profession (N = 138) | |
| Surgeon | 85 (61.6) |
| Anesthetists | 47 (34.1) |
| Others | 6 (4.3) |
| Number of year of practice (N = 116) | |
| Mean (SD) | 15.6 (10.1) |
| Range | 1–40 |
| Number of interventions/procedures by year (N = 102) | |
| Median (Mean, SD) | 500 (833, 1325) |
| Range | 20–8000 |
| Type of employment (N = 139) | |
| Public sector | 109 (78.4) |
| *non-university hospital* | *91 (83.5)* |
| *university hospital* | *18 (16.5)* |
| Private sector | 30 (21.6) |
| *private practice* | *21 (70.0)* |
| *private hospitals/clinics* | *9 (30.0)* |
| Postgraduate training in another country (N = 121) | |
| yes | 41 (33.9) |
| no | 80 (66.1) |
| Language of the questionnaire | |
| German | 128 (84.2) |
| French | 23 (15.1) |
| Italian | 1 (0.7) |

[a]Total of percentage exceed 100% due to surrounding.

## Implementation of the SSC

At the time of the survey, a SSC similar to the one proposed by the WHO was used by 65% of the respondents, the implementation being slightly higher in the public health sector than in the private sector (73% vs. 56%, respectively; p = 0.048). The median year of SSC adoption was 2009 (2007 and before, n = 5; 2008, n = 19; 2009, n = 44; 2010, n = 16; missing values, n = 68).

The implementation of the SSC within hospitals and clinics was supported by all institutional health care authorities (general management, surgery, anaesthesiology and nursing managers), although participants noted stronger support from anaesthesia departments and less support from nursing departments (Table 2). No differences were observed between the private and the public sectors.

## Perceived compliance to the SSC

As shown in Table 3, the "sign in" (91.5%) and "time out" (96.0%) sections of the SSC were largely included in the checklist used by respondents in their hospitals/clinics. According to respondents, the "sign in" and "time out" were completed "very often or quasi systematically" (89.9% and 82.5%, respectively). In contrast, the "sign out" was included only half the time in the checklist, and 45.2% of respondents described it as "never or rarely" completed. The proportion of "never or rarely" applied differed between the private and the public sectors (17% vs. 61%, respectively; p = 0.012). Additional sections to the WHO SCC were reported by 27% respondents, with no differences being observed between the private and the public sectors.

**Table 2.** Institutional support to the implementation of the Surgical Safety Checklist (Switzerland, 2010).

| *"In your opinion, to what extent was the implementation of the checklist supported by..."* | No support or little support | Medium support | Strong support or very strong | Mean* (SD) |
|---|---|---|---|---|
| the chief executive management in your hospital/clinic (N = 73) | 6.8% | 15.1% | 78.1% | 4.27 (0.96) |
| the chairman and consultants of the department of surgery (N = 89) | 5.6% | 19.1% | 75.3% | 4.24 (0.95) |
| the chairman and consultants of department of anesthesiology (N = 86) | 3.5% | 5.8% | 90.7% | 4.56 (0.81) |
| the head nursing department and operating theater manager (N = 81) | 22.2% | 11.1% | 66.7% | 3.84 (1.27) |

* No support = 1, Little support = 2, Medium support = 3, Strong support = 4, Very strong support = 5.

## Opinions regarding the SSC and its impact

The majority of respondents agreed that the SCC was a valuable tool for improving intraoperative safety (89.5%), developing a safety culture among surgical teams (75.4%) and fostering team communication (68.8%) (Table 4). In line with these perceptions, respondents largely disagreed with the opinion that the SCC is "a waste of time" (68.8%), "brings no added value to existing safety procedures" (61.5%) and "has not demonstrated its efficacy in the scientific literature" (53.7%). Opinions were less positive for the items "SSC facilitates teamwork" and "eliminates hierarchy (during the controls) between healthcare professionals"(43.3% disagreed).

Respondents who did not use the SCC tended to express more negative opinions regarding the SCC (compared to respondents using the SSC). The SSC was more often significantly perceived as "a waste of time", "bringing no extra value to existing safety procedures", and having "not demonstrated its efficacy in the scientific literature" (Table 5). The SCC was also more frequently perceived as "a waste of time" in the private sector than in the public sector. Age, gender, clinical experience, and training abroad did not influence judgement towards the SCC (data not shown). Likewise, attitudes towards the SCC among surgeons and anaesthetists were similar, except that anaesthetists agreed more often that the SCC eliminates interprofessional hierarchy (Table S1).

## Discussion

Since 2007, the implementation of the SSC has achieved relative worldwide success [16,21,32,33] and the objective of this study was to explore the situation in Switzerland and to answer a burning question: Is Switzerland keeping up? We found that 65% of respondents were already using a SSC in their hospital/clinic in the year of 2010, an encouraging result, suggesting that a majority of Swiss hospital and clinics are convinced of the importance of the SSC. Another Swiss survey conducted one year later (2011) found an implementation rate of 74% [19], but used another design for the questionnaire administration and was conducted among another population (directors of adult departments in operative medicine); however, this survey obtained a response rate (30%) similar to ours. More recently, a survey conducted in December 2012 among members of the Foederatio Medicorum Chirurgicorum Helvetica found an implementation rate of 79% (of a surgical checklist based on the WHO-checklist, on the Universal Protocol or other) [31], but was also impeded by a low response rate (23%). These results clearly indicate that the implementation of the SSC has evolved favourably in Switzerland; however, the low participation rate, potentially causing bias, stresses the need for additional research in this area.

Importantly, the median year of implementation was 2009. Considering that the SSC was launched worldwide in 2007 and in Europe in January 2009 [34], this suggests that most Swiss hospital and clinics have been responsive within a very short time to the campaign of "Safer Surgery Saves Lives".

Another encouraging result is the perceived positive reaction of hospitals' authorities towards the implementation of the SSC.

**Table 3.** Content of the Surgical Safety Checklist (SSC) implemented in the hospital's respondent and perceived compliance rate to the SSC (Switzerland, 2010).

| | Context of the SSC implemented in the hospital's respondent: | Perceived compliance rate to the SSC[a] | | | | |
|---|---|---|---|---|---|---|
| | % | Never (0%) or rarely (1–29%) | Partially (30–59%) | Very often (60–90%) or quasi systematically (>90%) | Mean* (SD) | Missing |
| Sign In (N = 94) | 91.5% | 4.5% | 5.6% | 89.9% | 4.6 (0.9) | 1 |
| Time Out (N = 101) | 96.0% | 8.2% | 9.3% | 82.5% | 4.4 (1.0) | 4 |
| Sign Out (N = 87) | 49.4% | 45.2% | 8.2% | 46.6% | 3.0 (1.8) | 14 |
| Other section (N = 45) | 26.7% | 10.0% | 0% | 90.0% | 4.6(1.0) | 2 |

[a]"Please indicate if these checklist sections are applied either never, rarely, partially, very often, or quasi systematically within *your surgical/anaesthetic team* (i.e., the one with which you operate most often)".

* Never = 1, Rarely = 2, Partially = 3, Very often = 4, Quasi systematically = 5.

**Table 4.** Attitudes toward the Surgical Safety Checklist (Switzerland, 2010).

| *The checklist...* | Don't agree at all or don't agree | Partially agree | Fully agree or agree | Mean* (SD) |
|---|---|---|---|---|
| improves the safety of procedures (anaesthetic and surgical) (N = 143) | 5.6% | 4.9% | 89.5% | 4.5 (0.9) |
| is a waste of time (N = 138) | 68.8% | 15.9% | 15.2% | 2.1 (1.2) |
| improves team communication (related to safety) (N = 141) | 12.1% | 19.1% | 68.8% | 3.8 (1.1) |
| brings no extra value to existing safety procedures already in place in my hospital/clinic before its implementation (N = 130) | 61.5% | 20.8% | 17.7% | 2.3 (1.2) |
| helps to develop a safety culture in surgical teams (N = 138) | 10.1% | 14.5% | 75.4% | 4.0 (1.1) |
| has not demonstrated its efficacy in the scientific literature (N = 95) | 53.7% | 24.2% | 22.1% | 2.4 (1.3) |
| facilitates teamwork (N = 136) | 21.3% | 33.1% | 45.6% | 3.4 (1.1) |
| eliminates (during the controls) hierarchy between healthcare professionals (N = 127) | 43.3% | 31.5% | 25.2% | 2.7 (1.2) |

*Don't agree at all = 1, Don't agree = 2, Partially agree = 3, Agree = 4, Fully agree = 5.

Indeed, institutional support was seen as globally positive, across all kinds of authorities (management, surgery, anaesthesiology, and nursing). At most, we observed differences between perceptions of managerial support in anaesthesia and nursing. In anaesthesia, the support was perceived as strong or very strong by more than nine out of ten respondents, while in nursing it was "only" two out of three. Most notably, we did not find significant differences between private and public healthcare institutions. Comparison of this result with existing literature is limited as they are few studies examining institutional support of SSC's implementation. We found only one French study showing that the SSC was supported by medical department and management in more than 80% [35].

## Perceived compliance to the SSC

Most of the international literature about the compliance to the SSC in high-income countries show a relative heterogeneity: self-reported compliance rates vary between 38% and 96% [20,23,28,30,36], whereas administrative audits have shown compliance rates between 66% and 100% [26,27,37–40] and observational studies have shown that the SSC was initiated between 80% and 99% [24,41–45]. But most of these compliance studies assessed the overall compliance without distinguishing the three parts of the SSC (Sign In, Time Out and Sign Out). Our results went further by assessing the compliance for each section and showed different perceived rates: almost 90% of respondents rated the SSC being applied by their surgical/anaesthetic team as "very often or quasi systematically" for the Sign In and 83% for the Time Out; however, the compliance with the Sign Out was rated applied "very often or quasi systematically" by only 47% of respondents. In other words, when implemented in hospitals and clinics, the SSC seems differently applied according to its content: before skin incision (Sign In and Time Out), the SSC seems conscientiously followed by both surgical and anaesthetic teams. However, at the end of the interventions, the compliance rate is perceived lower, a result similar to observational studies [24,46]. This lack of compliance with the Sign Out could be rooted in the different perceptions of when to initiate this phase (toward the end

**Table 5.** Attitudes towards the SSC among respondents working in hospitals with or without the SSC and those working in the public or private sector (Switzerland, 2010).

| | Respondents working in hospitals | | | | | |
|---|---|---|---|---|---|---|
| *Proportion of "Fully agree or agree" with the following items: The checklist...* | with checklist (N = 97) | without checklist (N = 48) | p-value* | public hospitals (N = 109) | private hospitals (N = 30) | p-value* |
| improves the safety of procedures | 91.7% | 86.7% | 0.556 | 90.6% | 84.0% | .469 |
| is a waste of time | 10.8% | 23.3% | 0.005 | 9.9% | 36.0% | .003 |
| improves team communication | 73.4% | 60.0% | 0.140 | 67.0% | 69.2% | .828 |
| brings no extra value to existing safety procedures already in place in my hospital/clinic | 14.0% | 23.8% | 0.020 | 16.7% | 24.0% | .394 |
| helps to develop a safety culture in surgical teams | 70.7% | 86.4% | 0.493 | 71.6% | 84.6% | .215 |
| has not demonstrated its efficacy in the scientific literature | 16.4% | 31.3% | 0.030 | 19.4% | 31.6% | .347 |
| facilitates teamwork | 45.6% | 47.7% | 0.816 | 43.0% | 44.0% | .928 |
| eliminates hierarchy between healthcare providers | 24.7% | 27.5% | 0.197 | 24.7% | 26.1% | .893 |

* Chi-square test or Fisher exact test if at least one cell had a frequency of 10 or less.

of the procedure, the surgeon operator could ask to initiate the Sign Out, although the "last stitch" and the dressing might not have been completed), as noted by an observational study of team interactions during the application of the SSC [24].

Most notably, we observed no difference in compliance between the private and the public sectors. This result is discordant with a study conducted in a central American country [47], where the compliance rate was higher among private hospitals.

Although the compliance rate reported in the current study is encouraging, it should be noted that routine could reduce it over time. Indeed, a qualitative observational study assessed the compliance rate to 5 new items into the checklist already in use in an healthcare organisation and results showed that compliance rate with the introduced items was high (between 75 and 86%) –a result similar to studies examining the compliance in settings where the checklist was recently implemented [24,41–45] – while compliance with the existing (well-established) items was relatively low (between 12% and 72%) [28].

## Perceptions of the SSC

Opinions of the respondents toward the SSC are generally positive. The SSC is perceived as an instrument, that could improve patient safety in hospitals, a result similar to other studies [20,21,23,48].

Some studies have pointed out that time pressures were a hindrance to compliance with the SSC, for examples in US [49] and French [26] contexts. In Switzerland, our study revealed that the SSC was not perceived as a waste of time. This is confirmed by observational studies which found that checking the items of the SSC is not time-consuming: the duration of the Time Out phase was between mean of 36[s] [24] and median of 60[s] [46].

Another barrier reported in the literature pointed out that some items of the SSC could unnecessarily duplicate existing procedures of control [26]. In our survey, more than six out of ten respondents disagreed with the opinion that the SSC brought no extra values to existing safety procedures in their hospital. This finding suggests that the SSC is perceived, overall, as a complementary tool in safety procedures rather than a duplicate.

A majority of respondents expressed the opinion that the SSC was a tool which could improve communication within the teams. According to the literature, OR teams think the SSC improves the communication within the team [20,25,47,50] or between interprofessional teams [30] though some teams disagree [23], and a recent systematic review of surgical team member' perceptions concluded that the SSC was positively perceived for communication [51]. However, the real impact of the introduction of the SSC on safety communication between OR teams' member remains much less evident [52].

We expected to see differences in the perceptions of the SSC between respondents working in hospital using the SSC versus those not. Some differences were found: among respondent working without SSC, the SSC was more often perceived as a waste of time, bringing no extra value to existing safety procedures and not having demonstrated its efficacy. Differences among most other items showed the same pattern of results, but were not significant, most likely because of a lack of power to detect differences due to small sample sizes (with SSC = 97, without SSC = 48). Of notable exception, respondents working with and without SSC were both not very convinced that the SSC facilitates teamwork, and eliminates the hierarchy between healthcare providers.

## Strengths and limitations

The current study did not assess barriers to the successful implementation of the SSC, a topic that has already been investigated [53]. The major limitation of our study is the low participation rate. It raises concern with the implementation and the compliance rates and with the assessment of perception agreements, which could be biased. Other Swiss studies examining the SSC [19,31] are impeded by the same problem. We hypothesize that respondents were more interested in the SSC and our compliance rates may be overestimated. Lower than desired participation rates in surveys are common in health services research [54] and time trends suggest a decline in response rates over time [55,56]. Nevertheless recent evidence from methodological studies indicates that non-response bias is not always systematic [57].

The topic of the present study could be potentially sensitive for some respondents and may have altered their response, causing information bias (or social desirability bias). We think that the design used for collecting data (anonymous questionnaire distributed during a congress) may have limited this effect, but it is not sure that confidentiality may affect information bias [58].

Finally, we should keep in mind that compliance with the SSC was self-reported and, thus, may have been overestimated in comparison with its actual use [59].

# Conclusion

In conclusion, the implementation of the SSC in Switzerland has been largely adopted in the majority of hospitals and clinics. The perceived compliance with the SSC and the perception of the SSC are rated positively overall. As determination of prevalence could be impeded by selection bias due to low participation rate, further research should be conducted to confirm these results.

# Supporting Information

**Table S1** Attitudes towards the SSC among surgeons and anesthetists.

# Acknowledgments

We thank the Chairmen of the Swiss Society of Surgery and the Swiss Society of Anesthesiology and Reanimation, respectively Dr. Othmar Schöb and Dr. Tiziano Cassina, for their authorization and their support to conduct the survey at the 97th Annual Meeting of the Swiss Society of Surgery, Interlaken, 26th-28th of May 2010. We address a special thank to Dr. Valentin Neuhaus, University Hospital of Zurich, for his kind support during the data administration. The data collection during the Meeting was conducted with the help of the following medical students from the University of Geneva: Pierre Starkov, Charlotte Vitos, Nicolas Broc, Rebecca Hertzog, Milena Alec, Jennifer Rubli, Doriane Ischer. Finally, we thank Dr. Ebrahim Khabiri, University Hospital of Geneva, for his contribution during the design of the study.

# Author Contributions

Conceived and designed the experiments: SC ML PF AD PB DC PC. Performed the experiments: SC ML. Analyzed the data: SC ML. Contributed reagents/materials/analysis tools: SC ML. Contributed to the writing of the manuscript: SC ML PF AD PB DC PC.

## References


1. Pearse RM, Moreno RP, Bauer P, Pelosi P, Metnitz P, et al. (2012) Mortality after surgery in Europe: a 7 day cohort study. The Lancet 380: 1059–1065.
2. Fuller RL, McCullough EC, Bao MZ, Averill RF (2009) Estimating the costs of potentially preventable hospital acquired complications. Health Care Financ Rev 30: 17–32.
3. Hallett JW Jr, Textor SC, Kos PB, Nicpon G, Bower TC, et al. (1995) Advanced renovascular hypertension and renal insufficiency: trends in medical comorbidity and surgical approach from 1970 to 1993. J Vasc Surg 21: 750–759; discussion 759–760.
4. Kirksey M, Chiu YL, Ma Y, Della Valle AG, Poultsides L, et al. (2012) Trends in in-hospital major morbidity and mortality after total joint arthroplasty: United States 1998–2008. Anesth Analg 115: 321–327.
5. Malyar N, Furstenberg T, Wellmann J, Meyborg M, Luders F, et al. (2013) Recent trends in morbidity and in-hospital outcomes of in-patients with peripheral arterial disease: a nationwide population-based analysis. Eur Heart J 34: 2706–2714.
6. Millar WJ, Cole CW, Hill GB (1995) Trends in mortality and hospital morbidity due to abdominal aortic aneurysms. Health Rep 7: 19–27, 21–30.
7. Buljac-Samardzic M, Dekker-van Doorn CM, van Wijngaarden JD, van Wijk KP (2010) Interventions to improve team effectiveness: a systematic review. Health Policy 94: 183–195.
8. Haller G, Garnerin P, Morales M-A, Pfister R, Berner M, et al. (2008) Effect of crew resource management training in a multidisciplinary obstetrical setting. International Journal for Quality in Health Care 20: 254–263.
9. Suva D, Haller G, Lübbeke A, Hoffmeyer P (2012) Differential Impact of a Crew Resource Management Program According to Professional Specialty. American Journal of Medical Quality 27: 313–320.
10. World Health Organization (2008) World Alliance For Patient Safety – Safe Surgery Saves Lives. Geneva: WHO. Available: http://www.who.int/patientsafety/safesurgery/en/index.html.
11. World Health Organization WHO Guidelines for Safe Surgery 2009. Geneva: WHO, Available: http://whqlibdoc.who.int/publications/2009/9789241598552_eng.pdf. Accessed 2009 May 11.
12. Haynes AB, Weiser TG, Berry WR, Lipsitz SR, Breizat A-HS, et al. (2009) A Surgical Safety Checklist to Reduce Morbidity and Mortality in a Global Population. N Engl J Med 360: 491–499.
13. Borchard A, Schwappach DL, Barbir A, Bezzola P (2012) A Systematic Review of the Effectiveness, Compliance, and Critical Factors for Implementation of Safety Checklists in Surgery. Ann Surg 256: 925–933.
14. Ko H, Turner TJ, Finnigan MA (2011) Systematic review of safety checklists for use by medical care teams in acute hospital settings - limited evidence of effectiveness. BMC Health Serv Res 11: 211.
15. NHS (2009) WHO Surgical Safety Checklist.
16. Cabarrot P, Bataillon R, Le Moign R (2011) Check-list «Sécurité du patient au bloc opératoire». Quels acquis, quelles perspectives, un an après son implantation en France. Ann Fr Anesth Reanim 30: 469–474.
17. Nugent E, Hseino H, Ryan K, Traynor O, Neary P, et al. (2013) The surgical safety checklist survey: a national perspective on patient safety. Ir J Med Sci 182: 171–176.
18. World Health Organization Global support for Safe Surgery Saves Lives Geneva: WHO: Available: http://www.who.int/patientsafety/safesurgery/endorsements_received/en/index.html. Accessed 2012 Jun 1.
19. Kaderli R, Hertig RC, Laffer U, Businger AP (2012) Surgical Safety Checklists in Operative Medicine in Switzerland. Archives of Clinical Experimental Surgery 1: 158–167.
20. Abdel-Galil K (2010) The WHO Surgical Safety Checklist: are we measuring up? Br J Oral Maxillofac Surg 48: 397–398.
21. Patterson P (2009) In survey, about half of ORs are using the WHO checklist. OR Manager 25: 1, 6–8.
22. Fargen KM, Velat GJ, Lawson MF, Firment CS, Mocco J, .et al. (Published Online First: 6 July 2012 doi:10.1136/neurintsurg-2012-01043) Enhanced staff communication and reduced near-miss errors with a neurointerventional procedural checklist. J Neurointerv Surg.
23. Gueguen T, Coevoet V, Mougeot M, Pierron A, Blanquart D, et al. (2011) [Deployment of the checklist "Patient safety in the operating room" in two Lorraine hospitals. Performances and difficulties]. Ann Fr Anesth Reanim 30: 489–494.
24. Cullati S, Le Du S, Raë A-C, Micallef M, Khabiri E, et al. (2013) Is the Surgical Safety Checklist successfully conducted? An observational study of social interactions in the operating rooms of a tertiary hospital. BMJ Quality & Safety 22: 639–646.
25. Bohmer AB, Wappler F, Tinschmann T, Kindermann P, Rixen D, et al. (2012) The implementation of a perioperative checklist increases patients' perioperative safety and staff satisfaction. Acta Anaesthesiol Scand 56: 332–338.
26. Fourcade A, Blache JL, Grenier C, Bourgain JL, Minvielle E (2012) Barriers to staff adoption of a surgical safety checklist. BMJ Qual Saf 21: 191–197.
27. Paugam-Burtz C, Guerrero O (2011) Check-list sécurité au bloc opératoire: le bilan après un an de déploiement à l'hôpital Beaujon. Ann Fr Anesth Reanim 30: 475–478.
28. Spence J, Goodwin B, Enns C, Dean H (2011) Student-observed surgical safety practices across an urban regional health authority. BMJ Qual Saf 20: 580–586.
29. Rodrigo-Rincón MI, Tirapu-León B, Zabalza-López P, Martín-Vizcaino MP, de La Fuente-Calixto A, et al. (2011) Percepción de los profesionales sobre la utilización y la utilidad del listado de verificación quirúrgica. Rev Calid Asist 26: 380–385.
30. Kearns RJ, Uppal V, Bonner J, Robertson J, Daniel M, et al. (2011) The introduction of a surgical safety checklist in a tertiary referral obstetric centre. BMJ Qual Saf 20: 818–822.
31. Mascherek AC, Schwappach DL, Bezzola P (2013) Frequency of use and knowledge of the WHO-surgical checklist in Swiss hospitals: a cross-sectional online survey. Patient Safety Surgery 7: 36.
32. Kelly JJ, Farley H, O'Cain C, Broida RI, Klauer K, et al. (2011) A survey of the use of time-out protocols in emergency medicine. Jt Comm J Qual Patient Saf 37: 285–288.
33. Sivathasan N, Rakowski KR, Robertson BF, Vijayarajan L (2010) The World Health Organization's 'Surgical Safety Checklist': should evidence-based initiatives be enforced in hospital policy? JRSM Short Rep 1: 40.
34. World Health Organization (2009) Safe Surgery Saves Lives European Workshop - 15 January 2009. Geneva: WHO. Available: http://www.who.int/patientsafety/events/09/150109/en/index.html.
35. De Thomasson E, Bonfait H, Delaunay C (2013) La check-list au bloc opératoire: quelques raisons d'espérer! Risques & qualité 10: 156–161.
36. Makary MA, Mukherjee A, Sexton JB, Syin D, Goodrich E, et al. (2007) Operating Room Briefings and Wrong-Site Surgery. J Am Coll Surg 204: 236–243.
37. Hani D, Sedani PK, Hardee P, Bridle C, Ali N, et al. (2010) P49 Implementing of the WHO Surgical Safety Checklist' in an outpatients setting - an audit. Br J Oral Maxillofac Surg 48: S37–S37.
38. Cunat C, Flatin V, Viale JP (2011) [Implementation strategy of the HAS French surgical check-list in a university hospital]. Ann Fr Anesth Reanim 30: 484–488.
39. Rateau F, Levraut L, Colombel AL, Bernard JL, Quaranta JF, et al. (2011) [Check-list "Patient Safety" in the operating room: one year experience of 40,000 surgical procedures at the university hospital of Nice]. Ann Fr Anesth Reanim 30: 479–483.
40. Fishpool S, Pope R, Roberts C, Anthony R (2010) Re: The World Health Organisation surgical safety checklist. Clin Otolaryngol 35: 439–439.
41. Johnston G, Ekert L, Pally E (2009) Surgical Site Signing and "Time Out": Issues of Compliance or Complacence. J Bone Joint Surg Am 91: 2577–2580.
42. Khoshbin A, Lingard L, Wright JG (2009) Evaluation of preoperative and perioperative operating room briefings at the Hospital for Sick Children. Can J Surg 52: 309–315.
43. Vats A, Vincent CA, Nagpal K, Davies RW, Darzi A, et al. (2010) Practical challenges of introducing WHO surgical checklist: UK pilot experience. BMJ 340: b5433-.
44. Aveling E-L, McCulloch P, Dixon-Woods M (2013) A qualitative study comparing experiences of the surgical safety checklist in hospitals in high-income and low-income countries. BMJ Open 3.
45. Rydenfält C, Johansson G, Odenrick P, Åkerman K, Larsson PA (2013) Compliance with the WHO Surgical Safety Checklist: deviations and possible improvements. International Journal for Quality in Health Care 25: 182–187.
46. Pickering SP, Robertson ER, Griffin D, Hadi M, Morgan LJ, et al. (2013) Compliance and use of the World Health Organization checklist in UK operating theatres. British Journal of Surgery 100: 1664–1670.
47. Delgado Hurtado JJ, Jimenez X, Penalonzo MA, Villatoro C, de Izquierdo S, et al. (2012) Acceptance of the WHO Surgical Safety Checklist among surgical personnel in hospitals in Guatemala city. BMC Health Serv Res 12: 169.
48. Papaconstantinou HT, Jo C, Reznik SI, Smythe WR, Wehbe-Janek H (2013) Implementation of a surgical safety checklist: impact on surgical team perspectives. The Ochsner Journal 13: 299–309.
49. Bragg K, Schlenk EA, Wolf G, Hoolahan S, Ren D, et al. (2012) Time out! Surveying surgical barriers. Nursing Management 43: 38–44.
50. Calland JF, Turrentine FE, Guerlain S, Bovbjerg V, Poole GR, et al. (2011) The surgical safety checklist: lessons learned during implementation. Am Surg 77: 1131–1137.
51. McDowell DS, McComb SA (2014) Safety Checklist Briefings: A Systematic Review of the Literature. AORN Journal 99: 125–137.e113.
52. Haynes AB, Weiser TG, Berry WR, Lipsitz SR, Breizat A-HS, et al. (2011) Changes in safety attitude and relationship to decreased postoperative morbidity and mortality following implementation of a checklist-based surgical safety intervention. BMJ Quality & Safety 20: 102–107.
53. Thomassen O, Espeland A, Softeland E, Lossius HM, Heltne JK, et al. (2011) Implementation of checklists in health care; learning from high-reliability organisations. Scand J Trauma Resusc Emerg Med 19: 53.
54. Shanafelt TD, Boone S, Tan L, Dyrbye L, Sotile W, et al. (2012) BUrnout and satisfaction with work-life balance among us physicians relative to the general us population. Archives of Internal Medicine 172: 1377–1385.
55. Morton LM, Cahill J, Hartge P (2006) Reporting Participation in Epidemiologic Studies: A Survey of Practice. American Journal of Epidemiology 163: 197–203.
56. Galea S, Tracy M (2007) Participation Rates in Epidemiologic Studies. Annals of Epidemiology 17: 643–653.

57. Ziegenfuss JY, Shah ND, Fan J, Van Houten HK, Deming JR, et al. (2012) Patient Characteristics of Provider Survey Respondents: No Evidence of Nonresponse Bias. Eval Health Prof 35: 507–516.
58. Perneger TV, Cullati S, Rudaz S, Agoritsas T, Schmidt RE, et al. (2014) Effect of numbering of return envelopes on participation, explicit refusals, and bias: experiment and meta-analysis. BMC Med Res Methodol 14: 6.
59. Rydenfält C, Ek Å, Larsson PA (2013) Safety checklist compliance and a false sense of safety: new directions for research. BMJ Quality & Safety.

4

# Anaesthetic Tricaine Acts Preferentially on Neural Voltage-Gated Sodium Channels and Fails to Block Directly Evoked Muscle Contraction

**Seetharamaiah Attili, Simon M. Hughes***

Randall Division of Cell and Molecular Biophysics, Guy's Campus, King's College London, London, United Kingdom

**Abstract**

Movements in animals arise through concerted action of neurons and skeletal muscle. General anaesthetics prevent movement and cause loss of consciousness by blocking neural function. Anaesthetics of the amino amide-class are thought to act by blockade of voltage-gated sodium channels. In fish, the commonly used anaesthetic tricaine methanesulphonate, also known as 3-aminobenzoic acid ethyl ester, metacaine or MS-222, causes loss of consciousness. However, its role in blocking action potentials in distinct excitable cells is unclear, raising the possibility that tricaine could act as a neuromuscular blocking agent directly causing paralysis. Here we use evoked electrical stimulation to show that tricaine efficiently blocks neural action potentials, but does not prevent directly evoked muscle contraction. Nifedipine-sensitive L-type $Ca_v$ channels affecting movement are also primarily neural, suggesting that muscle $Na_v$ channels are relatively insensitive to tricaine. These findings show that tricaine used at standard concentrations in zebrafish larvae does not paralyse muscle, thereby diminishing concern that a direct action on muscle could mask a lack of general anaesthesia.

**Editor:** Steven Barnes, Dalhousie University, Canada

**Funding:** SMH is a Medical Research Council Scientist (www.mrc.ac.uk) with Programme Grant G1001029 support, which funded this study. Additional support to SMH that contributed to the work came from a Biotechnology and Biological Sciences Research Council (www.bbsrc.ac.uk) project grant BB/K0101151/1 and UK-India Partnering Award grant. The funders had no role in study design, data collection and analysis, decision to publish, or preparation of the manuscript.

**Competing Interests:** The authors have declared that no competing interests exist.

* Email: simon.hughes@kcl.ac.uk

## Introduction

In the $18^{th}$ century, Luigi Galvani laid the foundations of biophysics by discovering that electrical stimuli can trigger muscular contraction, transmit to muscles via nerves and are also generated by animals themselves [1]. Since that time, neurons and skeletal muscle have been shown to be electrically excitable; electrical action potentials in neurons trigger further action potentials in muscle fibres that lead to contraction. Voltage gated ion channels are key to the generation of action potentials (reviewed in [2]). Neuron and muscle have subtly different electrical properties, each employing distinct voltage-gated channels. Normally, an action potential propagates rapidly along the neural axon, stimulating the release of the neurotransmitter, which in turn elicits an action potential in the muscle fibre plasma membrane. This second action potential propagates via the transverse-tubule system deep into the fibre, where the dihyropyridine receptor (DHPR) acts as a voltage sensor that causes release of $Ca^{++}$ from sarcoplasmic reticulum into the cytoplasm. Increased cytoplasmic $Ca^{++}$ concentration promotes actomyosin contractility [3,4]. Following Galvani, muscle contraction can be directly activated by external electric stimulation that triggers action, controlling not only immediate contraction events but also longer term muscle gene expression [5–8].

Excitability arises from the sequential opening and closing of voltage-gated $Na^+$, $Ca^{++}$ and $K^+$ channels [9,10]. In adult skeletal muscle, voltage-gated $Na^+$ ($Na_v$) channels initiate the action potential, rapidly activate and inactivate in a few milliseconds and have been widely studied [2,11]. In embryonic tissues, however, voltage–gated $Ca^{++}$ ($Ca_v$) channels can make a significant contribution to the action potential [12–14]. Additionally, L-type voltage-gated $Ca_V1.1$ channels play an essential role in calcium release in skeletal muscle through their role as components of the DHPR, which provides a voltage-sensitive mechanical link that triggers release of $Ca^{++}$ from the sarcoplasmic reticulum [12,15]. Drugs that target voltage-gated channels have proved invaluable in the clinic, but often have side effects due to their ability to bind more than one channel type [16]. Local anaesthetics, for example, inhibit the generation of neural action potentials by blocking the flow of ions through voltage-gated ion channels [17–19]. However, compounds such as lidocaine and bupivacaine can have side effects through, for example, cardiac depression.

The larvae of the zebrafish *Danio rerio* offer many advantages for drug screening and investigating the relationship between ion channel expression and nerve and muscle function *in vivo* [20,21]. The practical use of zebrafish often involves, however, the use of tricaine, which is a rapidly reversible general anaesthetic that supresses movement and thus permits visualisation and manipulation of the organism. Tricaine methanesulfonate (also known as 3-aminobenzoic acid ethyl ester or MS-222) is a preferred drug for aquatic anaesthesia in Norway [22] and in zebrafish experimentation by the U.K. Home Office [23] and is the only drug approved for use in fish by U.S. Food and Drug Administration (www.accessdata.fda.gov/scripts/animaldrugsatfda/). Previous reports have shown a suppressive effect of tricaine on zebrafish peripheral and central nervous system [24-26], but also adverse effects on physiology (summarised in [22]). Tricaine, at the normal concentrations used, has little effect on embryonic cardiac contractility, but the heart becomes more sensitive as animals mature [27]. The molecular and cellular targets of tricaine in zebrafish are not fully characterised. This is particularly important because the use of tricaine has recently been questioned on the grounds that fish sense and choose to avoid tricaine [23,28]. It would be of great concern if tricaine were to act directly to paralyse skeletal muscle, thereby preventing movement, as this might mask a lack of general anaesthesia.

Local anaesthetics of the amino amide class, to which tricaine belongs, are known to inhibit certain mammalian $Na_v$ channels e.g. [29]. Such channels are generally composed of alpha and beta subunits and are primarily defined by their large alpha subunit, which contains the voltage-sensing domain [2]. The zebrafish sodium channel (*scn*) gene family consists of four sets of duplicated alpha subunit genes. *scn1a* and *scn1Lab* form the $Na_v1.1$ channels expressed in cardiac muscle [30]. *scn4aa* and *scn4ab* contribute to $Na_v1.4$ channels and are expressed in skeletal muscle [30–32]. The expression of *scn12aa* and *scn12ab* (putatively forming $Na_v1.5$ channels) is transient in zebrafish muscle [31], but in mouse *Scn5a* is expressed in neonatal skeletal muscle and limbic system and in adult muscle after denervation [33]. *scn8aa* and *scn8ab* ($Na_v1.6$ channels) are expressed in brain eye, spinal cord, retina, and peripheral nervous system [30,31,34]. The zebrafish $Na_v$ channels targeted by tricaine are unclear.

Whether amino amide anaesthetics also inhibit zebrafish $Ca_v$ channels is unknown, but such effects have been reported in other species [35–38]. $Ca_v$ channels have similarities to $Na_v$ channels, in that their alpha subunits have clear structural and functional similarities [39]. Zebrafish somites make the first skeletal muscle and express L-type voltage gated calcium channels *cacna1sa* (CaV1.1)[40]. In contrast, the P/Q-type *cacna1a* is expressed in brain, neuronal cells and heart [40]. Thus, the channels and cell types inhibited by tricaine are not fully characterised.

We set out to investigate the tissue target(s) of tricaine in the zebrafish, particularly in muscle. We report the impact of tricaine on zebrafish skeletal muscle at early developmental stages. We also studied the impact of nifedipine, an L-type $Ca^{++}$ channel antagonist. Our findings show that, at the normal concentrations used for anaesthesia, tricaine does not prevent muscle contraction or interfere with excitation-contraction coupling.

## Materials and Methods

### Animals and Reagents

Danio rerio, either Tübingen wild type or $chrnd^{sb13}$ (here called '*fixe*') mutants [41] maintained on Tübingen background, were reared at 28.5°C according the standard procedures [42]. All experiments were performed at age of 3-3.5 days post-fertilization (dpf). Stock aliquots (2 ml) of 16 mM Tricaine (3-aminobenzoic acid ethyl ester methanesulphonate) in double distilled water at pH 7 were stored at -20°C. Agarose (Sigma Life Sciences) 2% in fish water was prepared and stored in fridge at 4°C. Aliquots (10 µl) of Nifedipine (Sigma-Aldrich) in dimethylsulfoxide (DMSO) at stock concentration of 100 mM were stored at −20°C. Tricaine and Nifedipine were thawed at room temperature each day of experiment prior to dilution.

### Electrical Stimulation

Fish larvae were subjected electrical stimulation at room temperature using a custom-built electric stimulation set-up (ESS) (Fig. 1A). To minimize damage to the fish, the ESS consists of two silver electrodes (0.5 mm , 99.9%, Arcos Organics, New Jersey, U.S.A.) arrayed parallel and 10 mm apart passing through the drilled holes of a 6-well tissue culture plate or a 60 mm petri dish. Chambers with electrodes were filled with 2% agarose gel, such that the silver electrodes are completely within the gel. A circular well of volume 0.5 mL was created by removing the agarose in the centre of the chamber between the two electrodes. Fish are placed carefully into the well with desired orientation. Care was taken not to expose the electrodes to the fish swimming in the well. The electrodes are connected to a stimulator (Grass S-88, Grass Instruments, U.S.A) that generated square wave pulse trains of indicated lengths. Polarity of electrodes was reversed between pulse trains to avoid electrolysis. A range of stimulation regimes was tested, with the aim of attaining a brief twitch response, and all experiments shown used a train of 200 20 V pulses, with 0.5 ms pulse duration (100 ms total train duration) once every 5 seconds (Fig. 1A).

### Drug treatments

For wash-out, fish were later transferred to a dish containing fresh fish water and were left there for over 30 minutes. Care was taken to exchange the fish water five times to remove residual tricaine.

### Data capture and analysis

Observations were made using a dissecting microscope (Leica MZ 16F, Germany). All videos were recorded using Olympus (DP70) camera with DP Controller software at a frame rate of 60 frames per second in total time of 25 seconds.

Fish tail displacement "*d*" was measured at the level of the last somite by superimposing images from video. Two images, before and after the onset of stimulation, were overlaid using Adobe Photoshop by false-colouring one image red and converting it to transparent mode.

### Ethics Statement

Fish were bred and experiments performed under licences from the UK Home Office and conform to all institutional, national and EU guidelines.

## Results

The performance of ESS was tested at a range of voltage and pulse train parameters to define a stimulation regime that was not toxic to the fish yet triggered motility. The response of fish to the external stimulus was immediate oscillatory swimming movement with the appearance of an escape response (Movie S1). Escape responses are under neural control either at spinal or higher levels [43]. Evoked movement was quantified by measuring tail tip displacement at the level of the last somite upon stimulation and was >1 mm in sentient fish (Fig. 1B,C). To determine whether electrical stimulation also acts directly on muscle cells, *fixe* mutant larvae, which lack functional acetylcholine receptors [41], were stimulated and gave a single strong contraction to each pulse train that subsequently relaxed (Movie S1). Maximal tail displacement was about 0.17 mm (Fig. 1D). Thus, electric stimulation evokes muscle fibre contraction directly.

Amino amide anaesthetics are known to hinder the generation of action potentials by blocking diffusion of ions through voltage-gated channels within excitable cells, thereby inhibiting the

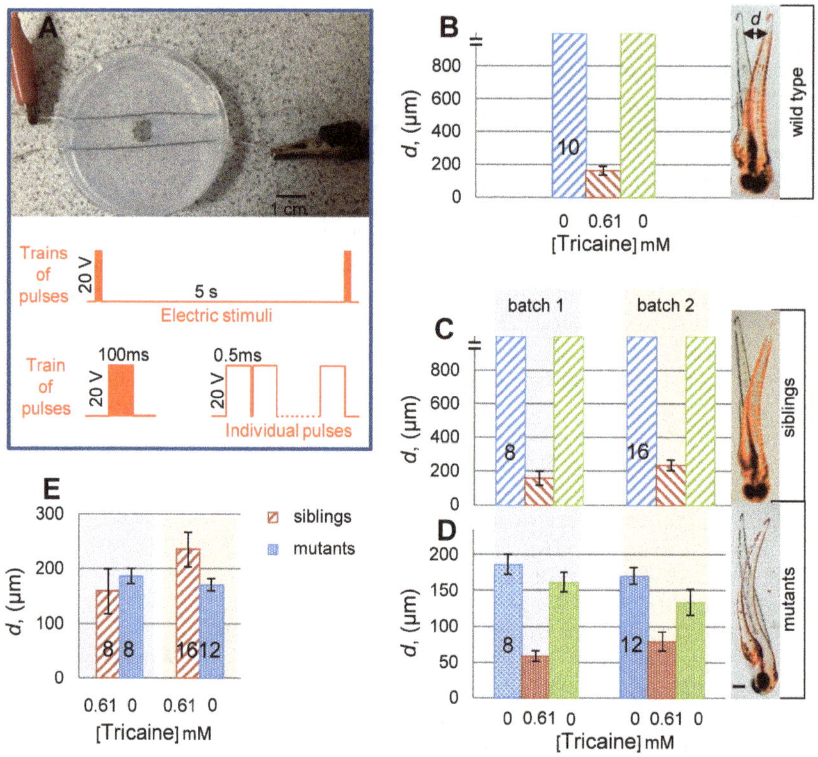


**Figure 1. Tricaine fails to block evoked muscle contractility. A.** The electrical stimulation set-up (ESS). Fish are placed within the central well aligned, when spontaneous motility permits, with their anteroposterior axis perpendicular to the electrodes. Schematic of the electric stimulus regime is shown below. **B-D.** Tail displacement (*d*) in embryos from wild type (B) or a *fixe* heterozygote incross sorted into motile siblings (C; *chrnd*$^{+/?}$ 97/132 = 73.5%) and immotile mutants (D; *chrnd*$^{sb13/sb13}$ 35/132 = 26.5%). Movement was quantified from videos as measured displacement (*d*) of tail as shown (B-D, right panels) in superimposed stills of single fish before stimulation (black image) and at maximum displacement (false-coloured red image). Unanaesthetized motile fish move extensively, generally out of the field of view (indicated by break in *Y*-axis). Fish were measured before tricaine exposure, after exposure to 0.61 mM tricaine for 30 min and after ≤30 minutes of tricaine washout into fish water. Note altered *Y*-scale in D compared to B,C. **E.** Comparison of mutants with tricaine-treated individuals reveals a striking similarity in displacement. Error bars are SEM. Numbers of embryos are shown on bars. Scale bars = 0.1 mm.

movement [18,44]. Adding tricaine to wild type or non-mutant *fixe* sibling larvae at the concentration widely used for anaesthetizing zebrafish (0.61 mM; 160 mg/L)[42] completely inhibited movement in response to touch, water flow or vibration (data not shown). However, tricaine did not block motility evoked by electrical stimulation (Movie S1). Strikingly, the contraction/relaxation timecourse and maximal displacement in anaesthetised fish was indistinguishable from that evoked in *fixe* mutants (Fig. 1E). The action of tricaine was fully reversible, as fish regained normal movement after washout of the anaesthetic (Fig. 1B,C). We conclude that tricaine anaesthesia does not prevent action potentials, excitation-contraction coupling or actomyosin contractility in zebrafish muscle fibres. We observed no difference in measured movements between wild type and non-mutant *fixe* siblings; we continued our experiments with *fixe* siblings.

Given that both tricaine and loss of acetylcholine receptors had the same effect of blocking the neurally-induced escape response but not electric stimulation-evoked motility, we predicted no effect of adding tricaine to *fixe* mutants. Strikingly, however, we consistently observed a reduction in evoked motility (Movie S1 and Fig. 1D). Again, the effect was reversible upon washout of tricaine. These observations confirmed that muscle fibres are resistant to the suppression of action potentials by tricaine, but further suggested that tricaine does act weakly on muscle fibre ion channels, at least those present in immotile *fixe* mutants. To test this hypothesis, higher doses of tricaine were applied to wild type or *fixe* sibling larvae. Motility gradually declined at successively higher doses until it was essentially inhibited by 3.2 mM tricaine (Fig. 2A and data not shown). In high dose tricaine, *fixe* mutants did not move detectably in response to stimulation, whereas their siblings still showed very slight twitches that caused negligible tail displacement (Movies S1). Thus, tricaine can directly inhibit striated muscle contraction, but functionally denervated muscle appears more sensitive to tricaine than muscle in unmanipulated larvae.

Why is muscle resistant to doses of tricaine that act as a general anaesthetic? One hypothesis is that the voltage-gated channels in skeletal muscle are distinct from those inhibited by tricaine in the nervous system. As $Na_v$ channels are known to be major targets of tricaine in neurons [18], we asked whether action potentials in larval muscle are $Ca^{++}$-based and thus have reduced sensitivity to tricaine. Nifedipine is a calcium channel blocker used to test the role of $Ca_v$ channels in generation of action potential [45]. Application of Nifedipine (0.1 mM) reduced the movement of unanaesthetised fish (data not shown). At higher concentrations (0.5 mM) nifedipine reduced movement significantly but less effectively than tricaine (Fig. 2B). Fish incubated in both 0.5 mM Nifedipine and 0.61 mM tricaine for 30 minutes showed no significant difference from fish treated with tricaine alone (Fig. 2B). When the drugs were washed out with fish water, movement returned to the level elicited by nifedipine alone, consistent with

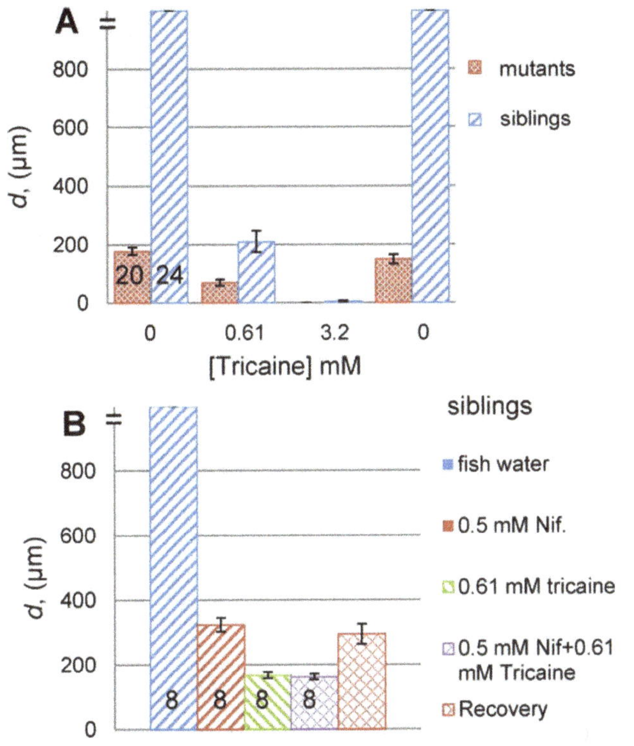


**Figure 2. Tricaine blocks muscle contraction at high concentrations. A.** Comparison of tail displacement (*d*) as a function of successively increasing tricaine concentration in *fixe* mutants and their siblings. In both cases, full movement is regained upon tricaine wash-out to fish water. **B.** Tail displacement in response to L-type $Ca_v$ channel blocker Nifedipine alone, tricaine alone, or both, and after wash-out of both drugs (right hand bar). Error bars are SEM. Numbers of embryos are shown on bars.

the known irreversible action of nifedipine [46,47]. Nifedipine did not reduce motility in *fixe* mutants (data not shown). These results suggest that nifedipine-sensitive L-type $Ca_v$ channels are functional in neurons of the motor pathway, but do not significantly contribute within the muscle itself.

## Discussion

There are four major results from the current study. First, a simple and custom built electric stimulation set-up shows that larval zebrafish muscle contraction can be directly evoked using external electric stimuli. Second, that tricaine anaesthesia at normal doses prevents movement by effectively inhibiting neural but not skeletal muscle action potentials. Thirdly, tricaine at higher concentrations also blocks muscle action potentials, probably via effects on $Na_v$ channels. Lastly, nifedipine-sensistive L-type voltage-gated calcium channels also act in the nervous system but appear to have little direct action within zebrafish muscle to promote contraction.

Movements in skeletal muscle can be elicited either by neurons (natural movement) or by external electrical stimulation (evoked movement, EES), in which muscle plasma membrane depolarization caused by the applied voltage triggers an action potential. In the current study, we show that EES can initiate contraction in mutants that lack the acetylcholine receptor delta subunits and therefore cannot receive natural input from motorneurons [41]. EES as used here triggers brief sub-tetanic contractions; ramping the voltage beyond 20 V caused more forceful movements (unpublished observations). EES will enable future studies of the impact of muscle electrical activity on gene expression and growth.

Amino amide anaesthetics are known to block $Na_v$ channels and thus block the conduction of action potentials in excitable cells [18]. Tricaine is the most commonly used anaesthetic agent for zebrafish. Tricaine is structurally similar to the anaesthetic agents procaine, bupivacaine and lidocaine. These anaesthetics also bind reversibly to $Na_v$ channels, blocking $Na^+$ movement through the channels, but can also affect other channels [38]. We were able to evoke muscle contraction in fish incubated in tricaine. The magnitude of contraction was similar to that evoked in mutants lacking transmission at the neuromuscular junction. We interpret these observations to show that tricaine does not prevent action potentials in skeletal muscle fibres, whereas action potentials in nerve cells are effectively prevented, leading to general anaesthesia. This finding is important for considerations of animal husbandry; although fish appear to detect and avoid tricaine [23,28], our data show that tricaine works preferentially at the neural, rather than muscular, level of control of movement. Although questions remain on the most appropriate agents for fish anaesthesia [22], our study shows that tricaine at standard concentrations does not act as a paralytic neuromuscular blocking agent in zebrafish.

Of the known $Na_v$ channel alpha subunit genes, only *scn4aa* and *scn4ab* are expressed in zebrafish skeletal muscle around 3 dpf [30-32]. It seems that channels made with these subunits ($Na_v1.4$) may be less sensitive to tricaine than those made with classical neural homologues, such as *scn1a* ($Na_v1.1$) and *scn8a* ($Na_v1.6$) subunits. The $Na_v1.5$ channel alpha subunit gene (*scn12ab* in zebrafish) appears to be expressed transiently in early developing slow muscle fibres, but may become restricted to cardiac muscle later [30,31]. The murine $Na_v1.5$ channel is up-regulated in skeletal muscle on denervation [48]. It is therefore possible that the effectiveness of tricaine in inhibiting evoked movement in *fixe* mutants reflects up-regulation of similar channels sensitive to tricaine in inactive somitic muscle. Indeed, mammalian $Na_v1.5$ appears several fold more sensitive than $Na_v1.4$ to lidocaine [29]. However, the ineffectiveness of tricaine to silence embryonic zebrafish heart demonstrates that the major cardiac $Na_v$ channel expressed at early stages (*scn12aa* [31]) is not particularly tricaine sensitive. Interestingly, the heart becomes more sensitive to tricaine as the fish matures, perhaps correlating with increasing predominance of expression of *scn12ab* in the myocardium [27,49]. Electrophysiological studies of isolated zebrafish channels are required to resolve these issues.

Higher concentrations of tricaine largely inhibit evoked muscle contraction, suggesting either that muscle action potentials can be prevented by this drug or that tricaine may affect channels involved in excitation-contraction coupling. The simplest explanation appears to be that the $Na_v1.4$ channels are inhibited by high dose tricaine. Alternatively, $Ca_v$ channels contain alpha subunits with structural similarity to $Na_v$ channels [2,12]. As developing muscle has been reported to have $Ca_v$ channels capable of supporting a $Ca^{++}$-based action potential [12], these could be targets of high dose tricaine. The *cacna1sa* channel thought to be a muscle-specific subunit of the DHPR is expressed in zebrafish somitic muscle [40]. So high dose tricaine might block excitation-contraction coupling directly.

We addressed the idea of $Ca^{++}$-based action potentials directly, but failed to find evidence in favour of this possibility. Specialised L-type $Ca_v$ channels can be blocked by nifedipine [50]. We found that nifedipine inhibits CNS function in zebrafish larvae, leading to reduced movement. However, nifedipine had no effect on the residual motility present in tricaine-treated larvae, indicating that neither evoked action potentials, nor the DHPR, were blocked by this drug. These findings argue that L-type $Ca_v$ channels are not responsible for the resistance of zebrafish muscle to normal doses of tricaine.

## Supporting Information

**Movie S1 Movement of wild type (wt), *fixe* mutants (*chrnd*$^{sb13/sb13}$) or *fixe* sibling (*chrnd*$^{sb13/+}$ *or chrnd*$^{+/+}$) fish in response to EES.** Fish were treated with the water control or tricaine at standard or fivefold dose, as indicated before each clip. A pulse train of 0.1 s duration was applied every 5 seconds. Movie is sped up about 2.5-fold for ease of viewing. Note increased movement in response to the first pulse, possibly reflecting the need for channel activation for tricaine to bind to $Na_v$ channels. Heartbeat shows all fish are alive. In '*fixe* + 5X tricaine' clip, heartbeat shows fish are alive but fail to respond to stimulation.

## Acknowledgments

We thank members of the Hughes lab for help and advice during the work.

## Author Contributions

Conceived and designed the experiments: SA SMH. Performed the experiments: SA. Analyzed the data: SA SMH. Contributed to the writing of the manuscript: SA SMH.

## References


1. Galvani A (1791) De viribus electricitatis in motu musculari commentarius. Bologna: Accademia delle Scienze. Eprint 2000 The International Centre for the History of Universities and Science (CIS), Università di Bologna.
2. Catterall WA (2014) Structure and function of voltage-gated sodium channels at atomic resolution. Experimental Physiology 99: 35–51.
3. Ebashi S, Endo M (1968) Calcium ion and muscle contraction. Prog Biophys Mol Biol 18: 123–183.
4. Matthews GG (2003) Cellular Physiology of Nerve and Muscle. Oxford: Blackwell Science Ltd.
5. Maffiuletti NA, Roig M, Karatzanos E, Nanas S (2013) Neuromuscular electrical stimulation for preventing skeletal-muscle weakness and wasting in critically ill patients: a systematic review. BMC Med 11: 137.
6. Salmons S, Sreter FA (1976) Significance of impulse activity in the transformation of skeletal muscle type. Nature 263: 30–34.
7. Pette D, Vrbová G (1999) What does chronic electrical stimulation teach us about muscle plasticity? Muscle Nerve 22: 666–677.
8. Windisch A, Gundersen K, Szabolcs MJ, Gruber H, Lomo T (1998) Fast to slow transformation of denervated and electrically stimulated rat muscle. J Physiol (Lond) 510: 623–632.
9. Hodgkin AL, Huxley AF (1952) A quantitative description of membrane current and its application to conduction and excitation in nerve. J Physiol 117: 500–544.
10. Armstrong CM, Hille B (1998) Voltage-gated ion channels and electrical excitability. Neuron 20: 371–380.
11. Chen R, Chung SH (2014) Mechanism of tetrodotoxin block and resistance in sodium channels. Biochem Biophys Res Commun 446: 370–374.
12. Catterall WA (2011) Voltage-Gated Calcium Channels. Cold Spring Harbor Perspectives in Biology 3.
13. Couchoux H, Allard B, Legrand C, Jacquemond V, Berthier C (2007) Loss of caveolin-3 induced by the dystrophy-associated P104L mutation impairs L-type calcium channel function in mouse skeletal muscle cells. The Journal of Physiology 580: 745–754.
14. Strube C, Tourneur Y, Ojeda C (2000) Functional expression of the L-type calcium channel in mice skeletal muscle during prenatal myogenesis. Biophys J 78: 1282–1292.
15. Lacinova L (2005) Voltage-dependent calcium channels. Gen Physiol Biophys 24 Suppl 1: 1–78.
16. Wang GK, Calderon J, Wang SY (2008) State- and use-dependent block of muscle Nav1.4 and neuronal Nav1.7 voltage-gated Na+ channel isoforms by ranolazine. Mol Pharmacol 73: 940–948.
17. Yamakage M, Namiki A (2002) Calcium channels - basic aspects of their structure, function and gene encoding; anesthetic action on the channels - a review. Canadian Journal of Anaesthesia-Journal Canadien D Anesthesie 49: 151–164.
18. Nau C, Wang GK (2004) Interactions of local anesthetics with voltage-gated Na+ channels. J Membr Biol 201: 1–8.
19. Butterworth JF, Strichartz GR (1990) Molecular mechanisms of local anesthesia: a review. Anesthesiology 72: 711–734.
20. Dahm R, Geisler R (2006) Learning from small fry: The zebrafish as a genetic model organism for aquaculture fish species. Marine Biotechnology 8: 329–345.
21. Skromne I, Prince VE (2008) Current perspectives in zebrafish reverse genetics: moving forward. Dev Dyn 237: 861–882.
22. Zahl I-H, Samuelsen O, Kiessling A (2012) Anaesthesia of farmed fish: implications for welfare. Fish Physiology and Biochemistry 38: 201–218.
23. Readman GD, Owen SF, Murrell JC, Knowles TG (2013) Do fish perceive anaesthetics as aversive? PLoS ONE 8: e73773.
24. Späth M, Schweickert W (1997) The effect of metacaine (MS-222) on the activity of the efferent and afferent nerves in the teleost lateral-line system. Naunyn-Schmiedeberg's Archives of Pharmacology 297: 9–16.
25. Svoboda KR, Linares AE, Ribera AB (2001) Activity regulates programmed cell death of zebrafish Rohon-Beard neurons. Development 128: 3511–3520.
26. Hedrick MS, Winmill RE (2003) Excitatory and inhibitory effects of tricaine (MS-222) on fictive breathing in isolated bullfrog brain stem. American Journal of Physiology - Regulatory, Integrative and Comparative Physiology 284: R405–R412.
27. Huang WC, Hsieh YS, Chen IH, Wang CH, Chang HW, et al. (2010) Combined Use of MS-222 (Tricaine) and Isoflurane Extends Anesthesia Time and Minimizes Cardiac Rhythm Side Effects in Adult Zebrafish. Zebrafish 7: 297–304.
28. Wong D, von Keyserlingk MAG, Richards JG, Weary DM (2014) Conditioned Place Avoidance of Zebrafish Danio rerio to Three Chemicals Used for Euthanasia and Anaesthesia. PLoS ONE 9: e88030.
29. Nuss HB, Tomaselli GF, Marbán E (1995) Cardiac sodium channels (hH1) are intrinsically more sensitive to block by lidocaine than are skeletal muscle (mu 1) channels. The Journal of General Physiology 106: 1193–1209.
30. Chopra SS, Stroud DM, Watanabe H, Bennett JS, Burns CG, et al. (2010) Voltage-gated sodium channels are required for heart development in zebrafish. Circ Res 106: 1342–1350.
31. Novak AE, Taylor AD, Pineda RH, Lasda EL, Wright MA, et al. (2006) Embryonic and larval expression of zebrafish voltage-gated sodium channel alpha-subunit genes. Dev Dyn 235: 1962–1973.
32. Venkatesh B, Lu SQ, Dandona N, See SL, Brenner S, et al. (2005) Genetic basis of tetrodotoxin resistance in pufferfishes. Curr Biol 15: 2069–2072.
33. Shang LL, Dudley SC Jr (2005) Tandem promoters and developmentally regulated 5'- and 3'-mRNA untranslated regions of the mouse Scn5a cardiac sodium channel. J Biol Chem 280: 933–940.
34. Catterall WA, Goldin AL, Waxman SG (2005) International Union of Pharmacology. XLVII. Nomenclature and structure-function relationships of voltage-gated sodium channels. Pharmacol Rev 57: 397–409.
35. Oyama Y, Sadoshima J, Tokutomi N, Akaike N (1988) Some properties of inhibitory action of lidocaine on the Ca2+ current of single isolated frog sensory neurons. Brain Res 442: 223–228.
36. Josephson IR (1988) Lidocaine blocks Na, Ca and K currents of chick ventricular myocytes. J Mol Cell Cardiol 20: 593–604.
37. Carmeliet E, Morad M, Van der Heyden G, Vereecke J (1986) Electrophysiological effects of tetracaine in single guinea-pig ventricular myocytes. J Physiol 376: 143–161.
38. Scholz A (2002) Mechanisms of (local) anaesthetics on voltage-gated sodium and other ion channels. Br J Anaesth 89: 52–61.
39. Catterall WA, Perez-Reyes E, Snutch TP, Striessnig J (2005) International Union of Pharmacology. XLVIII. Nomenclature and structure-function relationships of voltage-gated calcium channels. Pharmacol Rev 57: 411–425.
40. Sanhueza D, Montoya A, Sierralta J, Kukuljan M (2009) Expression of voltage-activated calcium channels in the early zebrafish embryo. Zygote 17: 131–135.
41. Etard C, Behra M, Ertzer R, Fischer N, Jesuthasan S, et al. (2005) Mutation in the delta-subunit of the nAChR suppresses the muscle defects caused by lack of Dystrophin. Dev Dyn 234: 1016–1025.
42. Westerfield M (2000) The Zebrafish Book-A guide for the laboratory use of zebrafish (Danio rerio).
43. Ritter DA, Bhatt DH, Fetcho JR (2001) In vivo imaging of zebrafish reveals differences in the spinal networks for escape and swimming movements. J Neurosci 21: 8956–8965.
44. Winlow W, Yar T, Spencer G, Girdlestone D, Hancox J (1992) Differential effects of general anaesthetics on identified molluscan neurones in situ and in culture. Gen Pharmacol 23: 985–992.
45. Toal CB, Meredith PA, Elliott HL (2012) Long-acting dihydropyridine calcium-channel blockers and sympathetic nervous system activity in hypertension: a literature review comparing amlodipine and nifedipine GITS. Blood Press 21 Suppl 1: 3–10.
46. Piriz J, Rosato Siri MD, Pagani R, Uchitel OD (2003) Nifedipine-Mediated Mobilization of Intracellular Calcium Stores Increases Spontaneous Neuro-

transmitter Release at Neonatal Rat Motor Nerve Terminals. Journal of Pharmacology and Experimental Therapeutics 306: 658–663.
47. Barry WH, Horowitz JD, Smith TW (1985) Comparison of negative inotropic potency, reversibility, and effects on calcium influx of six calcium channel antagonists in cultured myocardial cells. British Journal of Pharmacology 85: 51–59.
48. Rowan SL, Rygiel K, Purves-Smith FM, Solbak NM, Turnbull DM, et al. (2012) Denervation causes fiber atrophy and myosin heavy chain co-expression in senescent skeletal muscle. PLoS One 7: e29082.
49. Denvir MA, Tucker CS, Mullins JJ (2008) Systolic and diastolic ventricular function in zebrafish embryos: influence of norepenephrine, MS-222 and temperature. BMC Biotechnol 8: 21.
50. Nguemo F, Fleischmann BK, Gupta MK, Saric T, Malan D, et al. (2013) The L-type Ca2+ channels blocker nifedipine represses mesodermal fate determination in murine embryonic stem cells. PLoS One 8: e53407.

5

# Intraoperative and Anesthesia-Related Cardiac Arrest and Its Mortality in Older Patients: A 15-Year Survey in a Tertiary Teaching Hospital

**Juscimar C. Nunes[1], Jose R. C. Braz[1], Thais S. Oliveira[1], Lidia R. de Carvalho[2], Yara M. M. Castiglia[1], Leandro G. Braz[1]***

**1** Department of Anesthesiology, Botucatu Medical School, UNESP - Univ Estadual Paulista, Botucatu, São Paulo, Brazil, **2** Department of Biostatistics, Institute of Biosciences, UNESP - Univ Estadual Paulista, Botucatu, São Paulo, Brazil

## Abstract

***Background:*** Little information is known about factors that influence perioperative and anesthesia-related cardiac arrest (CA) in older patients. This study evaluated the incidence, causes and outcome of intraoperative and anesthesia-related CA in older patients in a Brazilian teaching hospital between 1996 and 2010.

***Methods:*** During the study, older patients received 18,367 anesthetics. Data collected included patient characteristics, surgical procedures, American Society of Anesthesiologists (ASA) physical status, anesthesia type, medical specialty team and outcome. All CAs were categorized by cause into one of four groups: patient's disease/condition-related, surgery-related, totally anesthesia-related or partially anesthesia-related.

***Results:*** All intraoperative CAs and deaths rates are shown per 10,000 anesthetics. There were 100 CAs (54.44; 95% confidence intervals [CI]: 44.68–64.20) and 68 deaths (37.02; 95% CI: 27.56–46.48). The majority of CAs were patient's disease-/condition-related (43.5; 95% CI: 13.44–73.68). There were six anesthesia-related CAs (3.26; 95% CI: 0.65–5.87) - 1 totally and 5 partially anesthesia-related, and three deaths, all partially anesthesia-related (1.63; 95% CI: 0.0–3.47). ASA I-II physical status patients presented no anesthesia-related CA. Anesthesia-related CA, absent in the last five years of the study, was due to medication-/airway-related causes. ASA physical status was the most important predictor of CA (odds ratio: 14.52; 95% CI: 4.48–47.08; $P<0.001$) followed by emergency surgery (odds ratio: 8.07; 95% CI: 5.14–12.68; $P<0.001$).

***Conclusions:*** The study identified high incidence of intraoperative CAs with high mortality in older patients. The large majority of CAs were caused by factors not anesthesia-related. Anesthesia-related CA and mortality rates were 3.26 and 1.63 per 10,000 anesthetics, with no anesthesia-related CA in the last five years of the study. Major predictors of intraoperative CAs were poorer ASA physical status and emergency surgery. All anesthesia-related CAs were medication-related or airway-related, which is important for prevention strategies.

**Editor:** Giovanni Landoni, San Raffaele Scientific Institute, Italy

**Funding:** The authors have no funding or support to report.

**Competing Interests:** The authors have declared that no competing interests exist.

* Email: lbraz@fmb.unesp.br

## Introduction

The global population is ageing. According to the World Health Organization, people ≥60 years old in developing countries, such as Brazil, are considered elderly [1]. A significant proportion of older people are living with chronic diseases, such as cardiovascular disease, cognitive impairments and a reduced physiological reserve, which remain a challenge for all areas of medicine [2].

Few studies on perioperative cardiac arrest (CA) and mortality carried out exclusively in geriatric patients undergoing all types of surgery have been published [3–6]. However, there are no studies on anesthesia-related CA and death exclusively in elderly patients. Therefore, little information is known about factors that influence intraoperative and anesthesia-related CA and death in older surgical patients.

A survey performed from 1996 to 2005 in a Brazilian general tertiary teaching hospital [7] and other studies that included patients of all age groups [8,9], found that the perioperative CA and mortality rates were higher in older adults than in young adults. Recognizing the importance of identification of high-risk patients to guide the planning, resourcing, and expert staffing required to enhance the safety and improve the anesthesia outcomes for older patients, our institution developed initiatives for the purpose of improving the care of surgical patients. This involved the organization of services for the care of older patients, including the operating room (OR) materials and equipments such as anesthesia workstations with ventilators to provide adequate ventilation and monitoring, and devices for temperature control, new drugs for anesthesia induction and increasing the number of adult intensive care beds.

The aim of this study was to evaluate the incidence, triggering factors, causes and outcome of intraoperative and anesthesia-related CA in older surgical patients over a 15-yr period in a Brazilian general tertiary teaching hospital.

## Methods

The project was approved by the Human Research Ethics Committee of the Botucatu Medical School (Ref: 3694-2010), who waived the requirement for written informed consent. This survey analyzed all reported CA in 18,367 consecutive anesthetics given to all older patients at least 60 years of age requiring anesthesia services at the Hospital of the Botucatu Medical School, *Universidade Estadual Paulista* (UNESP), São Paulo State, Brazil, a public tertiary teaching hospital, from January 1, 1996 to December 31, 2010. The UNESP hospital is a 450-bed tertiary-care referral facility with a catchment of 2 million people that performs approximately 7,000 surgeries per year on people of all age groups. The hospital has a 33-bed adult intensive care unit.

The basic safety monitoring protocol in the OR during regional and neuroaxial anesthesia and sedation included electrocardiogram, automatic non-invasive blood pressure and pulse oximetry. For general anesthesia were measured the core temperature, ventilation parameters, capnography and oxygen concentration. After 2005 the delivered nitrous oxide and halogenated anesthetic vapour concentrations were also measured. Critically ill patients received invasive blood pressure and central venous pressure monitoring. The same basic monitoring described for the OR was also used in the postanesthesia care unit (PACU).

Cardiac arrests and deaths in older patients in the OR and PACU were identified through an anesthesia database developed from a quality assessment form that is part of the mandatory documentation for each anesthetic procedure. The forms were completed by the anesthesia staff responsible for each administration of anesthetic. The recorded data included the date and location; patient characteristics; American Society of Anesthesiologists (ASA) physical status classification; surgical procedures (elective, urgent or emergency surgery); medical specialty team; anesthesia type (general, regional or monitored and supportive anesthesia care associated or not with local anesthesia in critically ill patients); outcome; and a 95-item checklist of airway, respiratory, cardiocirculatory, neurological, renal and miscellaneous events related to the OR or PACU stay.

Cardiac arrest was defined as the cessation of cardiac mechanical activity with loss of effective circulation determined by the absence of a palpable central pulse. The resuscitation was performed according to the interventions and protocols for Advanced Cardiovascular Life Support (ACLS) guidelines.

The anesthetist responsible for each case of CA was asked to review the case and provide a written summary for peer review. The medical and anesthesia records, the written summary, and, when applicable, the necropsy report were analyzed by the Anesthesia Cardiac Arrest Study Commission, which was composed of three authors who are faculty members in the Department of Anesthesiology (YMMC, JRCB and LGB). The triggering factors of CA and death were retrospectively assigned to one of four groups: (1) totally related to the surgery when a technical surgical problem was the only or the major contributory factor, (2) totally related to an older patient's disease or condition, (3) totally related to anesthesia when anesthesia was the only or the major contributory factor or (4) partially related to anesthesia when an older patient's condition/disease or surgical procedure was a factor additional to anesthesia in the CA or death. Unanimity was reached on the triggering factors in the majority of the CAs and deaths. Disagreements among the three members were resolved by discussion, and agreement was reached in all cases when at least two of the three members agreed on the triggering factors.

Some of the CAs in the current study were likely included in our previous study that examined perioperative CAs in all age groups from April 1996 to March 2005, but did not evaluate CAs in older patients exclusively [7]. Thus, only some of these older patients who experienced intraoperative CA (48) are included in the numerator in the present study whereas all of the older patients (6,796 who received anesthesia) are included in the denominator.

### Statistical analysis

The incidence (expressed per 10,000 anesthetics) and 95% confidence interval (CI) of intraoperative CA and mortality were calculated according to age, sex, ASA physical status, surgical procedures, anesthetic technique, surgical area and triggering factors. In these cases, the difference between rates were considered statistically significant if their respective 95% CIs did not overlap. Factors predicting intraoperative CA (age, sex, ASA physical status, surgical procedures and anesthesia technique) were analyzed with multivariate forward stepwise logistical regression with odds ratio and 95% CI reported. The conditional independence of all variables and stratifications was verified by the Cochran-Mantel-Haenszel test while the homogeneity of the odds ratio was validated by the Breslow-Day test. The statistical analysis was performed using the software Statistical Package for Social Sciences for Windows (version 17.1; SPSS Inc., Chicago, IL, USA). A $P$ value<0.05 was considered statistically significant.

## Results

Over the 15 years of the study, 18,367 older patients were anesthetized. One hundred CAs (54.44 per 10,000 anesthetics; 95% CI: 44.68–64.20) and 68 deaths (37.02 per 10,000 anesthetics; 95% CI: 27.56–46.48) were identified within the intraoperative period (OR and PACU). Thus, only 32% of the older patients who experienced intraoperative CA survived. The majority of CAs and deaths occurred in the OR (93% and 94.12%, respectively) compared with the PACU (7% and 5.88%, respectively).

The intraoperative CA and death incidence in older surgical patients increased with the ASA physical status classification, in emergency surgery (12:1 compared with elective surgery) (Table 1). General anesthesia (6.6:1 compared with neuroaxial anesthesia) and an older patient's disease/condition were important factors of intraoperative CA (13.4:1 compared with anesthesia and 5.7:1 compared with surgery) and death (Tables 2 and 3, respectively). Multiclinical (two or more surgical areas) per 10,000 anesthetics (1034; 95% CI: 706–1,362), cardiac (412; 95% CI: 158–665), vascular (124; 95% CI: 61–185), thoracic (58; 95% CI: 24–91) or gastroenterological surgery (56; 95% CI: 10–102) were also important CA factors.

Poorer ASA physical status (III–V), emergency surgery and general anesthesia were significant predictive factors of intraoperative CA and death in older patient (Tables 4 and 5, respectively). However, age and sex were not predictors of intraoperative CA or mortality (Tables 4 and 5, respectively).

Anesthesia-related CA was considered a contributing factor in 5 cases and a primary factor in 1 case. Furthermore, anesthesia was considered a contributing factor in all 3 anesthesia-related deaths

**Table 1.** Intraoperative cardiac arrest and death incidences among 18,367 anesthetics according to the characteristics of the older patients.

| | Anesthetics | Cardiac Arrests | | | Deaths | | |
|---|---|---|---|---|---|---|---|
| | *n* | *n* | Incidence per 10,000 | 95% CI | *n* | Incidence per 10,000 | 95% CI |
| **Age, yr** | | | | | | | |
| 60–74 | 13,546 | 71 | 52.41 | 40.25–64.57 | 48 | 35.43 | 25.42–45.44 |
| 75–90 | 4,586 | 28 | 61.05 | 38.50–83.60 | 19 | 41.43 | 22.84–60.02 |
| ≥91 | 235 | 1 | 42.55 | 0.00–125.77 | 1 | 42.55 | 0.00–125.77 |
| **Sex** | | | | | | | |
| Male | 9,716 | 56 | 57.64 | 36.07–79.21 | 35 | 36.02 | 24.11–47.93 |
| Female | 8,651 | 44 | 50.86 | 28.42–73.30 | 33 | 38.15 | 25.16–51.14 |
| **ASA physical status** | | | | | | | |
| I | 1,836 | 1 | 5.45 | 0.00–20.66 | 1 | 5.45 | 0.00–16.13 |
| II | 8,975 | 2 | 2.22 | 0.00–6.87 | 1 | 1.11 | 0.00–3.29 |
| III | 5,754 | 23 | 39.97 | 17.10–62.84 | 16 | 27.80 | 14.20–41.40 |
| IV | 1,660 | 54 | 325.30 | 194.81–455.79 | 36 | 216.86 | 146.80–286.94 |
| V | 142 | 20 | 1408.45 | 650.88–2166.02 | 14 | 985.91 | 495.58–1476.24 |
| **Surgical procedures** | | | | | | | |
| Elective | 11,531 | 27 | 23.41 | 10.78–36.04 | 21 | 18.21 | 10.43–25.99 |
| Urgent | 4,610 | 10 | 21.69 | 1.72–41.66 | 5 | 10.84 | 1.34–20.34 |
| Emergency | 2,226 | 63 | 283.01 | 173.32–392.70 | 42 | 188.67 | 132.15–245.19 |

CI = confidence interval.

**Table 2.** Intraoperative cardiac arrest and death incidences among 18,367 anesthetics in older patients according to anesthesia technique.

| | Anesthetics | Cardiac Arrests | | | Deaths | | |
|---|---|---|---|---|---|---|---|
| **Anesthesia technique** | ***n*** | ***n*** | **Incidence per 10,000** | **95% CI** | ***n*** | **Incidence per 10,000** | **95% CI** |
| General anesthesia | 10,541 | 86 | 81.58 | 56.70–106.48 | 57 | 54.07 | 40.07–68.07 |
| Regional anesthesia | | | | | | | |
| - Epidural/spinal | 6,520 | 8 | 12.27 | 0.04–24.50 | 5 | 7.66 | 0.95–14.39 |
| - Plexus block | 597 | 0 | 0.00 | 0.00–0.00 | 0 | 0.00 | 0.00–0.00 |
| Sedation | 488 | 0 | 0.00 | 0.00–0.00 | 0 | 0.00 | 0.00–0.00 |
| Other# | 221 | 6 | 271.49 | 10.54–532.44 | 6 | 271.49 | 57.22–485.76 |

CI = confidence interval;
#Monitored anesthesia and supportive care in ASA IV-V physical status patients.

(Table 3). With regard to the triggering factors, 50% of the older patients who experienced anesthesia-related CAs survived, compared with 28.6% in the cases of surgery-related CAs and 31.25% in those of patient condition-/disease-related CAs. All anesthesia-related CAs and deaths in older surgical patients occurred from 1996 to 2005 at rates of 5.42 (95% CI: 1.2–9.6) and 2.7 (95% CI: 0.0–5.7) per 10,000 anesthetics, respectively, against CA and mortality rates of zero per 10,000 anesthetics in the 2006–2010 period.

Additional information on the 94 intraoperative CAs and 65 deaths attributable to an older patient's disease/condition or surgery factors is provided in Table 6. Sepsis and multiple organ failure were the most common causes of CA, while a ruptured aneurysm was the most common cause of mortality.

Medication-related adverse events accounted for four (66.66%) anesthesia-related CAs, three of which were caused by cardiovascular collapse after neuroaxial anesthesia. Of these three patients, two ASA physical status IV older patients passed away in the OR during vascular surgery (lower limb amputation) while undergoing continuous epidural anesthesia. In the third patient, a 63-year-old male with an ASA physical status of III who suffered a femur fracture in a motor vehicle accident, and had multiple rib fractures, the CA occurred after the administration of a spinal anesthetic with hyperbaric bupivacaine (20 mg). Immediately after anesthesia induction, he developed hypotension and bradycardia, followed by cardiovascular collapse and CA. In this case, CA was attributed entirely to the anesthesia. Fortunately, the patient was successfully resuscitated and recovered completely. There was 1 case of fluid overload followed by acute pulmonary edema in the PACU after general anesthesia in a female patient with an ASA physical status of III and a medical history of chronic renal failure. This patient passed away.

Respiratory events accounted for two (33.33%) anesthesia-related CAs. In both cases, there was loss of airway and difficulty to intubate while the patients had significant underlying disease with an ASA physical status of III or IV. One patient with chronic obstructive pulmonary disease and *diabetes mellitus* had a cervical abscess and mediastinitis; intubation and ventilation were difficult after general anesthesia induction followed by hypoxemia, cardiovascular collapse and CA. The patient was successfully resuscitated and recovered. In another case, a patient, with atrial fibrillation after thoracoscopy to drain a pleural effusion, undergoing general anesthesia presented hypoventilation after tracheal extubation in the PACU followed by a difficult intubation, hypoxemia and CA. The patient was successfully resuscitated and recovered with myocardial infarction.

## Discussion

The main findings in this study were: (i) older patients continued to present high incidence of intraoperative CA with high mortality; (ii) anesthesia-related CA and mortality rates were 3.26 and 1.63 per 10,000 anesthetics, respectively; (iii) there was no anesthesia-related CA in ASA I–II physical status patients; (iv) there were no anesthesia-related CA and deaths rates in the last five years of the study; (v) the large majority of CAs (94%) and deaths (95.5%) that occurred during anesthesia were caused by factors not anesthesia-related, and (vi) ASA physical status and emergency surgery, but not age and sex, were significant predictors of intraoperative CA and death in older patients.

A study conducted in Thailand in older surgical patients reported a 24-hour perioperative death rate of 39.33 per 10,000 anesthetics [5]. Another Thai study reported 24-hour perioperative CA and death rates of 40.42 and 31.44 per 10,000 anesthetics,

**Table 3.** Intraoperative cardiac arrest and death incidences among 18,367 anesthetics in older patients according to triggering factor.

| | Cardiac Arrests | | | Deaths | | |
|---|---|---|---|---|---|---|
| **Triggering factor** | **n** | **Incidence per 10,000** | **95% CI** | **n** | **Incidence per 10,000** | **95% CI** |
| Patient's disease/condition | 80 | 43.55 | 13.44–73.68 | 55 | 29.94 | 22.05–37.85 |
| Surgery | 14 | 7.62 | 3.63–11.61 | 10 | 5.44 | 2.07–8.81 |
| Anesthesia | 6 | 3.26 | 0.65–5.87 | 3 | 1.63 | 0.00–3.4 |
| - Totally-related | 1 | 0.54 | - | 0 | 0.00 | - |
| - Partially-related | 5 | 2.72 | - | 3 | 1.63 | - |

CI = confidence interval.

respectively, in older patients who underwent non-cardiac surgery [3]. A previous survey of the perioperative CA rate in all age groups conducted at our institution revealed a higher incidence of perioperative CA in older patients of 70.62 per 10,000 anesthetics [7]. A few other studies conducted in developed countries in the last decade reported lower perioperative CA rates ranging from 10.73 to 16.08 per 10,000 anesthetics in older surgical patients [9,10]. A systematic review [11] and a meta-analysis [12] of the literature verified that perioperative mortality rates reported in surgical patients of all age groups were higher in developing than in developed countries.

It is difficult to compare the intraoperative CA and mortality rates in our study with the results of previous studies (Table 7) because of considerable differences in the methods and patient populations among studies [3,5–10,13–16]. There is no consensus in the literature regarding the definition of perioperative and anesthesia-related mortality [17].

Some perioperative CA studies excluded ASA V older patients [8], cardiac surgery [3,6,9,13,16] or trauma [9] and transplant surgeries [9,16]. Therefore, the inclusion of both all surgery types and poorer ASA physical status patients, resulting from certain pre-existing morbidities, certainly influenced our CA and death rates. Ninety-seven percent of the intraoperative CAs occurred in poorer ASA physical status (III–V) patients with sepsis and multiple organ failure being the most important causes (30.8%). Sepsis occurs at a high incidence in Brazil and other developing countries with high mortality [18].

The elderly are more predisposed to vascular disease than young persons. Thus, a ruptured aneurysm, or complications associated with cardiac surgery or intraoperative myocardial infarction were also important causes of intraoperative CA and death attributed to an older patient's disease/condition or surgical factors in the current study. Our study demonstrated that patients presenting a poorer ASA physical status (III–V) were more likely (14-fold) to suffer intraoperative CA than ASA I–II patients. Previous studies have shown a similar association of perioperative CA and mortality with poorer ASA physical status in the older individuals [3,5,6]. In our study, it was verified that many older patients arrived at the OR in poor health. Intraoperative CAs and deaths that occurred in some of these patients might have been

**Table 4.** Factors associated with intraoperative cardiac arrest in older patients.

| Factors | Odds Ratio | 95% CI | Estimated Coefficient | *P* value |
|---|---|---|---|---|
| **Age, yr** | | | | |
| 60–74 | 1.0 (Reference) | | | |
| 75–90 | 0.89 | 0.57–1.42 | −0.10 | 0.65 |
| ≥91 | 0.70 | 0.09–5.27 | −0.35 | 0.73 |
| **Sex** | | | | |
| Male | 1.0 (Reference) | | | |
| Female | 1.01 | 0.67–1.52 | 0.10 | 0.96 |
| **ASA physical status** | | | | |
| I–II | 1.0 (Reference) | | | |
| III–V | 14.52 | 4.48–47.08 | 2.67 | <0.001 |
| **Surgical procedures** | | | | |
| Nonemergency | 1.0 (Reference) | | | |
| Emergency | 8.07 | 5.14–12.68 | 2.09 | <0.001 |
| **Anesthesia technique** | | | | |
| No general anesthesia | 1.0 (Reference) | | | |
| General anesthesia | 4.31 | 2.21–8.41 | 1.46 | <0.001 |

ASA = American Society of Anesthesiologists; OR: odds ratio; CI = confidence interval.

**Table 5.** Factors associated with intraoperative mortality in older patients.

| Factors | Odds Ratio | 95% CI | Estimated Coefficient | *P* value |
|---|---|---|---|---|
| **Age, yr** | | | | |
| 60–74 | 1.0 (Reference) | | | |
| 75–90 | 0.91 | 0.56–1.59 | −0.09 | 0.75 |
| ≥91 | 1.07 | 0.14–8.16 | 0.07 | 0.97 |
| **Sex** | | | | |
| Male | 1.0 (Reference) | | | |
| Female | 0.858 | 0.52–1.40 | −0.15 | 0.54 |
| **ASA physical status** | | | | |
| I-II | 1.0 (Reference) | | | |
| III–V | 13.34 | 3.15–56.47 | 2.59 | <0.001 |
| **Surgical procedures** | | | | |
| Nonemergency | 1.0 (Reference) | | | |
| Emergency | 7.14 | 4.16–12.26 | 1.97 | <0.001 |
| **Anesthesia technique** | | | | |
| No general anesthesia | 1.0 (Reference) | | | |
| General anesthesia | 4.06 | 1.86–8.85 | 1.40 | <0.001 |

ASA = American Society of Anesthesiologists; OR: odds ratio; CI = confidence interval.

prevented by an adequate preoperative assessment. A study showed that perioperative death might have been prevented by anesthesia care in approximately 1 per 13,900 anesthetics [19]. These findings demonstrate a persistent need to improve the quantity and quality of resource utilization and access to healthcare, which are inadequate in Brazil and in other developing countries. In addition, it is necessary to adopt perioperative medical practices with demonstrable effectiveness, organize multidisciplinary discussion of adverse effects and implement of evidence-based safety protocols to improve perioperative patient care [20,21].

As demonstrated in our study and in others [3,5,6], the urgency of surgery is a well-established preoperative predictive factor for intraoperative CA and mortality in older patients. The risk of CA in emergency surgery is likely due to many factors, such as the impossibility of adequate evaluation and optimization of the patients before the surgery.

Despite the differences in methodology, studies [6–10,15] have suggested that anesthesia-related CA and mortality rates in older people are lower today than they were 40 years ago (35.91 per 10,000 anesthetics) [14]. Most studies performed in the last two decades in developed countries have reported in older patients anesthesia-related death rates ranging from 0.00 to 1.72 per 10,000 anesthetics [8,15,19], which represents an improvement of almost twenty-fold. Our study confirmed this trend (i.e., 1.63 anesthesia-related deaths per 10,000 anesthetics in its entire timeframe and zero per 10,000 anesthetics in its last five years in older patients). These data may be associated with the improvements achieved in the geriatric anesthesia safety in our institution in the recent years.

**Table 6.** Causes of intraoperative cardiac arrests and deaths attributed to an older patient's disease/condition or surgical factors.

| | Cardiac arrests | | Deaths | | Mortality |
|---|---|---|---|---|---|
| **Cause** | *n* | % | *n* | % | % |
| Sepsis and multiple organ failure | 29 | 30.85 | 14 | 21.53 | 48.27 |
| Ruptured aneurysm: abdominal, thoracic or cerebral | 21 | 22.34 | 19 | 29.23 | 90.48 |
| Complications associated with cardiac surgery including inability to wean from cardiopulmonary bypass | 19 | 20.22 | 15 | 23.08 | 78.95 |
| Intraoperative myocardial infarction | 6 | 6.38 | 4 | 6.15 | 66.66 |
| Trauma: motor vehicle accident, gunshot wound or stab wound with exsanguinating hemorrhage | 5 | 5.32 | 4 | 6.15 | 80.00 |
| Exsanguinating hemorrhage during surgery associated with primary disease | 5 | 5.32 | 3 | 4.62 | 60.00 |
| Pulmonary embolus | 3 | 3.19 | 3 | 4.62 | 100.0 |
| Complications associated with radical cancer surgery | 3 | 3.19 | 2 | 3.08 | 66.66 |
| Technical surgical complications | 3 | 3.19 | 1 | 1.54 | 33.34 |

**Table 7.** Previous studies of perioperative and anesthesia-related cardiac arrest and mortality in older patients.

| Investigators and publication | Time period and data source | Number of patients Time of CA/ death | Age (yr) | CA incidence per 10,000 anesthetics | | Mortality incidence per 10,000 anesthetics | |
|---|---|---|---|---|---|---|---|
| | | | | Perioperative | Anesthesia-related | Perioperative | Anesthesia-related |
| **Marx et al.** [14] | 1965–1969 | 4,176 | **>60** | **NR** | **NR** | **514.84** | **35.91** |
| **1973** | Teaching hospital | Death within 7 days | 61–70 | | | 442.02 | 20.40 |
| | USA | | 71–80 | | | 679.86 | 34.23 |
| | | | >81 | | | 821.91 | 684.93 |
| **Olsson & Hallen** [13]] | 1967–1984 | NR | **>60** | **NR** | **7.1** | **NR** | **NR** |
| **1988** | Teaching hospital | CA and death in OR | | | | | |
| | Sweden | Excluded: cardiac surgery | | | | | |
| **Aubas et al.** [15] | 1983–1987 | 34,633 | **≥55** | **NR** | **4.33** | **NR** | **1.44** |
| **1991** | Teaching hospital | CA and deaths in OR and PACU | 55–74 | | 2.67 | | 1.14 |
| | France | | 75–84 | | 8.86 | | 2.95 |
| | | | ≥85 | | 12.04 | | 0 |
| **Kubota et al.** [16] | 1962–1992 | 15,351 | **≥65** | **NR** | **0.65** | **NR** | **0** |
| **1994** | Teaching hospital | CA and death in OR | 65–70 | | 0 | | 0 |
| | Japan | Excluded: cardiac surgery | 70–80 | | 1.66 | | 0 |
| | | transplant cases | | | | | |
| | | | 80–90 | | 0 | | 0 |
| | | | 90–95 | | 0 | | 0 |
| **Biboulet et al.** [8] | 1989–1995 | 28,987 | **≥55** | **NR** | **2.75** | **NR** | **1.72** |
| **2001** | Teaching hospital | CA and death within 12 h | 55–74 | | 1.86 | | 0.46 |
| | France | Excluded: ASA V patients | 75–84 | | 1.83 | | 1.83 |
| | | | >84 | | 14.36 | | 14.36 |
| **Kawashima et al.** [10]] | 1999 | 208,568 | **≥66** | **10.73** | **NR** | **NR** | **0.33** |
| **2002** | Group of hospitals | CA and death within 7 days | 66–85 | 11.02 | | 6.56 | 0.25 |
| | Japan | | ≥86 | 6.66 | | 5.18 | 1.48 |
| **Braz et al.** [7] | 1996–2005 | 6,796 | **≥65** | **70.62** | **5.88** | **NR** | **2.94** |
| **2006** | Teaching hospital | CA and death in OR and PACU | 65–79 | 68.78 | 5.29 | | 1.76 |
| | Brazil | | ≥80 | 79.33 | 8.88 | | 8.88 |
| | | | | | | | |
| ***Rodanant et al.** [5] | 2003–2004 | 23,899 | **≥65** | **NR** | **NR** | **39.33** | **NR** |
| **2007** | Group of hospitals | Deaths within 24 h | | | | | |
| | Thailand | | | | | | |
| ***Tamdee et al.** [3] | 2003–2007 | 8,905 | **≥65** | **40.42** | **NR** | **31.44** | **NR** |
| **2009** | Teaching hospital | CA and death within 24 h | 65–75 | 22.87 | | | |
| | Thailand | Excluded: cardiac surgery | 76–85 | 67.22 | | | |

**Table 7.** Cont.

| Investigators and publication | Time period and data source | Number of patients Time of CA/ death | Age (yr) | CA incidence per 10,000 anesthetics | | Mortality incidence per 10,000 anesthetics | |
|---|---|---|---|---|---|---|---|
| | | | | Perioperative | Anesthesia-related | Perioperative | Anesthesia-related |
| | | | >86 | 148.51 | | | |
| ***Story et al.** [6] | 2004, 2007–2008 | 4,158 | **≥70** | **NR** | **NR** | **519.48** | **NR** |
| **2010** | Group of hospitals | Deaths within 30 days | 70–79 | | | 355.4 | |
| | Australia, New Zealand | Excluded: cardiac surgery | 80–89 | | | 695.6 | |
| | | | ≥90 | | | 1219.5 | |
| **Goswani et al.** [9] | 2005 – 2007 | 223,961 | **≥70** | **16.08** | **NR** | **NR** | **NR** |
| **2012** | Group of hospitals | CA in OR | | | | | |
| | USA | Excluded: cardiac surgery | | | | | |
| | | peripheral nerve block | | | | | |
| | | trauma cases | | | | | |
| | | transplant cases | | | | | |
| **Current study** | 1996–2010 | 18,367 | **≥60** | **54.44** | **3.26** | **37.02** | **1.63** |
| | Teaching hospital | CA and death in OR and PACU | 60–74 | 52.41 | 2.95 | 35.43 | 1.47 |
| | Brazil | | 75–90 | 61.05 | 4.36 | 41.43 | 2.18 |
| | | | ≥91 | 42.55 | 0 | 42.55 | 0 |

*Studies that included only older patients; CA: cardiac arrest; NR: not reported; OR: operating room; ASA = American Society of Anesthesiologists; PACU: postanesthesia care unit.

In contrast to our current study, many prior works have identified advanced age (>75 yr) as a risk factor for perioperative CA [3,6,8,15], and also did not find age itself to be an independent risk factor [10].

Sex was not a risk factor for intraoperative CA in our study. Sex is known to be a significant risk factor for perioperative CA and mortality in young men suffering from trauma [7]. In our study, trauma was the fifth highest cause of intraoperative CA and death in older surgical patients. The elderly are less predisposed to trauma and violence than young persons.

Our study showed that general anesthesia was a predictor of intraoperative CA. However, this may be attributable to the fact that many high-risk surgeries (cardiac, thoracic, vascular, gastro-enterological) in older patients were performed under general anesthesia. Another possible confounding factor in this case is that the anesthesiologist often prefers to give general anesthesia to the most fragile patients, independently of the type of surgery.

In our study, respiratory causes of anesthesia-related CA were less frequent (33%) than medication causes (67%). In a recent study in all age groups [22], the authors verified that 64% of anesthesia-related CAs were caused by airway complications. There were three cases of CA after the administration of neuroaxial anesthesia. After neuroaxial anesthesia, a condition in which the loss of sympathetically mediated vasoconstriction may decrease vascular resistance, and the loss of sympathetically mediated cardiac stimulation may diminish both the heart rate and stroke volume. The vasodilatation may permit the peripheral pooling of blood and lower the end-diastolic volume, stroke volume and cardiac output in older patients [23]. In the last five years of our study, we preferentially used isobaric bupivacaine for spinal anesthesia in older patients. This local anesthetic determines lower levels of sympathetic block with lower cardiovascular effects than hyperbaric bupivacaine in older patients [24].

There may have been some methodological weaknesses in our study. First, the data are derived from adverse events reported by faculty and residents. Underreporting is likely in this situation, even though filling out the form for each case was mandatory. To minimize the risk of underreporting CAs and deaths, the information was cross-checked with the operating theater records and hospital administration. Second, this study is representative of the experience in one tertiary referral center. Practices specific to our institution may have influenced our results and may not represent the entire spectrum of elderly patient care practices. A multi-institutional anesthesia database would not only provide useful insights into injury mechanisms, but would also facilitate the development of universally applicable strategies [25].

## Conclusions

Our study has identified high incidence of intraoperative CA with high mortality in older patients. The majority of CAs and deaths were caused by factors not related to anesthesia. Anesthesia-related CA and death rates were 3.26 and 1.63 per 10,000 anesthetics, respectively. Improvements achieved in anesthesia safety in the older patients in our institution allowed no anesthesia-related CA and mortality in the last five years of the study and no anesthesia-related CA in ASA I-II physical status older patients. Major predictor of CA and death was a preoperative indicator of health, the ASA physical status, followed by emergency surgery. The fact that all anesthesia-related CAs were associated with medication administration or airway management is important for the development of prevention strategies. The high fatality rate in older surgical patients due to poor physical status suggests that primary prevention might be the key to reducing mortality from intraoperative CA. These findings indicate the need to improve medical perioperative practices for older people with highly complex medical problems in a demonstrably effective manner in under-resourced settings.

## Acknowledgments

J. C. Nunes was granted a scholarship from CAPES/DINTER and T. S. Oliveira was granted a scholarship from PIBIC/CNPq. CAPES and CNPq are Brazilian governmental agencies dedicated to promoting scientific research.

## Author Contributions

Conceived and designed the experiments: JCN JRCB LGB. Performed the experiments: JCN JRCB LGB. Analyzed the data: JCN JRCB TSO LRDC YMMC LGB. Contributed to the writing of the manuscript: JCN JRCB TSO YMMC LGB.

## References

1. World Health Organization website. Available: http://www.who.int/features/factfiles/ageing/en/index.html. Accessed 2013 July 18.
2. Ward SA, Parikh S, Workman B (2011) Health perspectives: international epidemiology of ageing. Best Pract Res Clin Anaesthesiol 25: 305–317.
3. Tamdee D, Charuluxananan S, Punjasawadwong Y Tawichasri C, Kyokong O, et al. (2009) Factors related to 24-hour perioperative cardiac arrest in geriatric patients in a Thai university hospital. J Med Assoc Thai 92: 198–207.
4. Tuchinda L, Sukchareon I, Kusumaphanyo C, Suratsunya T, Hintong T, et al. (2010) The Thai Anesthesia Incident Monitoring Study (Thai AIMS): an analysis of perioperative complication in geriatric patients. J Med Assoc Thai 93: 698–707.
5. Rodanant O, Hintong T, Chua-in W, Tanudsintum S, Sirinanmd C, et al. (2007) The Thai anesthesia incidents study (THAI Study) of perioperative death in geriatric patients. J Med Assoc Thai 90: 1375–1381.
6. Story DA, Leslie K, Myles PS, Fink M, Poustie SJ, et al. (2010) Complications and mortality in older surgical patients in Australia and New Zealand (the REASON study): a multicentre, prospective, observational study. Anaesthesia 65: 1022–1030.
7. Braz LG, Módolo NS, do Nascimento P Jr, Bruschi BA, Castiglia YM, et al. (2006) Perioperative cardiac arrest: a study of 53,718 anesthetics over 9 yr from a Brazilian teaching hospital. Br J Anaesth 96: 569–575.
8. Biboulet P, Aubas P, Dubourdieu J, Rubenovitch J, Capdevila X, et al. (2001) Fatal and non fatal cardiac arrests related to anesthesia. Can J Anaesth 48: 326–332.
9. Goswami S, Brady JE, Jordan DA, Li G (2012) Intraoperative cardiac arrests in adults undergoing noncardiac surgery: incidence, risk factors, and survival outcome. Anesthesiology 117: 1018–1026.
10. Kawashima Y, Seo N, Morita K, Irita K, Iwao Y, et al. (2002) Anesthesia-related mortality and morbidity in Japan (1999). J Anesth 16: 319–331.
11. Braz LG, Braz DG, Cruz DS, Fernandes LA, Módolo NS, et al. (2009) Mortality in anesthesia: a systematic review. Clinics 64: 999–1006.
12. Bainbridge D, Martin J, Arango M, Cheng D (2012) Perioperative and anaesthetic-related mortality in developed and developing countries: a systematic review and meta-analysis. Lancet 380: 1075–1081.
13. Olsson GL, Hallen B (1988) Cardiac arrest during anaesthesia: A computer-aided study in 250,543 anaesthetics. Acta Anaesthesiol Scand 32: 653–664.
14. Marx GF, Mateo CV, Orkin LR (1973) Computer analysis of postanesthetic deaths. Anesthesiology 39: 54–58.
15. Aubas S, Biboulet P, Daures JP, du Cailar J (1991) Incidence and etiology of cardiac arrest occurring during the peroperative period and in the recovery room. A propos of 102,468 anesthesia cases. Ann Fr Anesth Reanim 10: 436–442.
16. Kubota Y, Toyoda Y, Kubota H, Ueda Y, Asad A, et al. (1994) Frequency of anesthetic cardiac arrest and death in the operating room at a single general hospital over a 30-year period. J Clin Anesth 6: 227–238.
17. Deshpande JK (2011) Cause and effect or conjecture? A call for consensus on defining "anesthesia-related mortality." Anesth Analg 112: 1259–1261.
18. Silva E, Cavalcanti AB, Bugano DD, Janes JM, Vallet B, et al. (2012) Do established prognostic factors explain the different mortality rates in ICU septic patients around the world? Minerva Anestesiol 78: 1215–1225.
19. Bishop MJ, Souders JE, Peterson CM, Henderson WG, Domino KB (2008) Factors associated with unanticipated day of surgery deaths in Department of Veterans Affairs hospitals. Anesth Analg 107: 1924–1935.

20. Pearse RM, Holt PJ, Grocott MP (2011) Managing perioperative risk in patients undergoing elective non-cardiac surgery. BMJ 343:d5759
21. Kehlet H, Wilmore DW (2008) Evidence-based surgical care and the evolution of fast-track surgery. Ann Surg 248: 189–198.
22. Ellis SJ, Newland MC, Simonson JA, Peters KR, Romberger DJ, et al. (2014) Anesthesia-related cardiac arrest. Anesthesiology 120: 829–838.
23. Rooke GA (2003) Cardiovascular aging and anesthetic implications. J Cardiothorac Vasc Anesth 17: 512–523.
24. Møller IW, Fernandes A, Edström HH (1984) Subarachnoid anaesthesia with 0.5% bupivacaine: effects of density. Br J Anaesth 56: 1191–1195.
25. Morray JP (2011) Cardiac arrest in anesthetized children: recent advances and challenges for the future. Pediatr Anesth 21: 722–729.

# 6

# Postoperative Pain Management among Surgically Treated Patients in an Ethiopian Hospital

**Tewodros Eyob Woldehaimanot[1]*, Tesfahun Chanie Eshetie[1], Mirkuzie Woldie Kerie[2]**

**1** Department of Pharmacy, Jimma University, Jimma, Ethiopia, **2** Department of Health Services Management, Jimma University, Jimma, Ethiopia

## Abstract

***Background:*** Incidence of postoperative pain has been reported to be between 47–100%. Ineffective postoperative pain management results in tangible and intangible costs. The purpose of this study was to assess the processes and outcomes of pain management in the surgical wards of Jimma University Specialized Hospital, Ethiopia.

***Methods and Findings:*** A prospective cross sectional study was conducted among 252 postoperative patients during February 13 to April 30, 2012. A contextually modified and validated (Cronbach's $\alpha$ coefficient of 0.78) American Pain Society Patient Outcome Questionnaire was used to assess pain experience of patients. Patients' charts were reviewed to assess the pattern of analgesic use. Incidence of postoperative pain was 91.4%, and remained high over 3 measurements (McNemar's; $p<0.05$), and 80.1% of the patients were undertreated. The mean pain intensity, and pain interference on functional status were $6.72\pm1.44$ and $5.61\pm1.13$ on a 10 point Numerical rating scale respectively; both being strongly correlated($r=0.86$: $p<0.001$). Pain intensity was varied by ethnicity, education and preoperative information (ANOVA; $P<0.05$). Only 50% of the patients were adequately satisfied with their pain management. As needed (*prn*), solo analgesic, null analgesic, and intramuscular orders were noted for 31.3%, 89.29%, 9.7% and 20.1% of the prescription orders respectively. Though under dose, diclofenac and tramadol were the top prescribed medications, and only 57% of their dose was administered. Linear regression model showed that the predictors of satisfaction were sex of an individual and pain interference with functional status.

***Conclusion:*** Despite patients' paradoxical high satisfaction with pain management, the majority of patients were inadequately and inappropriately treated. Thus, further research is needed to determine how best to break down current barriers to effective pain management.

**Editor:** Richard E. Burney, University of Michigan, United States of America

**Funding:** This research was conducted as a partial fulfillment for a Master of Science in Clinical Pharmacy awarded to the primary author Tewodros Eyob Woldehaimanot and it was solely sponsored by the hosting Jimma University. The funder had no role in study design, data collection and analysis, decision to publish, or preparation of the manuscript.

**Competing Interests:** The authors have declared that no competing interests exist.

* Email: teda.eyob@gmail.com

## Introduction

It has been repeatedly confirmed by studies in the past 3 to 4 decades that 20 to 80% of patients undergoing surgery suffer from inadequately treated pain [1,2] and pain is classified as a serious public health problem both in the developed [3] and in developing countries [4–6]. Despite this longstanding recognition of postoperative pain as a serious public health problem, and the increased knowledge and resources for treating pain, poorly controlled pain continues to pose a significant challenge to the management of patients in postoperative contexts [7–10].

In Africa, the issue of pain has been explored largely in relation to HIV/AIDS and cancer [11–13], even though pain from surgical procedures poses a far greater burden. A Human Rights Watch's report showed that only 10% of these group patients are able to receive optimal pain management [14]. Even though various workshops and African Union summits adopted pain relief as basic human right [13], shortage of clinicians, stringent legal towards morphine access, and lack of knowledge left millions of people to suffer because of inadequate pain control [13,15]. Ethiopia has almost nil morphine per capita which is on indicator of the equality of pain management [16].

In Ethiopia, a study conducted by the Ethiopian Public Health Association in 2005 showed that health care providers believes that pain was undertreated due to unstandardized practice, absence of medications and poor knowledge and attitude among professionals. The output of the survey was a step forward for the development of the 2007 National Pain Management Guideline [17]. The authors couldn't find any study to demonstrate the quality of postoperative pain management at the level of patients.

The present study was conducted to assess the quality of postoperative pain management in the surgical wards of Jimma University Specialized Hospital (JUSH) by examining the incidence, intensity and interference of pain. Satisfaction and attitude of patients plus the patterns of pharmacologic and non-pharmacologic interventions with regard to pain management were also examined. After the conduct of this research, the department of Anesthesia of the University in conjunction with anesthesiologists from UK has taken a step to prepare a pain assessment tool and treatment guide for use by the surgical ward's health care professionals.

## Materials and Methods

### Study setting and period

This study was conducted in the 3 surgical wards of JUSH during February 13 to April 30, 2012. The surgery department has 126 beds with a perceived 100% occupancy rate. Formal documentation of pain and preemptive analgesia are not common practices in this set up. Besides, anesthetists do not participate in the pain management of postoperative patients.

### Study design and Participants

Prospective cross sectional study design was used to determine the quality of postoperative pain management. Consecutive, hospitalized patients aged over 18 years and within 24 and 72 h of surgery were invited to participate in the study. Of the 280 approached patients over the study period, 252 were recruited for analysis (Figure 1). Patients who had difficulty of communicating, unconscious and had documented psychiatric illness were excluded from the study.

### Instruments and data collection methods

Based on the 1995 and 2010 versions of the American Pain Society Patient Outcome Questionnaire (APSPOQ), a contextually modified tool was prepared to collect data on patient satisfaction level, beliefs about pain and pain treatment, pain intensity, and effect of pain on function through face-to-face interview. These two tools are dependable and has been used extensively to survey pain in various contexts by multiple studies [4,10,18]. Both were designed by the American Pain Society (APS) and has incorporated a number of previously validated tools into its construction [19]. Over time and through its repeated usage and validation the APSPOQ has been translated into many languages other than English.

We predominantly used the 1995 version since it is extensively used and validated in both developed and developing countries. Initially three items, related to the use of non-pharmacological intervention and what perceived side effects patients come across, were picked from the 2010 version. After the pretest 2 items related to satisfaction with nurses' and doctors' were deleted since patients were not able to differentiate between a physician and a nurse. Similarly, the item that questioned patient's request for medication change was removed, since it resulted in unanimously similar response of 'No'. The item from the revised 2010 version of APSPOQ-R that assess the side effects of drugs was also erased because the side effects indicated were mainly related with strong opioids, which were not available in the study setting during the study period.

The final tool used in the current study had 13 items. The first item determines whether the patient experienced pain in the previous 24 hrs. The subsequent 3 items assess patients' pain intensity level on the 0–10 Numerical Rating Scale (NRS). Item 5 relates to the degree to which pain interferes with six activities of daily living (general activity, walking, sleep, deep breathing and coughing, relationships with others and mood) on the same scale as previous. The next 2 items measures patients' satisfaction with their overall pain management.

Then, 8$^{th}$ item enquire patients' alleged waiting time for analgesics when they ask for pain relief from 10 minutes or less to more than 60 minutes. If patients have pain at the time of

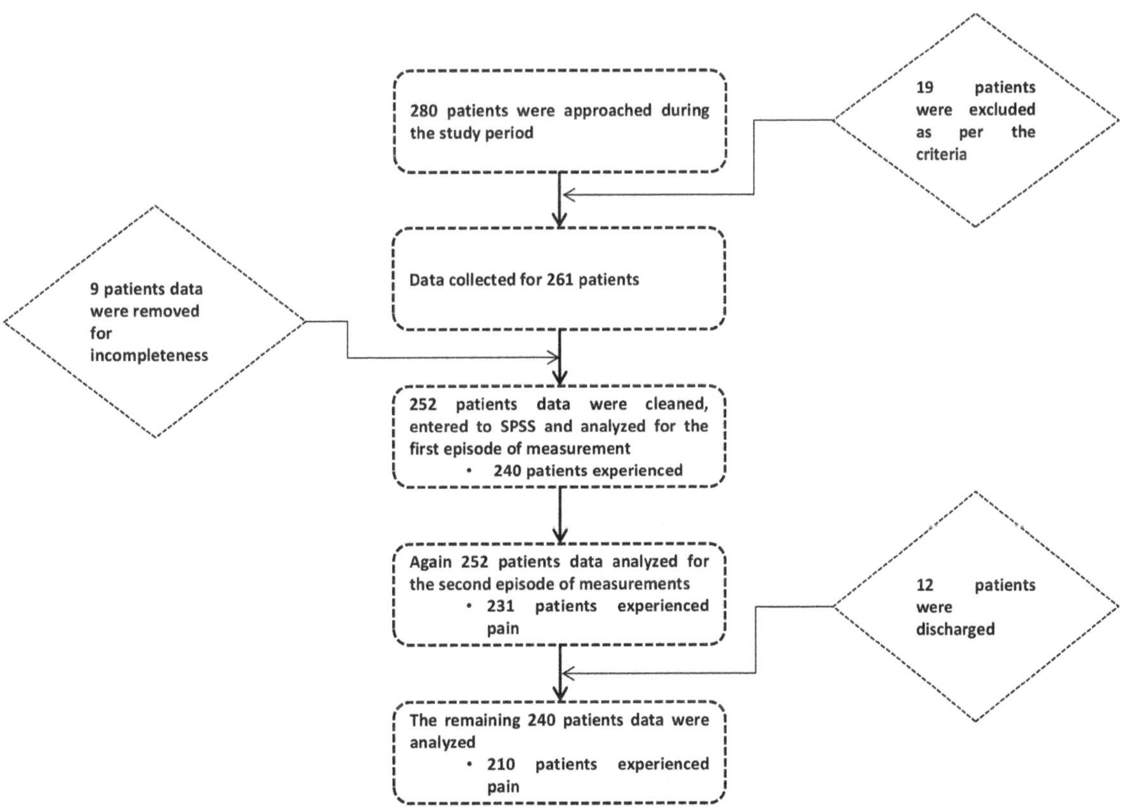


**Figure 1. Schematic representation of patient recruitment and data analysis.**

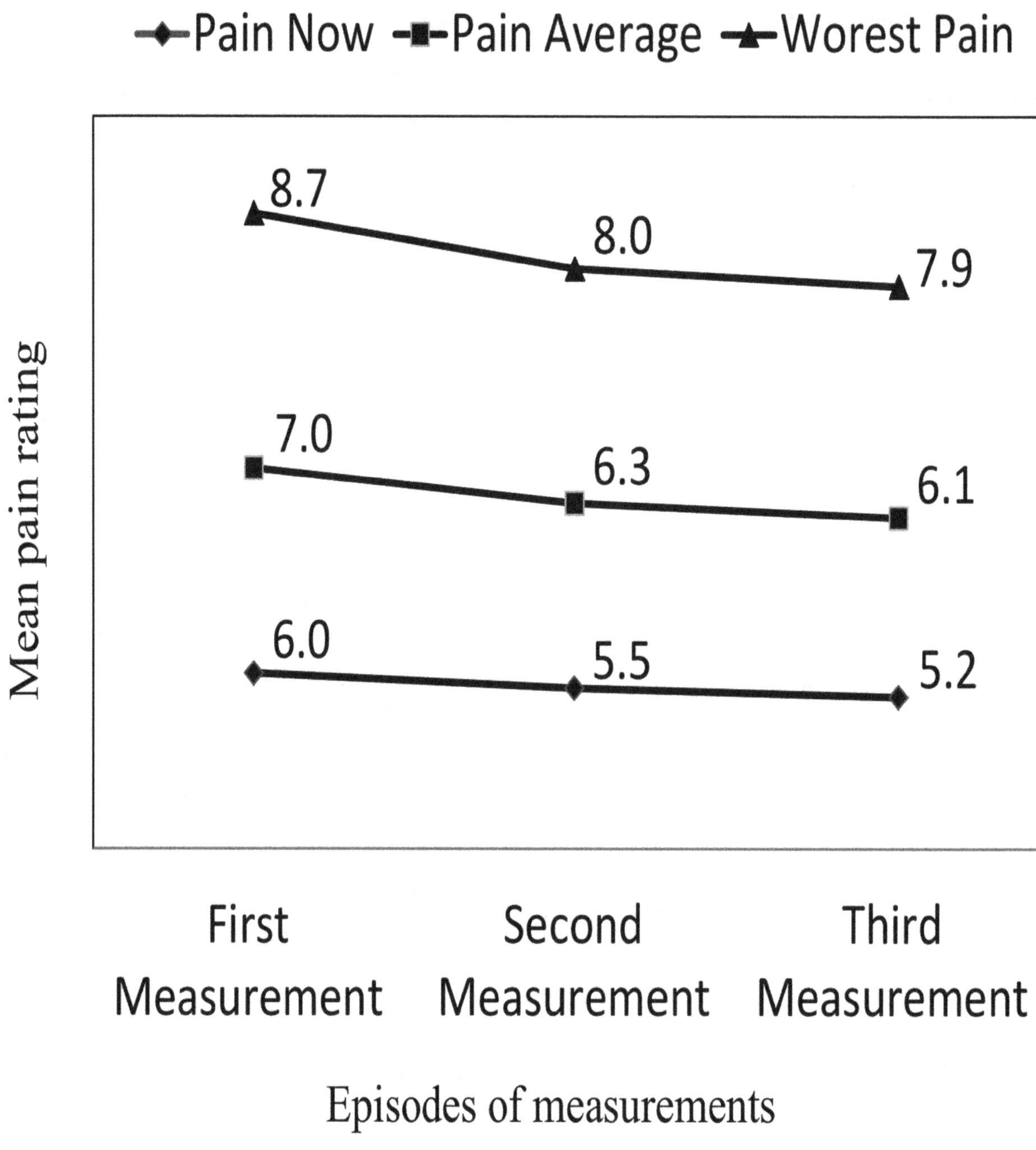


**Figure 2. Mean pain intensity rating over the three measurements.**

interview, they would be asked whether they like something stronger for pain relief in item 9. In the next item patients were asked about their agreement (attitude and belief) levels to statements (patient barrier statements) related to pain and pain management on a 6 point scale of 0 (do not agree at all) to 6 (agree very much); higher score to these statements indicates higher levels of patients barriers to pain management.

The 11th item relates to whether nurses or doctors inform patients about the importance of treating pain and reporting pain. The last two items assess patients experience with non-pharmacological management, and encouragement received from the health care professionals. Moreover, a structured data abstraction checklist was utilized to collect data on the pattern of pharmacological/non-pharmacological interventions and demographic characteristics of patients from the patient chart.

Those who were in a state to participate in the study were asked the first item. Patients with an experience of pain in the previous 24 hrs were interviewed with the APSPOQ in full, while patients with no experience in the previous 24 hrs were not asked the questions about pain intensity or the effect of pain on activities of daily living. Analgesics prescription and administration information for the previous 24 hrs were recorded for all participants by reviewing their medical records or interview of the patient and ward nurses. Satisfaction items were collected for the 1st 24 hrs. Items on attitude and belief towards pain were collected for the 2nd 24 hrs. While wait time, need for stronger dose, non-pharmacologic intervention were assessed for the 3rd 24 hrs. The items on medication profiles, pain presence, pain severity and pain interference were interviewed for all of the 3 assessment episodes.

## Ethical statement

Permission to conduct this study was obtained from the **Institutional Review Board, Jimma University**. The data collectors (3 medical interns) first assessed patients' ability to both comprehend the plain language information about the study and to participate in the study, by asking patients to repeat back the information provided. Patient's written informed consent to participate in the study was obtained after comprehensive explanation of the purpose and procedure of the study. Patients were informed about their rights to refuse or withdraw, and about confidentiality of the individual information obtained. Additionally, any personal information was de-identified before the final analysis. During data collection process, data of patients who were at any risk of complication due to pain were shared with their medical and nursing team for intervention.

## Data analysis

Data were coded, cleaned and entered into and analyzed using the Statistical Package for the Social Sciences (SPSS Inc., Chicago, IL, USA) version 19.0. Descriptive statistics were computed to summarize the participants' socio-demographic and clinical characteristics, patient satisfaction, and pain management processes (pharmacological and non-pharmacological interventions, patients request for pain relief and waiting time). The amount of analgesic patients received (mean dose ratio) was calculated as a proportion of dose administered to that of the total amount prescribed over the three episodes of measurements. The overall patients' agreement levels to barrier statements related to pain and pain management were calculated as mean scores for each sub items. ANOVA, McNemar's test, Pearson product moment were conducted to determine difference between groups, timed measurements, proportions, and link between variables accordingly.

The reliability of the APSPOQ used in this study was estimated by using the Cronbach's $\alpha$ coefficient. Reliability estimates for the various subscales were 0.93 for pain intensity (3 items), 0.88 for pain interference (6 items), and 0.79 for beliefs about pain (7 items). The overall reliably for all items was 0.78.

Principal component analysis was used to reduce the 3 items of pain intensity, 6 items of level of pain interference on patients' routines, and 7 items of barrier statements. The former two were measured over three days while the latter only at a point in time. The analysis was run independently for each the three factors. For the first two, the raw data matrix recoded so that the average of the three data point was taken during data reduction. However, the raw data matrix of the barrier statement was taken as it is since it was measured only once. Then, the appropriateness of the data was assessed using KMO's and Bartllet's test. The assessment of the Scree plot showed that only one component was enough for each category of measurement. Finally, the analysis for each was run again by setting the number of components to be one and the type of extraction Varimax. The generated scores were then used for subsequent analysis using ANOVA, correlations and linear regression.

To determine the adequacy of postoperative pain management Pain Management Index (PMI) was used. The PMI is based on a patient's level of worst pain intensity and is categorized into 0 (no pain), 1 (1–3: mild pain), 2 (4–6: moderate pain), and 3 (7–10: severe pain) [20]. The pain score is then subtracted from the most potent level of analgesic drug therapies prescribed: 0 (no analgesic drug), 1 (non-opioids), 2 (weak opioids), and 3 (strong opioids) [21]. The index can range from −3 to +3. Negative scores indicate inadequate orders for analgesic drugs. Although the PMI was designed to evaluate the appropriateness of cancer pain management, several studies of postoperative pain management have established it as a useful indicator of adequacy in evaluating the range and appropriateness of pain treatments for hospitalized postoperative patients [22–24]. For all of the analysis a p-value of 0.05 was taken as a cutoff point for statistical significance. In the text, mean values with its corresponding standard deviation is expressed as (mean±standard deviation).

# Results

## Patient characteristics

Of the approached 280 patients 252 (90%) were included in the final analysis (); 162 (64.3%) were males. Patients were between 19 and 81 (40.4±15.5) years. Majority of the participants (71.4%) were Muslim by religion; and Oromo (72.6%) by ethnicity. Approximately 49% of the patients had no any formal education. Only 9.5% of the patients demonstrated previous surgical history of any type. The patients stayed in the wards for 0 to 28 days (5.2±5.1) prior to their surgery. Surgical interventions were categorized according to approach, with the largest being abdominal 90 (35.7%). The majority, 228 (90.5%), received general anesthesia, while the remaining subjects received spinal anesthesia. A large proportion of subjects, 198 (78.6%), had scheduled surgical interventions. The mean duration of all the surgical procedures was 82.9±43.7 minute (Table 1).

## Principal component analysis

The principal component analysis generated one component for each group of items. The variations explained by the generated scores were 77%, 75% and 66% for pain intensity, interference and belief items respectively. The pain intensity component has the strongest correlation with the average pain item ($r = 0.91$), the interference one with mood ($r = 0.87$), while the barrier (belief) component with the addiction statement ($r = 0.82$).

## Incidence and severity of pain

When interviewed 240 (95.2%), 231 (91.7%), 210 (87.5%) of the patients had experienced pain in the 1st, 2nd, and 3rd previous 24 hrs respectively. The pain incidence of the first assessment was significantly higher than that of the second day (McNemar's; p = <0.05). The mean pain intensity for the three consecutive episodes were: (5.56±1.76), (6.46±1.33) and (8.16±1.23) for pain now, pain average, and pain worst pain respectively. A consistent and significant ($P<.001$) decrease in pain intensity was observed over time ().

Barrier to pain management ($r = -0.17$: $p<0.05$), age ($r = -0.20$: $p<0.001$) and duration of surgery ($r = -0.16$: $p<0.05$) were negatively and mildly correlated with pain intensity. Even though, it was not statistically significant, the ratio of drug administered and longer ward stay showed an inverse relation with pain intensity. In as much as the previous, patients who rated higher pain intensity were from the southern region of the country ($P<0.05$), more educated ($P<0.05$), and more pre-informed ($p<0.05$).

## Pain Interference with functional status

Mean of pain interference over the 3 days in decreasing order were: walking ability (6.77±1.44), general activity (6.57±0.98), mood (5.83±0.97), sleep (5.59±1.22), coughing and deep breathing (4.89±1.19), and relation with others (4.01±1.02). The overall mean over the 3 days was 5.61±1.13, and it decreased

**Table 1.** Demographic and clinical characteristics of participants (n = 252).

| Variables | N (%) |
|---|---|
| **Sex** | |
| Male | 162 (64.3) |
| Female | 90 (35.7) |
| **Religion** | |
| Muslim | 180 (71.4) |
| Christian | 48 (19.1) |
| Other* | 24 (9.5) |
| **Ethnic origin** | |
| Oromo | 183 (72.6) |
| Southern Ethiopia | 42 (16.7) |
| Others** | 27 (10.7) |
| **Educational status** | |
| Higher Education | 18 (7.1) |
| High School | 36 (14.3) |
| Elementary | 54 (21.4) |
| Basic | 21 (8.3) |
| Illiterate | 123 (48.8) |
| **Previous surgical history** | |
| No | 228 (90.5) |
| Yes | 24 (9.5) |
| **Surgical Procedures** | |
| Urological | 66 (26.2) |
| Abdominal | 90 (35.7) |
| Endocrine | 15 (6.0) |
| Orthopedics | 33 (13.1) |
| Thoracic | 6 (2.4) |
| Skin, Muscle& Soft Tissue | 42 (16.7) |
| **Category of surgery** | |
| Elective | 198 (78.6) |
| Emergency | 54 (21.4) |
| **Anesthesia type** | |
| General | 228 (90.5) |
| Spinal | 24 (9.5) |

*Includes: "Waqafata"; those without religion affiliations.
**includes: Tigrai, Amhara, Gambela.

significantly over time ($p<0.001$). Higher interferences were reported by individuals who; rated higher pain ($r=0.86$: $p<0.001$), spent shorter duration in surgical procedures, were younger, exhibited less hindering attitude, and were more educated ($p<0.05$).

## Attitude and belief (Indicators of barriers to adequate pain management from the patient side)

Patients were asked to rate on a 0 to 5 scale (0: do not agree at all, 5: agree very much) how much they agree with seven statements focused on common pain management misconceptions. The higher the rate on the likert scale, the greater the barrier (hindering attitude) to adequate pain management. Patients reported relatively higher levels of agreement with all 7 statements, with the highest level of agreement for the statement on addiction ($3.8\pm1.22$) (Table 2).

## Process of postoperative pain management and adequacy of management

Only few patients (2.5%) reported that they received pain medication within 15 minutes of complain of pain. However, a large number of patients (70.8%) never asked for pain medication during hospitalization. Despite the fact that only few patients requested for pain medication, 42.2% of the patients responded "Yes" when they were asked whether they want stronger medication for pain relief. Moreover, 14.2% of the patients reported that they never received the analgesics they requested (Table 3). Most patients, 91.2% (n = 230) reported that their

**Table 2.** Patients' agreement with barrier statements, sorted in increasing order.

| Statements | Mean ± SD |
|---|---|
| Pain medication should be 'saved' in case the pain gets worse | 2.3±1.0 |
| Complaints of pain could distract the doctor from treating my underlying illness | 2.4±0.9 |
| Good patients avoid talking about pain | 2.5±0.8 |
| It is easier to put up with pain than with the side effects that come with pain treatments | 2.8±1.4 |
| Pain medication cannot really control pain | 3.3±1.1 |
| The experience of pain is sign that the illness has gotten worse | 3.5±1.5 |
| People get addicted to pain medication very easily | 3.8±1.2 |

physicians or nurses haven't discussed with them the importance of pain management.

Even though the dominant pattern of analgesic prescriptions found in this study was scheduled one (68.7%); as needed (i.e., *prn*) orders for analgesics were noted in 31.1% of the orders. Analgesics that were prescribed with a fixed interval were administered 54% of the time; however, *prn* orders, irrespective of analgesic category, were only administered 5% of the time. The majority of patients were prescribed solo analgesics (89.29%). The remaining (10.71%) were prescribed dual analgesic: namely Diclofenac and Tramadol. It was also observed that forty five patients (10.1%) did not have prescription for any kind of specific analgesic. On average, the dose administered for Diclofenac was only 56.2% of the prescribed while for Tramadol it was 57.9% (Table 3).

The mean total daily dose (in mg) administered over the three measurements episodes were: 122.5±21.3, 88.8±14.2, 81.6±12.7 for Tramadol, and 101.4±19.3, 81.1±11.8, 64.9±9.5 for Diclofenac. The dose of the drugs administered decreased consistently and significantly over time ($P = .0001$). Change of prescription of pain medication was reported only in 3% of the cases. The most frequent non-pharmacological ways of managing pain were tolerating pain (84.4%), changing position (83.7%), and having family support (81.9%). Approximately, 83% of the participants did not receive support from the health care providers in this regard.

As PMI is a novel method for evaluating the range and appropriateness of pain treatments in term of prescription. It is used to determine adequacy of treatment. One hundred and ninety four participants (80.1%) received ineffective pain medication. The remaining 48 patients (19.9%) received adequate to good pain medication.

## Satisfaction with pain management

In response to questions about overall satisfaction with management of pain, 117 (50%) patients were satisfied or very satisfied. With a range of 1–6, the mean overall satisfaction with pain relief management was 4.22±1.51 for all patients. Though it was weak the only variable correlated with satisfaction level was pain interference ($r = -0.16$, $p<0.05$). Significant differences were between male and female ($P = 0.04$); female being less satisfied.

The only two variables shown to be associated with satisfaction and verified to be predictors of satisfaction ($F$ (2,225) = 5.311, $p = 0.006$, adjusted $R^2 = 0.16$) were sex of an individual and interference of pain with functional status. It was found that a unit increase in pain interference on functional status results in a 0.167 unit decrease in satisfaction level with pain management (B = –0167, 95%C:−0.852, −0.028). Similarly, females' satisfaction with pain management is lower than that of male by 0.137 (B = –0.137, 95%CI: −0.439, −0.057) (Table 4).

## Discussion

This study is the first to evaluate the quality of postoperative pain management in JUSH using the quality improvement standards recommended by APS [25]. In addition, it used multiple time measurements of the incidence, intensity and interference of pain, and the pattern of pharmacologic and non-pharmacologic interventions. Such kind of study does not require the same evidentiary and rigorous populations as is usually demanded of more general research as it is not primarily intended to generate new knowledge of widely generalizable or universal value [26]. Thus, the generated data could reliably show points of interventions to improve the quality of postoperative pain management and serve as a baseline for continuous audits to come.

Findings from this study should be interpreted and understood within the context of barriers of pain management in Africa, and postoperative pain management in Ethiopia, where, at the time of data collection, there was one national general guideline prepared by the Federal Ministry of Health (MOH) [17]. This guideline is expected to chaperon professionals to effectively manage postoperative pain. This guideline was prepared to be in tune with the World Health Organization (WHO) ladder of pain management.

In hospitals of most developing countries (Nigeria, Kenya, Uganda, South Africa, China, Columbia and Malaysia) pain management is derived from the medical staff's experience, and is not always consistent with recommendations from organizations such as the APS [11,12,15,27–30]. Postoperative pain medications are still prescribed on an as-needed basis, requiring patients to request pain medication, and interventions are implemented when patients are in severe pain [15]. In most acute care settings, pethidine and intramuscular injection are the commonest prescription orders, neither of which is recommended by pain management guidelines [25,29]. Maximum doses of paracetamol and non-steroidal anti-inflammatory drugs are rarely used unlike in the developed world [2,28–31]. The high cost of opioids in developing countries compounded this problem. The above mentioned challenges for better pain relief are also observed in our study.

The incidence and level of severity of pain reported in this study is higher than those from most Western and developing countries [2,10,22,24,32–34]. But, an earlier study done in China reported a 100% postoperative pain incidence [35]. Although, as expected, all pain intensity scores decreased over time, patients in this study continued to have an average pain score of greater than 6, and 79% had a worst pain score of greater than 6 on the third postoperative day. Besides, 34% of patients responded that they

**Table 3.** Processes of pain management.

| Variables | N (%) |
|---|---|
| **Waiting Time after requesting analgesics (n = 252)** | |
| Below 15 minute | 6(2.5) |
| Up to 30 minute | 4(1.7) |
| Up to 1 hour | 22(9.2) |
| Beyond 1 hour | 4(1.7) |
| Asked, Never received | 34(14.2) |
| Never asked | 170(70.8) |
| **Want stronger dose of medication (n = 252)** | |
| No | 133(57.8) |
| Yes | 97(42.2) |
| **Received pre-information (n = 252)** | |
| No | 230(91.3) |
| Yes | 22(8.7) |
| **Help to use non-pharmacological ways (n = 252)** | |
| Never | 200(83.3) |
| Sometimes | 31(12.9) |
| Often | 9(3.8) |
| **Name of prescribed medications (n = 279*)** | |
| None | 27 (9.7) |
| Diclofenac | 111 (39.8) |
| Tramadol | 120 (43) |
| Pethidine | 3 (1.1) |
| Unspecified | 18 (6.5) |
| **Route of administrations (n = 234§)** | |
| IV | 186 (79.5) |
| IM | 48 (20.5) |
| **Prescriber's qualifications (n = 244†)** | |
| Specialist | 42 (16.7) |
| Residents | 202 (80.2) |
| Unspecified | 8 (3.2) |
| **Frequency of medications (n = 234§)** | |
| BID | 43 (17.1) |
| *prn* | 79 (31.3) |
| QID | 40 (15.9) |
| TID | 90 (35.7) |

*N is 279, because 27 patients received two drugs.
§234 is the orders with medication regimen written.
†244 is patient cards with physician qualification written on.

**Table 4.** Regression model for patient characteristics and clinical outcomes as predictors of satisfaction.

| Variables | Coefficients | | | | |
|---|---|---|---|---|---|
| | Unstandardized | | Standardized | 95% CI for B | |
| | B | SE | B | Lower Bound | Upper Bound |
| Constant | 4.802 | 0.297 | | 4.218 | 5.386 |
| Interference of pain | −0.248 | 0.097 | −0.167 | −0.852 | −0.028 |
| Sex | −0.44 | 0.209 | −0.137 | −0.439 | −0.057 |

required stronger pain medications in the third postoperative day. Such troublesome level of postoperative pain may be explained by the high negative PMI scores and absence of strong opioids. Similarly, the inappropriate prescription and administration of analgesics plus only surgeon based care augment this too. Postoperative care delivered by multidisciplinary team including anesthesiologists/anesthetists in Acute Pain Service setups has shown a better outcome [36,37].

Age, attitude, information status and education are often considered indicators of the patient's perception of power [10,33]. In our study, less pain intensity was reported by the elderly and patients with poor attitude, and less educated and informed. This finding underpins that fact that these groups of patients are highly vulnerable and therefore needs greater attention. Similarly, increased duration of surgery was negatively correlated with pain intensity. This may be due to the fact that these groups of patients may receive higher amount of anesthesia, which may decrease pain perception.

The role of ethnic background (ethnic origin) to affect pain perception and satisfaction was mentioned in studies done in Singapore and Nigeria [15,38,39]. In our study, individuals from the southern part of the country were found to rate pain higher. This finding cannot be explained with the information at hand, thus we recommend further investigation to explore the matter. The fact that the amount of drug administered was found to affect pain intensity likely demonstrates the amount of drug prescribed was suboptimal from the very beginning.

The interference scores reported by the patients in this study were higher than those reported in other studies with more heterogeneous samples of hospitalized patients China, USA, and South America [32–34]. As with the case of pain intensity, mean pain interference scores also decreased over time. It was well correlated with pain intensity scores. Taking this correlation in to account, investigators of this study also came to the conclusion made by other studies that pain interference scores to be used as monitoring indicator of the quality of postoperative pain management [10,32]. However, future studies are non-optional to determine what specific pharmacologic and non-pharmacologic interventions can be implemented in decreasing pain intensity scores and its interferences.

The majority of patients never requested pain medication or changes in pain medication. In comparison to patients from other countries [33,34,40], the data showed that patients of the current setting were less likely to request pain medication even if they were suffering high levels of pain. This result, being harmonious with high level of barrier, may imply that patients were more passive in pain management or health care in general, and are less likely to verbalize their needs and concerns. A South African study conducted among 45 chronic patients showed that pain interference with quality of life was high among uninformed patients [11]. Due attention must be taken by the health care team in keeping patients well informed about the importance of pain relief.

Regarding adequacy of pain management, 80.1% of the population was poorly managed in the current study site. For comparison, 60.2% were inadequately treated for pain in Chinese population [34] whereas only 36% had inadequate treatment in a medical surgical sample in the United States [22]. In a secondary analysis of a large postoperative sample of the same study in United States after 3 years, reported an overall 30% rate of under treatment [41]. The negative PMI score represents a gross and minimum estimate of inadequate postoperative pain management. It would be reasonable to estimate that a mere presence and prescription of strong opioids would have minimized the negative PMI significantly.

The principal means the study participants used to cope with pain were tolerating pain, self-prayer, family help, and changing positions. This finding is consistent with findings from Chinese and Mexican population [24,34]. However the use of music, guided imagery, prayer by others, and other sophisticated methods which are commonly used by USA, Hispanic and Canadian samples are not available in our sample [22,32,42]. That fact that tolerating pain is opted for by our patients goes well with finding most agreed high with the barrier statements.

A paradoxical high satisfaction despite high pain intensity was observed in our study samples. But, the overall satisfaction of patients was lower than reported by most studies in developed and developing countries [2,8,32]. The main reasons identified by most studies for higher rate of satisfaction despite the presence of high pain intensity are the exceptionally good caring attitude of health care professional, presence of frequent pain assessment, high rate of preoperative pain education, and presence of good communication environment [10,32,40,43]. In our study, the majority of participants reported they had not received pain management education, and backing on the use of non-pharmacological methods was minimal. Similarly, the reason mentioned for dissatisfaction were overlooking of the clinician to patients' requests. All these together indicate low level of communication to patients which might explain the relatively lower satisfaction rate.

The correlates of satisfaction in our study were gender and interference of pain. Female's higher intensity of pain and dissatisfaction were also demonstrated by studies in Western countries [43–45] and eastern countries [33,35]. A south African study also reported this similar scenario [11]. The commonly proposed reason for this is that females are more socially acceptable to express pain and dissatisfaction [46,47], but it is yet to be determined as further studies are to be done in this area. Even though, expectation of pain and the perceived degree of pain relief were the most common predictors of satisfaction reported [26,48,49], gender and interference of pain were also reported in few instances [24,26]. Taken together, both streams of evidences well support that appropriate relief of pain with appropriate medications could bring optimal satisfaction.

Although this study is the first to use the APSPOQ in Ethiopia, to evaluate the quality of postoperative pain management in this setup, limitations that can affect generalizability need to be noted. First, collection of data in a single site and from patients operated by a limited number of surgeons presents a limitation to the external generalizability of this study. Second, the majority of patients were male which might decrease pain intensity and interference ratings, because women are more likely to report higher pain and interference scores than men. Thirdly, the majority of the patients had similar socio-demographic characteristics which also affect variability of responses. Furthermore, there are known multifactorial influences related to setting of facility, patient's expectations, professionals' attitude and knowledge on pain experience that have not been explored in this study.

In conclusion, postoperative pain management was suboptimal among postoperative patients of the surgical wards in JUSH. This was evidenced by the high incidence of postoperative pain and its consequences. Unstandardized treatment use, poor patient attitude, shortage of pain clinicians, lack of strong opioids, and lack of knowledge might be background causes. Thus, further research is needed to determine how best to break down current barriers to effective pain management.

## Acknowledgments

The authors are greatly indebted to Dr. Tirsit Retta for organizing patient recruitment, the data gathering, and those individuals who involved in data collection. Patients who unreservedly gave the information needed also deserve due thanks. We are deeply thankful for our colleagues who patiently corrected our manuscript for grammatical and topographical errors.

## Author Contributions

Conceived and designed the experiments: TEW TCE MWK. Performed the experiments: TEW TCE MWK. Analyzed the data: TEW TCE MWK. Contributed reagents/materials/analysis tools: TEW TCE MWK. Wrote the paper: TEW TCE MWK.

## References

1. Marks RM, Sachar EJ (1973) Undertreatment of medical inpatients with narcotic analgesics. Ann Intern Med 78: 173–181.
2. Lorentzen V, Hermansen IL, Botti M (2011) A prospective analysis of pain experience, beliefs and attitudes, and pain management of a cohort of Danish surgical patients. Eur J Pain.
3. Stephens J, Laskin B, Pashos C, Pena B, Wong J (2003) The burden of acute postoperative pain and the potential role of the COX-2-specific inhibitors. Rheumatology (Oxford) 42 Suppl 3: iii40–52.
4. Lin CC (2000) Applying the American Pain Society's QA standards to evaluate the quality of pain management among surgical, oncology, and hospice inpatients in Taiwan. Pain 87: 43–49.
5. Klopper H, Andersson H, Minkkinen M, Ohlsson C, Sjostrom B (2006) Strategies in assessing post operative pain–a South African study. Intensive Crit Care Nurs 22: 12–21.
6. Shen Q, Sherwood GD, McNeill JA, Li Z (2008) Postoperative pain management outcome in Chinese inpatients. West J Nurs Res 30: 975–990.
7. Manias E, Bucknall T, Botti M (2005) Nurses' strategies for managing pain in the postoperative setting. Pain Manag Nurs 6: 18–29.
8. Helfand M, Freeman M (2009) Assessment and management of acute pain in adult medical inpatients: a systematic review. Pain Med 10: 1183–1199.
9. Botti M, Bucknall T, Manias E (2004) The problem of postoperative pain: issues for future research. Int J Nurs Pract 10: 257–263.
10. Dihle A, Helseth S, Kongsgaard UE, Paul SM, Miaskowski C (2006) Using the American Pain Society's patient outcome questionnaire to evaluate the quality of postoperative pain management in a sample of Norwegian patients. J Pain 7: 272–280.
11. Dekker A, Amon J, Le Roux K, Gaunt B (2012) "What is killing me most": chronic pain and the need for palliative care in the Eastern Cape, South Africa. J Pain Palliat Care Pharmacother 26: 334–340.
12. Selman L, Simms V, Penfold S, Powell R, Mwangi-Powell F, et al. (2013) 'My dreams are shuttered down and it hurts lots'-a qualitative study of palliative care needs and their management by HIV outpatient services in Kenya and Uganda. BMC Palliative Care 12: 35.
13. Powell RA, Radbruch L, Mwangi-Powell FN, Cleary J, Cherny N (2013) Failing to numb the pain: The untreated epidemic.
14. Human Rights Watch (2011) Global State of PainTreatment: Access to Medicines and Palliative Care. New York: Human Rights Watch.
15. Vijayan R (2011) Managing Acute Pain in the Developing World. Pain: Clinical Updates.
16. Cleary J, Powell RA, Munene G, Mwangi-Powell FN, Luyirika E, et al. (2013) Formulary availability and regulatory barriers to accessibility of opioids for cancer pain in Africa: a report from the Global Opioid Policy Initiative (GOPI). Annals of Oncology 24: xi14–xi23.
17. MoH (2007) National Pain Managment Guideline. Ethiopia: Bole Printing.
18. Cohen E, Botti M, Hanna B, Leach S, Boyd S, et al. (2008) Pain beliefs and pain management of oncology patients. Cancer Nurs 31: E1–8.
19. Daut RL, Cleeland CS, Flanery RC (1983) Development of the Wisconsin Brief Pain Questionnaire to assess pain in cancer and other diseases. Pain 17: 197–210.
20. Cleeland CS, Gonin R, Hatfield AK, Edmonson JH, Blum RH, et al. (1994) Pain and Its Treatment in Outpatients with Metastatic Cancer. New England Journal of Medicine 330: 592–596.
21. Donnelly AJ, Golembiewski JA (2009) Perioperative Care. In: Koda-Kimble MA, Young LY, Alldredge BK, Corelli RL, Guglielmo BJ et al., editors. Applied Therapeutics: The Clinical Use Of Drugs. 9 ed. Philadelphia: Lippincott Williams & Wilkins. pp. P.9p27.
22. McNeill JA, Sherwood GD, Starck PL, Nieto B (2001) Pain management outcomes for hospitalized Hispanic patients. Pain management nursing: official journal of the American Society of Pain Management Nurses 2: 25–36.
23. Sherwood GD, McNeill JA, Starck PL, Disnard G (2003) Changing acute pain management outcomes in surgical patients. AORN J 77: 374, 377–380, 384–390 passim.
24. Sherwood G, McNeill JA, Hernandez L, Penarrieta I, Petersen JM (2005) A multinational study of pain management among Hispanics. Journal of Research in Nursing 10: 403–423.
25. Gordon DB, Dahl JL, Miaskowski C, McCarberg B, Todd KH, et al. (2005) American pain society recommendations for improving the quality of acute and cancer pain management: American Pain Society Quality of Care Task Force. Arch Intern Med 165: 1574–1580.
26. Gordon DB, Polomano RC, Pellino TA, Turk DC, McCracken LM, et al. (2010) Revised American Pain Society Patient Outcome Questionnaire (APS-POQ-R) for Quality Improvement of Pain Management in Hospitalized Adults: Preliminary Psychometric Evaluation. J Pain 11: 1172–1186.
27. Size M, Soyannwo OA, Justins DM (2007) Pain management in developing countries. Anaesthesia 62 Suppl 1: 38–43.
28. Ogboli-Nwasor E, Sule ST, Yusufu LM (2012) Pattern of postoperative pain management among adult surgical patients in a low-resource setting. J Pain Res 5: 117–120.
29. Faponle AF, Soyannwo OA, Ajayi IO (2001) Post operative pain therapy: a survey of prescribing patterns and adequacy of analgesia in Ibadan, Nigeria. Cent Afr J Med 47: 70–74.
30. Ocitti EF, Adwok JA (2000) Post-operative management of pain following major abdominal and thoracic operations. East Afr Med J 77: 299–302.
31. Soyannwo OA (1999) Post-operative pain control–prescription pattern and patients' experience. West Afr J Med 18: 207–210.
32. Gordon DB, Pellino TA, Miaskowski C, McNeill JA, Paice JA, et al. (2002) A 10-year review of quality improvement monitoring in pain management: recommendations for standardized outcome measures. Pain Manag Nurs 3: 116–130.
33. Chung JW, Lui JC (2003) Postoperative pain management: study of patients' level of pain and satisfaction with health care providers' responsiveness to their reports of pain. Nurs Health Sci 5: 13–21.
34. Qu Shen, Sherwood GD, McNeill JA, Zheng Li (2008) Postoperative Pain Management Outcome in Chinese Inpatients. Western Journal of Nursing Research 30: 975–990.
35. Tsui SL, Lo RJ, Tong WN, Yang JC, O'Regan AM, et al. (1995) A clinical audit for postoperative pain control on 1443 surgical patients. Acta Anaesthesiol Sin 33: 137–148.
36. Colman I, Rothney A, Wright SC, Zilkalns B, Rowe BH (2004) Use of narcotic analgesics in the emergency department treatment of migraine headache. Neurology 62: 1695–1700.
37. Barak M, Poppa E, Tansky A, Drenger B (2006) The activity of an acute pain service in a teaching hospital: Five years experience. Acute Pain 8: 155–159.
38. Olayemi O, Morhason-Bello IO, Adedokun BO, Ojengbede OA (2009) The role of ethnicity on pain perception in labor among parturients at the University College Hospital Ibadan. J Obstet Gynaecol Res 35: 277–281.
39. Tan EC, Lim Y, Teo YY, Goh R, Law HY, et al. (2008) Ethnic differences in pain perception and patient-controlled analgesia usage for postoperative pain. J Pain 9: 849–855.
40. Bedard D, Purden MA, Sauve-Larose N, Certosini C, Schein C (2006) The pain experience of post surgical patients following the implementation of an evidence-based approach. Pain Manag Nurs 7: 80–92.
41. McNeill JA, Sherwood GD, Starck PL (2004) The hidden error of mismanaged pain: a systems approach. J Pain Symptom Manage 28: 47–58.
42. Anderson KO (2005) Role of cutpoints: why grade pain intensity? Pain 113: 5–6.
43. Breivik H (1998) Postoperative pain management: why is it difficult to show that it improves outcome? Eur J Anaesthesiol 15: 748–751.
44. Edwards HE, Nash RE, Yates PM, Walsh AM, Fentiman BJ, et al. (2001) Improving pain management by nurses: A pilot Peer Intervention Program. Nurs Health Sci 3: 35–45.
45. Yates P, Dewar A, Edwards H, Fentiman B, Najman J, et al. (1998) The prevalence and perception of pain amongst hospital in-patients. J Clin Nurs 7: 521–530.
46. James FR, Large RG, Bushnell JA, Wells JE (1991) Epidemiology of pain in New Zealand. Pain 44: 279–283.
47. Bendelow G (1993) Pain perceptions, emotions and gender. Sociology of Health & Illness 15: 273–294.
48. Dawson R, Spross JA, Jablonski ES, Hoyer DR, Sellers DE, et al. (2002) Probing the paradox of patients' satisfaction with inadequate pain management. J Pain Symptom Manage 23: 211–220.
49. Ward SE, Gordon DB (1996) Patient satisfaction and pain severity as outcomes in pain management: a longitudinal view of one setting's experience. J Pain Symptom Manage 11: 242–251.

7

# Activation of Markers of Inflammation, Coagulation and Fibrinolysis in Musculoskeletal Trauma

**Olav Reikerås[1]*, Pål Borgen[2]**

**1** Institute of Clinical Medicine, Rikshospitalet, Oslo University Hospital, Oslo, Norway, **2** Martina Hansens Hospital, Oslo, Norway

## Abstract

***Background:*** Traumatic injury induces changes in mediators of inflammation and coagulation, but the pivotal roles of inflammation and coagulation has not been precisely clarified. Therefore we have studied markers of inflammation and coagulation after a standardized musculoskeletal trauma like total hip replacement surgery.

***Methods:*** We allocated 21 patients aged 50 to 84 years who underwent total hip replacement surgery. Releases of TNF-α, IL-1β, IL-6, IL-8 and IL-10 and protrombin fragment F1.2 and plasmin-antiplasmin complex (PAP) were examined during surgery and up 6 days postoperatively, and systemic releases were compared to pre-operative values. Surgery induced significant increments in serum levels of IL-6 at 6 hours and at 1 day after surgery and in levels of IL-8 at 6 hours after surgery. There were no significant changes in serum levels of TNF-α, IL-1β or IL-10. There were significant increments in blood levels of F1.2 and PAP up to 6 days postoperatively with highest levels at 6 hours after surgery. There were only week correlations between IL-6 and IL-8 and F1.2 and PAP.

***Conclusion:*** Major musculoskeletal surgery causes changes of the inflammatory, coagulatory and fibrinolytic cascades in stable patients, but with no correlations between inflammation and coagulation and fibrinolysis.

**Editor:** Guillermo López Lluch, Universidad Pablo de Olavide, Centro Andaluz de Biología del Desarrollo-CSIC, Spain

**Funding:** The authors have no support or funding to report.

**Competing Interests:** The authors have declared that no competing interests exist.

* Email: olav.reikeras@ous-hf.no

## Introduction

Traumatic activation of inflammation and coagulation is recognized as a physiologic reaction to initiate healing and to act as a barrier to injury propagation and infection [1]. It arises from the interplay between various mediators produced at the site of injury, but with serious traumatic events, it can lead to a generalized state of inflammation referred to as the systemic inflammatory response syndrome with the potential to cause local and remote organ injury [2]. Inflammation and coagulation are intricately related processes that may considerably affect each other. A large number of inflammatory mediators, including cytokines have been shown to affect the coagulation cascade at several levels in monocyte and liver cells and promote inflammation in endothelial cells with structural and functional changes [3]. However, it has become increasingly clear, that vice versa, components of the coagulation system are able to markedly modulate the inflammatory response [3], [4]. Coagulation factors as well as anticoagulant proteins may activate specific cell receptors on mononuclear or endothelial cells, which may affect cytokine production or inflammatory cell apoptosis.

The entire pathophysiology of posttraumatic organ dysfunction is not fully understood, and an improved understanding of the pivotal roles of inflammation and coagulation seems important for directing appropriate patient care after traumatic injury [5]. To get insight into the physiological interactions between inflammation and coagulation following injury, we have studied markers of inflammation and coagulation and fibrinolysis after a standardized musculoskeletal trauma in the form of total hip replacement (THR).

## Methods

The study was approved by the Regional Ethics Committee of South East Norway (105-08012d 1.2007.1798. 1306./2058, 17679) and was performed in accordance with the ethical standards of the Declaration of Helsinki. We included 13 women and 8 men aged 60 to 84 years after written informed consent to participate in the study (Table 1). They all underwent primary cemented total hip arthroplasty (THA) due to osteoarthritis under spinal anesthesia with 5 mg/mL bupivacaine (Marcain; AstraZeneca, Södertälje, Sweden) injected at the lumbar level. The operation was performed in the lateral position, using a standardized posterior approach. Closed postoperative drainage was used for 24 hours. All patients were mobilized on the first postoperative day.

Thromboprophylaxis with low-molecular-weight heparin (Fragmin; Pharmacia & Upjohn, Stockholm, Sweden) and infectious prophylaxis with cephfalothin (Keflin; Eli Lilly, Indianapolis, IN., USA) were used. Voluven and Ringer's acetate (Fresenius KABI,

**Table 1.** Patients' characteristics. Values are mean ± standard deviation and (ranges).

| | | |
|---|---|---|
| Age (years) | 70.6±7.8 | (60–84) |
| Height (cm) | 170±8.2 | (155–192) |
| Weight (kg) | 78.6±11.8 | (63–108) |
| BMI | 26.8±3.6 | (22–33) |
| ASA classification | 1.9±0.4 | (1–2) |

Bad Homburg, Germany) were used as plasma substitutes. Postoperative analgesia was administered according to a standard protocol consisting of paracetamol and codeine sulphate (Paralgin forte; Weifa AS, Oslo, Norway) and ketobemidon (Ketorax; Jenahexal Pharma, Jena, Germany).

Patients with allergy to dalteparin, bleeding disorders, renal failure, hepatic disease, active treatment for malignancy, on-going antithrombotic treatment, history of deep vein thrombosis or pulmonary embolus, and patients experiencing major operations, traumas, stroke, or cardiac infarction the last 3 months before surgery were excluded. Patients were advised to stop antiplatelet medication and high-dose aspirin 1 week before surgery.

Hemoglobin, hematocrit, white blood counts, platelet counts, c-reactive-protein, creatinin, and liver enzymes were analyzed the day before surgery.

Blood samples were obtained from a peripheral vein at the following time points: before induction of anesthesia (T1), after induction of anesthesia, but before surgery (T2), at the end of surgery (T3), at 6 hours after surgery (T4), at the day after surgery (T5) and at 6 days after surgery (T6). Blood samples was kept on ice until it was separated by centrifugation at 2500 g for 20 min at 18 degrees C and stored at −80 degrees C until assayed. Analyzes of tumor necrosis factor α (TNF-α), interleukin 10 (IL-10) (R & D systems, MS, USA), IL-1β, IL-6 and IL-8 (CLB, the Netherlands) were performed by ELISA according to the manufacturers instruction.

Prothrombin fragment F1.2 and plasmin/α2-antiplasmin (PAP) were measured by ELISA by the use of commercial kit (Enzygnost F1.2 micro; Dade Behring, Marburg, Germany) following manufacturer's instructions.

Statistical analyses were performed using SPSS II software Version 19 (IBM Inc. USA). Data are presented by mean and standard deviation. Time dependent changes were performed by analysis of variance (ANOVA). If significant differences were indicated, we used the LSD post hoc test. Correlations and regression analyses were carried out, and $P \leq 0.05$ was considered significant.

## Results

The postoperative course was uneventful in all patients up to 6 days after surgery when they left the hospital. Before surgery CRP was 3.2±4.4 mg/L, at 3 days after surgery it was significantly increased to 83±53 mg/L ($p<0.001$), and it was still significantly increased at 6 days after surgery (46±31 mg/L) ($p<0.001$).

Surgery induced significant increments in serum levels of IL-6 at 6 hours after surgery ($p<0.001$) and at 1 day after surgery ($p<0.001$) and in levels of IL-8 at 6 hours after surgery ($p=0.004$) (Table 2). There were no significant changes in serum levels of TNF-α (0.947), IL-1β ($p=0.421$) or IL-10 (0.989).

There were significant increments in blood levels of F1.2 and PAP up to 6 days postoperatively ($p<0.001$) with highest levels at 6 hours after surgery. There were week correlations between serum levels of IL-6 and F1.2 and PAP ($r=0.194$ and 0.066, respectively) and IL-8 and F1.2 and PAP ($r=0.183$ and 0.193, respectively). By analyses of regression we found that serum levels of IL-6, IL-8, F1.2 or PAP were not significantly associated with age, sex and body mass index (BMI) ($p=0.636$, 0.131 and 0.811, respectively).

## Discussion

Severe trauma results in the release of mediators of inflammation and coagulation, and sustained alterations have been associated with systemic complications [6], [7]. But the magnitude and relevance of such alterations in trauma patients who are physiologically stable are not widely appreciated. An important aspect is the link between coagulation and inflammation [8]. In our study we defined the insult in terms of a standardized surgical procedure. We found significant inflammatory, coagulatory and fibrinolytic responses following a major musculoskeletal injury in otherwise stable patients. However, there were no correlations between the markers of inflammation on one hand and the markers of coagulation and fibrinolysis on the other hand.

The age of our patients ranged from 60 to 84 years, and both women and men were included. Differences in age and sex as well as in nutritional status may influence the inflammatory response. However, the operations were done electively, all patients were well nourished as indicated by BMI, and there were no correlations between age, gender and BMI. Furthermore, we found no associations between age, gender and BMI on one side and inflammatory markers on the other. Second, it may be questioned whether the inflammatory response was influenced by the anesthetic. We measured markers before and after anesthesia, but before surgery, and we could not find any significant changes as a result of anesthetic. But as there is a rather short time interval between anesthesia and surgery, we can not say with certainty that anesthesia do or do not have inflammatory effects. Third, we did not measure the biomarkers locally. An increased production of pro-inflammatory mediators at the site of tissue damage may contribute to systemic inflammation and trauma-mediated immunosuppression [9].

The proinflammatory cytokines TNF-α, IL-1β, IL-6 and IL-8 and the antiinflammatory IL-10 have been considered important markers of inflammatory activity [10]. Therefore we focused on these. However, chemotactic cytokines govern the migration of inflammatory leukocytes into damaged areas, and typical inflammatory chemokines like CCL2 and CCL3 are known to play a key-role in the posttraumatic immune response [11]. These cytokines were also analyzed in our study, but as there were no significant changes in the systemic levels of these, they were not reported. Also, investigations into the use of IL-1β and IL-10 as clinical markers of the inflammatory response to trauma have been equivocal [12]. TNF-α is produced by a variety of cells and acts to

**Table 2.** Changes in TNF-α, IL-1β, IL-6, IL-8, F 1.2 and PAP (pg/mL).

| | T1 | T2 | T3 | T4 | T5 | T6 | ANOVA |
|---|---|---|---|---|---|---|---|
| TNF-α | 0.8±1.7 | 0.9±1.5 | 0.6±1.0 | 0.7±0.8 | 0.6±0.9 | 0.8±1.0 | 0.854 |
| IL-1β | 8.3±18 | 9.2±19 | 4.2±11 | 4.0±11 | 3.9±12 | 11±20 | 0.602 |
| Il-6 | 8.0±12 | 7.3±9.4 | 15±27 | 39±34[a] | 40±31[a] | 21±27 | <0.001 |
| Il-8 | 8.9±4.3 | 9.1±4.4 | 9.9±4.7 | 19±23[b] | 9.8±4.6 | 15±67 | 0.019 |
| Il-10 | 20±51 | 22±53 | 14±37 | 17±40 | 16±37 | 15±35 | 0.992 |
| F 1.2 | 172±67 | 212±83 | 524±164[a] | 573±148[a] | 278±164[c] | 350±109[a] | <0.001 |
| PAP | 542±143 | 535±138 | 907±259[a] | 1039±276[a] | 559±112 | 842±113[a] | <0.001 |

Time points are before induction of anaesthesia (T1), after induction of anaesthesia, but before surgery (T2), at the end of surgery (T3), at 6 hours after surgery (T4), at the day after surgery (T5), and at 6 days after surgery (T6).
Values are mean ± standard deviation.
[a]p<0.001, [b]p=0.004, [c]p=0.013 in relation to T1.

increase the permeability of endothelial cells and the expression of adhesion molecules. But binding to its shed soluble receptors may interfere with measurement of serum levels [13]. Our results discount the value of the measurement of systemic TNF-α, IL-1β and IL-10 concentrations as acute markers of trauma and surgery.

In contrast, a direct relationship has been confirmed between elevated levels of IL-6 and IL-8 and degree of injury [14]. In a study evaluating clinical outcome in children following blunt trauma, serum IL-8 level at admission was identified as a most important determinant of postinjury mortality [15]. The increases in IL-8 in our study were short-lived at 6 hour after surgery and reflect that IL-8 is a chemokine that attracts polymorphonuclear neutrophil cells and macrophages into the wound site. Typically, at 24 h the neutrophil population is at its maximum, and the activity of these neutrophils may play a critical role in recovery. It has also been noted that systemic levels of IL-6 increase immediately following trauma and that patients with the most severe injuries have the highest levels [16]. A similar increase in venous levels of IL-6 during reamed intramedullary nailing of the femur was observed by Giannoudis et al. [17], and it is well accepted that elective surgical procedures cause an acute rise in venous levels of IL-6 in proportion to the magnitude and duration of the procedure [18]. Our observations on the systemic release of IL-6 concur with these investigations [19]. We found that IL-6 levels were increased at 6 and 24 h after surgery. This is in agreement with a previous study in stable trauma patients [20]. On the other hand, sustained high levels of IL-6 have been associated with increased severity of tissue injury and have correlated with subsequent development of post injury complications [18,21].

IL-6 is the principal regulator of most acute-phase protein genes and regulates local and systemic inflammatory responses, including the synthesis of hepatic acute-phase reactants like C-reactive protein [22], [23]. We found increases in CRP like in Il-6. It has been suggested that IL-6 might partly be responsible for inducing the coagulatory cascade [24], and a positive correlation between IL-6 and prothrombin F1.2 concentrations has been noted [20]. F1.2 and PAP are accepted as specific markers of activation of the coagulation and fibrinolytic systems [25], and the systemic levels of these markers indicate the magnitude of tissue injury [26], [27]. Our results demonstrate a perioperative induction of these markers. We assume that intramedullary pressure during instrumentation cause intravasation of medullary contents with high levels of procoagulant factors [28], [29]. The perioperative increases in F1.2 might also be caused by passage into the lung of platelets that aggregate around fat emboli, thus inducing a systemic coagulatory response [30].

The immediate elevations in F1.2 and PAP preceded the increases in IL-6. The profile of F1.2 and PAP was decreasing the first postoperative day and then increasing until the 6the postoperative day. We assume that an unbalanced consumption and replenishment of coagulant and fibrinolytic factors explain the decreases the first postoperative day, followed by a hypercoagulable state that was prolonged after cessation of the inflammatory state. These findings harmonize with others and indicate a continuing procoagulant state even beyond hospital discharge in several patients [31]. As there were no correlations, our findings do not support the idea of a direct interaction between the inflammatory and the coagulatory cascade system in stable patients undergoing a major musculoskeletal trauma.

## Conclusion

Our study in stable patients undergoing a major musculoskeletal trauma indicates inflammatory and coagulatory and fibrinolytic responses with highest levels during the first postoperative day. But the processes of inflammation on one hand and coagulation and fibrinolysis on the other hand do not seem to affect each other.

## Acknowledgments

Authors would like to acknowledge Stine Bjornsen, Institute of Clinical Medicine, Oslo University Hospital, Rikshospitalet.

## Author Contributions

Performed the experiments: OR PB. Analyzed the data: OR. Contributed reagents/materials/analysis tools: OR. OR PB. Conceived and designed the experiments: OR PB. Wrote the paper: OR.

## References


1. Tidball JG (2005) Inflammatory processes in muscle injury and repair. Am J Physiol Regul Integr Comp Physiol 288: R345–353.
2. Rankin JA (2004) Biological mediators of acute inflammation. AACN Clin Issues15:3–17.
3. Aird WC (2003) The role of the endothelium in severe sepsis and multiple organ dysfunction syndrome. Blood 101: 3765–3777.
4. Esmon CT (2005) The interactions between inflammation and coagulation. Br J Haematol 131:417–430.
5. Lee CC, Marill KA, Carter WA, Crupi RS (2001) A current concept of trauma-induced multiorgan failure. Ann Emerg Med 38:170–176.
6. Cheadle WG, Hershman SR, Wellhausen SR, Polk HC Jr (1991) HLA-DR antigen expression on peripheral blood monocytes correlates with surgical infection. Am J Surg 161:639–645.
7. Gando S, Kameue T, Matsuda N, Hayakawa M, Ishitani T, et al. (2002) Combined activation of coagulation and inflammation has an important role in multiple organ dysfunction and poor outcome after severe trauma. Thromb Haemost 88:943–949.
8. Levi M, van der Poll T, Buller HR (2004) Bidirectional relation between inflammation and coagulation. Circulation 109:2698–2704.
9. Bastian D, Tamburstuen MV, Lyngstadaas SP, Reikerås O (2008) Systemic and local cytokine kinetics after total hip replacement surgery. Eur Surg Res 2008; 41(4):334–340.
10. Easton R, Balogh ZJ (2013) Peri-operative changes in serum markers after trauma: A systematic review. Injury 45:934–941.
11. Neunaber C, Oestern S, Andruszkow H, Zeckey C, Mommsen P, et al. (2013) Cytokine productive capacity of alveolar macrophages and Kupffer cells after femoral fracture and blunt chest trauma in a murine trauma model. Immunol Lett 152:159–66.
12. Giannoudis P, Tan H, Perry S, Tzioupis C, Kanakaris N (2010) The systemic inflammatory response following femoral canal reaming using the reamer-irrigator-aspirator (RIA) device. Injury 41:S57–S61.
13. Sakamoto K, Arakawa H, Mita S, Ishiko T, Ikei S, et al. (1994) Elevation ofcirculating interleukin 6 after surgery: factors influencing the serum level. Cytokine 6: 181–186.
14. Mimasaka S, Funayama M, Hashiyada M, Nata M, Tsunenari S (2007) Significance of levels of IL-6 and IL-8 after trauma: A study of 11 cytokines post-mortem using multiplex immunoassay. Injury 38:1047–1051.
15. Ozturk H, Yagmur Y, Ozturk H (2008) The prognostic importance of serum IL-1beta, IL-6, IL-8 and TNF-alpha levels compared to trauma scoring systems for early mortality in children with blunt trauma. Pediatr Surg Int 24:235–239.
16. Gebhard F, Pfetsch H, Steinbach G, Strecker W, Kinzl L, et al. (2000) Brückner UB. Is interleukin 6 an early marker of injury severity following major trauma in humans? Arch Surg 135:291–295.
17. Giannoudis PV, Smith RM, Bellamy MC, Morrison JF, Dickson RA, et al. (1999) Stimulation of the inflammatory system by reamed and unreamed nailing of femoral fractures. J Bone Joint Surg (Br) 81: 356–361.
18. Flohe S, Lendemans S, Schade F, Kreuzfelder E, Waydas C (2004) Influence of surgical intervention on the immune response of severely injured patients Intensive Care med 30:96–102.
19. Pape H-C, Schmidt RE, Rice J, van Griensven, M das Gupta R, et al. (2000) Biochemical changes after trauma and skeletal surgery of the lower extremity: Quantification of the operative burden. Crit Care Med 28:3441–3448.
20. Pape HC, Grimme K, Van Griensven M, Sott AH, Giannoudis P, et al. (2003) Impact of intramedullary instrumentation versus damage control for femoral fractures on immunoinflammatory parameters: Prospective randomized analysis by the EPOFF Study Group. J Trauma 55:7–13.
21. Baigrie RJ, Lamont PM, Kwiatkowski D, Dallman MJ, Morris PJ (1992) Systemic cytokine response after major surgery. Br J Surg 79:757–760.
22. Horn F, Henze C, Heidrich K (2000) Interleukin-6 signal transduction and lymphocyte function. Immunobiology 202: 151–167.
23. Ramadori G, Christ B (1999) Cytokines and the hepatic acute-phase response. Semin Liver Dis 19: 141–155.
24. Gando S, Nakanishi Y, Tedo I (1995) Cytokines and plasminogen activator inhibitor-1 in posttrauma disseminated intravascular coagulation: Relationship to multiple organ dysfunction syndrome. Crit Care Med 23: 1835–1842.
25. Jorgensen LN, Lind B, Hauch O, Leffers A, Albrecht-Beste E, et al. (1990) Thrombin-antithrombin III-complex and fibrin degradation products in plasma: Surgery and postoperative deep venous thrombosis. Thromb Res 59: 69–76.
26. Kwan HC (1984) Role of fibrinolysis in disease processes. Semin Thromb Haemostas 10: 71–79
27. Dahl O, Aspelin T, Lyberg T (1995) The role of bone traumatization in the initiation of proximal DVT during cemented hip replacement surgery in pigs. Blood Coagul Fibrinolysis 6:709–717.
28. Riseborough EJ, Herndon J (1976) Alterations in pulmonary function, coagulation and fat metabolism in patients with fractures of the lower limbs. Clin Orthop Rel Res 115: 248–266.
29. Pape H-C, Regel G, Tscherne H (1998) Localinstrumentation after severe trauma in sheep. J Trauma 45: 720–728
30. Heim D, Regazzoni P, Tsakiris DA, Aebi T, Schlegel U, et al. (1995) Intramedullary nailing and pulmonary embolism: Does unreamed nailing prevent embolization? An in vivo study in rabbits. J Trauma 38:899–906
31. Arnesen H, Dahl OE, Aspelin T, Seljeflot I, Kierulf P, et al. (2003) Sustained prothrombotic profile after hip replacement surgery: the influence of prolonged prophylaxis with dalteparin. J Thromb Haemost 1:971–975.

# 8

# Ultrasound-Guided Transversus Abdominis Plane Block versus Continuous Wound Infusion for Post-Caesarean Analgesia: A Randomized Trial

**Michel Chandon[1], Agnès Bonnet[2], Yannick Burg[1], Carole Barnichon[2], Véronique DesMesnards-Smaja[1], Brigitte Sitbon[2], Christine Foiret[1], Jean-François Dreyfus[3], Jamil Rahmani[2], Pierre-Antoine Laloë[4], Marc Fischler[1], Morgan Le Guen[1]***

1 Department of Anesthesiology, Hôpital Foch, Suresnes, France, 2 Department of Anesthesiology, Institut Hospitalier Franco-Britannique, Levallois-Perret, France, 3 Department of Clinical Research and Innovation, Hôpital Foch, Suresnes, France, 4 Department of Health Education, Bradford Teaching Hospitals, Leeds, United Kingdom

## Abstract

***Objective:*** To compare the analgesic effect of ultrasound-guided Transversus Abdominis Plane (TAP) block versus Continuous Wound Infusion (CWI) with levobupivacaine after caesarean delivery.

***Methods:*** We recruited parturients undergoing elective caesareans for this multicenter study. Following written informed consent, they received a spinal anaesthetic without intrathecal morphine for their caesarean section. The postoperative analgesia was randomized to either a bilateral ultrasound guided TAP block (levobupivicaine = 150 mg) or a CWI through an elastomeric pump for 48 hours (levobupivacaine = 150 mg the first day and 12.5 mg/h thereafter). Every woman received regular analgesics along with oral morphine if required. The primary outcome was comparison of the 48-hour area under the curve (AUC) pain scores. Secondary outcomes included morphine consumption, adverse events, and persistent pain one month postoperatively.

***Results:*** Recruitment of 120 women was planned but the study was prematurely terminated due to the occurrence of generalized seizures in one patient of the TAP group. By then, 36 patients with TAP and 29 with CWI had completed the study. AUC of pain at rest and during mobilization were not significantly different: 50 [22.5–80] in TAP versus 50 [27.5–130] in CWI ($P = 0.4$) and 190 [130–240] versus 160 [112.5–247.5] ($P = 0.5$), respectively. Morphine consumption (0 [0–20] mg in the TAP group and 10 [0–32.5] mg in the CWI group ($P = 0.09$)) and persistent pain at one month were similar in both groups (respectively 29.6% and 26.6% (P = 0.73)).

***Conclusion:*** In cases of morphine-free spinal anesthesia for cesarean delivery, no difference between TAP block and CWI for postoperative analgesia was suggested. TAP block may induce seizures in this specific context. Consequently, such a technique after a caesarean section cannot be recommended.

***Trial Registration:*** ClinicalTrials.gov NCT01151943

**Editor:** Kristina Gemzell-Danielsson, Karolinska Institutet, Sweden

**Funding:** The authors have no support or funding to report.

**Competing Interests:** The authors have declared that no competing interests exist.

* Email: m.leguen@hopital-foch.org

## Introduction

Caesarean delivery is one of the most commonly performed surgical procedures and postoperative pain is a great concern for women [1]. Its severity may impair early postoperative maternal rehabilitation and recovery [2]. Opioids and non-steroidal anti-inflammatory drugs, as components of a multimodal analgesic regimen, achieve effective analgesia. However both systemic and neuraxial opioid administration are associated with frequent dose-dependent adverse effects including nausea, vomiting, pruritus, sedation, respiratory depression, hyperalgesia [3] and are transferred across the placenta to the fetus. Thus, alternatives such as peripheral nerve block or wound infiltration have been suggested especially for cases where general anesthesia is indicated or where intrathecal opioids are contra-indicated. Seeing that a single dose of local anesthetic wound infiltration only offers short-term analgesia in the postoperative period [4], a regional block or a continuous local anesthetic technique may provide better analgesia. Two recent meta-analyses have shown the efficacy of single shot bilateral Transversus Abdominis Plane (TAP) block [5,6] after caesarean section while another demonstrated the usefulness of local anesthetic agent with Continuous Wound Infiltration (CWI) during a few days [7]. The former has been improved by ultrasound guidance [8] and the latter by placement of a multi–

orifice catheter below the fascia [9]. To date, no prospective trial has directly compared the analgesic efficacy of these two techniques.

We therefore conducted a study to compare continuous delivery of local anesthetic using a wound catheter and ultrasound-guided bilateral TAP block after elective caesarean delivery during the first 48 postoperative hours.

## Results

The study began September 2010 and was prematurely stopped in July 2011 due to the occurrence of generalized convulsions a few minutes after a TAP block. This event required transient mechanical ventilation and was successfully treated using an intravenous lipid emulsion infusion. It has been considered to be the consequence of a partial systemic absorption of local anesthetic. An independent pharmaco-vigilance committee has recommended stopping the trial because this event if expected as every regional technique occurred with a high rate (1/40) that was higher than expected. Moreover, physiological changes of pregnancy may favor its occurrence and further research is required. Consequently, only 80 subjects were enrolled in the study, 39 were randomized to the CWI group and 41 to the TAP group. Ten patients did not complete the study in the CWI group and 5 in the TAP group as seen in the Consort diagram (Figure 1).

Demographic characteristics, as well as intraoperative parameters were similar (Table 1). The Intention to Treat analysis showed that pain at rest was low in the postoperative period in both groups with a median AUC of pain scores during 48 hours at 50 [22.5–80] in the TAP group and at 50 [27.5–130] in the CWI group ($P = 0.3$). During mobilization, pain was higher but similar in both groups with an AUC at 190 [130–240] in the TAP group and at 160 [105–262] in the CWI group ($P > 0.9$). The per-protocol analysis has given similar results with an AUC at rest at 70 [30–110] and 50 [22.5–120] ($P = 0.4$) and during mobilization at 190 [130–240] and 160 [112.5–247.5] respectively ($P = 0.5$) (Figure 2). The mixed model for repeated measures showed a non-significant group effect both for pain scores at rest ($P = 0.5$) and pain scores with movement ($P = 0.5$). In both cases the time factor was significant ($P_{rest} = 0.03$, $P_{movement} = 0.00002$) showing a significant change in the perception of pain along time. The time × group interaction is not significant ($P_{rest} = 0.6$, $P_{movement} > 0.9$) as we were unable to show a different time profile of effect for the two procedures.

No woman required rescue intravenous morphine administration in the post-anesthesia care unit. Oral morphine was not required by the third postoperative hour in the TAP Block group but was required in 2 cases in the CWI group ($P = 0.21$). Median oral morphine consumption was not significantly different between the groups: 0 [0–20] mg in the TAP group and 10 [0–32.5] mg in the CWI group ($P = 0.09$), with a large inter-individual variability. Seventeen patients of 36 (47%) in the TAP group compared to 16 patients out of 29 (55%) in the CWI group took oral morphine during the first 60 postoperative hours ($P = 0.7$).

Patients experienced nausea and vomiting more frequently in the TAP group ($P = 0.03$). No difference was reported concerning other opioid related adverse effects (pruritus and sedation). A wound complications were seen in 2 cases from the CWI group ($P = 0.19$). Patient satisfaction with pain relief did not significantly differ between groups (Table 2).

Median postoperative length of stay was similar in both groups (6 [5–7] days) ($P = 0.9$). Twenty seven patients in the TAP group (66%) and 19 patients (49%) in the CWI group responded to the postoperative interview. They reported similar rates of persistent wound pain and of neuropathic pain (Table 3).

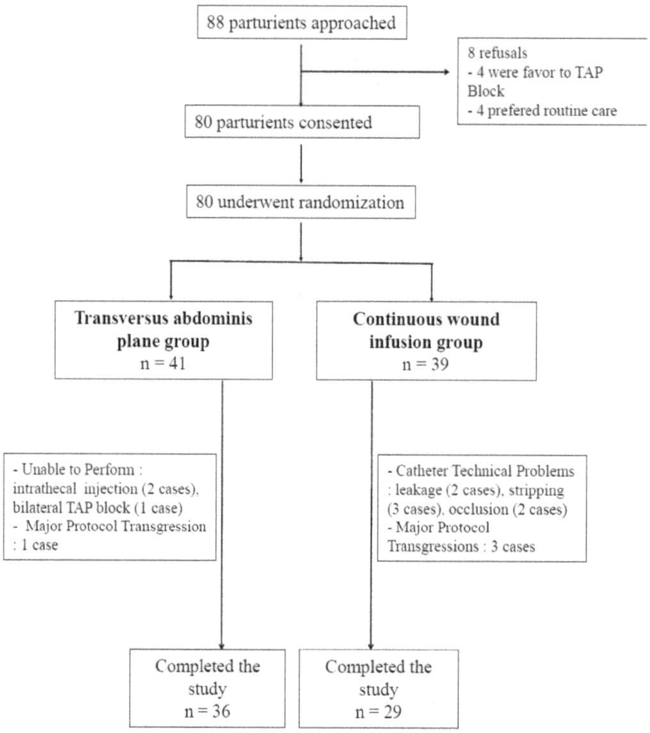


**Figure 1. Consort trial diagram.**

**Table 1.** Characteristics of study patients, presented as mean [1st and 3rd interquartile] and as numbers (%).

| | Transversus abdominis plane block Group | | Continuous wound infusion Group | |
|---|---|---|---|---|
| | ITT | PP | ITT | PP |
| | n = 41 | n = 36 | n = 39 | n = 29 |
| Age (yr) | 34 (30–37) | 33 (30–37) | 32 (30–37) | 32 (30–38) |
| Height (cm) | 164 (160–168) | 165 (160–169) | 165 (161–170) | 164 (160–170) |
| Weight (kg) | 72 (65–81) | 74 (68–82) | 73 (68–81) | 74 (68–81) |
| Surgical time (min) | 40 (34–48) | 40 (35–50) | 45 (37–50) | 45 (40–60) |
| Surgical difficulties (%) | 7 (17.0) | 7 (19.4) | 11 (28.2) | 9 (31.0) |
| Previous abdominal surgery (%) | 19 (46.3) | 19 (52.7) | 25 (64.1) | 17 (58.6) |

ITT: *Intent to Treat* Analysis (all included patients); PP: *Per Protocol* Analysis (patients who completed the study protocol).

## Discussion

The occurrence of generalized seizures occurring a few minutes after an ultrasound guided TAP block led to the premature study termination. Consequently this randomized trial was underpowered to detect any significant difference in term of analgesia between continuous wound infiltration and TAP block in cases of scheduled caesarean delivery under spinal anesthesia.

Local anesthetic agent wound infiltration has been proposed after various surgical procedures and a meta-analysis by Gupta et al. demonstrated that wound catheters provided no significant analgesia at rest or on activity, except in patients undergoing gynecological and obstetric surgery [13]. Another meta-analysis by Bamigboye and Hofmeyr confirmed the interest of this technique after caesarean section [7].

Efficacy of a wound infiltration technique using a local anesthetic/non-steroidal anti-inflammatory drug mixture [14] is increased when the catheter tip is placed below the fascia [9]. The safety of wound infiltration was demonstrated by Gupta et al. in their meta-analysis: low incidence of side effects and above all no statistically significant differences for wound infection, wound erythema, and hematoma when compared with control patients, except for a lower risk for wound breakdown in patients receiving a local anesthetic [13]. In our study, technical problems were frequently encountered - 7 cases (17.9%) - with inadvertent stripping of the catheter in the operating theatre or during the transfer from operating table to bed, leakage, and occlusion despite cautious during patient mobilization. Even though they claimed global satisfaction with the technique, several women stated that it was uncomfortable to have a wound catheter and an elastomeric pump for forty hours post-operatively; however, we did not systematically study this point.

On the other hand, TAP block techniques are gaining wide acceptance, especially with ultrasound guidance [8]. Results from two meta-analyses are contradictory. The first one concluded that there is only limited evidence to suggest that usage of perioperative TAP block reduces opioid consumption and pain scores after abdominal surgery when compared with no intervention or placebo [15]. A more recent meta-analysis concluded that TAP block is safe, reduces postoperative morphine requirements, nausea and vomiting and possibly the severity of pain after abdominal surgery [16]. If there is some doubt regarding its indication after abdominal surgery, conversely, two meta-analyses have shown efficacy of bilateral TAP block after caesarean section

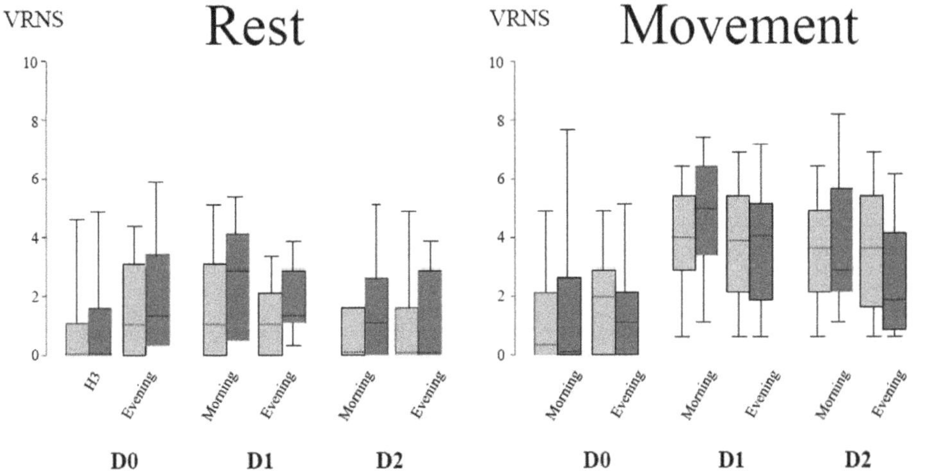


**Figure 2. Pain scores at D0 (3rd postoperative hour and evening), D1 (morning and evening) and D2 (morning and evening).** Results are represented by box plot. The horizontal solid line gives the median value and the upper and lower limit give the interquartile range. At last, the 5 and 95th percentiles correspond to the limit of the whiskers. Left panel: pain scores at rest. Right panel: pain scores during mobilization. VRNS: verbal response numerical scale pain score.

**Table 2.** Side effects and Satisfaction, presented as numbers (%).

| | Transversus Abdominis Plane block Group | Continuous wound infusion Group | *P* value |
|---|---|---|---|
| | n = 36 | n = 29 | |
| Nausea and vomiting | 6 (16.7) | 0 (0) | 0.03 |
| Pruritus | 7 (19.4) | 6 (20.7) | >0.9 |
| Gastrointestinal function reestablishment at 48 h | | | |
| Flatus | 33 (91.7) | 24 (82.7) | >0.9 |
| Faeces | 12 (33.3) | 8 (27.6) | >0.9 |
| Sedation* | 5 (13.9) | 4 (13.8) | >0.9 |
| Surgical wound complication** | 0 (0) | 2 (6.9) | 0.18 |
| Satisfaction Scores | | | >0.9 |
| 1 or 2 | 35 (97.2) | 27 (93.1) | |
| 3 or 4 | 1 (2.8) | 1 (3.4)*** | |

*cases with mild to moderate sedation,
**slight oozing from the scar and scar haematoma,
***one missing data.

[5,6]. These meta-analyses did not report major adverse events. We are only aware of one previous published case of convulsions which occurred 3 hours after a TAP block in a patient that had had a laparoscopy-assisted myomectomy [17].

This study showed no significant difference between local anesthetic agent wound infiltration and TAP block especially in terms of postoperative analgesia but it must be outlined that there was a wide inter-individual variability in the dose of oral morphine showing that both techniques have variable efficacy. Adverse effects and pain persisting at one month concerned 25 to 30% of the patients, a value higher than that reported in the literature (14–18%), were similar in both groups [2,18]. Previously described risk factors such as pre-existing pain, acute postoperative pain, a young age and general anesthesia cannot explain these results. The short follow-up time (one month versus 3 months in literature) and modalities of study and interview (prospective series with DN4 interview) may have affected our findings. Finally, designing this study with a morphine-free spinal anesthetic, most likely had an effect on immediate to intermediate pain scores.

The limitations of the study are as follows. We did not include the whole sample of 120 patients as initially planned by the statistical analysis because of the occurrence of a major undesirable event in the TAP group. Furthermore, several patients were excluded from analysis as described above. It can be postulated that the study is underpowered; however it is unlikely that a significant difference between groups could have been found with a complete set of patients. A second major limitation is due to the fact that our study was not blinded and that patients systematically received paracetamol, ketoprofen, and nefopam. This could reduce the difference between the studied loco-regional techniques but represents our routine postoperative care. Conversely, our use of intrathecal bupivacaine with sufentanil instead of a longer acting opioid such as morphine avoids a supplementary confounding factor in our analysis of the analgesic effect and side effects. This is important as a recent study showed that TAP block is associated with greater supplemental morphine requirements and higher pain scores than intrathecal morphine after caesarean section [19].

In conclusion, our randomized trial was prematurely ended do to the occurrence of a severe adverse event following a TAP block demonstrating that local anesthetic toxicity can occur even with continuous ultrasound guidance. Despite the fact that our study is consequently underpowered, a difference in term of analgesic efficacy between TAP block and wound infiltration seems improbable regarding our results. As a consequence, use of TAP block after caesarean cannot be recommended before further pharmacological studies on the relationship between adverse effect to local anesthetic and pregnancy.

## Methods

This multicenter randomized clinical open trial with parallel arms was approved by an Ethic Committee (Comité de Protection des Personnes, Hôpital A. Paré, Boulogne Billancourt, France) and by the French national regulatory office (Agence Française de Sécurité Sanitaire des Produits de Santé). The trial was registered

**Table 3.** Main results obtained from the a follow-up postal standardized questionnaire, presented as numbers (%).

| | Transversus Abdominis Plane block Group | Continuous wound infusion Group | *P* value |
|---|---|---|---|
| | n = 27 | n = 19 | |
| Incidence of pain in the scar area (VRNS) | 8 (29.6) | 4 (26.6) | 0.73 |
| Neuropathic pain* | 2 (7.4) | 4 (26.6) | 0.21 |

VRNS: Verbal Response Numerical Scale,
*defined as score of 4 or above on the DN4 questionnaire [11].

on ClinicalTrials.gov as NCT01151943. The protocol for this trial and supporting CONSORT checklist are available as supporting information; see Checklist S1 and Protocol S1.

Parturients were eligible if they were scheduled for an elective caesarean delivery at term with a low transverse incision (Joel-Cohen incision) under spinal anesthesia. Other criteria of inclusion were American Society of Anesthesiologists physical status 1 or 2 and a singleton fetus >37 weeks of gestation. Non-inclusion criteria were women in active labour, age<19 or >40 years old, height< 155 cm, weight<50 kg or a Body Mass Index>35 kg/m$^2$ and women with contra-indication to any of the study protocol analgesics (paracetamol, ketoprofen, nefopam and levobupivacaine). Exclusion criteria were conversion from spinal to general anesthesia owing to inadequate intraoperative analgesia, failure of the neuraxial technique, failure to site the multi-hole catheter (CWI group) and failure to visualize the intrafascial space (TAP group).

Some weeks (from 4 to 10) before the caesarean delivery, a pre-anesthetic visit was performed during which oral and written information about spinal anesthesia and the study protocol were given. Written informed consent was then obtained either the day before or on the day of surgery. Upon admission to the operative room, every parturient received a standard monitoring including electrocardiogram, non-invasive arterial pressure, and pulse oximetry. At this moment, randomization was performed using a computer-generated set of scratch cards with blocks of 6 and a ratio 1:1 for each arm, and patients were assigned to one of the two groups for postoperative analgesia TAP or CWI. Intrathecal anesthesia was standardized with a dural puncture at level L3–L4 and administration of 0.5% hyperbaric bupivacaine (8 mg if height<1.60 m, 10 mg otherwise) plus sufentanil 5 µg. After the block was established, the caesarean section was performed. In the TAP group, a trained anesthesiologist performed US-guided TAP block just after completion of surgery [10] injecting 20 mL of levobupivacaine 0.375% (150 mg) bilaterally. TAP block is a regional anesthetic technique that blocks the abdominal wall neural afferents (T6-L1) into the neurofascial plane between the internal oblique and transversus abdominis muscles. A bilateral injection is required after cesarean section. Ultrasound allows real-time identification the three layers of abdominal muscles: external oblique, internal oblique, and transversus abdominis and visualization the spread of the local anesthetic. The quality of the detachment of the two muscle fascia spreading was recorded by the investigator but no attempt by checking sensory level was made to verify that the TAP block was working. In the CWI group, prior to skin closure, the surgeon inserted under aseptic conditions a multihole catheter (Painfusor Baxter 15 cm), previously tested with a bolus of saline to check catheter patency. The catheter was placed below the fascia between the unclosed parietal peritoneum and the underside of the transversalis fascia before its closure, along the full length of the wound [9]. The catheter was then connected to an elastomeric pump (Infusor LV5 Baxter) containing 250 mg levobupivacaine in 200 mL solution set to deliver 5 mL per hour, i.e. 150 mg the first 24 postoperative hours. For ethical reasons, patients and investigators were not blinded. Oral paracetamol (1 gram), ketoprofen (50 mg) and nefopam (20 mg), four times a day completed the multimodal analgesia plan.

In the post-anesthesia care unit, intravenous morphine was titrated if required (verbal response numerical scale (VRNS) pain score ≥4 on a scale ranging from 0 = no pain to 10 = unbearable. VRNS pain scores ≥4 were managed with oral morphine (morphine sulfate, 10 mg per tablet; Mundipharma, Paris, France) in the post-natal ward. Ondansetron and symptomatic treatment of vomiting was available if required. For the purpose of the study, nurses, not involved in the study, from the mobile pain unit assessed patients 3 hours post-cesarean delivery, in the evening (between 18:00 and 22:00, allowing for a time interval of 6 to 12 hours since the first assessment) of the operative day (D0), in the morning (around 9:00) and the evening (between 18:00 and 20:00) of the first (D1) and second (D2) postoperative days. They collected also every adverse event of the techniques for safety concern. During the assessment, the women were asked to rate pain with VRNS at rest and when moving (from supine to sitting position in bed), to report any pruritus and any nausea or vomiting (absent or present). The level of sedation (1 = awake and alert, 2 = mild sedation or asleep but easily roused, 3 = moderate sedation, and 4 = unable to rouse) was also reported. For the purpose of statistical analysis, sedation was present if a woman had a score of two or more. Satisfaction with pain control was recorded immediately before the patient left hospital with a VRNS (1 = very satisfied, 2 = satisfied, 3 = dissatisfied, 4 = very dissatisfied). Gastrointestinal function on the second postoperative day (flatus and faeces), and length of stay at hospital were also recorded.

One month post−delivery, the women were interviewed by phone by an investigator blinded to the patient's group assignment. Women were asked if there was any pain in the scar area. In case of a positive answer, the incidence of neuropathic pain was evaluated using the DN4 questionnaire, such a diagnosis being made if the score was equal or greater than 4 on a 0–10 scale [11]. A consultation for chronic postoperative pain could be organized 3 months after the delivery.

## Statistical analysis

The primary outcome was pain over the 48 h postoperative period, i.e. period of local anesthetic in the CWI group, at rest and during mobilization using the area under the curves (AUC) of pain scores. This method allows a better precision in analgesic efficacy than individual pain score reports. AUC was calculated by the trapezoidal method [12] considering that the first measurement was made 3 hours after surgery, the second one 9 hours after the first one and the following ones every 12 hours thereafter. Secondary outcomes included the time to the first rescue dose of morphine, the total morphine requirements during the first postoperative 48 hour period, adverse events, patients' satisfaction, length of hospital stay, and prevalence of neuropathic postoperative pain.

The study was designed to detect a between means ratio of 1.25 in either direction for the AUC, with 85% power allowing for an attrition rate of 10%. The coefficient of variation of the means was hypothesized to be 0.4. With a bilateral significance level of 0.05, the sample size was calculated at 60 patients per group. The Intention to Treat population included all patients that were randomized to the study whatever the treatment they actually received and the Per-Protocol population includes subjects who completed the follow-up in each group.

Since the AUC pain scores were skewed and not normalized by a logarithmic transformation, nonparametric tests (Mann-Whitney) were used for group comparisons. Categorical variables, expressed as numbers with frequencies (%) were compared using Chi−square and Fisher's exact tests as appropriate. Continuous variables and pain scores are reported as median with [interquartile range]. A mixed model for repeated measures with two primary factors (pain control method: CWI or TAP and time) and an interaction term was fitted. The Akaike criterion was used to select the most appropriate model. P values <0.05 were considered statistically significant. No interim analysis was planned. Statistical analysis was performed using NCSS (Versions 8 and 9, Kaysville, USA).

## Supporting Information

**Checklist S1** CONSORT Checklist.

**Protocol S1** Trial Protocol.

## Author Contributions

Conceived and designed the experiments: MC JFD MF MLG. Performed the experiments: MC AB YB CB VDS BS CF JR MLG. Analyzed the data: YB JFD PAL MF MLG. Contributed reagents/materials/analysis tools: JFD. Wrote the paper: YB PAL MF MLG.

## References


1. Carvalho B, Cohen SE, Lipman SS, Fuller A, Mathusamy AD, et al. (2005) Patient preferences for anesthesia outcomes associated with cesarean delivery. Anesth Analg 101: 1182–7.
2. Lavand'homme P. (2006) Postcesarean analgesia: effective strategies and association with chronic pain. Curr Opin Anaesthesiol 19: 244–8.
3. Angst MS, Clark JD. (2006) Opioid-induced hyperalgesia: a qualitative systematic review. Anesthesiology 104: 570–87.
4. Corsini T, Cuvillon P, Forgeot A, Chapelle C, Seffert P, et al. (2013) [Single-dose intraincisional levobupivacaine infiltration in caesarean postoperative analgesia: a placebo-controlled double-blind randomized trial]. Annales francaises d'anesthesie et de reanimation 32: 25–30.
5. Abdallah FW, Chan VW, Brull R. (2012) Transversus abdominis plane block: a systematic review. Reg Anesth Pain Med 37: 193–209.
6. Mishriky BM, George RB, Habib AS. (2012) Transversus abdominis plane block for analgesia after Cesarean delivery: a systematic review and meta-analysis. Can J Anaesth 59: 766–78.
7. Bamigboye AA, Hofmeyr GJ. (2010) Caesarean section wound infiltration with local anaesthesia for postoperative pain relief - any benefit? S Afr Med J 100: 313–9.
8. Hebbard P, Fujiwara Y, Shibata Y, Royse C. (2007) Ultrasound-guided transversus abdominis plane (TAP) block. Anaesthesia and intensive care 35: 616–7.
9. Rackelboom T, Le Strat S, Silvera S, Schmitz T, Bassot A, et al. (2010) Improving continuous wound infusion effectiveness for postoperative analgesia after cesarean delivery: a randomized controlled trial. Obstet Gynecol 116: 893–900.
10. Hebbard PD, Barrington MJ, Vasey C. (2010) Ultrasound-guided continuous oblique subcostal transversus abdominis plane blockade: description of anatomy and clinical technique. Reg Anesth Pain Med 35: 436–41.
11. Bouhassira D, Attal N, Alchaar H, Boureau F, Brochet B, et al. (2005) Comparison of pain syndromes associated with nervous or somatic lesions and development of a new neuropathic pain diagnostic questionnaire (DN4). Pain Mar 114: 29–36.
12. Matthews JN, Altman DG, Campbell MJ, Royston P. (1990) Analysis of serial measurements in medical research. Bmj 300: 230–5.
13. Gupta A, Favaios S, Perniola A, Magnuson A, Berggren L. (2011) A meta-analysis of the efficacy of wound catheters for post-operative pain management. Acta Anaesthesiol Scand 55: 785–96.
14. Lavand'homme PM, Roelants F, Waterloos H, De Kock MF. (2007) Postoperative analgesic effects of continuous wound infiltration with diclofenac after elective cesarean delivery. Anesthesiology 106: 1220–5.
15. Charlton S, Cyna AM, Middleton P, Griffiths JD. (2010) Perioperative transversus abdominis plane (TAP) blocks for analgesia after abdominal surgery. Cochrane Database Syst Rev 12: CD007705.
16. Johns N, O'Neill S, Ventham NT, Barron F, Brady RR, et al. (2012) Clinical effectiveness of transversus abdominis plane (TAP) block in abdominal surgery: a systematic review and meta-analysis. Colorectal disease: the official journal of the Association of Coloproctology of Great Britain and Ireland 14: e635–42.
17. Sakai T, Manabe W, Kamitani T, Takeyama E, Nakano S. (2010) [Ropivacaine-induced late-onset systemic toxicity after transversus abdominis plane block under general anesthesia: successful reversal with 20% lipid emulsion]. Masui 59: 1502–5.
18. Nikolajsen L, Sorensen HC, Jensen TS, Kehlet H. (2004) Chronic pain following Caesarean section. Acta Anaesthesiol Scand 48: 111–6.
19. Loane H, Preston R, Douglas MJ, Massey S, Papsdorf M, et al. (2012) A randomized controlled trial comparing intrathecal morphine with transversus abdominis plane block for post-cesarean delivery analgesia. Int J Obstet Anesth 21: 112–8.

9

# Lidocaine, Dexmedetomidine and Their Combination Reduce Isoflurane Minimum Alveolar Concentration in Dogs

**Carlos M. Acevedo-Arcique[1], José A. Ibancovichi[1]*, Julio R. Chavez[1], Eduardo Gutierrez-Blanco[3], Rafael Moran-Muñoz[1], José M. Victoria-Mora[2], Francisco Tendillo-Cortijo[4], Martín Santos-González[4], Pedro Sanchez-Aparicio[1]**

**1** Department of Anaesthesia and Analgesia, Faculty of Veterinary Medicine, Universidad Autónoma del Estado de México, Toluca, State of Mexico, Mexico, **2** Department of Orthopaedic Surgery and Trauma, Faculty of Veterinary Medicine, Universidad Autónoma del Estado de México, Toluca, State of Mexico, Mexico, **3** Department of Animal Health and Preventive Medicine, Faculty of Veterinary Medicine, Universidad Autónoma de Yucatán, Merida, State of Yucatan, Mexico, **4** Hospital Universitario Clínica Puerta de Hierro, Madrid, España


## Abstract

The effects of intravenous (IV) lidocaine, dexmedetomidine and their combination delivered as a bolus followed by a constant rate infusion (CRI) on the minimum alveolar concentration of isoflurane ($MAC_{ISO}$) in dogs were evaluated. Seven healthy adult dogs were included. Anaesthesia was induced with propofol and maintained with isoflurane. For each dog, baseline MAC ($MAC_{ISO/BASAL}$) was determined after a 90-minute equilibration period. Thereafter, each dog received one of the following treatments (loading dose, CRI): lidocaine 2 mg $kg^{-1}$, 100 µg $kg^{-1}$ $minute^{-1}$; dexmedetomidine 2 µg $kg^{-1}$, 2 µg $kg^{-1}$ $hour^{-1}$; or their combination. MAC was then determined again after 45- minutes of treatment by CRI. At the doses administered, lidocaine, dexmedetomidine and their combination significantly reduced $MAC_{ISO}$ by 27.3% (range: 12.5–39.2%), 43.4% (33.3–53.3%) and 60.9% (46.1–78.1%), respectively, when compared to $MAC_{ISO}/_{BASAL}$. The combination resulted in a greater $MAC_{ISO}$ reduction than the two drugs alone. Their use, at the doses studied, provides a clinically important reduction in the concentration of ISO during anaesthesia in dogs.


**Editor:** Douglas Thamm, Colorado State University, United States of America

**Funding:** The resources of this study were awarded by the Autonomous University of State of Mexico through the research project number 2762/2009. The funders had no role in study design, data collection and analysis, decision to publish, or preparation of the manuscript.

**Competing Interests:** The authors have declared that no competing interests exist.

* Email: ibanvet@gmail.com

## Introduction

The end-tidal partial pressure of inhalant anaesthetics required to prevent movement in 50% of individuals exposed to a supramaximal noxious stimulus (i.e. minimum alveolar concentration, MAC) represents an index of potency of anaesthetic agents [1]. The MAC of contemporary inhalant anaesthetics has been previously reported in dogs and after the administration of different opioids, sedatives, tranquilisers and local anaesthetics [2,3,4]. Clinically, one of the main issues concerning inhalant anaesthesia is the progressive cardiovascular depression related to the delivery of high concentrations. Drugs such as lidocaine (local anaesthetic) and dexmedetomidine (sedative) decrease the MAC of inhaled anaesthetics and may also reduce the risk of cardiopulmonary depression by means of decreasing the inhalant anaesthetic requirements during anaesthesia [5,6,7]. In addition, the combination of these agents with different pharmacological mechanisms of action may provide better analgesia and an even a greater inhalant-sparing effect [2,8,9,10,11]. Lidocaine (LIDO) is an amide local anaesthetic that can be administered intravenously (IV) via a bolus or constant rate infusion (CRI) to provide perioperative analgesia, sedation and anti-arrhythmic effects. In dogs, lidocaine decreases the MAC of inhaled anaesthetics by 18.7% to 43.3% in a dose-dependent manner [2,3,5,7,9,12,13]. Dexmedetomidine (DEX) is the active enantiomer of the racemic mixture medetomidine. DEX is a potent $\alpha_2$ adrenoceptor agonist; it is approximately eight times more selective toward $\alpha_2$ adrenoceptors than clonidine [14] and at least two times as potent as medetomidine [15]. It has a high $\alpha_2$: $\alpha_1$ selectivity ratio (1620:1) compared with xylazine (160:1), clonidine (220:1), and romifidine (340:1) [16]. DEX is widely used in small animal anaesthesia to provide sedation, anxiolysis and analgesia [6]. DEX bolus, CRI and epidural administration has been shown to reduce the anaesthetic requirement for the induction and maintenance of general anaesthesia in dogs [4,6,17]. To the best of our knowledge, the effect of a LIDO-DEX combination administered by bolus followed by CRI on the $MAC_{ISO}$ has not been reported in dogs. The purpose of this study was to evaluate the $MAC_{ISO}$-sparing effect of LIDO, DEX and their combination in dogs. Bearing in mind their different mechanisms of action, the authors hypothesised that the combination LIDO-DEX would reduce $MAC_{ISO}$ to a greater extent than the two drugs alone.

## Materials and Methods

This study was approved by the Animal Research Ethics Committee for Animal Experimentation (protocol number 2267/2009) of the Faculty of Veterinary Medicine, Universidad Autónoma del Estado de México.

### Animals

Seven adult (1 to 2 years old) mixed-breed neutered dogs (three male and four female; mean ± SD body weight of 18.1±9 kg) were included in a prospective randomised blinded cross-over experiment with a two-week washout period between treatments. A computer generated random numbers table was used to assign treatments. Each dog was studied on three separate occasions, receiving one treatment at one time. The treatments were assigned in random order. Dogs were considered to be healthy based on medical history, physical examination, complete blood count and serum biochemical analysis and urinalysis. Food, but not water, was withheld 8 hours prior to each anaesthetic procedure.

### Anaesthesia and instrumentation

A 20-gauge catheter was aseptically placed into the cephalic vein, and connected to a resealable male luer injection port (BD-luer loK; Becton Dickinson and Company, NJ, USA). Anaesthesia was induced with IV administration of propofol to effect (4–6 mg $kg^{-1}$; Fresofol 1%; Fresenius Kabi, Australia). After intubation was performed with an appropriately sized, cuffed endotracheal tube, dogs were connected to a rebreathing system. Anaesthesia was maintained with isoflurane (ISO) (Forane; Baxter Laboratories, USA) and oxygen flow rates were set at 100 mL $kg^{-1}$ $minute^{-1}$ after induction; 10 minute later, the oxygen flow was reduced to 50 mL $kg^{-1}$ $minute^{-1}$. Intermittent positive pressure ventilation (IPPV) was instituted (Fabius Dräger Medical; Lübeck, Germany), and the respiratory rate and inspiratory peak airway pressure were adjusted to maintain eucapnia (end-tidal carbon dioxide tension [$PECO_2$] 33–45 mmHg, 4.4–5.9 kPa). Dogs were then placed in lateral recumbency and a 20-gauge catheter (Introcan; B-Braun, Brazil) was aseptically introduced into the dorsal pedal artery for direct blood pressure monitoring and the collection of arterial blood to determine blood gases. A thermistor was advanced to the thoracic portion of the oesophagus for body temperature monitoring. A circulating warm-water blanket was used to maintain body temperature at 37.5–38.5°C. An electrolyte solution (saline 0.9%; Solution DX-CS; Pisa Farmaceutica, Mexico) was administered at 3 mL $kg^{-1}$ $hour^{-1}$ throughout anaesthesia by the use of an infusion pump (Colleague; Baxter Healthcare Corporation Medication Delivery, IL, USA).

Heart rate and rhythm were obtained by a continuous lead II ECG trace (Surgivet; Smith Medical Inc., Waukesha, WI, USA). Systolic, mean and diastolic arterial blood pressures (SAP, MAP and DAP, respectively) were continuously monitored via a blood pressure transducer system (BD DTX Plus; Becton Dickinson and Company) connected to the dorsal pedal artery. Before each experiment, the transducers was zeroed, calibrated and levelled to the heart position. Zeroing was performed by exposing the transducer to atmospheric pressure and levelled to the heart position. The calibration was performed using a mercury manometer as the gold standard.

Pulse oximetry ($SpO_2$) was measured by pulse oximetry (Advisor; Surgivet) with a sensor attached to the dog's tongue. Inspired ISO (FIIso) and end-tidal (FEIso) concentrations, $PECO_2$ and respiratory rate ($f_R$) values were continuously measured with an infrared gas analyser (Dräger Vamos; Dräger Medical, Lübeck, Germany). The gas analyser was calibrated before starting each experiment with a standard gas mixture provided by the manufacturer. For blood gas analysis (pH, $PaO_2$ and $PaCO_2$), 0.5 mL of blood were obtained from the catheter placed in the dorsal metatarsal artery immediately before the first noxious stimulation and another one after determining the MAC. The inspired oxygen fraction and temperature were corrected (GEM Premier 3000; Instrumentation Laboratory, UK). The gas analyser was calibrated before each experiment by using two aqueous buffered bicarbonate solutions containing precise concentrations of carbon dioxide and oxygen (GEM CVP Solutions 1–2: Instrumentation Laboratory, UK).

### MAC determination

Following propofol induction, the dogs were anaesthetised for at least 90 min as an initial equilibration period at an $ET_{ISO}$ of 1.8% to minimise the effects of propofol. The determination of $MAC_{ISO/BASAL}$ for each dog was started after the initial equilibration period. Once the $MAC_{ISO/BASAL}$ was determined, the dogs received a bolus followed by CRI treatment of lidocaine, or dexmedetomidine, or their combination. The CRI of drugs (LIDO, DEX and LIDO-DEX) was maintained for 45 min allowing for an adequate, theoretical plasma drug equilibration time based on prior investigations [3,18]; after this period, the isoflurane treatment MAC ($MAC_{ISO/T}$) was determined and the CRI of drugs was stopped.

Determinations of MAC were carried out using well-established techniques [3]. Noxious stimulation was applied by clamping a paw at the fourth digit. The clamping technique was performed with 24-cm sponge forceps (with protective plastic tubing on each jaw) clamped to the first notch until gross purposeful movement was detected or a period of 60 sec elapsed [19]. A positive motor response was considered if jerking or twisting motion of the head or if movement of extremities was observed. A negative response included a lack of movement of the head and limbs, muscle rigidity, shivering, tail movement, swallowing, chewing or an increase in spontaneous respiratory efforts during controlled ventilation [19,20]. When a positive response was elicited, the $ET_{ISO}$ was increased by 10% and maintained at this concentration for at least 20 min, and the noxious stimulus procedure was repeated. When a negative response was detected, the $ET_{ISO}$ was decreased by 10% and maintained at this concentration for at least 20 minute, and the noxious stimulus procedure was repeated. The procedure was continued until purposeful movement ceased (after an increase in the anaesthetic concentration) or returned (after a decrease in the anaesthetic concentration). The isoflurane MAC was calculated as the mean value between the highest $ET_{ISO}$ at which the purposeful movement was detected and the lowest $ET_{ISO}$ at which the purposeful movement was not detected. In each dog, the MAC basal and MAC treatment were evaluated in duplicate and averaged.

The isoflurane MAC values were corrected to sea level by multiplying the barometric pressure of the location/760 mmHg by the obtained MAC value. The mean barometric pressure was obtained from the official city meteorological station for the altitude at which the experiment was performed (2,680 meters above sea level) and was 556 mmHg. After determining the MAC of the treatments, the CRI of the drugs was discontinued; the dogs were disconnected from the anaesthesia machine, and extubated when the swallowing reflex was present. After recovery, the dogs were administered 4 mg $kg^{-1}$ of carprofen (Rimadyl, Pfizer Animal Health BV, Capelle a/d I Jssel, The Netherlands) subcutaneously every 24 h for two days.

**Table 1.** Mean ± SD of minimum alveolar concentration of isoflurane ($MAC_{ISO}$) before ($MAC_{ISO/BASAL}$) and after one of the following treatments ($MAC_{ISO/T}$): lidocaine (LIDO), dexmedetomidine (DEX), or the combination LIDO-DEX in dogs ($n = 7$).

| Treatment | $MAC_{ISO/BASAL}$ | $MAC_{ISO/T}$ | % Change in $MAC_{ISO}$ (% range) |
|---|---|---|---|
| LIDO | 1.28±0.16%. | 0.93±0.11* | 27.3 (12.5–39.2)* |
| DEX | 1.58±0.28%. | 0.90±0.17* | 43.4 (33.3–53.3)* |
| LIDO-DEX | 1.46±0.21%. | 0.57±0.18*# | 60.9 (46.1–78.1)*# |

The percentage (%) change in $MAC_{ISO}$ after treatment was calculated from [($MAC_{ISO}$ after treatment − $MAC_{ISO/BASAL}$)/$MAC_{ISO/BASAL}$] X 100.
*Statistically different from $MAC_{ISO/BASAL}$ ($p<0.05$).
#Statistically different from the rest of the treatments ($p<0.05$).

## Experimental protocol

Each dog was anaesthetised on three separate occasions with a two-week washout interval between treatments. Following $MAC_{BASAL}$ determination, the dogs were assigned to one of the following three treatments in a randomised cross-over study design:

Group LIDO: Lidocaine (Lidocaine 2%; Pisa, Mexico) IV loading dose (LD) of 2 mg $kg^{-1}$ followed by a CRI of 100 µg $kg^{-1}$ $minute^{-1}$;

Group DEX: Dexmedetomidine (Dexdomitor; Orion, Finland) IV LD of 2 µg $kg^{-1}$ followed by a CRI of 2 µg $kg^{-1}$ $hour^{-1}$;

Group LIDO-DEX: Lidocaine IV LD of 2 mg $kg^{-1}$ followed by a CRI of 100 µg $kg^{-1}$ $minute^{-1}$, and dexmedetomidine IV LD of 2 µg $kg^{-1}$ followed by a CRI of 2 µg $kg^{-1}$ $hour^{-1}$.

Loading doses were diluted up to a final volume of 3 mL with sterile water and administered IV over 1 minute. Treatments were diluted up to 60 mL with saline 0.9% and delivered as a CRI accordingly. All CRIs were started immediately after bolus administration using a syringe infusion device (Colleague; Baxter Healthcare, IL, USA).

## Statistical analysis

Statistical analysis was performed using SigmaStat 3.5 (Systat Software Inc., Point Richmond, CA, USA). The Shapiro-Wilk test was used for the assessment of data normality. Data are reported as mean ± standard deviation (SD). A repeated-measures ANOVA was used to the evaluate percentage change in $MAC_{ISO}$, and $MAC_{ISO}$ values before ($MAC_{BASAL}$) and after treatment, time to MAC determination and extubation time. ANOVA was used to compare MAC values between treatments. A *post hoc* Tukey test was used where appropriate. Values were considered statistically different when $p<0.05$.

## Results

The mean ± SD $MAC_{ISO/BASAL}$ of all treatments was 1.44±0.04%. $MAC_{ISO/T}$ values are shown in Table 1. $MAC_{ISO/BASAL}$ values were not significantly different among treatments. At the doses administered, LIDO, DEX and LIDO-DEX significantly decreased $MAC_{ISO}$ by 27.3% (range, 12.5–39.2%), 43.4% (33.3–53.3%) and 60.9% (46.1–78.1%) ($p = 0.001$, $p = 0.013$, $p = 0.013$), respectively, when compared to $MAC_{ISO/BASAL}$. The $MAC_{ISO}$ was significantly lower after LIDO-DEX when compared with LIDO or DEX treatments alone ($p = 0.001$ and $p = 0.013$, respectively). The time to $MAC_{ISO/BASAL}$ determination was 172±24 min, 194±17 min and 181±18 min for LIDO, DEX and LIDO-DEX, respectively; these values were not significantly different between groups. The time for $MAC_{ISO}$ determination after LIDO, DEX and LIDO-DEX were 168±26 min, 152±10 min and 163±15 min, respectively. These values were not significantly different when the groups were compared. Extubation time was 9.0±1 min, 9.7±1 min and 10.6±1 min for groups LIDO, DEX and LIDO-DEX, respectively ($p = 0.057$). Anaesthetic recovery was uneventful in all dogs. Blood gas values were not significantly different between groups

**Table 2.** Mean ± SD of cardiovascular parameters and other variables measured immediately before the MAC determination of isoflurane ($MAC_{ISO/BASAL}$) and immediately before the final MAC of isoflurane ($MAC_{ISO/T}$) determination during constant rate infusion of lidocaine (LIDO), dexmedetomidine (DEX), or the combination LIDO-DEX.

| | | Treatment | | |
|---|---|---|---|---|
| Variables | ISO/BASAL | LIDO | DEX | LIDO-DEX |
| Heart rate (beats $min^{-1}$) | 107±4 | 97±7 | 74±7 | 62±7# |
| Systolic blood pressure (mmHg) | 102±18 | 103±15.8 | 106±10.4 | 128±12.6# |
| Diastolic blood pressure (mmHg) | 64±12.4 | 63±11.3 | 64±11.3 | 72±8.3 |
| Mean arterial pressure (mmHg) | 78±13.4 | 77±12.6 | 79±9.7 | 93±9.9 |
| Pulse oximetry values ($SpO_2$%) | 97±0.3 | 97±0.5 | 97±0.5 | 96±0.5 |
| Oesophageal temperature (°C) | 37.8±0.1 | 38±0.1 | 38.1±0.1 | 38.3±0.1 |
| pH | 7.33±0.028 | 7.36±0.032 | 7.31±0.021 | 7.31±0.021 |
| $PaCO_2$ (mmHg) | 36.8±2.63 | 35.0±3.1 | 35.1±4.24 | 36.1±3.46 |
| $PaO_2$ (mmHg) | 503.2±28.19 | 487.6±36.14 | 486.5±50 | 501.33±22.85 |

#Statistically different to baseline and to the rest of the treatments ($p<0.05$).

for pH, $PaCO_2$ or $PaO_2$. Other data are reported in Table 2. HR was significantly lower in DEX ($p<0.001$) and LIDO-DEX ($p< 0.001$) when compared with baseline. HR was significantly lower in LIDO-DEX when compared with LIDO ($p = 0.009$) and DEX ($p = 0.002$). SAP was significantly higher in LIDO-DEX than under basal conditions (p = 0.04), LIDO ($p = 0.004$) and DEX ($p = 0.04$).

## Discussion

The results of this study are consistent with previous reports that showed a decrease in $MAC_{ISO}$ after the administration of lidocaine or dexmedetomidine [3,4,21,22]. In addition, the combination LIDO-DEX produced a greater effect than the two drugs alone, in accordance with the hypothesis of this study. The range of MAC values reported here for isoflurane (1.28–1.58%) was similar to that shown in previous studies (1.34–1.57%) [2,3,4,17]. One reason for small discrepancies among MAC studies is subjectivity in the interpretation regarding what constitutes movement after the application of a noxious stimulus. However, bias was minimised by the use of the same anatomical site and the same noxious stimulation in all dogs. In addition, a single observer was employed to determine gross movement during the MAC determination. Nevertheless, MAC values recorded in this study may have been subject to small errors [23]. LIDO is a sodium channel blocker that reduces inhalant MAC by unknown mechanisms [3]. IV administration of lidocaine has been shown to reduce $MAC_{SEVO}$ in dogs [7,9] and $MAC_{ISO}$ in several species in a dose-dependent manner. Cardiovascular changes such as slight non-significant increases in blood pressure have been observed in different species, but are considered to be of minimal clinical relevance [2,3,8,24,25], in agreement with the results obtained in our study. The design of the present study was not able to demonstrate that a significant reduction in $MAC_{ISO}$ after LIDO administration was associated with significant changes in heart rate or blood pressure.

In the present study, a lidocaine CRI of 100 $\mu g\ kg^{-1}\ minute^{-1}$ reduced $MAC_{ISO}$ by approximately 27%, which is similar to the results in previous reports. When LIDO was administered to dogs (LD of 2 $mg\ kg^{-1}$ followed by a CRI of 50 or 200 $\mu g\ kg^{-1}\ minute^{-1}$), the drug reduced the $MAC_{ISO}$ by 18.7% and 43.4%, respectively [3]. Lidocaine CRI (LD 1.5 mg kg followed by 250 $\mu g\ kg^{-1}\ minute^{-1}$) reduced ISO requirements by 34–44% in dogs undergoing unilateral mastectomy, which may be of clinical relevance [5].

Dexmedetomidine is the most selective $\alpha_2$ adrenergic agonist commonly used in the clinical setting due to its sedative and analgesic effects [6,26], as well as for its ability to reduce the anaesthetic requirements for the induction and maintenance of general anaesthesia [4,6]. In the present study, at the dose administered, DEX decreased $MAC_{ISO}$ by 43.4%, similar to what was observed in a previous study [4]. DEX reduced $MAC_{ISO}$ by 18% and 59% after an LD of 0.5 $\mu g\ kg^{-1}$ followed by CRI at 0.5 $\mu g\ kg^{-1}\ hour^{-1}$, and an LD of 3 $\mu g\ kg^{-1}$ followed by CRI at 3 $\mu g\ kg^{-1}\ hour^{-1}$, respectively [4]. DEX increases systemic blood pressure, presumably as a result of $\alpha_2$-mediated vasoconstriction [4]. Baroreflex-mediated bradycardia is commonly observed due to increased vagal tone, decreased sympathetic tone and peripheral vasoconstriction [27,28]. According to our results, DEX alone did not increase the blood pressure as expected; even when $MAC_{ISO}$ after DEX CRI was significantly lower than $MAC_{ISO/BASAL}$, only a slight increase in arterial blood pressure was recorded. However, there was a significant increase in SAP and a decrease in HR with the combination LIDO-DEX when compared with $MAC_{ISO/BASAL}$. This finding may be related to significantly decreased isoflurane concentrations, as reported previously [3,7]. The dosage regimens reported here are commonly used during surgery in dogs when the provision of analgesia, sedation and limitation of the stress response is required [6,11,17].

The combination of LIDO and DEX produced a statistically significant reduction in $MAC_{ISO}$, of 60.9%. Even though a mathematical reduction in $MAC_{ISO}$ of almost 70% could be expected (27% LIDO plus 43% DEX), the design of the current study did not make it possible to determine if an additive or synergistic effect between LIDO and DEX was present. Some pharmacological variables such as chemical drug interactions involving pH and the degree of ionisation, which were not considered in this study, may have influenced the effect of the drug combination. However, it is clear that some combined effect was observed, since the combination of drugs produced $MAC_{ISO}$ reductions that were greater than when LIDO or DEX was administered alone. Indeed, the combination of different analgesic drugs has been shown to reduce inhalant anaesthetic requirements in the clinical setting. Based on the results of the present study, it can be concluded that the combination of LIDO and DEX may be used to substantially decrease ISO requirements in dogs undergoing surgery.

In conclusion, this study showed that, at the doses administered, LIDO and DEX reduced $MAC_{ISO}$ in the same trend as reported by previous studies. The combination of these treatments resulted in a greater $MAC_{ISO}$ reduction than the two drugs alone. Their use, at the doses studied, provides a clinically important reduction in the concentration of ISO during anaesthesia in dogs. Further study is needed to clarify the interaction of LIDO and DEX with ISO and their cardiovascular effects.

## Author Contributions

Conceived and designed the experiments: CMA-A EG-B RM-M JMV-M PS-A FT-C MS-G JAI. Performed the experiments: CMA-A JRC EG-B RM-M PS-A FT-C MS-G JAI. Analyzed the data: CMA-A EG-B JRC RM-M JAI. Contributed reagents/materials/analysis tools: CMA-A EG-B RM-M JRC JAI. Wrote the paper: CMA-A EG-B RM-M PS-A JAI.

## References

1. Eger EI, Saidman LJ, Brandstater B (1965) Minimum alveolar anesthetic concentration: a standard of anesthetic potency. Anesthesiology 26: 756–763.
2. Muir WW, Wise AJ, March PA (2003) Effects of morphine, lidocaine, ketamine, and morphine-lidocaine-ketamine drug combination on minimum alveolar concentration in dogs anesthetized with isoflurane. Am J Vet Res 64: 1115–1160.
3. Valverde A, Doherty TJ, Hernandez WD (2004) Effect of intravenous lidocaine on isoflurane minimum alveolar concentration in dogs. Vet Anesth Analg 31: 264–271.
4. Pascoe PJ, Raekallio M, Kuusela E, McKusick B, Granholm M (2006) Changes in the minimum alveolar concentration of isoflurane and some cardiopulmonary measurements during three continuous infusion rates of dexmedetomidine in dogs. Vet Anaesth Analg 33: 97–103.
5. Steagall PV, Teixeira Neto FJ, Minto BW, Campagnol D, Correa MA (2006) Evaluation of the isoflurane-sparing effects of lidocaine and fentanyl during surgery in dogs. J Am Vet Med Assoc 15: 522–527.
6. Uilenreef JJ, Murrell JC, McKusick BC, Hellebrekers LJ (2008) Dexmedetomidine continuous rate infusion during isoflurane anaesthesia in canine surgical patients. Vet Anaesth Analg 35: 1–12.
7. Matsubara LM, Oliva VL, Gabas DT, Oliveira GC, Casseteri ML (2009) Effect of lidocaine on the minimum alveolar concentration of sevoflurane in dogs. Vet Anaesth Analg 36: 407–413.
8. Doherty TJ, Redua MA, Queiroz-Castro P, Egger C, Cox SK, et al. (2007) Effect of intravenous lidocaine and ketamine on the minimum alveolar concentration of isoflurane in goats. Vet Anaesth Analg 34: 125–131.

9. Wilson J, Doherty TJ, Egger CM, Fidler A, Cox S, et al. (2008) Effects of intravenous lidocaine, ketamine, and the combination on the minimum alveolar concentration of sevoflurane in dogs. Vet Anaesth Analg 35: 289–296.
10. Aguado D, Benito J, Gómez de Segura IA (2011) Reduction of the minimum alveolar concentration of isoflurane in dogs using a constant rate of infusion of lidocaine-ketamine in combination with either morphine or fentanyl. Vet J 189: 63–66.
11. Gutierrez-Blanco E, Victoria-Mora JM, Ibancovichi-Camarillo JA, Sauri-Arceo CH, Bolio-Gonzalez ME, et al. (2013) Evaluation of the isoflurane-sparing effects of fentanyl, lidocaine, ketamine, dexmedetomidine, or the combination lidocaine-ketamine-dexmedetomidine during ovariohysterectomy in dogs. Vet Anaesth Analg 40: 599–609.
12. MacDougall LM, Hethey JA, Livingston A, Clark C, Shmon CL, et al. (2009) Antinociceptive, cardiopulmonary, and sedative effects of five intravenous infusion rates of lidocaine in conscious dogs. Vet Anaesth Analg 36: 512–522.
13. Columbano N, Secci F, Careddu GM, Sotgiu G, Rossi G, et al. (2012) Effects of lidocaine constant rate infusion on sevoflurane requirement, autonomic responses, and postoperative analgesia in dogs undergoing ovariectomy under opioid-based balanced anesthesia. Vet J 193: 448–455.
14. Kamibayashi T, Maze M (2000) Clinical uses of alpha-2-adrenergic agonists. Anesthesiology 93: 1345–9
15. Kuusela E, Raekallio M, Anttila M, Falck I, Molsa S, et al. (2000) Clinical effects and pharmacokinetics of medetomidine and its enantiomers in dogs. J Vet Pharmacol Ther 1: 15–20.
16. Virtanen R, Ruskoaho H, Nyman L (1985) Pharmacological evidence for the involvement of alpha-2 adrenoceptores in the sedative effect of detomidine, a novel sedative-analgesic. J Vet Pharmacol Ther 8: 30–7.
17. Campagnol D, Teixeira Neto FJ, Giordano T, Ferreira TH, Monteiro ER (2007) Effects of epidural administration of dexmedetomidine on the minimum alveolar concentration of isoflurane in dogs. Am J Vet Res 68: 1308–1318.
18. Gómez-Villamanos RJ, Palacios C, Benítez A, Granados MM, Domínguez JM, et al. (2008) Effect of medetomidine infusion on the anaesthetic requirements of desflurane in dogs. Res Vet Sci 84: 68–73.
19. Valverde A, Morey TE, Hernandez J, Davies W (2003) Validation of several types of noxious stimuli for use in determining the minimum alveolar concentration for inhalation anesthetics in dogs and rabbits. Am J Vet Res 64: 957–962.
20. Quasha AL, Eger EI 2nd, Tinker JH (1980) Determination and applications of MAC. Anesthesiology 53: 314–34.
21. Weitz JD, Foster SD, Waugaman WR, Katz RL, Bloor BC (1991) Anesthetic and hemodynamic effects of dexmedetomidine during isoflurane anesthesia in a canine model. Nurse Anesth 2: 19–27.
22. Bloor BC, Frankland M, Alper G, Raybould D, Weitz J, et al. (1992) Hemodynamic and sedative effects of dexmedetomidine in dog. J Pharmacol Exp Ther 263: 690–697.
23. Shaughnessy M, Hofmeister E (2014) A systematic review of sevoflurane and isoflurane minimum alveolar concentration in domestic cats. Vet Anaesth Analg 41: 1–13.
24. Pypendop BH, Ilkiw JE (2005) The effects of intravenous lidocaine administration on the minimum alveolar concentration of isoflurane in cats. Anesthesiology 53: 315–334.
25. Dzikiti TB, Hellebrekers LJ, van Dijk P (2003) Effects of intravenous lidocaine on isoflurane concentration, physiological parameters, metabolic parameters and stress-related hormones in horses undergoing surgery. J Vet Med. A Physiol Pathol Clin Med 50: 190–195.
26. Lin G, Robben JH, Murrell JC, Aspegrén J, McKusick BC, et al. (2008) Dexmedetomidine constant rate infusion for 24 hours during and after propofol or isoflurane anaesthesia in dogs. Vet Anaesth Analg 35: 141–153.
27. Badoer E, Head GA, Korner PI (1983) Effects of intracisternal and intravenous alpha-methyldopa and clonidine on haemodynamics and baroreceptor-heart rate reflex properties in conscious rabbits. J Cardiovasc Pharmacol 5: 760–767.
28. Murrell JC, Hellebrekers LJ (2005) Medetomidine and dexmedetomidine: a review of cardiovascular effects and antinociceptive properties in the dog. Vet Anaesth Analg 32: 117–127.

# 10

# The Accuracy of the New Landmark Using Respiratory Jugular Venodilation and Direct Palpation in Right Internal Jugular Vein Access

**Hyungseok Seo, Dong-Min Jang, Jung-Min Yi, Hong-Gi Min*, Jai-Hyun Hwang**

Department of Anesthesiology and Pain Medicine, Asan Medical Center, University of Ulsan College of Medicine, Seoul, Republic of Korea

## Abstract

***Background:*** Although ultrasonography is recommended in internal jugular vein (IJV) catheterization, the landmark-guided technique should still be considered. The central landmark using the two heads of the sternocleidomastoid muscle is widely used, but it is inaccurate for IJV access. As an alternative landmark, we investigated the accuracy of the new landmark determined by inspection of the respiratory jugular venodilation and direct IJV palpation in right IJV access by ultrasonography.

***Methods and Findings:*** Thirty patients were enrolled. After induction of anesthesia, the central landmark was marked at the cricoid cartilage level (M1) and the alternative landmark determined by inspection of the respiratory jugular venodilation and direct palpation of IJV was also marked at the same level (M2). Using ultrasonography, the location of IJV was identified (M3) and the distance between M1 and M3 as well as between M2 and M3 were measured. The median (interquartile range) distance between the M2 and M3 was 3.5 (2.0–6.0) mm, compared to 17.5 (12.8–21.3) mm between M1 and M3. ($P<0.001$) The dispersion of distances between M2 and M3 was significantly smaller than between M1 and M3. ($P<0.001$) The visibility of respiratory jugular venodilation was associated with CVP more than 4 mmHg. Limitations of the present study are that the inter-observer variability was not investigated and that the visibility of the alternative landmark can be limited to right IJV in adults.

***Conclusion:*** The alternative landmark may allow shorter distance for the right side IJV access than the central landmark and can offer advantages in right IJV catheterization when ultrasound device is unavailable.

***Trial Registration:*** Clinical Research Informational Service KCT0000812

**Editor:** Francesco Cappello, University of Palermo, Italy

**Funding:** The authors have no support or funding to report.

**Competing Interests:** The authors have declared that no competing interests exist.

* Email: anesthminhg@gmail.com

## Introduction

Internal jugular vein (IJV) catheterization is commonly performed in clinical practice for central vein access. The central landmark, defined by the apex of the triangle between the two heads of the sternocleidomastoid muscle, is frequently used for IJV catheterization [1]. However, the complications of the central landmark-guided IJV catheterization occur in more than 15% of patients and the central landmark itself was reported to be inaccurate for IJV access [2,3]. Ultrasonography can reduce the incidence of complications and improves success rate in central venous catheterization (CVC) [4–8].

Although ultrasound-guided CVC is recommended as a standard technique, several reasons such as the limited availability of ultrasound machine, lack of training, or longer procedure time can hinder the widespread use of ultrasound device in CVC [6,9–11]. Particularly in emergency situation, which requires urgent CVC without ultrasound device, the landmark-guided technique can be useful and required to be practiced.

Because the central landmark has been known to be inaccurate [3], respiratory jugular venodilation, the pulse-like skin elevation which develops due to IJV dilatation following intrathoracic pressure change in patients receiving positive pressure ventilation, has been suggested as a new landmark especially for right IJV catheterization in patients receiving mechanical ventilation [12]. Additionally, IJV can be palpated directly, which is helpful to identify the IJV location and to increase the accuracy of IJV access.

In the present study, we hypothesized that the alternative landmark determined by the inspection of respiratory jugular venodilation and direct IJV palpation would be closer to the IJV than the central landmark during mechanical ventilation. Although the shorter distance does not mean the better outcomes, better accuracy could reduce the incidence of complications in situation where ultrasonography is limited. For the identification of IJV location, we used ultrasonography and measured the distance between each of the two landmarks and the IJV.

## Subjects and Methods

The protocol for this trial and supporting TREND checklist are available as supporting information; see Checklist S1 and Protocols S1 and S2.

### Subjects

Thirty adult patients admitted to the Asan Medical Center for elective urologic surgery between Jan 8 2013 and Jul 1 2013 were enrolled in the study (Figure 1). Patients were excluded from the study if they were aged <20 years, overweight (BMI>30 kg/m$^2$), underweight (BMI<18.5 kg/m$^2$), with known pulmonary or cardiovascular disorders, or at risk from internal jugular venous catheterization because of limited cervical motion or lesions in head and neck area. In patients who are indicated to receive IJV catheterization and not excluded from the study, randomly sampled patients by operation schedule were participated. Blinding was not accomplished in the present study. The study protocol was approved by the Asan Medical Center Institutional Review Board (approval number: 2012-0859) and registered with the Clinical Research Informational Service, which is the primary registry of WHO International Clinical Trials Registry Platform (KCT 0000812, http://cris.nih.go.kr). Authors obtained the verbal informed consent from all patients participated in the present study. Because authors measured the distance between surface landmark non-invasively and CVC was performed in the standard manner under ultrasonography with no other interventions, ethics committees approved that our study agreed that verbal consent was sufficient. None of the patients were premedicated before the surgery.

### Anesthesia and measurement protocols

Staff anesthesiologists who have fully experienced for both landmark and ultrasound-guided technique were randomly performed IJV catheterization. General anesthesia was induced with thiopental sodium 5 mg/kg, followed by sevoflurane inhalation. Rocuronium bromide 0.6 mg/kg was administered to facilitate tracheal intubation. Anesthesia was maintained with sevoflurane, 50% oxygen and nitrous oxide mixture. Mechanical ventilation was performed with tidal volume of 8 ml/kg, respiratory rate of 10, without positive end-expiratory pressure to maintain end tidal carbon dioxide at 35–40 mmHg. Peak airway pressure was monitored not to exceed 20 cm $H_2O$ during CVC.

After induction of anesthesia, patients were placed in a supine, slightly head-down position (approximately 15 degrees) with right arm adduction and the head slightly (approximately less than 15 degrees) turned to the left for the right IJV access. A pillow or facial mask was placed on the left side of the patient's head to prevent extreme head rotation and overlapping of the IJV and common carotid artery. The central landmark (M1), defined as the apex of the triangle composed of two heads of the sternocleidomastoid muscle and the clavicle, was marked on the line at the level of the cricoid cartilage (Figure 2). At the same cricoid cartilage level containing the central landmark, the alternative landmark (M2) was sought and marked by inspection of the respiratory jugular venodilation, which was identified as a pulse-like skin elevation synchronised with the inspiration phase of positive pressure ventilation [12] and by IJV palpation. After determining the two landmarks, the IJV was identified at the same cricoid cartilage level by using the ultrasound device (S-Nerve, Sonosite Inc., Washington, USA) with a 7.5 MHz linear probe and a cross-sectional view of the IJV was obtained. The ultrasound probe was placed vertical to the skin and adjusted to locate the midpoint of the IJV transverse diameter at the center of the sonographic view. The location of the ultrasound-identified IJV (M3) was marked at the center of the ultrasound probe. As a primary outcome, the distances between M1 and M3, M2 and M3, were measured by a flexible ruler and compared each other. For secondary outcomes, factors associated with the visible respiratory jugular venodilation were investigated.

After sterile skin preparation, the ultrasound-guided CVC was performed by an experienced anesthetist. Before insertion of the puncture needle, the depth and diameter of the IJV, and the diameter of the carotid artery were measured in the same sonographic field of view. After IJV catheterization, the correct catheter location and complications including posterior wall hematoma and pneumothorax was identified by ultrasonography.

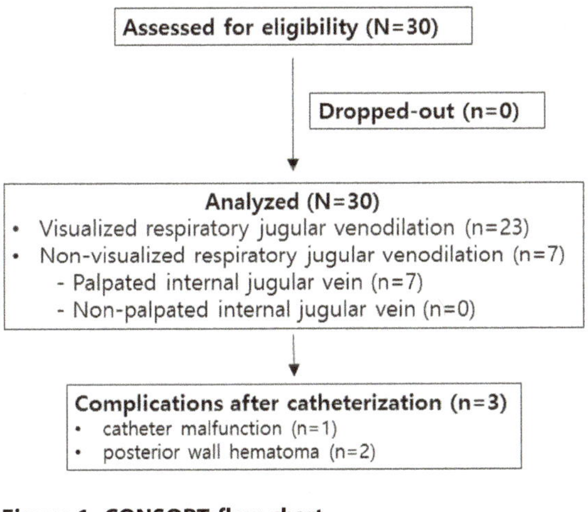


**Figure 1. CONSORT flow chart.**

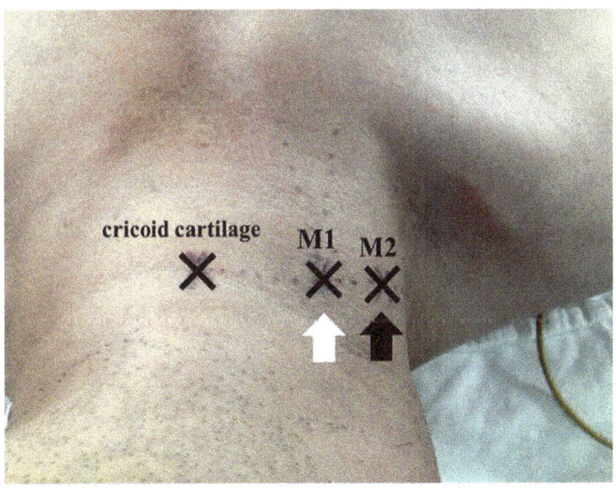


**Figure 2. Anatomical location of the two landmarks in the patient.** M1 is the central landmark (white arrow), determined by the apex of the triangle between the two heads of the sternocleidomastoid muscle. M2 is the alternative landmark (black arrow), determined by the inspection of respiratory jugular venodilation and direct internal jugular vein palpation.

Central venous pressure (CVP) was also measured after IJV catheterization.

## Sample size calculation and statistical analysis

The pilot data showed that the mean (sd) distances from the central landmark and the alternative landmark to the ultrasound-identified puncture site were 14.3 (3.9) mm and 4.6 (4.2) mm, respectively. We considered the alternative landmark to be within 5.0 mm of the ultrasound-identified puncture site. Assuming a type I error of 0.05 and a desired power of 0.90, 30 patients were required in the present study. Data are presented as mean (sd) in the table and median (interquartile range, IQR) in Figure 2. Statistical analyses were performed using SPSS 13.0 (SPSS Inc. Chicago, IL, USA). A normality test was performed using the Shapiro-Wilk test. Differences in distances were analysed using Mann-Whitney rank sum test. F-test was performed to investigate the difference of the dispersion. Receiver operator characteristic (ROC) curve analysis was performed to determine the predictabilities of CVP, the depth of IJV, and IJV diameter to detect the respiratory jugular venodilation. $P<0.05$ was considered to be statistically significant.

## Results

Thirty patients receiving scheduled urologic surgery were enrolled and none of the patients was excluded. The patient characteristics and anatomic variables are shown in Table 1. Respiratory jugular venodilation was identified in 23 patients (76.7%). In the remaining seven patients, the alternative landmark was identified by direct IJV palpation at the cricoid cartilage level. After the ultrasound-guided IJV catheterization, a case of catheter malfunction and two cases of posterior wall hematoma which are not related with inadvertent arterial puncture developed. There were no complications such as arterial puncture, hemothorax or pneumothorax in all of the patients.

The median [interquartile range] distance between M1 (the central landmark) and M3 (the location of ultrasound-identified IJV) was 17.5 [12.8–21.3] mm and the distance between M2 (the alternative landmark) and M3 was 3.5 [2.0–6.0] mm, ($P<0.001$) (Figure 3). The dispersion of measured distances between M2 and M3 was significantly smaller than between M1 and M3 (F statistic = 8.25, $P<0.001$).

ROC curve analysis showed that CVP >4 mmHg was associated with visible respiratory jugular venodilation, demonstrating 91.3% sensitivity and 71.4% specificity. The area under the curve of CVP was 0.89 ($P = 0.002$) (Figure 4). The depth of IJV and IJV diameter was not associated with the visibility of jugular venodilation.

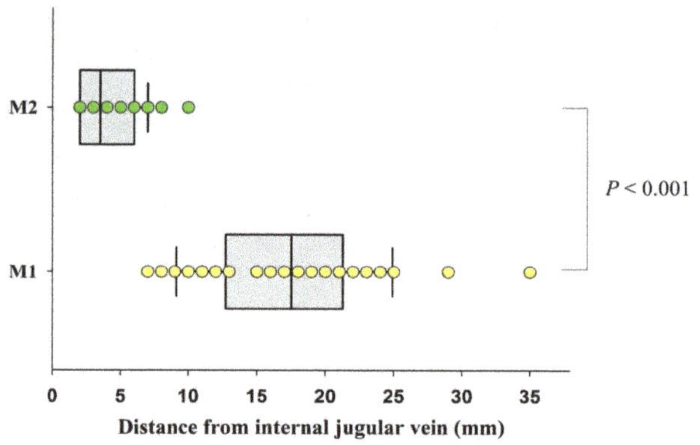


**Figure 3. Comparison of distances between M1 and M2 from the ultrasound-identified IJV.** Individual and median (interquartile range) distances between M1 and M2 from the ultrasound-identified IJV. For effective representation of the distance, the axes were inverted. The line in the middle box represents the median value and the lateral borders of the box represent interquartile ranges. Individual values are represented as dots (*yellow dots* in M1 and *green dots* in M2). M1, the central landmark; M2, the alternative landmark; IJV, internal jugular vein.

## Discussion

In the present study, we demonstrated that the alternative landmark identified by the inspection of respiratory jugular venodilation and direct IJV palpation was closer to the ultrasound-identified IJV than the central landmark determined by the external anatomy landmark method. Additionally, the visibility of jugular venodilation correlated with CVP >4 mmHg.

A number of techniques for IJV catheterization and the central landmark have been described so far [1,13–15]. The central landmark is the apex of the triangle defined by the two heads of the sternocleidomastoid muscle and the clavicle, when the patient's head is turned away from the catheterization site. However, it has been associated with more frequent complications than ultrasound-guided CVC [6,16,17], and the inaccuracy of the central landmark might contribute to the risk of arterial puncture and failure to find IJV [3]. The ultrasound-guided CVC is beneficial in improving success rate and reducing the incidence of complications such as arterial puncture, pneumothorax, and catheter-associated blood stream infection [16,17]. Therefore, the use of real-time ultrasound-guided CVC has been commonly recommend in clinical practice [4,5,7,8,11].

Although ultrasound-guided CVC has been recommended as a standard practice, some studies have shown that the use of

**Table 1.** Patient demographics and sonographic variables.

| Patient demographics | Values |
|---|---|
| Age (years) | 60.4 (11.2) |
| Sex (Male:Female ratio) | 20:10 |
| Body mass index (kg/m$^2$) | 24.1 (2.6) |
| **Sonographic variables** | |
| Depth of internal jugular vein from skin (mm) | 8.6 (3.0) |
| Diameter of internal jugular vein (mm) | 11.4 (3.1) |
| Diameter of common carotid artery (mm) | 7.7 (2.0) |

Values are expressed as mean (sd) and ratio.

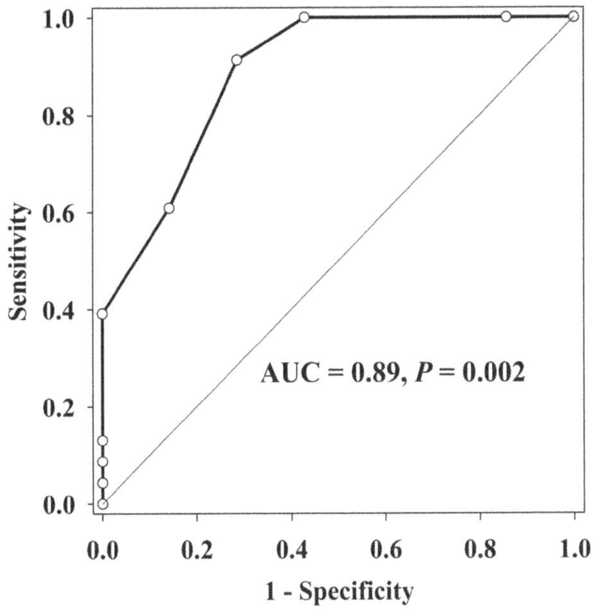


**Figure 4. ROC curve of the central venous pressure for the visible respiratory jugular venodilation.** Area under the curve is given inside the ROC curve. ROC curve, receiver operator characteristic curve.

ultrasound during CVC still remains limited in clinical practice. The limited availability and the physician's perceived utility of ultrasound devices contribute to their limited use [9,10,18]. In addition to these limiting factors, there is a potential risk of operators losing the skills necessary for the landmark technique. In emergency situations when CVC should be performed without time delay, the landmark technique might be beneficial because it requires less time for preparation and vein puncture. Moreover, the complication rate was reported to be similar between landmark technique and ultrasound-guided technique [19,20]. For these reasons, the landmark technique in CVC should still be considered as a clinically acceptable practice, despite the recommendation of ultrasound-guided CVC as a standard practice. Additionally, Health Technology Assessment also recommends that training for CVC using the landmark technique should be given in addition to the training for ultrasound-guided CVC [6].

However, ultrasonography revealed that the central landmark was unreliable for accessing the IJV and head rotation during the central landmark guided CVC increased the overlap of the carotid artery and IJV, leading to increased inadvertent arterial puncture [21,22]. These findings suggest that the alternative landmark can be considered to access IJV in landmark-guided CVC, especially when ultrasound is not available.

Before the inspection of the respiratory jugular venodilation, we standardized the CVC protocol. Patients were maintained with supine, slightly head-down position to increase IJV diameter [23,24]. Respiratory jugular venodilation, which is the increase in IJV diameter caused by intrathoracic pressure change synchronized with respiration, can be easily observed in patients receiving positive pressure ventilation, and it reflects the location of IJV more accurately than the central landmark, particularly in right side IJV catheterization [12,25]. When jugular venodilation was visible, the success rate of IJV catheterization at first attempt and arterial puncture incidence was 79% and 0.6% respectively, compared to 42.9% and 9.5% when jugular venodilation was not visible [12]. Since respiratory jugular venodilation represents the change in IJV diameter, it can indicate the location of the right IJV directly. Additionally, direct palpation may help to identify the location of the right IJV and it may increase the accuracy of IJV identification in combination with the inspection of jugular venodilation. We observed jugular venodilation in 77% of the patients and palpated the IJV directly in patients lacking the visible jugular venodilation. The median distance of the alternative landmark from the IJV was 3.5 mm, suggesting that the position of the alternative landmark is nearly identical to the position of IJV because the mean IJV diameter was 17.5 mm. In addition to the small median value, the small range of the distance from ultrasound-identified IJV also supports the notion that the alternative landmark is more accurate for accessing the IJV than the central landmark in CVC.

The respiratory jugular venodilation was visible in more than 75% of ventilated patients, however, its visibility was not associated with the level of the operator's experience or the IJV size, but with the extent of the dynamic change of IJV during the respiratory cycle [26]. In the present study, the ROC curve analysis showed the visibility of jugular venodilation was associated with the CVP and the CVP of more than 4 mmHg could predict the visible jugular venodilation (area under curve = 0.89, $P = 0.002$). This finding suggests that low CVP status would be less influenced by intrathoracic pressure change during mechanical ventilation, leading to small dynamic change of IJV.

The alternative landmark-guided IJV catheterization has several limitations. First, the variability of the alternative landmark between different investigators was not compared. Since there is no exact definition of the findings of the jugular venodilation and IJV palpation, the location of the alternative landmark might be influenced by investigator's experience. However, it was technically difficult to keep blinding between investigators in the present study design and the use of an ultraviolet ray-sensitive pen might be helpful for the blinding. Second, the respiratory jugular venodilation cannot be observed in all cases. In normal spontaneous breathing, respiratory movement with negative interpleural pressure can collapse internal jugular vein, thus respiratory jugular venodilation can be observed in patients receiving positive pressure ventilation [27]. Although it is commonly observed in approximately 80% of ventilated patients, there is a lack of evidence for its efficacy in paediatric patients. Moreover, respiratory jugular venodilation is not clearly identified in left IJV, because the left IJV is relatively far from the right atrium. Therefore, the efficacy of the alternative landmark can be limited to right IJV access in adult patients receiving positive pressure ventilation. Third, we did not investigate the effectiveness of the alternative landmark, such as the success rate at first attempt and the incidence of arterial puncture, in IJV catheterization. Although the distance of the alternative landmark from the IJV is shorter than that of the central landmark, the shorter distance might not mean better. To compare the efficacy between the two landmarks in IJV catheterization, a further study should be required. However, there can be an ethical problem of not using ultrasonography in CVC because the ultrasound-guided technique is currently recommended as a standard procedure. Although we performed IJV catheterization under ultrasonography guidance, previous research of IJV catheterization using jugular venodilation with 30 degrees left-turned head position and needle directed caudad with 60 degrees of puncture angle, revealed increase of the success rate at first attempt and decrease the arterial puncture incidence [12].

In summary, the alternative landmark identified by respiratory jugular venodilation and IJV palpation may allow more accuracy for the right side IJV access than the central landmark identified by the sternocleidomastoid muscle. To reduce the complications related to CVC, ultrasound-guided technique is inevitable. But, for access to right internal jugular vein when an ultrasound device is not available, better accuracy can reduce complication rate and the alternative landmark-guided technique may offer advantages.

## Supporting Information

**Checklist S1 Trend Statement Checklist.**

**Data S1 Clinical Research Data.**

**Protocol S1 Clinical Research Protocol (English).**

**Protocol S2 Clinical Research Protocol (Korean).**

## Author Contributions

Conceived and designed the experiments: HS HGM JHH. Performed the experiments: HS JMY HGM. Analyzed the data: HS DMJ JMY HGM. Contributed reagents/materials/analysis tools: HS DMJ HGM. Contributed to the writing of the manuscript: HS HGM JHH.

## References


1. English IC, Frew RM, Pigott JF, Zaki M (1969) Percutaneous catheterisation of the internal jugular vein. Anaesthesia 24: 521–531.
2. McGee DC, Gould MK (2003) Preventing complications of central venous catheterization. N Engl J Med 348: 1123–1133. doi:10.1056/NEJMra011883.
3. Bailey PL, Whitaker EE, Palmer LS, Glance LG (2006) The accuracy of the central landmark used for central venous catheterization of the internal jugular vein. Anesth Analg 102: 1327–1332. doi:10.1213/01.ane.0000202467.10465.12.
4. Feller-Kopman D (2007) Ultrasound-guided internal jugular access: a proposed standardized approach and implications for training and practice. Chest 132: 302–309. doi:10.1378/chest.06-2711.
5. Shojania KG, Duncan BW, McDonald KM, Wachter RM, Markowitz AJ (2001) Making health care safer: a critical analysis of patient safety practices. Evid Rep Technol Assess (Summ): i–x, 1–668.
6. Calvert N, Hind D, McWilliams RG, Thomas SM, Beverley C, et al. (2003) The effectiveness and cost-effectiveness of ultrasound locating devices for central venous access: a systematic review and economic evaluation. Health Technol Assess 7: 1–84.
7. Balls A, LoVecchio F, Kroeger A, Stapczynski JS, Mulrow M, et al. (2010) Ultrasound guidance for central venous catheter placement: results from the Central Line Emergency Access Registry Database. Am J Emerg Med 28: 561–567. doi:10.1016/j.ajem.2009.02.003.
8. Froehlich CD, Rigby MR, Rosenberg ES, Li R, Roerig PL, et al. (2009) Ultrasound-guided central venous catheter placement decreases complications and decreases placement attempts compared with the landmark technique in patients in a pediatric intensive care unit. Crit Care Med 37: 1090–1096. doi:10.1097/CCM.0b013e31819b570e.
9. Jefferson P, Ogbue MN, Hamilton KE, Ball DR (2002) A survey of the use of portable ultrasound for central vein cannulation on critical care units in the UK. Anaesthesia 57: 365–368.
10. Bailey PL, Glance LG, Eaton MP, Parshall B, McIntosh S (2007) A survey of the use of ultrasound during central venous catheterization. Anesth Analg 104: 491–497. doi:10.1213/01.ane.0000255289.78333.c2.
11. Matera JT, Egerton-Warburton D, Meek R (2010) Ultrasound guidance for central venous catheter placement in Australasian emergency departments: potential barriers to more widespread use. Emerg Med Australas 22: 514–523. doi:10.1111/j.1742-6723.2010.01347.x.
12. Hayashi H, Ootaki C, Tsuzuku M, Amano M (2000) Respiratory jugular venodilation: a new landmark for right internal jugular vein puncture in ventilated patients. J Cardiothorac Vasc Anesth 14: 40–44.
13. Chatrath RR, Stock JG, Jones OD (1983) Internal jugular catheterisation in small children. The use of a posterior approach. Anaesthesia 38: 380–383.
14. Oda M, Fukushima Y, Hirota T, Tanaka A, Aono M, et al. (1981) The para-carotid approach for internal jugular catheterization. Anaesthesia 36: 896–900.
15. Rao TL, Wong AY, Salem MR (1977) A new approach to percutaneous catheterization of the internal jugular vein. Anesthesiology 46: 362–364.
16. Denys BG, Uretsky BF, Reddy PS (1993) Ultrasound-assisted cannulation of the internal jugular vein. A prospective comparison to the external landmark-guided technique. Circulation 87: 1557–1562.
17. Karakitsos D, Labropoulos N, De Groot E, Patrianakos AP, Kouraklis G, et al. (2006) Real-time ultrasound-guided catheterisation of the internal jugular vein: a prospective comparison with the landmark technique in critical care patients. Crit Care 10: R162. doi:10.1186/cc5101.
18. Girard TD, Schectman JM (2005) Ultrasound guidance during central venous catheterization: a survey of use by house staff physicians. J Crit Care 20: 224–229. doi:10.1016/j.jcrc.2005.06.005.
19. Miller AH, Roth BA, Mills TJ, Woody JR, Longmoor CE, et al. (2002) Ultrasound guidance versus the landmark technique for the placement of central venous catheters in the emergency department. Acad Emerg Med 9: 800–805.
20. Atkinson P, Boyle A, Robinson S, Campbell-Hewson G (2005) Should ultrasound guidance be used for central venous catheterisation in the emergency department? Emerg Med J 22: 158–164. doi:10.1136/emj.2003.011288.
21. Hong JY, Koo BN, Kim WO, Choi E, Kil HK (2010) Effect of head rotation on overlap and relative position of internal jugular vein to carotid artery in infants and children: a study of the anatomy using ultrasonography. J Crit Care 25: 360 e369–360 e313. doi:10.1016/j.jcrc.2009.12.005.
22. Wang R, Snoey ER, Clements RC, Hern HG, Price D (2006) Effect of head rotation on vascular anatomy of the neck: an ultrasound study. J Emerg Med 31: 283–286. doi:10.1016/j.jemermed.2005.12.026.
23. Valdueza JM, von Munster T, Hoffman O, Schreiber S, Einhaupl KM (2000) Postural dependency of the cerebral venous outflow. Lancet 355: 200–201.
24. Bazaral M, Harlan S (1981) Ultrasonographic anatomy of the internal jugular vein relevant to percutaneous cannulation. Crit Care Med 9: 307–310.
25. Devine PJ, Sullenberger LE, Bellin DA, Atwood JE (2007) Jugular venous pulse: window into the right heart. South Med J 100: 1022–1027; quiz 1004. doi:10.1097/SMJ.0b013e318073c89c.
26. Hayashi H, Ootaki C, Tsuzuku M, Amano M (2000) Respiratory jugular venodilation: its anatomic rationale as a landmark for right internal jugular vein puncture as determined by ultrasonography. J Cardiothorac Vasc Anesth 14: 425–427. doi:10.1053/jcan.2000.7939.
27. Hamilton DR, Sargsyan AE, Garcia K, Ebert DJ, Whitson PA, et al. (2012) Cardiac and vascular responses to thigh cuffs and respiratory maneuvers on crewmembers of the International Space Station. J Appl Physiol (1985) 112: 454–462. doi:10.1152/japplphysiol.00557.2011.

# 11

# Efficacy of Tricaine Methanesulfonate (MS-222) as an Anesthetic Agent for Blocking Sensory-Motor Responses in *Xenopus laevis* Tadpoles

**Carlana Ramlochansingh, Francisco Branoner, Boris P. Chagnaud, Hans Straka***

Department Biology II, Ludwig-Maximilians-University Munich, Planegg, Germany

**Abstract**

Anesthetics are drugs that reversibly relieve pain, decrease body movements and suppress neuronal activity. Most drugs only cover one of these effects; for instance, analgesics relieve pain but fail to block primary fiber responses to noxious stimuli. Alternately, paralytic drugs block synaptic transmission at neuromuscular junctions, thereby effectively paralyzing skeletal muscles. Thus, both analgesics and paralytics each accomplish one effect, but fail to singularly account for all three. Tricaine methanesulfonate (MS-222) is structurally similar to benzocaine, a typical anesthetic for anamniote vertebrates, but contains a sulfate moiety rendering this drug more hydrophilic. MS-222 is used as anesthetic in poikilothermic animals such as fish and amphibians. However, it is often argued that MS-222 is only a hypnotic drug and its ability to block neural activity has been questioned. This prompted us to evaluate the potency and dynamics of MS-222-induced effects on neuronal firing of sensory and motor nerves alongside a defined motor behavior in semi-intact *in vitro* preparations of *Xenopus laevis* tadpoles. Electrophysiological recordings of extraocular motor discharge and both spontaneous and evoked mechanosensory nerve activity were measured before, during and after administration of MS-222, then compared to benzocaine and a known paralytic, pancuronium. Both MS-222 and benzocaine, but not pancuronium caused a dose-dependent, reversible blockade of extraocular motor and sensory nerve activity. These results indicate that MS-222 as benzocaine blocks the activity of both sensory and motor nerves compatible with the mechanistic action of effective anesthetics, indicating that both caine-derivates are effective as single-drug anesthetics for surgical interventions in anamniotes.

**Editor:** Michael Klymkowsky, University of Colorado, Boulder, United States of America

**Funding:** The authors CR FB BPC and HS acknowledge financial support from the German Science Foundation (CRC 870, TP B12), the German Federal Ministry of Education and Research under the Grant code 01 EO 0901, the Munich Center for Neurosciences - Brain and Mind (MCN) and the Graduate School for Systemic Neurosciences (GSN). The funders had no role in study design, data collection and analysis, decision to publish, or preparation of the manuscript.

**Competing Interests:** The authors have declared that no competing interests exist.

* Email: straka@lmu.de

## Introduction

Anesthetics have transformed modern medicine and basic biological research on vertebrate species by their ability to reversibly relieve pain, decrease body movements and render the animal unconscious during surgical interventions [1,2]. While there are numerous potent, surgery-specific choices of anesthetics for use in mammals for which the mechanisms of action are well known [3], there is only a limited number of approved drugs for anesthesia in anamniote vertebrates such as fish and amphibians [4,5,6]. However, the increasing use of model species such as zebrafish, *Xenopus* or axolotl for systemic research approaches requires reliable and potent anesthetic drugs for which the sites and mechanisms of action are determined. Currently, the anesthetic of choice for fish and amphibian species is Tricaine methanesulfonate (MS-222), which is a sulfonated analog of benzocaine. Even though the pharmacological mechanism of benzocaine and its derivates are known on a cellular and subcellular level [7,8], the precise mechanistic action and site(s)/ extent of pharmacological impact on neuronal tissue on a systemic level *in vivo* remains relatively unclear and thus a distinction from related substances is elusive. This distinction, however, is of particular importance because a drug's classification strongly influences administration and usage policies in both medicine and basic research approaches that require approved animal protocols. Usually, during general surgical anesthesia in mammals a combination of several drugs cover analgesic, paralytic and anesthetic effects [9], while benzocaine and its derivates, as single substances, might cover all aspects during general anesthesia in fish and amphibians [5]. Assuming that caine-derivates potentially access all neuronal and myocytic elements during systemic applications, benzocaine or MS-222 could simultaneously block pain sensation [10], paralyze the animal by muscle relaxation and exert a general anesthesia [5] through a block of $Na^+$-conductances [8] of cellular elements comprising the neuromuscular system (brain and muscles).

Benzocaine has been shown to effectively block the generation of action potentials through reversible interactions with voltage-dependent $Na^+$-channels [1,4,5]. Consequently, this drug would be sufficient for anesthesia, analgesia and paralysis e.g. during surgical interventions in anamniote species, provided that the action potential initiation is blocked in all excitable cells, such as neurons and myocytes. Although MS-222 is a derivative and likely achieves its effect by a similar reversible suppression of action potentials, a complete understanding of the extent of this mechanism at the systemic level is still absent. As the current anesthetic of choice for fish and amphibians [5], MS-222 should block the action potential generation in both sensory and motor systems as well as in central nervous circuits. The sulfate moiety of tricaine (MS-222), which otherwise has a similar structure as benzocaine, renders the former drug much more hydrophilic [11]. The increased solubility has facilitated the employment as an anesthetic for poikilothermic vertebrates such as fish and amphibians [12,13] because it allows administration simply by submerging these animals in an aqueous solution of the drug. This is at variance with benzocaine, which requires an organic solvent for its solubility [1]. After submergence in MS-222 (0.01–0.08%), a dose-dependent loss of the righting reflex and response to nociceptive stimuli was observed in leopard frogs [1] and decreased reactions to noxious stimuli have been reported in koi fish [10]. The impact on motor activity as well as on nociception suggests that along with the anesthetic effect, MS-222 as a single drug is well suited for surgical interventions in anamniote vertebrates. However, the potency of this drug on the spike discharge of distinct neuronal populations or on the activity of identified neural networks responsible for the mediation of a defined sensory-motor behavior still remains to be determined.

Here, we describe the dose-dependent effect of MS-222 on spontaneous and evoked activity in afferent sensory (vestibular, lateral line) as well as in motor (extraocular) nerves in *Xenopus laevis* tadpoles. In semi-intact *in vitro* preparations with functional sensory organs and motor effectors [14] the anesthetic impact and pharmacological capacity of MS-222 was determined at the input and output stage of a well defined sensory-motor behavior in comparison to benzocaine and pancuronium (a pure paralytic).

## Material and Methods

### Animals

*Xenopus laevis* tadpoles were obtained from the in house animal breeding facility at the Biocenter-Martinsried (Ludwig-Maximilians-University Munich). Tadpoles were kept in tanks filled with 17–18°C non-chlorinated water at a 12/12 light/dark cycle and were fed daily with finely ground algae. A total of 89 animals at developmental stages 53–57 [15] were used for experimentation. Experiments were performed *in vitro* on isolated, semi-intact preparations and comply with the National Institute of Health publication entitled "Principles of animal care", No. 86–23, revised 1985. Permission for these experiments was granted by the governmental institution, Regierung von Oberbayern/Government of Upper Bavaria (55.2-1-54-2532.3-59-12).

### Isolated semi-intact in vitro preparation

In all experiments, tadpoles were anesthetized in 0.05% MS-222 (Pharmaq Ltd., UK) in frog Ringer (75 mM NaCl, 25 mM $NaHCO_3$, 2 mM $CaCl_2$, 2 mM KCl, 0.5 mM $MgCl_2$, and 11 mM glucose, pH 7.4) and decapitated at the level of the upper spinal cord. For experiments on the lateral line system, the spinal cord was cut at the same segmental level, however, the entire tail musculature and skin remained intact. As previously described [16], the skin covering the dorsal head (Fig. $1A_1$) was removed, the soft skull tissue opened and the forebrain disconnected (dotted white line in Fig. $1A_2$). This surgical procedure anatomically preserved the bilateral vestibular endorgans within the otic capsule (inner ear; Fig. $1B_{1,2}$), the central nervous system (brain) and the extraocular motor innervation and eye muscles (Fig. 1C) for prolonged *in vitro* experimentation [14]. The functionally persisting central nervous system, intact vestibular sensory periphery, afferent connections and efferent projections to the eye muscles along with spatio-temporally appropriate contractions of the latter allowed an *in vivo*-like activation of vestibulo-ocular reflexes (VOR) during natural motion patterns (Fig. 1D,E) under controlled *in vitro* conditions [17,14]. This isolated preparation is thus highly suitable for pharmacological studies because it combines the advantages of *in vitro* experiments for bath application of defined drug concentrations with the possibility to quantitatively determine the impact of a particular drug on sensory and motor behavior, otherwise only possible under *in vivo* conditions.

### Neuronal activity and behavioral measurements

Spontaneous and evoked neural activity was recorded from selected sensory and motor nerves along with motion-triggered eye movements (Fig. 1F-H) [16]. After the isolation and completion of the final dissection that gave access to individual target nerves (vestibular, posterior lateral line, trochlear) all preparations were rinsed in freshly oxygenated Ringer solution (Carbogen: 95% $O_2$, 5% $CO_2$), transferred to a small tank (volume 40–50 ml) and maintained for 24 hours at 6–8°C to ensure complete wash-out of MS-222 after the different preparations had been generated (description, see below).

*Vestibular nerve (N.VIII)*

Both N.VIII were transected at the entrance into the brainstem, leaving the peripheral part of each nerve along with the ganglion of Scarpa and the sensory innervation of individual vestibular endorgans in the otic capsule intact (Fig. $1B_{1,2}$). The brain was removed to facilitate the visibility and access to the cut surface of the N.VIII for electrophysiological recordings. The next day, the preparation was mechanically secured to the Sylgard floor of a recording chamber that was mounted onto a two-axis turntable (Fig. 1D) in the center of the horizontal and vertical rotation axes. The spike discharge of vestibular nerve afferent fibers was recorded by targeting glass suction electrodes with a micromanipulator to the central portion of the fasciculated cut end of the N.VIII (Fig. 1G).

**Lateral line nerve.** The posterior lateral line nerve was severed at the entrance into the brain. This made the peripheral portion of the nerve, connected to the sensory periphery of the lateral line system, accessible for electrophysiological recordings. A large part of the peripheral sensory target area of the posterior lateral line nerve (neuromasts on the skin of the dorsolateral part of the head and rostral tail) remained intact and allowed natural stimulation through induction of water waves along the body surface. Electrophysiological recordings were made on the following day from the posterior lateral line nerve with individually adjusted glass suction electrodes.

**Trochlear nerve (N.IV).** The skin surrounding the eyes was removed and the identified nerve branch innervating the superior oblique (SO) eye muscle, i.e. the trochlear nerve (Fig. 1C) was disconnected from its target muscle. After 24 hours the preparation was fixed to the Sylgard floor in the recording chamber, which was mounted in the center of the rotation axes of the turntable as described above (Fig. 1D,E). Individually adjusted glass suction electrodes were used for the electrophysiological recordings as in earlier studies (Fig. 1F) [18,16].

**Electrophysiological recordings of nerve activity.** Spontaneous and sensory stimulus-evoked multiple-unit spike discharge of the vestibular, lateral line and trochlear nerve before, during and after drug application were recorded

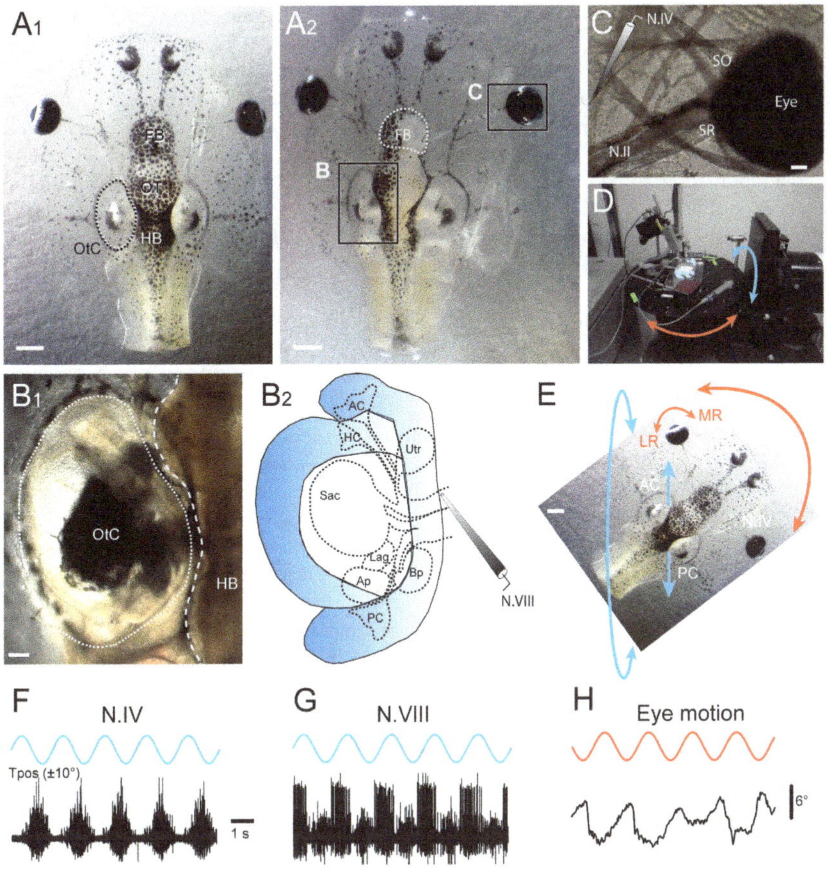


**Figure 1. Semi-intact *Xenopus laevis* preparation with functional sensory and motor elements for *in vitro* pharmacological experimentation.** ***A-C,*** Photomicrographs, depicting an isolated head of a *Xenopus laevis* tadpole before (***A₁***) and after opening of the dorsal cranium (***A₂***) and removal of the skin to disconnect the forebrain (FB, white dotted line in ***A₂***) and to make the brainstem, otic capsule (OtC in **A₁**,***B₁,₂***) and extraocular neuromuscular system (i.e. N.IV motor innervation of the SO eye muscle in ***C***) accessible for extracellular single- and multiple-unit recordings and bath-application of drugs; further removal of the entire hindbrain (HB, white dashed line in ***B₁***) yielded access to the peripheral part of the N.VIII for electrophysiological recordings of afferent fibers innervating the different vestibular sensory endorgans in the otic capsule (***B₂***). ***D,E,*** A computer-controlled turntable (***D***) allowed spatially specific application of sinusoidal rotational stimuli of semi-intact preparations in the horizontal (red arrows) and vertical planes (e.g. left AC - right PC, blue arrows in ***E***). ***F,G,*** Typical multiple-unit discharge modulation, recorded from N.IV (trochlear nerve, ***F***) and the anterior branch of N.VIII (vestibular nerve, ***G***) during 5 cycles of rotation (0.5 Hz) in the AC - PC plane, illustrated in ***E***. ***H,*** *In vitro* optical motion recording of the left eye (***E***) during 5 cycles of rotation in the horizontal plane (0.5 Hz). Scale bar is 1 mm in ***A₁,₂*** and 0.2 mm in ***B₁,C;*** calibration bar and positional excursion amplitude of the rotational stimulus in ***F*** also apply to ***G,H;*** AC, PC, anterior, posterior vertical semicircular canal; LR, MR, SR, lateral, medial, superior rectus eye muscle; SO, superior oblique eye muscle; OT, optic tectum, Tpos, table position.

extracellularly (EXT 10-2F; npi electronics, Germany) with glass suction electrodes, digitized at 10–20 kHz (CED 1401, Cambridge Electronic Design, UK) and stored on computer for offline analysis. Glass microelectrodes for extracellular recordings were made with a horizontal puller (P-87, Sutter Instruments Co., USA) and were individually broken at the tip to fit the respective nerve diameters.

**Eye motion.** After isolation of the preparation and maintenance in oxygenated Ringer solution for 24 hours, the recording chamber with the preparation secured to the Sylgard floor was mounted on the two-axis turntable in the center of the rotation axes (Fig. 1D,E). Sinusoidal rotations around the vertical axis triggered oppositely directed compensatory eye movements in the horizontal plane, illustrating the activation of an angular VOR [19]. Even though this *in vitro* preparation is isolated, it is still capable of expressing effective motor reactions upon sensory stimulation, such as compensatory eye movements during vestibular stimulation on motion simulators with spatio-temporal characteristics identical to those observed in intact animals [14,18]. Eye movements were recorded non-invasively (Fig. 1H) with a video camera (Grasshopper B/W, Point Grey Research Inc, Canada) and a zoom objective (Optem Zoom 70XL, Qioptiq Photonics GmbH & Co KG, Germany) with an adequate lens (M25×0.75+0.25). This system was mounted on top of the experimental setup to visualize the motion of one or both eyes from above during vestibular stimulation at a video capture frame rate of 30 Hz with the respective software (FlyCap2 v2.3.2.14.).

During all electrophysiological and eye motion recordings, preparations were continuously superfused with oxygenated Ringer solution at a rate of ~2 ml/min. The temperature of the bath solution was controlled and maintained at 17±0.5°C throughout the experiments.

## Sensory stimulation

Motion stimuli for modulating vestibular (N.VIII) nerve afferent and trochlear (N.IV) motor nerve activity were delivered with a computer-controlled motorized two-axis turntable (Fig. 1D; Acutronic Switzerland Ltd.), suitable to cause natural motion-dependent activation of the vestibular endorgans. The stimulus consisted of sinusoidal rotations around the horizontal axis at a frequency of 0.5 Hz and position amplitude of ±10° (blue arrows in Fig. 1E) corresponding to a peak table velocity of ±30°/s. The recording chamber with the isolated preparation in the center was positioned on the turntable such that the plane of the turntable rotation (roll stimulation) caused a maximal discharge modulation of the vestibular afferent activity in a particular experiment. During trochlear motor nerve recordings, the roll motion stimulation occurred along the ipsilateral posterior/contralateral anterior semicircular canal plane to maximize spike discharge modulation of these extraocular motoneurons [19]. For eliciting horizontal VOR-associated eye movement behavior, the motion stimulus consisted of a vertical-axis rotation at a frequency of 0.5 Hz and a positional excursion of ±10° corresponding to a peak table velocity of ±30°/s and specifically activated the bilateral horizontal semicircular canals (red arrows in Fig. 1E).

Water waves, produced with a vibrating sphere (diameter 3 mm) were used to activate lateral line hair cells of neuromasts on the skin surface. The sphere was positioned with a micromanipulator lateral to the tail of the animal and controlled by a piezo drive (PX 1500, Piezosystem Jena, Germany). The vibrating sphere was cyclically displaced along the rostro-caudal body axis at the level of the tail at a distance of ~1 mm from the skin surface at a frequency of 10 Hz, a displacement of ±150 µm for a period of 10 s. Spike discharge activity in the posterior lateral line nerve, innervating the respective neuromasts, was measured for a period of 10 s prior and during stimulation.

### Pharmacological agents

The drugs, MS-222 (Pharmaq Ltd., UK), benzocaine and pancuronium (both from Sigma-Aldrich, France), were administered to the preparation using bath application of the respective substance in oxygenated Ringer solution at a rate of ~2 ml/min, at a temperature of 17°C [17]. MS-222 at four different concentrations (0.0025, 0.005, 0.01 and 0.05%) and pancuronium (0.12 mg/ml) were dissolved in frog Ringer. In contrast, benzocaine was dissolved in 0.003% dimethylsulfoxide (DMSO, Sigma-Aldrich, France) before dilution in frog Ringer (final concentrations 0.0025, 0.005, 0.01 and 0.05%). All drug solutions were buffered to a pH 7.4 with $NaHCO_3$. A drug-related reduction of the spontaneous and evoked responses in similar isolated preparations usually occurred after 3–5 min and reached steady state after 15 min [20]. The wash-out of the different drugs was determined for a period of up to four hours in some experiments and revealed a dose- and drug-dependent recovery of the resting rate and stimulus-induced discharge modulation.

### Analysis

Eye motion profiles and parameters were extracted from the captured video sequences using a custom video-processing algorithm written in Matlab [21]. To calculate the motion of the eye, an ellipse was drawn around the eyeball and the angle between the minor axis of the ellipse and the longitudinal axis of the head was calculated in each frame of a given video sequence. Based on the frame rate (30 Hz), the change in eye position over time was computed. The generation of peri-stimulus time histograms for a single cycle of sinusoidal vertical-axis turntable rotation was used to calculate the eye motion gain (ratio eye/table motion) of the VOR. This value was determined before (control), during and after drug application (wash-out) to measure the impact of the different substances. Electrophysiological recordings were analyzed with Spike2 software using customized scripts to create peri-stimulus time histograms (PSTH). The PSTH values were grouped into control, 5 and 15 min exposure and wash-out after drug removal. All values were for comparative reasons normalized to control values obtained prior to the drug application. The normalized values were statistically analyzed using one-way ANOVA and post-hoc tests (Dunnett and Tukey's; GraphPad Prism software) to assess significance levels. Averaged results were expressed as means ± standard error of the mean (SEM). Graphical presentations were made with the aid of commercially available computer software (GraphPad Prism; Igor Pro; Illustrator, Adobe Systems).

## Results

### Effect of MS-222, benzocaine and pancuronium on eye motion

Application of sinusoidal rotational stimuli to isolated semi-intact *in vitro* preparations of *Xenopus* tadpoles with a motion simulator (Figs. 1A,D,E, 2A) activates a robust vestibulo-ocular reflex behavior with characteristics comparable to those observed *in vivo* [14,18]. Accordingly, non-invasive video recordings of compensatory eye movements during sinusoidal rotation (0.5 Hz; ±10°) around the vertical axis in control animals revealed conjugate movements of both eyes in the opposite direction to the turntable motion (Figs. 1H, 2B,C) with a gain (ratio eye/table motion) of 0.25±0.04 ($n = 20$), typical for the horizontal angular VOR (aVOR) in larval *Xenopus* at this developmental stage [18].

Following bath application of pancuronium (0.12 mg/ml), a paralytic drug [22], the evoked eye movements were gradually reduced, reached ~50% of the control values after 5 min and were essentially abolished ($n = 4$) after 15 min (Fig. 2D,G,J). The block of the response was long-lasting as indicated by the absence of any recovery of the responses 1 hour after the beginning of the wash-out of the drug (Fig. 2D,G,J). As expected from the pharmacological mechanism of pancuronium as a competitive nicotinic acetylcholine receptor antagonist [22], vestibular-evoked extraocular muscle activity was consistently blocked for an extended period in isolated *Xenopus* tadpole preparations.

Bath application of benzocaine (0.05%), a reversible blocker of voltage-dependent $Na^+$ channels [8] exhibited a very potent and rapid effect on the evoked aVOR behavior (Fig. 2E,H,J). Motion-triggered eye movements during sinusoidal turntable rotation were essentially blocked 5 min after the initial application in all preparations ($n = 5$) and were consistently extinguished 15 min after adding the drug to the bath solution (Fig. 2E,H,J). At a concentration of 0.05%, no recovery was seen 1 hour after wash-out (Fig. 2E,H,J) and the block usually persisted for several hours. The faster onset of the effect, relative to pancuronium, is likely due to the ubiquitous accessibility of $Na^+$ channels in all neurons along the VOR pathway in this preparation, thereby blocking the activity at the sensory periphery in the inner ear, the central vestibular and extraocular motor nuclei as well as the eye muscles, in agreement with the expected pharmacological impact of this drug.

Bath application of MS-222 at a concentration of 0.05% exhibited a slightly slower time course and lower potency of blocking the elicited aVOR behavior compared to benzocaine (Fig. 2E,F,H-J). Nonetheless, five minutes after bath application of MS-222 (0.05%), vestibular-evoked eye movements were reduced by ~90% ($n = 5$) and completely blocked 15 min after adding the drug to the bath solution (Fig. 2F,I,J). No detectable recovery of the aVOR behavior was seen after 1 hour wash-out at this concentration, however, a partial recovery was observed 3 hours after removal of MS-222 from the bath (Fig. 2F,I,J). The effect of this drug on the evoked aVOR behavior was dose-dependent as

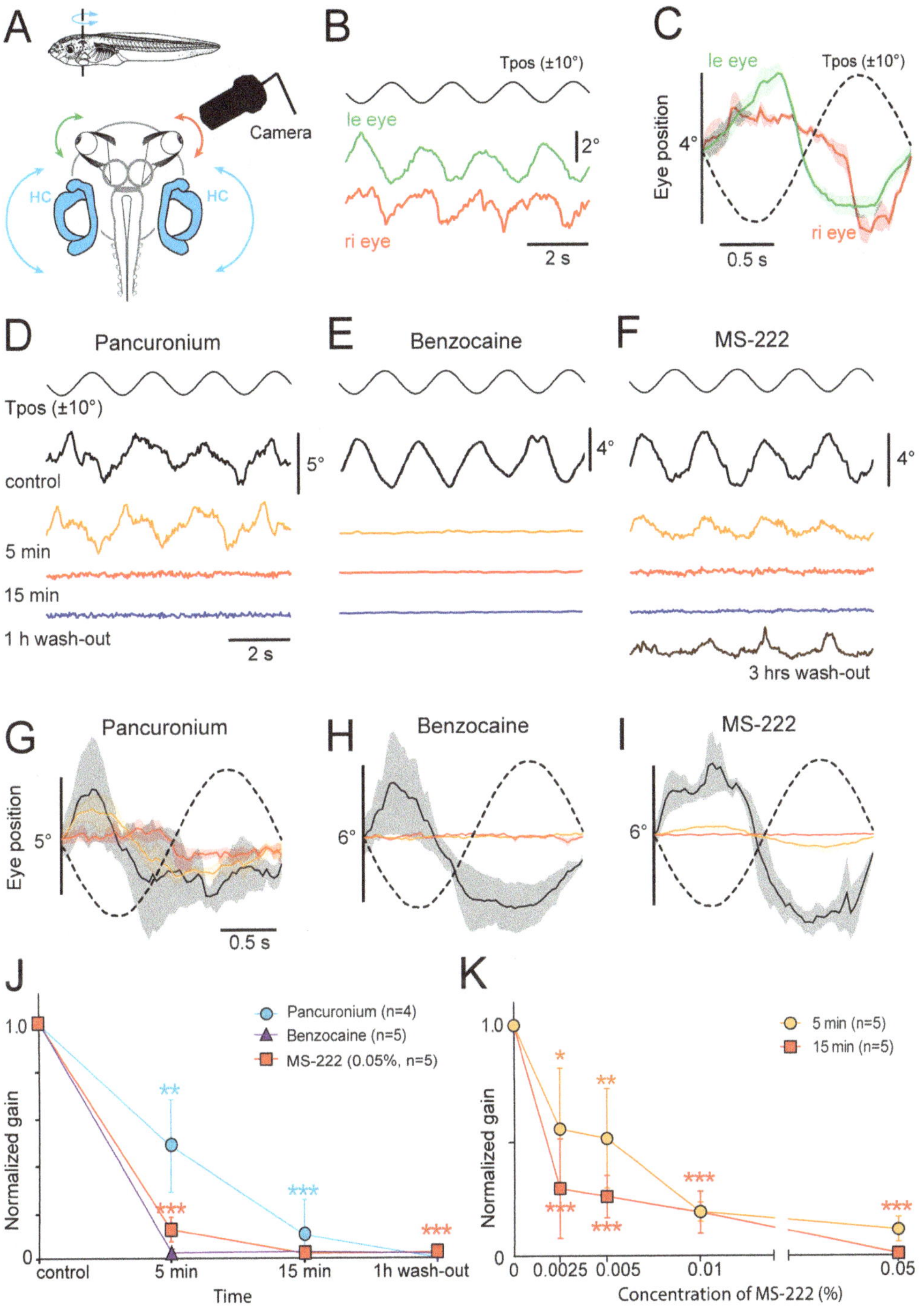


**Figure 2. Effect of pancuronium, benzocaine and MS-222 on the horizontal aVOR in *Xenopus* tadpoles.** ***A***, Schematic of the experimental setting depicting the semi-intact preparation, horizontal sinusoidal turntable positional changes (Tpos; 0.5 Hz, ±10°) and video capture of eye motion. ***B,C***, Single sweeps of co-aligned horizontal positional oscillations of the left (green) and right (red) eye, extracted from video sequences during turntable rotation (***B***) and average responses (± SEM, shaded areas; $n=8$) over a single cycle (***C***); note that table and eye motion are oppositely directed in agreement with aVOR behavior. ***D-I***, Effect of bath-applied pancuronium (0.12 mg/ml, ***D,G***), benzocaine (0.05%, ***E,H***) and MS-222 (0.05%, ***F,I***) on single sweeps of horizontal sinusoidal turntable motion (Tpos)-evoked eye movements (***D-F***) and average response (± SEM, shaded areas; $n=8$, respectively) over a single cycle (dashed line; ***G-I***); recordings (same color code in ***G-I***) were obtained before (Control, black traces), 5 min (orange traces) and 15 min (red traces) after onset of drug application as well as 1 hour (blue traces, ***D-F***) and 3 hours after beginning of the wash-out (brown trace, ***F***). ***J***, Progression of pharmacological influence on eye motion gain (ratio of eye/table motion magnitude) after application/wash-out of pancuronium, benzocaine and MS-222. ***K***, Dose-response curve of MS-222 impact on the gain of rotation-induced eye motion 5 and 15 min after drug application; the significance of difference in ***J,K*** is indicated: *, $p \leq 0.01$; **, $p \leq 0.001$; ***, $p \leq 0.0001$, with respect to control values. Calibration bars in ***D,G*** also apply to ***E,F*** and ***H,I***, respectively.

indicated by the more pronounced effects of increasing concentrations on the response, both 5 and 15 min after wash-in of the drug (Fig. 2K). While a significant reduction of the eye motion amplitude was caused at all concentrations, a complete block of the responses 15 min after application was only achieved at a concentration of 0.05% MS-222 (Fig. 2K).

## Effect of MS-222, benzocaine and pancuronium on spontaneous and evoked extraocular motor activity

In order to comparatively evaluate the effect of the different paralytic and anesthetic drugs on motor commands that generate aVOR behavior, the neuronal discharge of the respective motoneurons was recorded from the trochlear nerve during natural vestibular stimulation (Fig. 3A). After disconnecting the trochlear nerve from its target superior oblique extraocular muscle, extracellular multiple-unit spike activity was recorded at rest and during horizontal-axis roll stimulation in the plane of the ipsilateral posterior/contralateral anterior vertical semicircular canal (Fig. 3A,$B_1$). A rotation along this plane optimally activates this eye muscle [18]. In the absence of table rotation the rate of the multiple-unit trochlear nerve (N.IV) activity was ~15 Hz (14.6±2.6 Hz; $n=14$). During sinusoidal turntable motion (0.5 Hz; ±10°) in the roll plane, the extraocular motor nerve discharge was modulated with a dynamic characteristic that matched the expected motor command signal for compensatory eye movements in isolated preparations with intact neuromuscular connections [18]. The average peak discharge modulation rate during roll motion stimulation was ~140 Hz (140.6±21.4 Hz; $n=14$), with the peak firing rate occurring slightly before the table position tilted in the direction of the ipsilateral posterior semicircular canal (Fig. $3B_{1,2}$,$C_{1,2}$).

Bath application of pancuronium (0.12 mg/ml; $n=4$), had neither a significant effect on the spontaneous trochlear nerve firing rate ($p=0.918$) nor on the discharge modulation during turntable motion ($p=0.975$) compared to controls (Fig. $3B_{1,2}$). The insensitivity of the extraocular motor nerve discharge to pancuronium (Fig. $3B_2$), at variance with the suppression of eye movements by this drug during the same stimulus (Fig. 2D,G,J) complies with the absence of nicotinic acetylcholine receptors in central VOR pathways [19]. This shows that the observed block of aVOR behavior (Fig. 2D,G) was caused by the impact of pancuronium on the synaptic transmission at the neuromuscular synapse between extraocular motoneurons and eye muscles.

Bath application of benzocaine, in contrast to pancuronium, blocked the spontaneous multiple-unit discharge as well as the modulated activity of the trochlear nerve during roll motion stimulation (Figs. $3C_{1,2}$, 4A,B). Following application of benzocaine (0.05%; $n=5$) to the bath solution, the spontaneous multiple-unit firing (Fig. 4A) as well as the discharge modulation during sinusoidal roll motion (Figs. $3C_{1,2}$, $4B_{1,2}$) ceased rapidly and caused a complete and long-lasting block of the spike activity in the nerve in all experiments after 5 min (Figs. $3C_{1,2}$,E, $4B_{1,2}$). During wash-out, both the spontaneous activity as well as the vestibular-evoked modulation of the trochlear nerve discharge remained suppressed for more than 1 hour and only reappeared gradually thereafter (Fig. 4A,B).

Bath application of MS-222 (0.05%; $n=5$) was similarly effective in blocking the trochlear nerve activity (Fig. 3D) as benzocaine. After adding MS-222 to the bath solution, the spontaneous multiple-unit firing rate gradually ceased, reached ~10% of the control value after 5 min and was completely blocked after 15 min for a prolonged period (Fig. $3D_1$,E). In contrast to the relatively rapid blocking effect of this drug on the resting rate in the absence of motion, the peak discharge during roll motion stimulation diminished more slowly and reached ~60% of the control value after 5 min but was completely blocked after 15 min in all experiments (Fig. $3D_{2,3}$,E). During wash-out of MS-222, the spontaneous discharge as well as the motion-evoked firing rate modulation depth recovered slowly and reached 20 and 50%, respectively, of the initial magnitudes after 1 hour (insets in Fig. $3D_{1,3}$) and was generally re-established after 4 hours.

In order to comparatively assess the potency and dynamics of the benzocaine and MS-222-induced reduction of the spontaneous and evoked trochlear nerve discharge, the suppressive influence on motor activity was tested after bath-application of the two drugs at four different concentrations (Fig. 3E). Since benzocaine was dissolved in DMSO, a control application of this solvent in the absence of benzocaine was performed and found to have no influence on the spontaneous and motion-evoked trochlear nerve firing rate ($p=0.880$; Fig. 4A,B). Comparison of the dose-dependency indicated that benzocaine is more potent than MS-222 with regard to spontaneous activity since application of the former drug achieved a complete block of the nerve discharge at lower concentrations compared to the latter (Fig. 3E). However, both drugs effectively and reliably suppressed the spontaneous and evoked extraocular motor activity in a similar time-dependent and reversible manner, consistent with the expected mechanistic action of this class of anesthetic drugs.

## Effect of MS-222 on spontaneous and evoked sensory nerve activity

The clear, dose-dependent and reversible suppressive effect of MS-222 on spontaneous and sensory-evoked extraocular motor responses is likely due to drug actions at multiple levels along the VOR pathway. However, in order to evaluate and isolate the potential suppressive effect of this drugs on the discharge of sensory fibers, a series of experiments was conducted that determined the potency and dynamics of this drug on mechanoreceptor-related (vestibular, lateral line) afferent sensory activity.

**Lateral line nerve activity.** The activity of sensory fibers in the posterior lateral line nerve (PLLN) was recorded as multiple-unit spike discharge in the absence of hydrodynamic stimulation and during induced oscillatory translational motion to lateral line neuromasts on the tail with a sphere (Fig. 5A). The spontaneous firing without sensory stimulation (Fig. $5B_1$) was rather variable between different preparations with an average rate of ~70 Hz (69.5±17.7 Hz; $n=11$), depending on the number of simultaneously sampled units in a given recording. Generation of oscillatory translational water waves across the innervated skin area at 10 Hz (sphere displacement ±150 μm) evoked a rhythmic bursting that was strictly phase-locked to the cyclic stimulus (dashed lines in Fig. $5C_1$) with a peak firing rate of ~140 Hz (143.2±24.2 Hz; $n=19$). Bath application of 0.05% MS-222 (Fig. $5B_1$,$C_1$) significantly reduced the spontaneous as well as the sensory stimulus-evoked firing after 5 min ($p\leq0.0001$, $n=5$) and caused a complete block of the multiple-unit nerve discharge after 15 min (Fig. $5B_2$,$C_2$). The impact of MS-222 was more pronounced on the spontaneous compared to the sensory stimulus-coupled firing, however, the discharge was blocked completely under both conditions (Fig. 5D; n=11). During wash-out, there was recovery of the spontaneous and evoked firing rate after 1 hour (Fig. $5B_{1,2}$,$C_{1,2}$).

**Vestibular nerve afferent activity.** The activity of vestibular sensory afferents in the N.VIII was recorded as multiple-unit spike discharge in the absence of body motion and during sinusoidal horizontal-axis roll stimulation (Fig. 5E). The spontaneous (Fig. $5F_1$) multiple-unit N.VIII afferent firing rate of ~15 Hz (14.7±6.5 Hz; $n=19$) was modulated cyclically

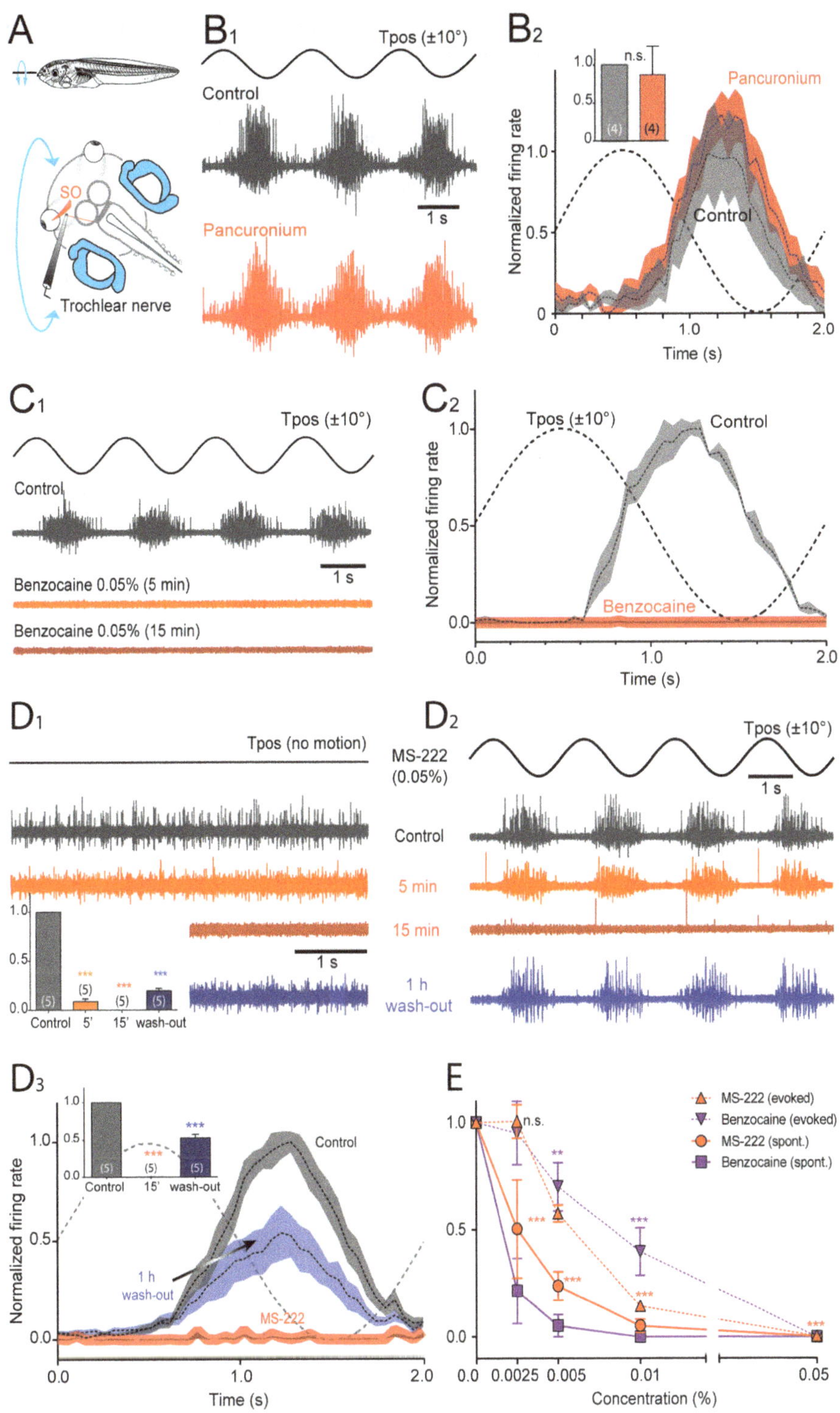


**Figure 3. Effect of pancuronium, benzocaine and MS-222 on extraocular motoneuronal discharge in *Xenopus* tadpoles.** *A*, Schematic of the experimental setting depicting the semi-intact preparation, roll-axis turntable positional changes ($T_{pos}$, 0.5 Hz, ±10°) and extracellular recordings of spontaneous and motion-evoked multiple-unit discharge of the superior oblique (SO) eye muscle-innervating trochlear nerve. ***B-D***, Single sweeps of sinusoidal roll motion (Tpos)-evoked discharge modulation ($B_1$,$C_1$,$D_2$), spontaneous firing of the trochlear nerve ($D_1$) and average firing rate modulation (± SEM, shaded areas) over a single cycle (dashed line; $B_2$,$C_2$,$D_3$) before (Control, gray traces and plots), 5 min (orange traces and plots), 15 min (red traces and plots) and after wash-out (blue traces and plots) of bath-applied pancuronium (0.12 mg/ml, ***B***), benzocaine (0.05%, ***C***) and MS-222 (0.05%, ***D***); inset in $B_2$ shows relative peak firing rates before (gray) and after pancuronium application (red); insets in $D_{1,3}$ show relative resting rates ($D_1$) and peak firing rates during roll motion stimulation ($D_3$) before and during drug application and after wash-out; number of experiments in parentheses in insets; while no significant change (*n.s.*, $p = 0.975$) of the peak firing rate occurred after adding pancuronium to the bath (***B***), benzocaine (***C***) and MS-222 (***D***) blocked the motor responses entirely (***, $p \leq 0.0001$). ***E***, Dose-response curve of benzocaine and MS-222 ($n = 20$, respectively) on spontaneous and motion-triggered peak modulation values of multiple-unit trochlear motor spike discharge.

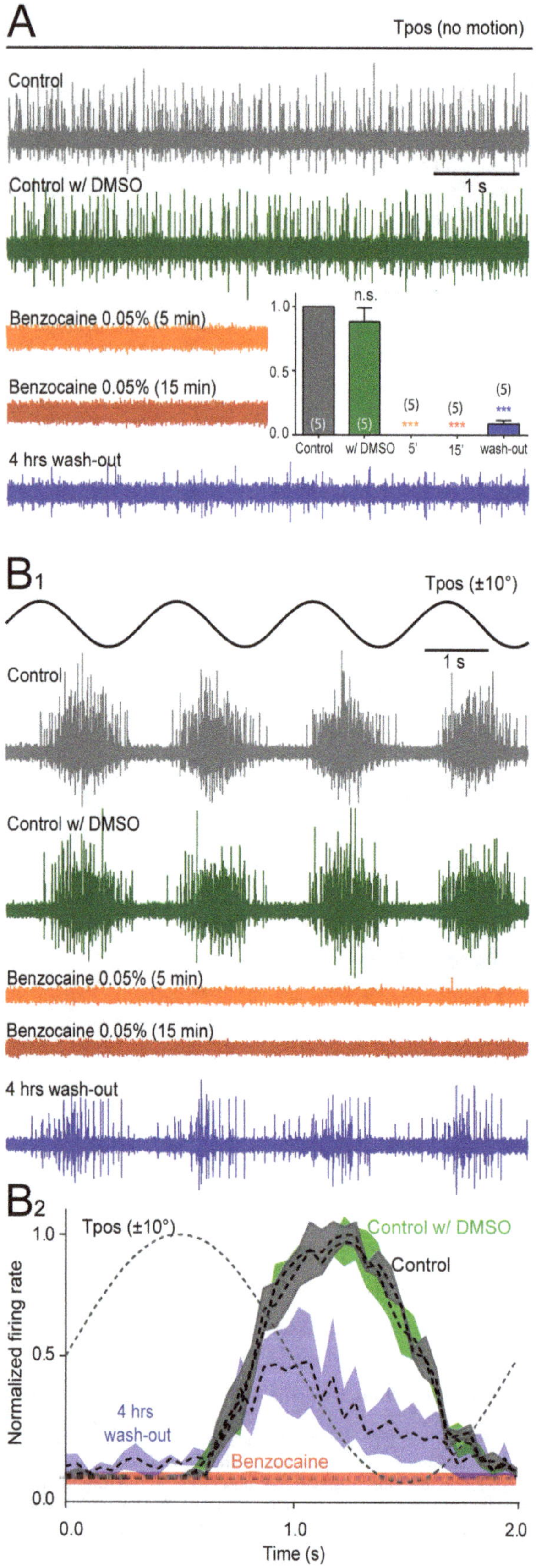


**Figure 4. Effect of benzocaine on extraocular motoneuronal discharge in *Xenopus* tadpoles.** ***A-B***, Single sweeps of spontaneous (***A***), roll motion (Tpos)-evoked (***B₁***) multiple-unit discharge of the superior oblique (SO) eye muscle-innervating trochlear nerve and average firing rate modulation (± SEM, shaded areas; ***B₂***) over a single cycle (dashed line; ***B₂***) before (Control, gray traces and plot), 10 min after application of dimethylsulfoxide (Control w/DMSO, green traces and plot), 5 min (orange traces) and 15 min after application of benzocaine (0.05%; red traces) and four hours after wash-out (blue traces and plot); inset in ***A*** show relative resting rates before (gray), in the presence of DMSO (green), benzocaine (orange and red, complete block) and after wash-out (blue); number of experiments in parentheses; while no significant change (*n.s.*, $p = 0.880$) of the peak firing rate occurred after adding DMSO to the bath, benzocaine (0.05%) blocked the motor responses entirely (***, $p \leq 0.0001$).

(Fig. 5G$_1$) during sinusoidal turntable motion (0.5 Hz, ±10°), reaching an average peak firing rate of ~70 Hz (71.4±17.2 Hz; $n = 19$). Since the N.VIII contains fibers from semicircular canal and otolith organs (Fig. 1B) with in part opposite directional sensitivities (i.e. anterior-posterior vertical canal, utricle), the multiple-unit peak response in the example shown in Fig. 5F,G was in phase with a horizontal-axis table rotation in the ipsi- as well as the contraversive direction ($^{\#}$ and $^{\#\#}$, respectively, in Fig. 5G$_{1,2}$). Application of 0.05% MS-222 (Fig. 5F,G) caused a gradual decrease of the resting rate and roll motion-evoked vestibular afferent firing to 20–30% of the control values after 5 min ($p \leq 0.0001$, $n = 5$) and a complete block of the spike activity after 15 min (Fig. 5F$_{1,2}$,G$_{1-3}$). This effect on the sensory nerve discharge was reversible, however the recovery was only partial after 1 hour wash-out reaching 20–30% of the control value (Fig. 5F,G). Determination of the dose-response curve of MS-222 ($n = 19$) for blocking spontaneous and roll motion-evoked vestibular afferent firing yielded a similar efficacy and dependency as observed for the corresponding lateral line activity (Fig. 5D).

## Discussion

Bath application of MS-222 and benzocaine, at variance with pancuronium, reversibly suppressed spontaneous and naturally evoked extraocular motor commands as well as responses in mechanosensory nerves in semi-intact *Xenopus* preparations in a dose-dependent manner, compatible with a specific block of voltage-dependent $Na^+$-channels by both caine-derivates. The complete block of the discharge in sensory nerves by benzocaine and MS-222, along with the suppression of motoneuronal activity and muscle contractions indicates that these drugs have an analgesic, sedative and paralytic capacity and thus can be used as a single-drug anesthetic for surgical interventions in anamniotes. While the pharmaco-dynamics and efficacy of benzocaine and MS-222 were comparable, the use of an aqueous solution of the latter drug simplifies the anesthesia in fish and amphibians.

### Semi-intact in vitro preparations of Xenopus tadpoles for pharmacological studies of drug-related effects on neural processing and behavioral performance

The outcome of the present study was greatly facilitated by the employment of an isolated semi-intact preparation of *Xenopus* tadpoles that allowed *in vitro* neuropharmacology of a reactive sensory-motor behavior [14]. This preparation combines the advantage of *in vitro* drug testing such as the use of precise concentrations of substances and defined application onsets with the advantage of *in vivo* pharmacology with a specific behavioral readout. Classical pharmacological studies in contrast, are either performed *in vitro* on cell cultures (e.g. [23]), isolated parts of

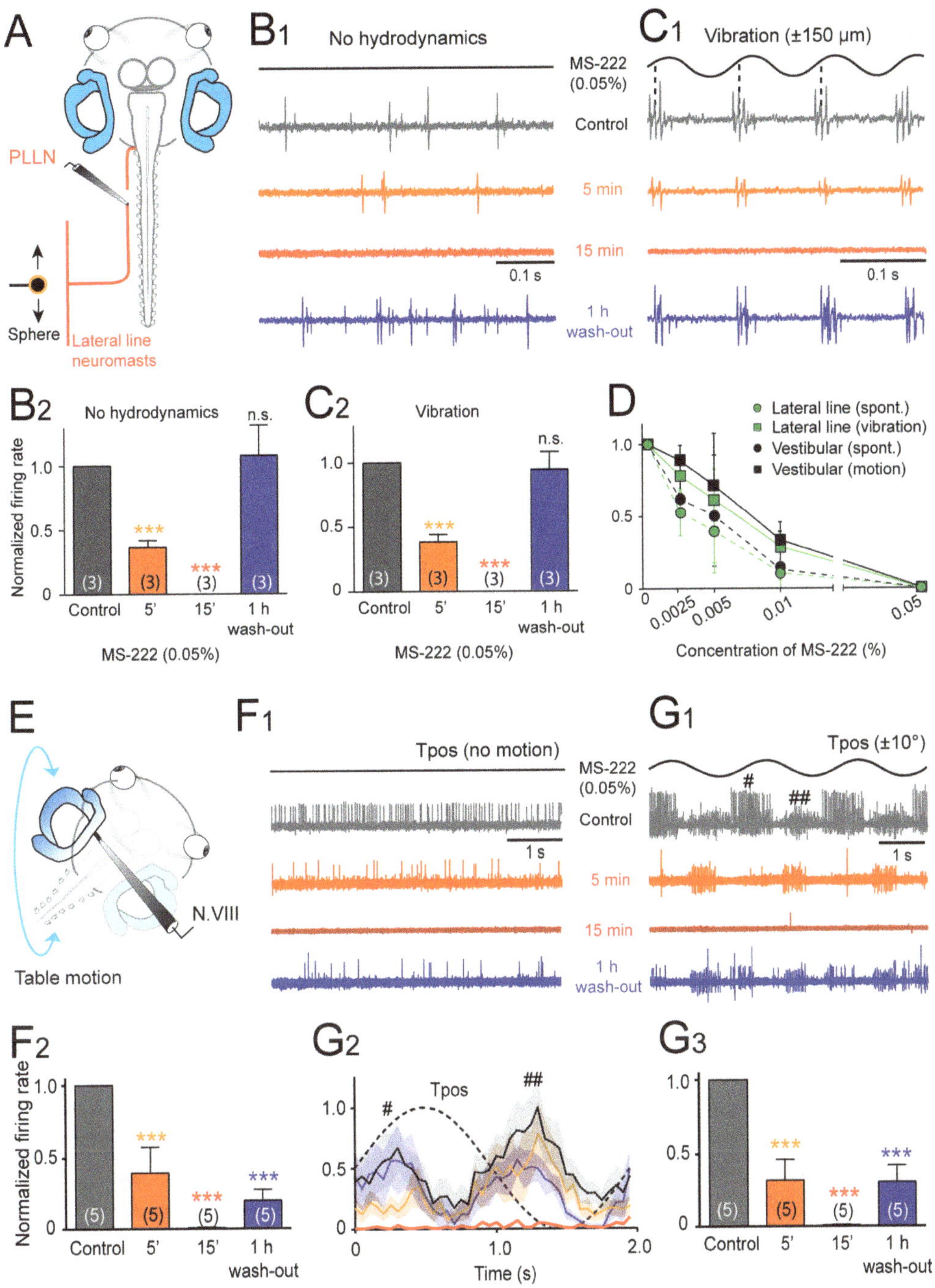


**Figure 5. Effect of MS-222 on the spike discharge of mechanoreceptor sensory afferent fibers in *Xenopus* tadpoles.** ***A***, Schematic of the experimental setting depicting the semi-intact preparation, vibrational stimulation of lateral line neuromasts (10 Hz, ±150 µm) and extracellular recordings of the multiple-unit discharge of the peripheral portion of the posterior lateral line nerve (PLLN). ***B,C***, Single sweeps of spontaneous (***$B_1$***) and vibration-evoked discharge modulation (***$C_1$***) in the PLLN before (Control, gray traces and plots), 5 min (orange traces and plots) and 15 min after bath-application (red traces and plots) and after wash-out (blue traces and plots) of MS-222 (0.05%); relative resting (***$B_2$***) and peak firing rates (***$C_2$***) before, during and after wash-out show the reversible drug effect; number of experiments in parentheses. ***D***, Dose-response curve of MS-222 on multiple-unit spontaneous and sensory stimulus-evoked spike discharge modulation in mechanosensory (lateral line and vestibular) nerve fibers. ***E***, Schematic of the experimental setting depicting the semi-intact preparation, roll-axis turntable positional changes ($T_{pos}$, 0.5 Hz, ±10°) and extracellular recordings of the multiple-unit discharge of the peripheral portion of N.VIII (vestibular). ***F,G***, Single sweeps of spontaneous (***$F_1$***) and roll motion-evoked discharge modulation (***$G_1$***) of the N.VIII and average firing rate modulation (± SEM, shaded areas; *n*=8, respectively) over a single cycle (dashed line; ***$G_2$***) before (Control, gray traces and plots), 5 min (orange traces and plots) and 15 min after bath-application (red traces and plots) and after wash-out (blue traces and plots) of MS-222 (0.05%); $^{\#,\#\#}$ in ***$G_{1,2}$*** indicate activated responses in different nerve fibers by either direction of the sinusoidal roll motion; relative resting (***$F_2$***) and peak firing rates (***$G_3$***) before, during and after wash-out show a complete block and partially reversed drug effect; number of experiments in parentheses; ***, $p \leq 0.0001$; *n.s.*, not significant.

specific organs (e.g. [24]), or *in vivo* by behavioral pharmacology in the intact animal (e.g. [25]). Even though, each of the different methodological approaches has its advantages, all suffer from a variety of drawbacks, including difficulties in consolidating results from both approaches on concentration dependency, mechanistic principles or target sites of a specific drug. Neuroactive drugs usually influence the synaptic transmission or its modulation or impair the generation of action potentials. *In vitro* tests of such drugs, potentially interfering with single cell or network computations, typically employ cell cultures or slice preparations with limited residual interconnectivity between different cell groups [24]. While these studies allow evaluating dose-response curves or mechanistic principles, any inference on the behavioral impact of a particular drug remains difficult and requires additional *in vivo* studies. On the other side, a direct and unrestricted access to the central nervous system following systemic application of a neuroactive substance in intact animals is often prevented by the blood-brain barrier, thus impeding the assessment of behaviorally relevant effects of certain drugs.

While anamniote vertebrate species (fish, amphibians) are considered excellent model systems for drug discovery and testing [26,25], isolated semi-intact preparations of larval or adult amphibians in particular combine many advantages of *in vivo* and *in vitro* approaches [20,14]. The possibility to exploit specific behavioral paradigms, such as locomotion, respiration, vocalization or eye motion *in vitro* [27,28,18] and to record respective outputs as real or fictive motor behavior offers an unprecedented access to the underlying sensory-motor transformations for pharmacological impairment. This is of particular advantage for the evaluation of sites, mechanisms and concentration-dependency of general anesthetic drugs such as the caine-derivates in the current study. The unrestricted access to the central nervous system and the possibility to quantify a behavioral readout in an isolated preparation allowed precisely estimating the impact of the drugs on the spike activity of excitable cells, synaptic transmission and the generation of motor commands within a defined behavioral context. In addition, the intact sensory systems in *Xenopus in vitro* preparations faciliated a direct evaluation of the anesthetic drug effects on the encoding of spontaneous and evoked sensory signals at the first neuronal level. The reduction of spike amplitude and eventual block of the firing is compatible with the known mechanistic impact of caine derivates on voltage-gated $Na^+$ channels [8,29]. The block of $Na^+$ conductances in all cells with excitable membranes (neurons and myocytes) also includes nociceptive sensory afferents, and thus, the employment of an isolated preparation of *Xenopus* tadpoles with intact sensory and motor systems for pharmacological studies provides indirect evidence for the analgesic potency of MS-222, supporting the ubiquitous use of this drug as single substance anesthetic for surgical interventions in fish and amphibians [6].

## Adequate anesthesia/sedation of anamniote vertebrates for surgical interventions

A number of different pharmacological substances, traditionally classified as anesthetics or hypnotic drugs, have been used previously to sedate anamniote vertebrate species for surgical interventions [1]. While anesthetic drugs such as MS-222 or benzocaine block action potentials in excitable cells, typical hypnotic drugs such as benzodiazepines or barbiturates have only indirect antagonizing effects on the spike discharge activity of neurons and neuronal networks. Both of the latter classes of drugs bind to respective sites of the $GABA_A$ receptor, thereby potentiating the effect of GABA [30]. The consequence of a facilitation of the GABAergic inhibition is a sedative or hypnotic effect through a general reduction of neuronal excitability throughout the brain. A concomitant antagonizing influence of barbiturates on the glutamatergic AMPA receptor has been shown to further depress neuronal activity throughout the brain, thereby enhancing the sedative effect [31]. Despite the additional weak effect on nociception, barbiturates, however fail to offer a complete and reliable analgesia and therefore should not be used for surgical interventions in the absence of other analgesic compounds since anamniote vertebrates also possess pain receptors and pathways that are classically involved in the central nervous processing and perception of noxious stimuli [6,32].

Apart from barbiturates and benzodiazepines, a number of anesthetic gases, such as metoxyflurane, halothane or isofluorane [33,34] or injectable drugs including propofol, ketamine or tiletamine [35,36,37,38] have previously been used for sedation in various anamniotes. Most of these sedatives however produce a variable depth and duration of anesthesia with an often unknown or unreliable analgesic effect [6]. While the detailed mode of action for most of these substances remains still unknown, all appear to exert their action through a more or less pronounced interference with various neurotransmitter or neuromodulator systems such as GABA, glycine, glutamate/NMDA or opiate receptors. A block or impairment of the neuronal transmission to various, partly unknown degrees however is inadequate for a reliable achievement and maintenance of a sufficiently deep and long anesthesia including analgesia and muscle relaxation. Thus, based on the broad mode of action that suppress the generation of action potentials in all nerve cells and muscle fibers, local anesthetics such as caine derivates (MS-222, benzocaine) are considerably more reliable and therefore more appropriate for the anesthesia in anamniote vertebrates for surgical interventions.

## MS-222 as potent single-substance anesthetics for anamniotes

In the current experiments on semi-intact *in vitro* preparations, MS-222 induced a complete block of eye motion, underlying extraocular motor commands but most importantly sensory nerve activity after 15 minutes of bath application. Accordingly, MS-222 exhibited classic sedative characteristics similar to ideal anesthetics, which are able to reversibly decrease body movements (paralytic), remove sensation (sedative/hypnotic) and relieve pain (analgesic), particularly during surgical interventions. Most local anesthetics have a similar mechanism of action and consist of a gradual reduction and finally complete block of action potentials [29]. The impairment of spike activity usually starts with small unmyelinated fibers and gradually blocks increasingly larger fibers, which in turn elicit a loss of sensation followed by a loss of motor function and CNS depression [1]. Since pain signals are transmitted in amphibians by small fibers, namely myelinated A-delta and unmyelinated C type fibers [39], there is a distinct advantage for MS-222 to block nociception in these animals at very early stages of drug exposure. Additionally, the duration of the MS-222 anesthesia is concentration/dose- and time-dependent. The concentration of MS-222 gradually increases in cells and tissue depending on the gradient. Since there is a higher extracellular concentration of MS-222, a large amount of the drug is absorbed, causing an increase in the drug effects. Similarly, the duration of exposure positively affects the extent of drug effect; the longer the exposure the longer the anesthetic effect lasts. Due to the accumulation of the drug in tissue and organs, there is a longer elimination time leading to an increased length of recovery time. However, when MS-222 is compared to another caine-derivate, benzocaine, its recovery time is considerably shorter. Since benzocaine is a lipophilic drug [40], it particularly sequesters in fatty tissue from where it is only released slowly and therefore its effects are not as readily reversible as those of MS-222. Thus, this makes MS-222 a very good choice of anesthetics, especially when experimentation requires a quick recovery of physiological function. On the other hand, MS-222 being highly water-soluble can present a problem for drug absorption, as it can be difficult for the drug to cross cell membranes given that they are not very permeable to ionized hydrophilic molecules. Fortunately, amphibians are equipped to readily absorb hydrophilic drugs in solution when submerged since they are capable of aqueous exchange across their gills and skin, at times through aquaporins [12,41]. In fact, the water-solubility of MS-222 in contrast to benzocaine, which requires an organic solvent, is highly beneficial for a simple use in anamniote species. Nonetheless, both drugs have their distinct advantages as anesthetics in fish and amphibians and depending on the particular experimental condition and eco-physiological circumstance, the one or the other might be more appropriate, respectively. With respect to previous estimations of MS-222 for anesthesia, this drug has been proven in the current study to be an excellent single-drug anesthetic that includes appropriate analgesia and muscle relaxation for surgical interventions. MS-222 is thus well suited in particular for multiple anesthesia of individual animals or an employment in novel isolated anamniote experimental *in vitro* preparations [14], given the fact it completely blocks the spike discharge in muscle fibers, motoneurons and sensory neurons.

## Acknowledgments

The authors are grateful for the help of Alexander Knorr with the Matlab software scripts for eye motion analysis and Dr. Tobias Kohl for Spike2 software scripts. The authors thank Haike Dietrich and Sara Hänzi for critically reading the manuscript.

## Author Contributions

Conceived and designed the experiments: CR HS. Performed the experiments: CR FB BPC. Analyzed the data: CR FB BPC. Contributed reagents/materials/analysis tools: CR FB BPC HS. Contributed to the writing of the manuscript: CR FB BPC HS.

## References


1. Cakir Y, Strauch SM (2005) Tricaine (MS-222) is a safe anesthetic compound compared to benzocaine and pentobarbital to induce anesthesia in leopard frogs (*Rana pipiens*). Pharmacol Rep 57: 467–474.
2. Stedman TL (1995) Stedman's medical dictionary. 26th ed. Baltimore: Williams & Wilkins.
3. Parker BM (2006) Anesthetics and anesthesia techniques: impacts on perioperative management and postoperative outcomes. Cleve Clin J Med 73 (Suppl 1): S13.
4. Lalonde-Robert V, Beaudry F, Vachon P (2012) Pharmacologic parameters of MS222 and physiologic changes in frogs (*Xenopus laevis*) after immersion at anesthetic doses. J Am Assoc Lab Anim Sci 51: 464–468.
5. Zahl IH, Samuelsen O, Kiessling A (2012) Anaesthesia of farmed fish: implications for welfare. Fish Physiol Biochem 38: 201–218.
6. Guénette SA, Giroux MC, Vachon P (2013) Pain perception and anesthesia in research frogs. Exp Anim 62: 87–92.
7. Bai CX, Glaaser IW, Sawanobori T, Sunami A (2003) Involvement of local anesthetic binding sites on IVS6 of sodium channels in fast and slow inactivation. Neurosci Lett 337: 41–45.
8. Butterworth JFT, Strichartz GR (1990) Molecular mechanisms of local anesthesia: a review. Anesthesiology 72: 711–734.
9. Nair G, Kim M, Nagaoka T, Olson D, Thulé P, Pardue M, et al. (2011) Effects of common anesthetics on eye movement and electroretinogram. Doc Ophthalmol 122: 163–176.
10. Stockman J, Weber III ESP, Kass PH, Pascoe PJ, Paul-Murphy J (2013) Physiologic and biochemical measurements and response to noxious stimulation at various concentrations of MS-222 in Koi (*Cyprinus carpio*). Vet Anaesth Analg 40: 35–47.
11. Stoskopf M, Posner LP (2008) Anesthesia and analgesia in laboratory animals 2nd ed. San Diego: Academic Press.
12. Palmer LM, Mensinger AF (2004) Effect of the anesthetic tricaine (MS-222) on nerve activity in the anterior lateral line of the oyster toadfish, *Opsanus tau*. J Neurophysiol 92: 1034–1041.
13. Sladky KK, Swanson CR, Stoskopf MK, Loomis MR, Lewbart GA (2001) Comparative efficacy of tricaine methanesulfonate and clove oil for use as anesthetics in red pacu (*Piaractus brachypomus*). Am J Vet Res 62: 337–342.
14. Straka H, Simmers J (2012) *Xenopus laevis*: an ideal experimental model for studying the developmental dynamics of neural network assembly and sensory-motor computations. Dev Neurobiol 72: 649–663.
15. Nieuwkoop PD, Faber J (1994) Normal table of *Xenopus laevis* (Daudin): a systematical and chronological survey of the development from the fertilized egg till the end of metamorphosis. New York: Garland.
16. Lambert FM, Combes D, Simmers J, Straka H (2012) Gaze stabilization by efference copy signaling without sensory feedback during vertebrate locomotion. Curr Biol 22: 1649–1658.
17. Straka H, Dieringer N (1993) Electrophysiological and pharmacological characterization of vestibular inputs to identified frog abducens motoneurons and internuclear neurons *in vitro*. Eur J Neurosci 5: 251–260.
18. Lambert FM, Beck JC, Baker R, Straka H (2008) Semicircular canal size determines the developmental onset of angular vestibuloocular reflexes in larval *Xenopus*. J Neurosci 28: 8086–8096.
19. Straka H, Dieringer N (2004) Basic organization principles of the VOR: lessons from frogs. Prog Neurobiol 73: 259–309.
20. Biesdorf S, Malinvaud D, Reichenberger I, Pfanzelt S, Straka H (2008) Differential inhibitory control of semicircular canal nerve afferent-evoked inputs in second-order vestibular neurons by glycinergic and GABAergic circuits. J Neurophysiol 99: 1758–1769.
21. Beck JC, Gilland E, Baker R, Tank DW (2004) Instrumentation for measuring oculomotor performance and plasticity in larval organisms. Methods Cell Biol 276: 385–413.
22. Su PC, Su WH, Rosen AD (1979) Pre- and postsynaptic effects of pancuronium at the neuromuscular junction of the mouse. Anesthesiology 50: 199–204.
23. Ramlochansingh C, Taylor RE, Tizabi Y (2011) Toxic effects of low alcohol and nicotine combinations in SH-SY5Y cells are apoptotically mediated. Neurotox Res 20: 263–269.
24. Drexler B, Hentschke H, Antkowiak B, Grasshoff C (2010) Organtypic cultures as tools for testing neuroactive drugs - link between *in-vitro* and *in-vivo* experiments. Curr Med Chem 17: 4538–4550.
25. Rihel J, Schier AF (2012) Behavioral screening for neuroactive drugs in zebrafish. Dev Neurobiol 72: 373–385.
26. Wheeler GN, Brändli AW (2009) Simple vertebrate models for chemical genetics and drug discovery screens: lessons from zebrafish and *Xenopus*. Dev Dyn 238: 1237–1308.
27. Combes D, Merrywest SD, Simmers J, Sillar KT (2004) Developmental segregation of spinal networks driving axial- and hindlimb-based locomotion in metamorphosing *Xenopus laevis*. J Physiol 559: 17–24.
28. Zornik E, Kelley DB (2008) Regulation of respiratory and vocal motor pools in the isolated brain of *Xenopus laevis*. J Neurosci 28: 612–621.
29. Arnolds DEW, Zottoli SJ, Adams CE, Dineen SM, Fevrier S, et al. (2002) Physiological effects of tricaine on supramedullary/dorsal neurons of the Cunner, *Tautogolabrus adspersus*. Biol Bull 203: 188–189.
30. Simmonds MA, Turner JP (1987) Potentiators of responses to activation of gamma-aminobutyric acid (GABAA) receptors. Neuropharmacology 26: 923–930.
31. Lodge D, Johnson KM (1990) Noncompetitive excitatory amino acid receptor antagonists. Trends Pharmacol Sci 11: 81–86.
32. Stoskopf MK (1994) Pain and analgesia in birds, reptiles, amphibians and fish. Invest Ophthalmol 35: 775–780.
33. Wass JA, Kaplan HM (1994) Methoxyflurane anesthesia for *Rana pipiens*. Lab Anim Sci 24: 669–671.
34. Smith JM, Stump KC (2000) Isoflurane anesthesia in the African clawed frog (*Xenopus laevis*). Contemp Top Lab Anim Sci 39: 39–42.
35. Letcher J, Durante R (1995) Evaluation of use of tiletamine/zolazepam for anesthesia of bullfrogs and leopard frogs. J Am Vet Med Assoc 207: 80–82.
36. Lafortune M, Mitchell MA, Smith JA (2001) Evaluation of medethomidine, clove oil and propofol for anesthesia of leopard frogs, *Rana pipiens*. J Herpetological Med Surg 11: 13–18.
37. Gentz EJ (2007) Medicine and surgery in amphibians. ILAR 48: 255–259.
38. Guénette SA, Beaudry F, Vachon P (2008) Anesthetic properties of propofol in African clawed frogs (*Xenopus laevis*). J Am Assoc Lab Anim Sci 45: 35–38.
39. Stevens CW (2011) Analgesia in amphibians: preclinical studies and clinical applications. Vet Clin North Am Exot Anim Pract 14: 33–44.
40. Machin KL (1999) Amphibian pain and analgesia. J Zoo Wild Med 30: 2–10.
41. Hasegawa T, Sugawara Y, Suzuki S, Tanaka S (2004) Spatial and temporal expression of the ventral pelvic skin aquaporins during metamorphosis of the tree frog, *Hyla Japonica*. J Membrane Biol 199: 119–126.

12

# Binocular Flash Suppression in the Primary Visual Cortex of Anesthetized and Awake Macaques

**Hamed Bahmani[1,2], Yusuke Murayama[1], Nikos K. Logothetis[1,3], Georgios A. Keliris[1,2]***

**1** Max Planck Institute for Biological Cybernetics, Tübingen, Germany, **2** Bernstein Center for Computational Neuroscience, Tübingen, Germany, **3** Imaging Science and Biomedical Engineering, University of Manchester, Manchester, United Kingdom

## Abstract

Primary visual cortex (V1) was implicated as an important candidate for the site of perceptual suppression in numerous psychophysical and imaging studies. However, neurophysiological results in awake monkeys provided evidence for competition mainly between neurons in areas beyond V1. In particular, only a moderate percentage of neurons in V1 were found to modulate in parallel with perception with magnitude substantially smaller than the physical preference of these neurons. It is yet unclear whether these small modulations are rooted from local circuits in V1 or influenced by higher cognitive states. To address this question we recorded multi-unit spiking activity and local field potentials in area V1 of awake and anesthetized macaque monkeys during the paradigm of binocular flash suppression. We found that a small but significant modulation was present in both the anesthetized and awake states during the flash suppression presentation. Furthermore, the relative amplitudes of the perceptual modulations were not significantly different in the two states. We suggest that these early effects of perceptual suppression might occur locally in V1, in prior processing stages or within early visual cortical areas in the absence of top-down feedback from higher cognitive stages that are suppressed under anesthesia.

**Editor:** Samuel G. Solomon, University College London, United Kingdom

**Funding:** This study was supported by the Max Planck Society and the Bernstein Center for Computational Neuroscience, Tuebingen (grant number FKZ 01GQ1002). The funders had no role in study design, data collection and analysis, decision to publish, or preparation of the manuscript.

**Competing Interests:** The authors have declared that no competing interests exist.

* Email: georgios.keliris@tuebingen.mpg.de

## Introduction

Visual information is processed across a distributed network of interconnected visual areas [1]. The primary visual cortex (V1), being hierarchically the first cortical area receiving information from the eyes through the thalamus, constitutes a cornerstone of the visual system [2,3,4,5,6]. Although V1 has been studied extensively and is arguably the best-understood area in the cerebral cortex, its role in visual awareness remains controversial and has been a subject of intense debate [7,8,9,10,11,12,13].

The use of visual stimuli that induce ambiguous perception has been established as a classical paradigm to identify the neural circuits subserving subjective perception [14,15,16,17,18]. Under these conditions, a single interpretation of the external world cannot be unambiguously achieved. When the brain is presented with such stimuli, typically only one possible interpretation is perceived at a time and after a few seconds the percept switches abruptly to another [18]. Notably, such perceptual alternations occur while the sensory input is kept constant, thus offering a clear dissociation of sensory stimulation and subjective awareness [9,11,14,19,20,21]. Some celebrated examples of such perceptual phenomena include binocular rivalry (BR) and binocular flash suppression (BFS) [22,23,24,25,26,27,28]. Based on many psychophysical studies over decades, the primary visual cortex (V1) was implicated as an important candidate for the site of perceptual suppression during BR [29,30,31,32,33]. However, neurophysiological evidence obtained in monkeys did not corroborate this hypothesis but instead found only a small percentage of neurons that modulated their activity in parallel with the subjective perception of the animals [10,19,34,35,36,37]. In contrast, studies using functional magnetic resonance imaging (fMRI) in humans found that V1 is indeed modulated to a large extent by the subjective percept [12,13,38,39,40].

Possible explanations for this discrepancy include differences in the stimulus configurations, the species tested, and the experimental methodology. In addition, a major difference between many of these studies is the extent to which the subject is involved in attending and consciously reporting the bistable alternations [41,42,43]. Such higher cognitive processes could be based on different mechanisms from those subserving local processes and are only observable in V1 when the subject is awake and behaving [44,45].

In order to disentangle these two processes and investigate the role of the local processing during multistable stimulation, we performed and compared BFS experiments in anesthetized and awake, passively fixating macaques. We conjectured that any effects preserved under anesthesia, in the absence of cognitive feedback from central processes, might reflect local interactions critically involved in the initiation of competition during incongruent stimulation. We found comparable modulations in neural activity as reflected in the multi-unit activity (MUA) and local field potentials (LFPs) in both anesthetized and awake passively fixating animals. Our results suggest that the small significant modulations observed under these non-attentive conditions are arising from circuit mechanisms in early visual areas. It remains to be shown if top-down feedback to V1 engaged during active behavior would elicit larger modulations comparable to the ones previously reported by fMRI.

## Materials and Methods

### Ethics Statement

The experimental and surgical procedures were performed with great care and in full compliance with the German Law for the Protection of Animals, the European Community guidelines for the care and use of laboratory animals (EUVS 86/609/EEC), and the recommendations of the Weatherall report for the use of non-human primates in research (http://www.mrc.ac.uk/Utilities/Documentrecord/index.htm?d=MRC003440). The regional authorities (Regierungspräsidium Tübingen) approved our experimental protocol (Nr. KY1/02) and the institutional representatives for animal protection supervised all procedures. Animals were kept in large cages located adjacent to the training and experimental facilities. Space in these cages allows swinging and jumping, and enrichment equipment such as toys was changed frequently. Group housing was maintained to increase the quality of life by rich visual, olfactory, auditory and social interaction and stimulation for play. Balanced nutrition and regular veterinary care and monitoring, were provided. Chamber implantation and an anatomical scan were performed while the animals were under general anesthesia and aseptic conditions. To alleviate post-surgical pain we administered analgesics for a week after the surgery (see also surgical procedures below). Animals were not sacrificed after the experiments.

### Subjects

Four adult monkeys (*Macaca mulatta*) where used for anesthetized (N = 2; B01 and D01, 6 years old, weighing 10 and 8 kg respectively) and awake (N = 2; D98 and F03, aged 12 and 9 years, weighing 16 and 11 kg respectively) electrophysiological recordings.

### Surgical procedures

Recording chambers were positioned over the operculum in area V1 according to stereotaxic coordinates. This was aided by high-resolution magnetic resonance anatomical imaging. The anatomical scan and recording chamber implantation were done while the animals where under general anesthesia. Details of the procedure can be found elsewhere [37,46].

### Visual stimulation and data acquisition

**Anesthetized experiments.** Data was recorded from two monkeys (B01 and D01) in separate sessions (two sessions for monkey B01, three sessions for monkey D01) under general anesthesia. The procedure is described in detail previously [46]. Balanced anesthesia was maintained with isoflurane (end-tidal 0.3%) and fentanyl (3 µg/kg/hr). Muscle relaxation was achieved with mivacurium chloride (3–6 mg/kg/hr). Physiological parameters were monitored and maintained within the normal physiological range [46].

Visual stimuli were presented binocularly using a SVGA fiber optic system (Avotec, Silent Vision) with a resolution of 800×600 pixels at 60 Hz frame rate. To focus the eyes on the stimulus plane, animals were fitted with eye-lenses (Woehlk-Contact-Linsen). The eyepieces of the presentation system were positioned by using a modified fundus camera (Zeiss RC250) which ensures the alignment of the stimulus center with the fovea of each eye [46]. The size of stimuli varied between 6° to 9° radius in different sessions.

Intracortical recordings were conducted with the Eckhorn multielectrode arrays [47,48]. This allowed us to simultaneously monitor and record from up to 13 sites. Electrodes were $Pt_{90}W_{10}$ wire (20 µm diameter) with a glass coating (80 µm external diameter) and were guided into the brain through the overlying dura mater. During the recordings, a custom-made adaptor was used to distribute the electrodes against the dura in a 4×4 square array, with an inter-electrode spacing of 2.5 mm which separated the neighboring electrode pairs by 2.5 mm, while the pairs on opposite corners had a physical separation of 10.6 mm.

Data collection was controlled by an industrial PC (Advantech) running under the QNX operating system (QNX Software Systems). The broadband signals from each channel were amplified by a factor of 8000 and band-pass filtered between 1 Hz and 5 kHz (Alpha Omega Engineering). The signals were then individually digitized at a rate of 20.83 kHz on a 16-bit analog to digital board (PCI-6052E; National Instruments) and stored on a PC for further analysis using custom software written in MATLAB (The Mathworks Inc.).

**Awake experiments.** Two other animals (D98 and F03) were used in the awake sessions. We recorded spiking activity as well as local field potentials (LFP) from V1 of both monkeys by custom made tetrodes guided to the brain by manually adjustable microdrives (Crist Instrument Co.). We also recorded from a chronically implanted array of tetrodes inside a form-specific titanium chamber over the operculum of one of the monkeys (D98). The recording chambers were from either medical-grade titanium or polyether ether ketone (TECAPEEK; Ensinger GmbH). Details have been described elsewhere [37,49]. The animals were implanted with a scleral search coil [50,51] and their eye movements were monitored online.

Visual stimuli were sinusoidal gratings with different orientations and a typical size of 1°–2° in diameter, displayed using a dedicated graphics workstation (TDZ 2000; Intergraph Systems) running an OpenGL-based stimulation program. Dichoptic presentation of the visual stimuli was through a custom-made stereoscope with two LCD monitors at both sides running at a resolution of 1280×1024 and a 60 Hz refresh rate. After eye calibration and alignment of the displays, a coarse receptive field mapping was performed to position the stimulus for the experiments. The multi-unit responses were put through a sound amplifier (Grass Technologies) so that the experimenter could evaluate the gross location of the receptive fields and the preferences of the multi-unit responses towards different orientations and sizes. Details have been described previously [37].

Multi-unit activity was sampled at 32 kHz, digitized (12 bits), and stored using the Cheetah data acquisition system (Neuralynx) and was defined as the events that exceeded a predefined threshold (25 µV) of the filtered (600 Hz–6 kHz) and digitized signal. LFP signals were recorded after filtering the raw signal using analog band-pass filtering (1 Hz–475 Hz) and digitized at 2 kHz (12 bits).

### Experimental design

To study the relationship between neural activity and perceptual modulations, we used the paradigm of binocular flash suppression (BFS). During this paradigm, a visual stimulus presented to one eye is suppressed from awareness as a result of presenting a different stimulus, referred to as *flash*, to the other eye at the location corresponding to the image to the first eye [26].

In anesthetized experiments, monkeys were presented with blank screen for two seconds in the beginning of each trial. Subsequently, one of the two stimuli was presented alone to either the left or the right eye for two seconds, followed by the onset (flash) of the second stimulus at the corresponding retinal location in the contralateral eye and the simultaneous presentation of both incongruent stimuli for another two seconds until the end of the trial. The two stimuli have been chosen to elicit maximal differences in neural activity based on the average responses to a battery of natural and generic images (N = 50) that were presented to the animal prior to the BFS experiment. The time course of an example trial is depicted in Figure 1A for two stimuli used in our experiments. Figure 1C shows all four possible configurations of BFS conditions (1–4) as well as two control conditions termed physical alternation (5–6). For these conditions, the stimuli are presented congruently across the two eyes producing the same perceptual sequence (in awake conditions) and are used as controls.

The same paradigm was used in awake experiments. The monkeys had to passively fixate on a central fixation point in order to initiate the BFS trial. A fixation point (0.2°) appeared in the center of the screen for 300 milliseconds followed by flash

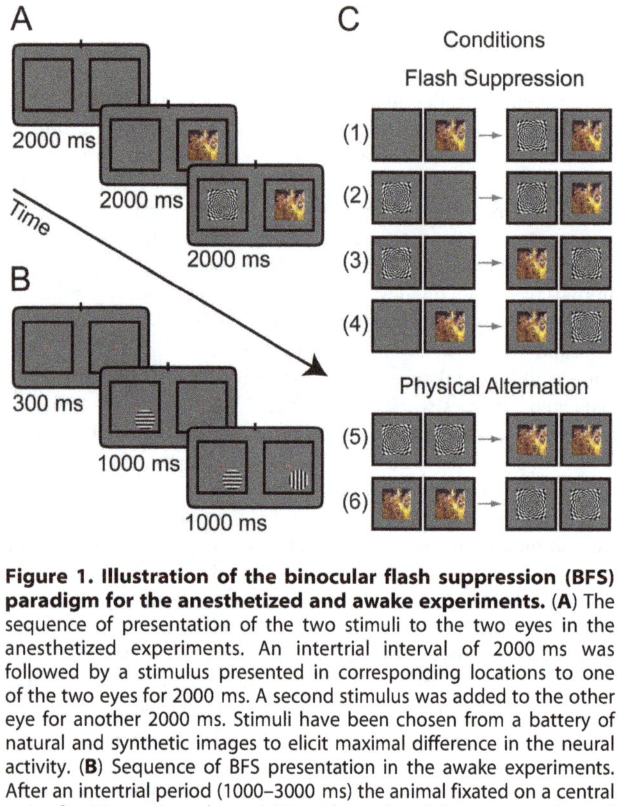


**Figure 1. Illustration of the binocular flash suppression (BFS) paradigm for the anesthetized and awake experiments. (A)** The sequence of presentation of the two stimuli to the two eyes in the anesthetized experiments. An intertrial interval of 2000 ms was followed by a stimulus presented in corresponding locations to one of the two eyes for 2000 ms. A second stimulus was added to the other eye for another 2000 ms. Stimuli have been chosen from a battery of natural and synthetic images to elicit maximal difference in the neural activity. **(B)** Sequence of BFS presentation in the awake experiments. After an intertrial period (1000–3000 ms) the animal fixated on a central point for 300 ms in order to initiate the trial and then monocular and binocular stimuli followed similar to **A**. Stimulus presentation times were 1000 ms and the stimuli were static sinusoidal gratings with orthogonal orientations optimized to elicit maximal (preferred orientation) and minimal (non-preferred orientation) responses in the recorded channels. The position of the stimuli was chosen to cover the receptive fields of the recorded sites and the sizes of the stimuli were 1°–3°. The animal fixated within a window with radius 0.5° around a small point throughout the trial to receive juice reward. Unsuccessful trials were aborted and not further analyzed. **(C)** Different possible configurations of BFS and control conditions. Left and right columns present the monocular and binocular periods respectively. Note that the four different flash suppression conditions can be split in two pairs (1–2 and 3–4) with identical stimulus presentation across the different eyes albeit different perceptual outcomes depending on the initial monocular stimulus (see methods). Physical alternation conditions (5–6) demonstrate an identical perceptual experience albeit without binocular conflict and serve as controls.

suppression stimulation similar to anesthetized condition but with a duration of one second for each period (Fig. 1B). Stimuli were static sinusoidal gratings with orthogonal orientations optimized to elicit maximal differences between the responses to the two orientations. The sizes of the stimuli were 1°–3°, covering the receptive fields of the recorded sites. A drop of juice was delivered to the animal if it maintained the fixation throughout the trial. For more details see [37].

### Statistical and data analysis

We used custom programs written in Matlab (The Mathworks Inc.) for data analysis. Statistical significance ($P<0.05$) of physical and perceptual modulations was assessed by using a nonparametric Wilcoxon rank sum test for equal medians. For all the comparisons, we excluded the first 500 ms after the flash to avoid initial transient biases. We then calculated the preference and modulation indices by using discriminability index ($d'$). This was defined as:

$$d' = \frac{\mu_A - \mu_B}{\sqrt{(\sigma_A^2 + \sigma_B^2)/2}}$$

Where $\mu$ and $\sigma$ are the mean response and the standard deviation of the conditions put in the comparison. In this paper, we report the $d'$ indices for either pairs of binocularly presented identical stimuli (referred to as sensory preference $d'_{sens}$) or incongruent stimuli (referred to as perceptual preference $d'_{perc}$). Bigger values of $d'$ indices indicate larger discriminability of responses and thus larger preference to one of the conditions being compared.

To estimate the time-courses of neural adaptation to prolonged presentation of the preferred stimulus we fitted exponentials of the form $y = a + b \cdot e^{-t/\tau}$ to the data of the monocular period.

## Results

### Perceptual modulation of multi-unit activity

We recorded neural activity from V1 of four macaques being either under general anesthesia (B01 and D01), or awake, passively fixating (D98 and F03). This allows the comparison of neural activity in the anesthetized and awake brains during the BFS task, which in awake conditions, ensures robust perceptual suppression of a monocular stimulus upon asynchronous presentation of a second stimulus to the other eye (see Materials and Methods for details). Recordings were performed with the Eckhorn multi-electrode arrays and custom made tetrodes. Unless otherwise specified, statistical tests were performed using a Wilcoxon two-sided rank sum test with a critical value of 0.05.

During anesthetized experiments, we recorded multi-unit activity from 33 electrode penetrations in two monkeys. In monkey B01, 13 electrodes were used in a single experimental session while in monkey D01, 10 electrodes were used in two separate sessions. From the total of 33 MUAs in two monkeys, 31 (94%) were visually responsive. Out of these, 29 showed significant tuning to the physical alternation conditions as measured by the $d'$ index (see Materials and Methods). Twenty multi-unit sites (two non-tuned during physical alternation) showed significant modulations across at least one pair of binocular incongruent conditions with the same stimulus configuration. Note that these conditions elicit different percepts in awake subjects and we will refer to them as "perceptual" modulations but keep in mind that the animal was anesthetized. Some examples of significantly modulating sites are presented in Figure 2. On average, the magnitude of the perceptual modulations was substantially smaller $\bar{d}'_{perc} = 0.40 \pm 0.05 < \bar{d}'_{sens} = 1.75 \pm 0.18$

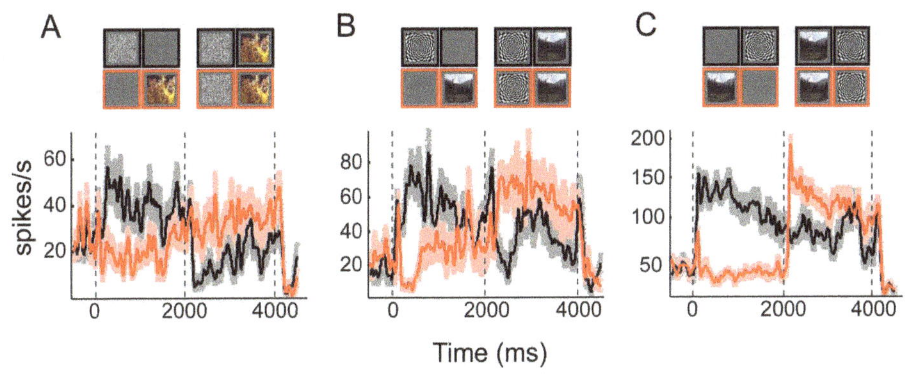


**Figure 2. Examples of multi-unit modulations during binocular flash suppression in anesthetized monkeys (A–C).** The spike-density functions of three example multi-units are shown (A from monkey B01, B–C from monkey D01). Upper diagrams on each panel demonstrate the conditions with corresponding color outlines as the spike density functions below. The conditions contrasted in each case had the same stimulus during the binocular period but notably predict different percepts in awake subjects. Note the significant modulations during the binocular (same stimulus) conditions that are, however, smaller than the preference during the monocular presentation. The shaded areas represent SEM across trials. Time zero was defined to be the onset of the monocular stimuli.

[$\mu$+SEM] in comparison to the physical alternation period ($p = 1.8\times10^{-8}$, one-tailed two-sample T-test, N = 31 visually responsive sites).

For awake experiments, we analyzed the spiking activity recorded from two other animals (D98 and F03). Analysis of the single unit activity of these two animals has been published elsewhere [37]; here we report multi-unit activity (MUA) and compare it with MUA from the anesthetized experiments. From a total of 393 multi-units, 364 were visually responsive (92%) and 275 units showed sensory tuning to the visual stimuli. Perceptual modulations were found in 88 of these sites. As in the anesthetized, the magnitude of the perceptual modulations was substantially smaller $\bar{d}'_{perc} = 0.25 \pm 0.01 < \bar{d}'_{sens} = 1.52 \pm 0.08$ [$\mu$+SEM] in comparison to the physical alternation period ($p \approx 0$, one-tailed two-sample T-test, N = 364 visually responsive sites).

## Comparison between the two conscious states

To study the effect of unconsciousness (during anesthesia) on perceptual modulations during flash suppression, we compared the spiking activity in anesthetized monkeys with those of their awake counterparts. Differences between the two conditions could potentially be also attributed to differences in experimental design and indirect influences of anesthesia (but see Discussion).

Figure 3 compares the activity for the population of multi-units across the two conscious states. A small but significant modulation was present in both the anesthetized and awake states during the flash suppression period (Fig. 3B, D). Furthermore, the relative amplitudes of the perceptual modulations as measured by the ratio of perceptual to sensory $|d'|$ were not significantly different for the two states. This was on average 28% and 25% of the sensory modulation in anesthetized and awake conditions respectively (across significantly modulating sites in both animals in each conscious state, N = 84 in awake and N = 18 in anesthetized). The close similarity between the relative amplitude of modulations in the two conditions suggests similar mechanisms for these two states.

Table 1 summarizes the numbers and percentages of significant modulations for both conscious states. We tested if the proportion of perceptually modulating sites (PM) was significantly different in anesthetized and awake macaques (two-sampled t-test between proportions, t-value 4.924, $p < 10^{-5}$). This was on average 65% in anesthetized (20/31 recorded units with a 95% C.I. of 48–81%,

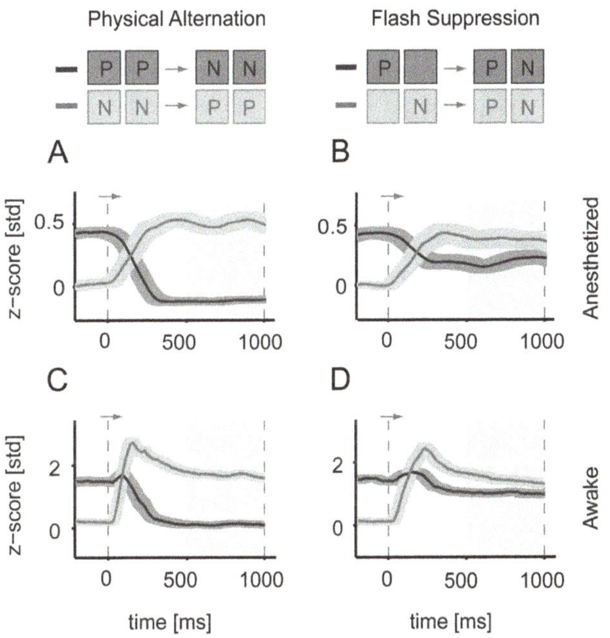


**Figure 3. Population responses of neurons during physical alternation and binocular flash suppression conditions in anesthetized (A,B) and awake (C,D) monkeys.** Different conditions are depicted on top of the panels with corresponding shaded outlines as the spike density functions below. Eyes are presented with preferred (P) and non-preferred (N) stimuli. Left group on the top are the two conditions of physical alternation and rightward the two flash suppression conditions eliciting the same perceptual sequence. (**A**) Population activity in z-scores during physical alternation conditions and (**B**) during binocular flash suppression in anesthetized monkey for all visually responsive multi-units (N = 31) in anesthetized experiments. Prior to averaging, conditions were sorted to preferred (P) and non-preferred (N) according to the responses during the monocular presentation. (**C,D**) the same as **A** and **B**, but in awake passively fixating monkeys. In all four panels, dark lines represent the responses to the preferred stimulus followed by non-preferred stimulus after the flash. Lighter gray lines represent the responses to the non-preferred stimulus first followed by the responses to the preferred in the second period. The shaded areas around the lines represent SEM across sites. Time zero was defined to be the time of the flash or switch of the stimuli.

**Table 1.** Numbers and percentages of significant modulations.

| | | Anesthetized | Awake |
|---|---|---|---|
| T | Total # of multi-units/recorded sites | 33 | 393 |
| VR | Visually responsive (% of T) | 31 (94%) | 364 (92%) |
| SM | Sensory stimulus modulation (% VR) | 29 (94%) | 275 (76%) |
| PM | Perceptual stimulus modulation (% VR) | 20 (65%) | 88 (24%) |
| PaS | Perceptual & sensory (% PM) | 18 (90%) | 84 (95%) |
| xP | Only perceptual (% PM) | 2 (10%) | 4 (5%) |

The absolute numbers and respective percentages of significant modulations are presented for multi-unit activities (MUA) in the two conscious states. In the first row (T) the total numbers of multi-units/recorded-sites are reported. The second row (VR) presents the number (percentage) of sites that showed significant visual responses. The third row (SM) presents the number of sites that were responding differentially two the different congruent stimuli (sensory modulation) and the fourth row (PM) the number of sites that showed differential responses under the different perceptual conditions (under the same stimulus) as a percentage of visually responsive units/sites. Note the significant difference in PM between the two conditions. In the last two rows, PaS presents the numbers of perceptually modulating sites that showed, in addition, sensory modulations and xP presents the numbers of sites that showed exclusively perceptual modulations.

Bernoulli distribution), which was higher than the average of 24% in awake macaques (88/364 recorded units with 95% C.I. of 20–29%, Bernoulli distribution).

## Flash suppression and adaptation

Neural adaptation is an inherent potential complication of the binocular flash suppression (BFS). The different history of stimulation leading to the two alternative percepts can introduce differences in the level of adaptation in the neural populations encoding the competing stimuli. However, a simple model of adaptation cannot explain the responses of V1 neurons during BFS. To examine this, we estimated the time course of adaptation of the first stimulus (preferred) for the whole duration of a trial by fitting an exponential to the data during the monocular presentation (see Materials and Methods). We found that the parallel presentation of the non-preferred stimulus during BFS introduces additional suppression compared to the estimated level of activity predicted by adaptation (Fig. 4). The time constants of adaptation ($\tau$) were $\tau_{aw} = 225$ ms for the awake while for the anesthetized adaptation was slower with $\tau_{an} = 546$ ms. These results demonstrate that interocular and/or stimulus interactions beyond adaptation are taking place and contribute to the perceptual modulations during incongruent stimulation. Similar interactions were also present at the level of single neurons reported in a previous study (see figure 10 in [37]).

## Modulations of the local field potentials

We acquired local field potentials from 33 recording sites in three anesthetized experiments. Similar to the awake results reported previously [37], the power of the gamma frequency range of the LFP (24–90 Hz) showed an increase shortly after the stimulus onset. Also, a preference for the stimulus was observed in 26 recording sites during congruent stimulation. During the incongruent presentation, however, only one third of recording sites (11/33) showed a significant difference in perceptual modulation. Similar to the MUAs, this difference was substantially smaller than sensory tuning of the LFPs (Fig. 5).

Lower frequency LFP power (1–12 Hz) showed a significant increase in oscillatory activity after stimulus onset in only 14 of 33 recording sites. Sensory tuning to the stimulus was observed in the same fraction of recording sites (14). During the dichoptic phase (perceptual suppression), this difference was significant in only 4 recording sites of one of the animals (B03). These results indicate that perceptual modulations of the lower band of the LFP in V1 are essentially absent in anesthetized conditions, similar to the awake passively fixating animals reported previously [37].

## Discussion

The neural correlates of visual awareness have been attracting scientists' interest for decades. In particular, the role of primary visual cortex (V1) in perceptual rivalry has been a subject of intense debate [7,8,52]. On one hand, psychophysical data and the hierarchical position of V1 in the visual system initially suggested that perceptual suppression is resolved at the level of V1 through interocular competition between the two monocular channels [29,32,33]. Electrophysiological recordings from multiple visual areas in the brain including V1, on the other hand, provided evidence for competition happening at higher visual areas presumably between internal representations of stimuli rather than information from monocular channels in V1 [10,14,19,36]. In a comprehensive review, Blake and Logothetis discussed supporting evidence for each of these alternatives and proposed a hybrid model of rivalry which involves both mechanisms of local and global processing at different hierarchical levels [11]. This model gained further support by a number of psychophysical and computational studies [53,54,55,56].

Local and global processing in V1 could be based on different mechanisms. Feedback signals from extrastriate visual areas modulate V1 activity extensively. The density of such feedback projections is as much as or larger than the feedforward afferents [57]. For example, top-down attention is a process that could be mediated via such projections and has been shown to modulate V1 activity [58,59,60,61,62]. In a series of fMRI studies in human, perceptual suppression has also been found to strongly modulate BOLD activity in primary visual cortex [12,13]. In addition, we have shown previously that the activity of some single cells in V1 also shows significant modulations during perceptual suppression induced by BFS [37]. However, only a small proportion of neurons in V1 showed these effects and importantly the amplitude of perceptual modulations was very small in comparison to the sensory preference. One possible explanation for the difference between the strength of modulations in area V1 of human and monkeys is the extent to which the subjects were asked to consciously attend to the stimuli [41,63]. It is conceivable that the effects recorded by fMRI in humans reflect top-down modulations mediated by changes in attentional state and/or the active employment of the subject in the task instead of directly reflecting the competition happening at the level of V1 circuitry

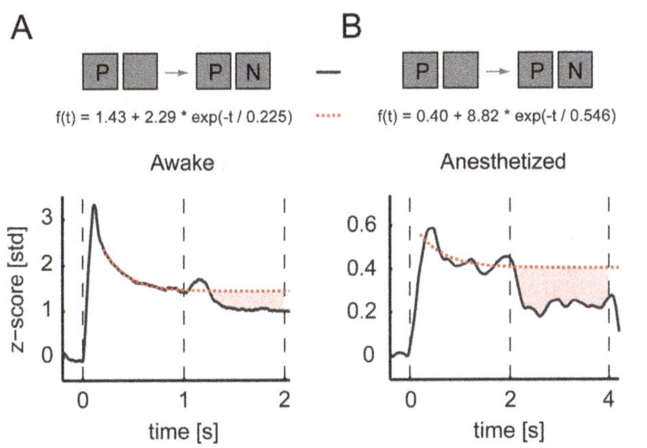


**Figure 4. Effects of adaptation.** (**A**) The suppression caused by the presence and perception of the non-preferred stimulus (N) compared with a modeled (red-dashed line) continuous presentation of the preferred stimulus (P) in awake experiments and (**B**) in anesthetized experiments. Shaded red areas indicate the additional suppression caused by interocular and/or stimulus interactions beyond adaptation.

[39,41,64,65]. On the contrary, most monkey electrophysiology studies used paradigms with animals passively fixating not directly being engaged in reporting the perceptual transitions.

Two studies that did require the monkeys to report their subjective perception also reported small percentages of neurons showing spike rate modulations [10,35]. Note, however, that these studies used different stimulus paradigms and could potentially underestimate the effects. The first study by Leopold and Logothetis, 1996 used binocular rivalry (BR). Although BR has many advantages over BFS, the variability in the animal reaction times is expected to smooth the average triggered responses thereby underestimating the effect. The second study by Wilke et al., 2006 used generalized flash suppression (GFS) that notably involves no direct interocular interaction of corresponding retinal locations. Critically, the effectiveness of GFS depends on parameters like the distance of the surround stimuli to the target, the density etc. (see [66]). The authors adjusted the parameters so that the target would disappear only in about 50% of the trials. This means that the suppression-inducing stimulus was not as potent as in the case of BFS, for which suppression happens essentially in 100% of the trials [37], and therefore could also underestimate the effect.

In the present study, we compared neural activity in V1 during binocular flash suppression in anesthetized and awake monkeys to shed light on the mechanisms of perceptual suppression. Some aspects of global processing such as the attentive and conscious analysis of a scene have been observed in V1 only in awake and perceiving animals [64,67,68]. We conjectured that if the small effects observed in previous electrophysiological studies are due to influences from central processes these modulations should be eliminated under anesthesia. However, we found significant modulations of the multi-unit activity recorded in V1 of anesthetized macaques during binocular flash suppression. These modulations were small, albeit comparable to those observed in passively fixating awake animals. This suggests that these effects are arising from early processes that initiate the competition between monocular channels and do not necessarily need consciousness.

The effects of anesthesia on consciousness are controversial. Anesthesia disrupts cortical integration [69] which is associated

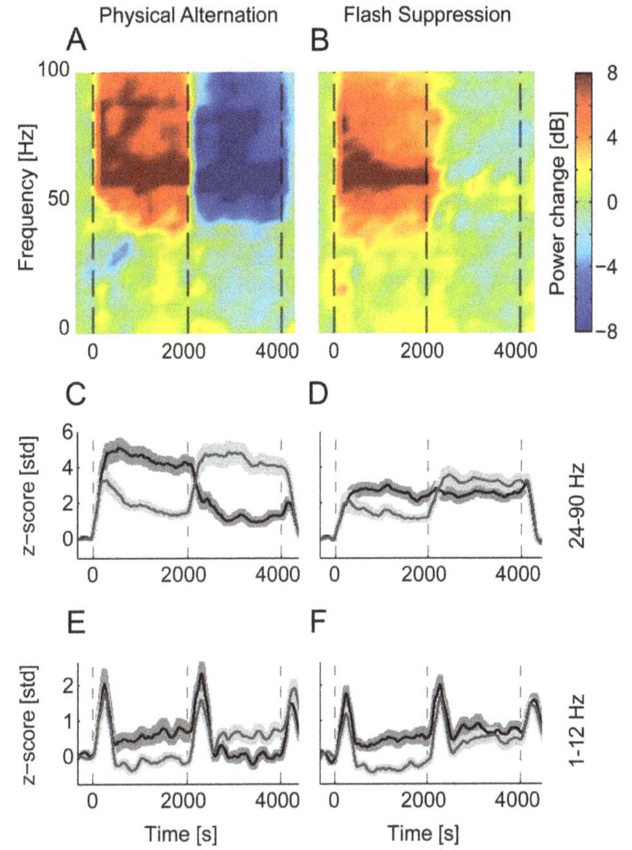


**Figure 5. Population average of the local field potentials (LFP) of all visually responsive sites (anesthetized experiments).** (**A**) The average difference in the spectrogram between the two conditions during physical alternation periods and (**B**) during flash suppression conditions. Spectrograms are plotted only for frequencies below 100 Hz. (**C,D**), Time domain band-passed average of the gamma-band frequencies (24–90 Hz) for physical alternation and flash suppression conditions. (**E,F**), Time domain average of the lower frequency bands (1–12 Hz), during physical and perceptual alternations, respectively.

with unconsciousness. In particular, it abolishes contextual and attentional modulation of firing, presumably mediated by feedback connections [70]. In this study, we employed an optimized protocol for balanced anesthesia that allows robust and reproducible activation of primary visual cortex and a number of extrastriate visual areas, including areas in the superior temporal sulcus [46]; however, cognitive signals like top-down attention and post-perceptual feedback to early visual areas were presumably suppressed in this state. Given the similarly small magnitudes of perceptual modulation during the awake, passively fixating condition and the anesthetized condition, we suggest that such cognitive signals from task-related central processes are a key ingredient of the larger modulations that have been observed in human V1 by fMRI.

Furthermore, we found that the proportion of perceptually modulating sites during wakefulness was significantly lower than that under anesthesia. We note that this result should be interpreted with caution as the difference could be attributed to several potential confounds such as stimulus differences and biases in electrode positioning. Another possible explanation is that processing during awake stimulation conditions might be actively reducing perceptual modulations e.g. by decorrelating the neuronal ensembles involved in the competition. For example, neuromodulatory processes like attention have been shown to decrease correlated variability in neuronal populations [71,72,73]. Such active gain mechanisms can largely change spiking correlations [74]. Such processes can enrich the information carried by neuronal populations in V1 and at the same time reduce bottom-up competition as reflected in perceptual modulations in multi-unit sites. Alternatively, this difference could be arising from factors that are not inherently related to perception.

In a recent study, Wilke and colleagues demonstrated that the low frequencies of the LFP in the thalamus show robust perceptual modulations only if the animals are actively reporting their percept and are eliminated when the animals passively fixate [75]. Similarly, our previous study in passively fixating animals found negligible perceptual modulations of the LFP at this frequency range [37]. Here, we found that lower frequency LFPs in anesthetized V1 were also not predictive of the percept consistent with the hypothesis that active engagement of the animal in the task might be necessary. Given the relationship between the BOLD signal and the LFP [76], it is conceivable that strong BOLD activation in V1 during binocular rivalry in humans is more likely related to the feedback from higher cognitive central stages. However, differences in the nature of the read-out signals could be still a possible explanation for these differences.

Our results confirm that V1 is involved in the process of perceptual suppression during interocular incongruent stimulation and we suggest that it plays a role in initiating the competition. This process is independent of the feedback from higher areas when the subject is not consciously involved in the task. It remains to be shown if a more pronounced and robust modulation of V1 is present during an active task, which can be eliminated under anesthesia or a no-task, passive fixation condition.

## Acknowledgments

We thank Drs. David Leopold and Andreas Tolias for their help in the experimental design and data acquisition. Joachim Werner and Axel Oeltermann provided excellent technical support. This work was supported by the Max-Planck Society and the Bernstein Center for Computational Neuroscience, Tuebingen (BMBF; FKZ: 01GQ1002).

## Author Contributions

Conceived and designed the experiments: GAK NKL YM. Performed the experiments: GAK YM. Analyzed the data: HB GAK. Contributed reagents/materials/analysis tools: HB GAK YM NKL. Wrote the paper: HB GAK.

## References

1. Felleman DJ, Van Essen DC (1991) Distributed hierarchical processing in the primate cerebral cortex. Cereb Cortex 1: 1–47.
2. Hubel DH, Wiesel TN (1962) Receptive fields, binocular interaction and functional architecture in the cat's visual cortex. J Physiol 160: 106–154.
3. Hubel DH, Wiesel TN (1977) Ferrier lecture. Functional architecture of macaque monkey visual cortex. Proc R Soc Lond B Biol Sci 198: 1–59.
4. Gilbert CD (1993) Circuitry, architecture, and functional dynamics of visual cortex. Cereb Cortex 3: 373–386.
5. Angelucci A, Bressloff PC (2006) Contribution of feedforward, lateral and feedback connections to the classical receptive field center and extra-classical receptive field surround of primate V1 neurons. Prog Brain Res 154: 93–120.
6. Sincich LC, Horton JC (2005) The circuitry of V1 and V2: integration of color, form, and motion. Annu Rev Neurosci 28: 303–326.
7. Crick F, Koch C (1995) Are we aware of neural activity in primary visual cortex? Nature 375: 121–123.
8. Pollen DA (1995) Cortical areas in visual awareness. Nature 377: 293–295.
9. Logothetis NK (1998) Single units and conscious vision. Philos Trans R Soc Lond B Biol Sci 353: 1801–1818.
10. Leopold DA, Logothetis NK (1996) Activity changes in early visual cortex reflect monkeys' percepts during binocular rivalry. Nature 379: 549–553.
11. Blake R, Logothetis NK (2002) Visual competition. Nat Rev Neurosci 3: 13–21.
12. Tong F, Engel SA (2001) Interocular rivalry revealed in the human cortical blind-spot representation. Nature 411: 195–199.
13. Polonsky A, Blake R, Braun J, Heeger DJ (2000) Neuronal activity in human primary visual cortex correlates with perception during binocular rivalry. Nat Neurosci 3: 1153–1159.
14. Leopold DA, Logothetis NK (1999) Multistable phenomena: changing views in perception. Trends Cogn Sci 3: 254–264.
15. Logothetis NK (1999) Vision: a window on consciousness. Sci Am 281: 69–75.
16. Rock I (1995) Perception: Scientifc American Library.
17. Rock I, Hall S, Davis J (1994) Why do ambiguous figures reverse? Acta Psychol (Amst) 87: 33–59.
18. Attneave F (1971) Multistability in perception. Sci Am 225: 63–71.
19. Logothetis NK, Schall JD (1989) Neuronal correlates of subjective visual perception. Science 245: 761–763.
20. Pitts MA, Nerger JL, Davis TJ (2007) Electrophysiological correlates of perceptual reversals for three different types of multistable images. J Vis 7: 6.
21. Ramachandran VS, Anstis SM (1985) Perceptual organization in multistable apparent motion. Perception 14: 135–143.
22. DuTour M (1760) Discussion d'une question d'optique [Discussion on a question of optics]. Memoires de Mathematique et de Physique Presentes par Divers Savantes. Paris: Academie des Sciences.
23. Wheatstone C (1838) On some remarkable, and hitherto unobserved, phenomena of binocular vision. Philos Trans R Soc Lond B Biol Sci 128: 371–394.
24. Breese BB (1899) On inhibition. Psychol Rev 3: 1–65.
25. Breese BB (1909) Binocular Rivalry. Psychol Rev 16: 410–415.
26. Wolfe JM (1984) Reversing ocular dominance and suppression in a single flash. Vision Res 24: 471–478.
27. Tsuchiya N, Koch C (2005) Continuous flash suppression reduces negative afterimages. Nat Neurosci 8: 1096–1101.
28. Tsuchiya N, Koch C, Gilroy LA, Blake R (2006) Depth of interocular suppression associated with continuous flash suppression, flash suppression, and binocular rivalry. J Vis 6: 1068–1078.
29. Blake R (1989) A neural theory of binocular rivalry. Psychol Rev 96: 145–167.
30. Abadi RV (1976) Induction masking–a study of some inhibitory interactions during dichoptic viewing. Vision Res 16: 269–275.
31. Cogan AI (1987) Human binocular interaction: towards a neural model. Vision Res 27: 2125–2139.
32. Blake R, Tadin D, Sobel KV, Raissian TA, Chong SC (2006) Strength of early visual adaptation depends on visual awareness. Proc Natl Acad Sci U S A 103: 4783–4788.
33. Lehky SR (1988) An astable multivibrator model of binocular rivalry. Perception 17: 215–228.
34. Gail A, Brinksmeyer HJ, Eckhorn R (2004) Perception-related modulations of local field potential power and coherence in primary visual cortex of awake monkey during binocular rivalry. Cereb Cortex 14: 300–313.
35. Wilke M, Logothetis NK, Leopold DA (2006) Local field potential reflects perceptual suppression in monkey visual cortex. Proc Natl Acad Sci U S A 103: 17507–17512.
36. Sheinberg DL, Logothetis NK (1997) The role of temporal cortical areas in perceptual organization. Proc Natl Acad Sci U S A 94: 3408–3413.
37. Keliris GA, Logothetis NK, Tolias AS (2010) The role of the primary visual cortex in perceptual suppression of salient visual stimuli. J Neurosci 30: 12353–12365.
38. Yuval-Greenberg S, Heeger DJ (2013) Continuous flash suppression modulates cortical activity in early visual cortex. J Neurosci 33: 9635–9643.
39. Maier A, Wilke M, Aura C, Zhu C, Ye FQ, et al. (2008) Divergence of fMRI and neural signals in V1 during perceptual suppression in the awake monkey. Nat Neurosci 11: 1193–1200.
40. Lee SH, Blake R (2002) V1 activity is reduced during binocular rivalry. J Vis 2: 618–626.
41. Watanabe M, Cheng K, Murayama Y, Ueno K, Asamizuya T, et al. (2011) Attention but not awareness modulates the BOLD signal in the human V1 during binocular suppression. Science 334: 829–831.
42. Zhang P, Jamison K, Engel S, He B, He S (2011) Binocular rivalry requires visual attention. Neuron 71: 362–369.
43. Brascamp JW, Blake R (2012) Inattention abolishes binocular rivalry: perceptual evidence. Psychological Science 23: 1159–1167.
44. Lamme VA, Spekreijse H (2000) Modulations of primary visual cortex activity representing attentive and conscious scene perception. Front Biosci 5: D232–243.
45. Lamme VAF, Zipser K, Spekreijse H (1998) Figure-ground activity in primary visual cortex is suppressed by anesthesia. Proceedings of the National Academy of Sciences of the United States of America 95: 3263–3268.
46. Logothetis NK, Guggenberger H, Peled S, Pauls J (1999) Functional imaging of the monkey brain. Nat Neurosci 2: 555–562.

47. Leopold DA, Murayama Y, Logothetis NK (2003) Very slow activity fluctuations in monkey visual cortex: Implications for functional brain imaging. Cerebral Cortex 13: 422–433.
48. Eckhorn R, Thomas U (1993) A new method for the insertion of multiple microprobes into neural and muscular tissue, including fiber electrodes, fine wires, needles and microsensors. J Neurosci Methods 49: 175–179.
49. Tolias AS, Ecker AS, Siapas AG, Hoenselaar A, Keliris GA, et al. (2007) Recording chronically from the same neurons in awake, behaving primates. Journal of Neurophysiology 98: 3780–3790.
50. Robinson DA (1963) A Method of Measuring Eye Movement Using a Scleral Search Coil in a Magnetic Field. IEEE Trans Biomed Eng 10: 137–145.
51. Judge SJ, Richmond BJ, Chu FC (1980) Implantation of magnetic search coils for measurement of eye position: an improved method. Vision Res 20: 535–538.
52. Crick F, Koch C (2003) A framework for consciousness. Nat Neurosci 6: 119–126.
53. Dayan P (1998) A hierarchical model of binocular rivalry. Neural Comput 10: 1119–1135.
54. Brascamp JW, Knapen TH, Kanai R, van Ee R, van den Berg AV (2007) Flash suppression and flash facilitation in binocular rivalry. J Vis 7: 12 11–12.
55. Silver MA, Logothetis NK (2007) Temporal frequency and contrast tagging bias the type of competition in interocular switch rivalry. Vision Res 47: 532–543.
56. Bhardwaj R, O'Shea RP, Alais D, Parker A (2008) Probing visual consciousness: rivalry between eyes and images. J Vis 8: 2 1–13.
57. Douglas RJ, Martin KAC (1991) A Functional Microcircuit for Cat Visual-Cortex. Journal of Physiology-London 440: 735–769.
58. Mehta AD, Ulbert I, Schroeder CE (2000) Intermodal selective attention in monkeys. II: Physiological mechanisms of modulation. Cerebral Cortex 10: 359–370.
59. Mehta SD, Ulbert I, Schroeder CE (2000) Intermodal selective attention in monkeys. I: Distribution and timing of effects across visual areas. Cerebral Cortex 10: 343–358.
60. Buracas GT, Boynton GM (2007) The effect of spatial attention on contrast response functions in human visual cortex. Journal of Neuroscience 27: 93–97.
61. Corbetta M, Miezin FM, Dobmeyer S, Shulman GL, Petersen SE (1990) Attentional Modulation of Neural Processing of Shape, Color, and Velocity in Humans. Science 248: 1556–1559.
62. Huk AC, Ress D, Heeger DJ (2001) Neuronal basis of the motion aftereffect reconsidered. Neuron 32: 161–172.
63. Koch C, Tsuchiya N (2012) Attention and consciousness: related yet different. Trends in Cognitive Sciences 16: 103–105.
64. Guo K, Benson PJ, Blakemore C (2004) Pattern motion is present in V1 of awake but not anaesthetized monkeys. European Journal of Neuroscience 19: 1055–1066.
65. Lee SH, Blake R, Heeger DJ (2007) Hierarchy of cortical responses underlying binocular rivalry. Nature Neuroscience 10: 1048–1054.
66. Wilke M, Logothetis NK, Leopold DA (2003) Generalized flash suppression of salient visual targets. Neuron 39: 1043–1052.
67. Lamme VAF, Zipser K, Spekreijse H (1998) Figure-ground activity in primary visual cortex is suppressed by anesthesia. Proc Natl Acad Sci U S A 95: 3263–3268.
68. Lamme VAF, Spekreijse H (2000) Modulations of primary visual cortex activity representing attentive and conscious scene perception. Frontiers in Bioscience 5: D232–D243.
69. Alkire MT, Hudetz AG, Tononi G (2008) Consciousness and anesthesia. Science 322: 876–880.
70. Super H, Spekreijse H, Lamme VAF (2001) Two distinct modes of sensory processing observed in monkey primary visual cortex (V1). Nat Neurosci 4: 304–310.
71. Cohen MR, Maunsell JHR (2009) Attention improves performance primarily by reducing interneuronal correlations. Nat Neurosci 12: 1594-U1148.
72. Mitchell JF, Sundberg KA, Reynolds JH (2009) Spatial Attention Decorrelates Intrinsic Activity Fluctuations in Macaque Area V4. Neuron 63: 879–888.
73. Ecker AS, Berens P, Keliris GA, Bethge M, Logothetis NK, et al. (2010) Decorrelated Neuronal Firing in Cortical Microcircuits. Science 327: 584–587.
74. Ramalingam N, McManus JNJ, Li W, Gilbert CD (2013) Top-Down Modulation of Lateral Interactions in Visual Cortex. Journal of Neuroscience 33: 1773–1789.
75. Wilke M, Mueller KM, Leopold DA (2009) Neural activity in the visual thalamus reflects perceptual suppression. Proc Natl Acad Sci U S A 106: 9465–9470.
76. Goense JBM, Logothetis NK (2008) Neurophysiology of the BOLD fMRI signal in awake monkeys. Current Biology 18: 631–640.

# 13

# The Conditioned Place Preference Test for Assessing Welfare Consequences and Potential Refinements in a Mouse Bladder Cancer Model

**John V. Roughan[1]*, Claire A. Coulter[1], Paul A. Flecknell[1], Huw D. Thomas[2], Kenneth J. Sufka[3]**

**1** Comparative Biology Centre, The Medical School, University of Newcastle, Newcastle upon Tyne, United Kingdom, **2** Northern Institute for Cancer Research, The Medical School, University of Newcastle, Newcastle upon Tyne, United Kingdom, **3** Research Institute of Pharmaceutical Sciences and Departments of Psychology and Pharmacology, Peabody Building, University of Mississippi, Oxford, Mississippi, United States of America

## Abstract

Most pre-clinical analgesic efficacy assays still involve nociceptive testing in rodents. This is despite concerns as to the relevance of these tests for evaluating the pain-preventative properties of drugs. More appropriate methods would target pain rather than nociception, but these are currently not available, so it remains unknown whether animal pain equates to the negatively affective and subjective/emotional state it causes in humans. Mouse cancer models are common despite the likelihood of substantial pain. We used Conditioned Place Preference (CPP) testing, assessments of thermal hyperalgesia and behaviour to determine the likelihood that MBT-2 bladder cancer impacts negatively on mouse welfare, such as by causing pain. There was no CPP to saline, but morphine preference in tumour bearing mice exceeded that seen in tumour-free controls. This occurred up to 10 days before the study end-point alongside reduced body weight, development of hyperalgesia and behaviour changes. These effects indicated mice experienced a negative welfare state caused by *malaise* (if not pain) before euthanasia. Due to the complexity of the assessments needed to demonstrate this, it is unlikely that this approach could be used for routine welfare assessment on a study-by-study basis. However, our results show mice in sufficiently similar studies are likely to benefit from more intensive severity assessment and re-evaluation of end-points with a view to implementing appropriate refinements. In this particular case, a refinement would have been to have euthanased mice at least 7 days earlier or possibly by provision of end-stage pain relief. CPP testing was found to be a helpful method to investigate the responses of mice to analgesics, possibly on a subjective level. These findings and those of other recent studies show it could be a valuable method of screening candidate analgesics for efficacy against cancer pain and possibly other pain or disease models.

**Editor:** Bradley Taylor, University of Kentucky Medical Center, United States of America

**Funding:** The study was funded by the UK National Centre for the 3Rs (NC3Rs): http://www.nc3rs.org.uk/, Grant Number G0900763, PI: JV Roughan. The funder had no role in study design, data collection and analysis, decision to publish, or preparation of the manuscript.

**Competing Interests:** The authors have declared that no competing interests exist.

* Email: j.v.roughan@ncl.ac.uk

## Introduction

An array of nociceptive tests are used to determine the potential efficacy of new analgesics, and laboratory rats and mice are overwhelmingly the most widely used test subjects. These tests are typically classified according to the duration and intensity of the noxious stimulus and the nature of the response. Acute or phasic nociceptive assays that apply heat or mechanical stimulation (e.g. the tail-flick and Hargreaves tests; von Frey, respectively), due to the largely reflexive nature of the responses obtained, are considered less appropriate than tonic or sub-chronic tests (e.g. formalin or carrageenan) that elicit significant and persistent inflammation [1]. However, the inadequacies of both are well known [2]. Despite the development of animal simulations of persistent pain syndromes (e.g. arthritic or neuropathic pain), concerns prevail as to their clinical relevance. These ultimately stem from a continuing lack of understanding of how animal pain equates to the human experience; being a multidimensional phenomenon including both sensory and affective emotional state changes (collectively termed 'life quality' changes). Theoretically at least, animal pain and analgesic assays that inform on changes in these states should afford greater translational validity. This need has driven recent calls for the development of more clinically relevant *in-vivo* models [3,4] providing a more systems-based approach [5]. This rationale explains why affective (subjective) state assessment is increasingly being considered as a more relevant approach to establishing the welfare consequences of models where animals could be exposed to pain [6–8]. Cancer models are one research area where considerably more knowledge on how extensively pain impacts on welfare may be long overdue.

A large and steadily increasing number of animals (mainly mice) are used in cancer testing (471,000 in the UK in 2012; a 16% increase on the previous year [9]) with only minimal knowledge regarding potentially negative impacts on welfare. However, the guidelines that are meant to minimise suffering in these studies [10,11] do not incorporate any evaluation of changes in underlying subjective state, and obtaining evidence of cancer pain in rodents has relied heavily on assessing underlying nociceptive changes [12–15], and it seems this is still the case today [16–19]. Our group has extensively assessed changes in naturalistic behaviours as a means of assessing post-operative pain in rodents and other species using both manual [20–26] and automated methods [27–30], or used a combination of both types of analysis [31]. However, such behaviour analysis has rarely been used to assess the effects of cancer, and those few studies that cite 'pain behaviour' actually mean nociceptive or nocifensive behaviours (i.e. withdrawal or guarding) rather than true spontaneous (e.g. home-cage) behaviour (see for example [14,32]). Whichever method of data collection is used, establishing links between outcome and causation in behavioural studies is difficult because many factors can contribute to the observed changes. Changes could occur as an indirect result of procedural influences (e.g. anaesthesia, hypothermia, dehydration) or factors linked to these such as fear and associated anxiety. Nevertheless, establishing whether and when pain arises in cancer studies would have significant consequences. Firstly it would encourage a more rigorous approach to ethical decision making by enabling researchers to apply more effective cost-benefit analyses when determining if end-points are justified. Improving welfare standards in this manner would also be beneficial to studies because unalleviated pain may also jeopardise model validity. Preventing pain has been shown to be beneficial to validity in at least one cancer trial [33] and possibly other *in-vivo* research applications [34]. Cancer pain is also an area where advances in human treatments are urgently required. Pain is the most common and feared consequence of cancer and between 30–60% of oncology patients continue to report pain prior to, throughout and following treatment [35]. Indeed, it seems the outlook remains bleak despite 40 years of attempts to address the problem [36]. Clearly, cancer pain management needs to be refined, and animal cancer models provide an ideal platform for parallel progress on welfare advancement and drug discovery. Despite this, cancer models are not generally used to screen potential analgesics, with only rare exceptions [13,37]. This may be because most cancer studies have alternative aims, but could also be due to a lack of appropriate assessment methods; i.e. those that accommodate subjective aspects.

Conditioned Place Preference (CPP) testing is widely used to evaluate the psychoactive (affective) properties of drugs in animals [38], but usually to identify abuse liability by humans. Animals are conditioned by being confined in one 'place' and pairing that with drug treatment, whereas in another place they are given only a placebo. As the 'places' have distinctly different cues (usually in colour or texture) animals progressively associate the drugs' affect with the place where they experienced it. If this is a rewarding experience, either due to the drugs' positively or negatively reinforcing (analgesic) effects, animals typically spend longer in, or visit the drug-paired place more frequently. Provision of analgesia is a positive experience in painful humans, so if the same applies to animals then CPP studies have potential for evaluating both the aversive properties of pain and the analgesic effects of drugs. The approach has increasingly been applied to research on pain following the first demonstration that arthritis causes enhanced CPP to morphine and the N-methyl-D-aspartate antagonist MK-801 [39]. It was subsequently shown that a bradykinin $B_1$ receptor antagonist has therapeutic potential against chronic inflammatory pain [40]. A considerable time later, King et al. showed CPP is also an effective method for assessing analgesics against neuropathic pain [41]. Qu et al. illustrated the relevance of CPP to assessing subjective aspects of neuropathic pain in rats by showing that the rostral anterior cingulate cortex is essential to mediating pain affect [42]. Rutten et al. were also able to use CPP to dissociate between the positively and negatively rewarding consequences of analgesics with opioid-like affects compared to other mechanisms in a rat inflammatory (carrageenan) model [43]. Davoody et al. then showed increased CPP to clonidine (an α-2 agonist) in rats using spinal cord injury as a centralised pain model [44]. Okun et al. utilised a similar approach to show CPP to several different drugs in an osteoarthritic model [45], and most recently, Park et al. showed absence of positive reinforcement (reward) to gabapentin in normal mice, but CPP in a polyneuropathic pain model caused by antineoplastic (cisplatin) treatment [46]. Collectively, these findings clearly demonstrate that the CPP paradigm is capable of providing animals with a means to report on their awareness of pain, and so could offer a more appropriate method of evaluating its centralised (affective/subjective) as opposed to nociceptive (effective) properties.

The notion that pain could be as complex in animals (at least in mammals) as it is in humans is underlined by the fact that no single measurement criterion can (so far) effectively evaluate it. Bateson et al. originally applied a multiple measures approach to scientific problem solving (later termed 'triangulation') [47], citing that although "evidence obtained by different approaches was ambiguous", "when the whole body of evidence was considered, much greater confidence could be placed on a particular meaning". In addressing the problem of animal suffering, and accepting that "we cannot directly observe an animals' feelings", Bateson recommended that "we should use a variety of tasks to gain confidence in conclusions" [48]. Accordingly, studies are now increasingly applying several different measures in an attempt to characterise pain more reliably [49,50]. In this study we adopted a comparable approach by assessing a standard welfare parameter (body weight) alongside peripheral hypersensitivity testing, monitoring spontaneous exploratory behaviour and conducting CPP testing. Despite several limitations, hyperalgesia (hypersensitivity) testing still provides a valuable secondary indicator of pain of various different modalities including cancer [12,16,19]. Behaviour changes are also a common response to pain, but data collection and analyses are often time consuming, especially if applied in studies that typically last several weeks; as is usually the case in cancer studies. Interpretation of these data can also be problematic because, as has already been described, there are always alternative explanations for any behavioural changes that are detected. One often cited possibility is that signs of incapacity in rodents could be hidden as an adaptive response to reduce the likelihood of predation; although to our knowledge this has never been shown unequivocally. To at least partly overcome the time limitation we used automated behaviour registration software (HomeCageScan; Clever Systems Inc., VA, USA (HCS)). This recognises a range (>20) mouse behaviours with comparable accuracy to manual analysis by a trained observer [27,28]. In this study we contrasted findings on hyperalgesia and behaviour changes with the results of CPP testing to assess the consequences of bladder cancer on the welfare of mice; applying the concept of triangulation. So far as we are aware, no previous attempt has been made to evaluate the CPP approach as described here during tumour development; with consecutive conditioning and testing cycles. We also sought to gauge (at least hypothetically) whether this could be a useful approach to screening candidate drugs for the treatment of cancer pain in humans. We found tumour mice gained less weight, developed hyperalgesia and showed behaviour changes that were time-linked to enhanced morphine seeking in tumour-bearing mice in the 7 days preceding euthanasia. We concluded that the most likely explanation for these changes was pain. If not due to pain, at the very least the results indicated negative impacts on welfare, possibly including *malaise*. Ordinarily mice would only be removed from studies after this time, indicating a likely need for end-point refinement in this mouse model of bladder cancer. Our method of applying CPP testing could also be a potentially useful method of testing the effectiveness of analgesics intended for cancer and other conditions, especially those where pain can escalate over time.

## Methods

### Ethics Statement

All work was conducted in accordance with the Animals (Scientific Procedures) Act 1986 and was subject to local ethical review. The experiments also adhered to the guidelines of the Committee for Research and Ethical Issues of the International Association for the Study of Pain (IASP). All procedures were approved by the UK Home Office (Project Licence PPL 60/4431).

### Subjects and Husbandry

All mice were female C3H/HeN, weighed 25 to 30 g on delivery (Charles River Laboratories Inc., UK) and had free access to a commercial pelleted diet (R&M no.3 SDS LTD., Whitham, UK) and tap water in groups of 10 for one week of acclimation. They were then housed singly (Macrolon 2 cages; North Kent Plastics, UK) for another week prior to enrolment. Sawdust and wood shavings were used as bedding and cages were supplemented with 'Sizzle Nest', an aspen chew-block and a cardboard tube (B & K Universal). Room temperature was maintained at 21±1°C with 15–20 air changes per hour under a 12-hour light cycle (lights off at 19:00 h). All testing was conducted between 10 am and 3 pm.

### Data Collection

The results of 3 studies using separate groups of mice are described; (1) Hargreaves (nociceptive testing) study, (2) Behaviour study and (3) Conditioned Place Preference (CPP) testing consisting of a Pilot dose ranging investigation and then a main study. The data obtained on studies 1 and 2 were from exploratory trials undertaken by colleagues of the Northern Institute for Cancer Research (NICR) using syngeneic MBT-2 (Mouse Bladder Tumour) cells derived from C3H/HeN/J mice (cells donated by Prof. Michael O'Donnell (University of Iowa, Iowa City, IA, USA) and Dr. William A. Larchian (EMH/Cleveland Clinic Prostate Centre, Cleveland, OH, USA)). The CPP data were obtained from mice specifically obtained for testing. Our colleague's objectives were; initially to characterise the growth profile of orthotopically implanted bladder tumours (Study 1) and then to refine the implant methodology (Study 2). However, both studies were an opportunity to collect supplemental data on pathological effects (possibly including pain) that would help in the design of the main (CPP) study; thereby reducing animal use to as low a level as possible.

### Hargreaves Study

This was a pilot study undertaken to establish the growth characteristics of orthotopically implanted MBT-2 cells that would inform on the eventual design of the CPP study. Group sizes were determined by NICR colleagues based on their study requirements. Mice were randomly allocated to three groups of 5 that underwent laparotomy for orthotopic implantation of 100 µl of Dulbecco's Phosphate Buffered Saline (DPBS), or the same volume of DPBS containing $2\times10^4$ or $2\times10^5$ MBT-2 cells. A fourth group of 5 mice were anaesthesia only controls. Eight mice that underwent surgery were randomly chosen to receive 5 mg/kg meloxicam (subcutaneously; s/c) to alleviate post-surgical pain [27], while the remainder received saline (0.3 mls s/c; n = 7). Anaesthesia was induced with 5% isoflurane in oxygen (5 l/min.) in a Perspex chamber. Mice then lay in dorsal recumbency on a heating blanket to maintain body temperatures between 34.5 and 37.5°C and anaesthesia was maintained with 1.5–2% isoflurane in oxygen (500 ml/min.). Depth was monitored by observing respiratory rates and regularly assessing toe-pinch reflexes. Simple eye ointment (Pliva Pharma Ltd., UK) was used to prevent corneal drying. Surgery was a 0.5 cm midline incision in the skin and muscles overlying the bladder. Once exposed, 0.1 ml of saline or the appropriate tumour cell suspension was injected intramuscularly into the bladder wall using an insulin syringe. The abdominal muscles and skin were closed separately using 5/0 polyglactin 910 ('Vicryl', Ethicon Ltd, Edinburgh, UK) and tissue glue ('Nexaband', Abbott laboratories, Chicago). Anaesthesia lasted approximately 10 minutes.

Thermal withdrawal latencies were obtained at baseline, and at 1 hour and 1 day (24 hours) following surgery, and then on days; 3, 7, 10, 14, 17, 21 and 24 using the Plantar Test (Model 37370; Ugo Basile, Italy) according to the method of Hargreaves [51]. Animals were placed in clear acrylic chambers on a glass floor and habituated for 10 minutes. An infra-red heat source was alternately applied to the mid-plantar area of each hind paw (70% of maximum heating capacity; equivalent to 253±7 mW/$cm^2$; 30 second cut-off). This provided a suitable range of response latencies in normal mice (~between 3 and 8 seconds). Three responses were obtained from each hind paw with a minimum interval of 1 minute between ipsilateral recordings. Data were only obtained from the anaesthesia control mice until day 3 when they were required elsewhere. Body weights were recorded daily until day 4, and then on nociceptive test days. As tumours were internal, growth stage was estimated by daily palpation by an experienced technician who graded tumours on a 3 point scale; from 1 (barely present) to 3 (obvious without handling). These inspections also included a record of activities associated with abdominal pain in rodents [21,31] and other signs of ill-health such as haematuria, lethargy, dehydration and poor coat and body condition.

### Behaviour Study

The behaviour data were collected as part of a follow-up study (again without additional animal use) to assess a potentially more refined (non-surgical) method of cell implantation [52]. Our colleagues sought to establish if tumour engraftment could be improved with this method, whereas we wished to evaluate the longer term effects of cancer growth on behaviour. As before, group sizes were pre-determined; 20 mice were allocated to the DPBS group and 20 to the tumour group. Anaesthesia was induced as previously described but in batches of 5 mice using a custom-made open-mask gas delivery system. The implant procedure has already been described, but briefly, the bladder of each mouse was accessed via a 27 gauge paediatric cannula placed in the urethra. Urine was voided by gentle supra-pubic pressure and aspiration, and the bladder mucosa conditioned with a mild acid rinse (50 µl of 0.1 M HCl) for 20 seconds. This was also aspirated and then neutralised with 50 µl 0.1 M KOH, and three DPBS washes. The bladder was emptied before instilling 50 µl of $5\times10^6$ MBT-2 cells or the same volume of DPBS via a syringe tied to the tail. The greater cell concentration was in anticipation of an unknown cell fraction being voided in urine following recovery. Cells were left *in-situ* for 30 minutes, following which the mice were placed in an incubator at 37°C for 20 minutes. Daily tumour development was monitored as before and body weights were also recorded daily. Mice were filmed individually for 10 minutes using a video camera (Sony DCR-HC96, Sony, Japan) positioned on a tripod 30 cm from the front of clear '1284'cages (35×20×14 cm; Techniplast, UK Ltd) containing only bedding (Aspen sawdust). The procedure for behaviour data collection was as previously

| | Block 1 | | | Block 2 | | | Block 3..... |
|---|---|---|---|---|---|---|---|
| Baseline | Day 1 | Day 2 | Day 3 | Day 4 | Day 5 | Day 6 | Day 7...... |
| Initial Preference Testing (15mins) | Conditioning 1 (am) Saline, S- | Conditioning 3 (am) Saline, S- | Preference 1 Drug Free | Conditioning 5 (am) Saline, S- | Conditioning 7 (am) Saline, S- | Preference 2 Drug Free | Repeat (am)... |
| | Conditioning 2 (pm) Saline/Mor2, S+ | Conditioning 4 (pm) Saline/Mor2, S+ | | Conditioning 6 (pm) Saline/Mor2, S+ | Conditioning 8 (pm) Saline/Mor2, S+ | | Repeat (pm).... |

**Figure 1. Timeline of CPP testing.** Successive blocks were each of two conditioning days where mice underwent morning S− (saline) and then afternoon S+ (morphine or saline) treatments and were confined for 45 minutes in the black or white chamber. The third day of each block was a drug free preference test, and 3 day cycle was repeated until euthanasia.

described [28] except that it was on alternate days before tumour detection, and then daily. Filming was always during the light phase but the time of day each mouse was filmed was randomised within the tumour and control groups.

## Conditioned Place Preference Studies

The CPP work was conducted in 2 stages. The first was a pilot study to explore development of CPP to morphine under repetitive conditioning and testing cycles, and to identify a morphine dose for the main CPP study. The chosen dose would be one that supported only modest place preference but retained sufficient analgesic properties to elicit negative reinforcement in tumour bearing mice. Numbers were determined using a retrospective power analysis on previous morphine CPP results across a range of dose rates in normal mice (1 and 5 mg/kg s/c) [53] that should also elicit significant analgesic effects [54,55]. Sample sizes of 8 or 10 were retrospectively found to achieve 79% or 91% power in detecting significant CPP to a drug (3 or 5 mg/kg morphine) versus placebo-paired compartment. The CPP apparatus consisted of black (steel rod floored) and white (steel grid floored) compartments separated by a grey (solid floored) start chamber. We used 4 identical testing units (Med Associates, St Albans, VT, USA; Model CPP-3013AT) equipped with automatically controlled guillotine doors and lights. Compartments housed infra-red arrays to automatically record compartment residence times and movements within and between the 3 compartments. An initial trial was used to determine the baseline compartment preference of each animal. For this they were placed into the central (grey) start chamber for 1 minute prior to turning on the lights and opening the guillotine doors. Preference testing was always conducted between 10 am and 2 pm. The relative time spent exploring the black and white compartments over a subsequent 15 minute trial was calculated as a proportion of the total test time (see CPP data analysis section). The mice were assigned for S+ (saline or morphine) conditioning in the compartment in which they spent proportionately the least amount of time (i.e. their non-preferred chamber), but no mice showed proportionate initial compartment preferences exceeding 0.6 (the CPP analysis section details the preference calculation method). The design was then counter-balanced such that the initial relative group preference approximated as closely as possible to 0.5 (i.e. equal numbers were assigned per group to the black (B) or white (W) S+ chambers). On this basis eight mice were allocated to each of 2 morphine groups spanning the likely range of effective analgesic dose rates (1 or 5 mg/kg s/c) and a representative group of 4 mice were saline controls. Once we reached the stage of cancer testing we knew the traditional CPP approach of repetitive conditioning trials followed by a single preference test would not be appropriate. This was because if pain occurred; we also wished to capture its onset. Informed by this, all CPP testing (including in the pilot study) consisted of repetitive 3 day blocks, with each block comprising 2 days of conditioning before a drug-free preference test each subsequent day (shown in Figure 1). For the pilot study the 4 controls received only saline (0.03 mls s/c) under both the S− and S+ conditions. Because of possible morphine 'carry-over' to afternoon S+ trials it was necessary that vehicle (S−) injections were always given in the morning and S+ (morphine or saline) in the afternoon. Morphine was obtained as morphine sulphate solution (30 mg/ml; NHS Supplies, UK) and was appropriately diluted with water for injection (wfi) to be administered subcutaneously in a volume of 0.03 mls. All injections were given immediately before placement into the allocated B or W compartment for a 45 minute conditioning period with the guillotine doors closed. Mice were returned to their home-cages immediately following each conditioning session. Four consecutive preference tests were undertaken for the pilot study (4 test blocks; Figure 1) precisely following the method used to determine the initial compartment preference.

The main CPP investigation began with a repeat of initial preference testing. Each mouse was assigned a B or W compartment for subsequent S−/S+ conditioning in the previously described manner (balancing numbers initially preferring the B or W compartment across the control and tumour groups). As before, mice were assigned to their initially non-preferred compartment as far as possible. Tumour mice were again implanted via the urethra with 50 µl DPBS containing $5\times10^6$ MBT-2 cells. Thirty mice were orthotopically implanted with tumour cells and ten were saline controls. These numbers were informed by our previous findings on numbers of graft failures following urethral implantation. We planned to balance the design (and further conserve animal usage) by assigning any such failures to control groups, but only if there were no palpable or other signs of tumour development after 21 days. Tumour absence was also confirmed *post-mortem*. Once the clinical inspections confirmed tumour growth, each mouse began CPP conditioning and a treatment matched non-tumour control entered the study simultaneously. The 3 day series of conditioning and test sessions then continued until mice were euthanased (see section on end-point determination). Experimental groups therefore formed a 2 (Drug)×2 (Treatment) factorial design that combined conditioning to morphine or 0.9% Saline in tumour or non-tumour mice. We selected an intermediate dose of morphine (2 mg/kg s/c) for the main study based on the findings of the pilot study. In the main CPP study preference tests were also 45 instead of 15 minutes, but the methodology was otherwise identical to that used in the pilot study. Due to time constraints and the potential confound of placement into other unfamiliar environments (effectively other 'places'), behaviour and hyperalgesia assessments were not undertaken as the CPP study progressed. However, the effect of late-stage analgesic treatment on behaviour was assessed as a potential refinement option. This meant that on euthanasia days mice were filmed for 20 minutes before and after injection of the conditioning dose of morphine (2 mg/kg s/c) and identical recordings were made from an equal number of controls on the last day of the study.

### End-point determination

Clinical inspections were conducted in all studies to determine if tumour-bearing mice needed to be withdrawn. These were in accordance with published guidelines [10,11] and with the advice of highly experienced animal care staff. Euthanasia was unavoidable once animals had a large palpable tumour or more than 15% body weight loss, and if either of these coincided with significant haematuria (indicated by blood stained fur and/or bedding). All mice including the controls underwent palpation. They were restrained in the manner that is usual for an intraperitoneal injection. The bladder region was then gently palpated between the thumb and forefinger, but with sufficient pressure to determine the earliest time of onset of tumour development as reliably as possible.

### Data Analysis

**Hargreaves study.** As response latencies were initially similar between the left and right hind-paws, all values were averaged to calculate the overall mean response latency at each recording time. The data met the requirements for parametric analysis so were examined using repeated measures ANOVA with 'Time' (10 levels) and 'Group' (4 levels; 2×tumour; 1×placebo and anaesthesia only) as within and between-subject's factors respectively. *Post-hoc* individual time and group comparisons were made and probability levels adjusted accordingly (*Bonferroni*). The body weight changes were also calculated as change from baseline and the same statistical methods applied. For greater clarity, the weight changes are depicted as absolute values at each time-point. Due to absence of nociceptive data in the non-surgery control mice after day 3 and body weight data after day 4 all analyses following these times included the surgery groups only. Finally, the effects of pre-surgery meloxicam were examined by comparing baseline response latencies to the 1 hour time point in the ANOVA; but with 'pre-treatment' (meloxicam or saline) as a between subject's factor (n = 7 (Saline) versus n = 8 (meloxicam)).

**Behaviour study.** The behaviour data were processed using HCS automated analysis software. The measures used were total distance travelled and five behaviour classes comprising different elements of the 20 individual behaviours the system recognised. These were: 1) Rearing (comprising 'Rear Up' (both partial and full bipedal extension) & the reciprocal activity 'Come Down'); 2) Active behaviour (including walking, running, jumping and climbing); 3) Abdominal Grooming, and 5) Resting (inactive periods). We summed the occurrences of behaviours within each class as the relative magnitude of class elements was sufficiently uniform. The mean frequency of each class was calculated for each mouse on each filming day. The relative duration of each class (duration/frequency) was also calculated to investigate the possibility that time spent engaging in each type of activity changed independently of its total occurrence. All behaviour data were tested and met the assumptions necessary for parametric analysis. Repeated measures ANOVA was used with 'Time' (Days) and 'Group' (Tumour versus Control) as the within and between subject's factors for each measurement. Calculations of body weight change from baseline following non-surgical tumour implantation were evaluated again with 'Time' and 'Group' (saline or tumour) as within and between subjects factors, also using repeated measures ANOVA. Multiple comparisons between individual times were again probability corrected (*Bonferroni*).

**Conditioned Place Preference Studies.** In both the pilot study and main CPP study the initial black or white compartment preferences were calculated as the proportionate time spent in each compartment. Where t = time, the Black (B) compartment preference (Bpref) was therefore calculated as tB/(tB+tW), and the White (W) compartment preference (Wpref) as tW/(tW+tB). Thus, a proportionate score of >0.5 indicated a greater preference for that chamber and this became the S+ condition. All subsequent calculations of chamber preference were made in the same way, and the proportion of time spent exploring the S+ chamber relative to S−(tS+/((tS+)+(tS−)) was the dependent measure over successive preference tests. We again used repeated measures ANOVA to compare S+ preference scores over successive tests in the pilot and main study with 'Time' and 'Group' as respective within and between subject's factors. The source of any individual group differences was again determined using *post-hoc* analyses and applying *Bonferroni* correction of probability levels.

## Results

All results are expressed as mean±1SEM. The electronic files pertaining to all analyses are publicly available at Dryad (http://datadryad.org/), or can be accessed by contacting the lead author.

### Hargreaves Study

Three mice in the 20 K group had palpable tumours (graded 1–2) at day 14, and three in the 200 K group reached this stage by day 10. Thereafter tumour burden gradually increased, and by day 21 tumours were apparent in all animals such that in several cases tumours could be identified without need for palpation. There was no indication of a need to euthanase any mice before the pre-scheduled study end-point on day 24. As expected, the anaesthesia controls showed no adverse effects, and aside from the first day following surgery the saline/surgery controls also appeared 'normal'. Figure 2a shows the mean change in Hargreaves withdrawal latencies (threshold to respond) in the tumour and control groups over the time course of the study. Thresholds were initially similar across the 4 groups; between 4.5 and 5.5 seconds; indicating equivalent nociceptive status initially. Although withdrawal occurred significantly earlier at the 1 hour time-point in the surgery groups (5±0.4 vs 3±0.3 seconds; ($F(1,13) = 16.6$, $p = 0.001$), by 24 hours these showed thresholds that were no longer significantly different from baseline. This was also the case in in the anaesthesia controls over their 3 post-treatment recording days. The surgery controls had also apparently recovered by day 3, and over the time course of the study their response thresholds remained relatively consistent; from 4.3±1.4 at baseline compared to 4.3±1.2 s on day 24. By contrast, mice implanted with tumours showed an overall increase in thermal sensitivity (thresholds/latency to respond reduced). These effects led to a significant overall '|Group' effect (Tumour vs Control; ($F(1,12) = 12.2$, $p = 0.001$) and 'Group x Time' interaction ($F(18,108) = 2.6$, $p = 0.001$). *Post hoc* analyses showed both tumour groups had significantly reduced thresholds compared to DPBS controls arising on day 14 ($p = 0.019$, 0.001, 20 K and 200 K vs. DPBS, respectively). This was maintained until day 21 in both groups, but by day 24 only the 200 K group showed significantly reduced response latencies relative to controls ($p = 0.002$). There were no significant effects of meloxicam (positive or otherwise) on either withdrawal thresholds or body weight (data therefore not shown).

As shown in Figure 2b Surgery/Saline mice were somewhat lighter initially, but not significantly so (~1.5 g). To account for this ANOVA with individual (*post-hoc*) comparisons was conducted on calculations of weight change from baseline over the first 3 days. Post-surgery losses averaged 1.7±0.3 g overall ($F(1,13) = 32.4$, $p<0.001$). Weights were maintained in the non-surgery mice. Both tumour (surgery) groups showed this weight loss from 1 to 3 days, with the greatest mean loss being 2.2±0.8 g in the 200 K tumour group on day 1. The 20 K and 200 K tumour groups both lost significantly more weight than the anaesthesia controls on post-surgical days 1 and 2 ($p = 0.01$, 0.003 (day 1); 0.01, 0.04 (day 2), 20, 200 K groups respectively). The same comparison between the surgery and anaesthesia controls was not significant, probably because the surgery controls were initially lighter. The surgery controls therefore lost seemingly less weight immediately, and had recovered more weight by day 3 than either the 20 K ($p = 0.038$) or 200 K tumour groups ($p = 0.018$). By day 4 there were no significant group differences. The pattern was then of increased weight until the end of the study. This resulted in a significant effect of 'Time' ($F(6,72) = 7.1$, $p = 0.002$). Groups showed only a modest (~1.5–2 g) increase in weight, although by the end of the study (days 17 to 24) there was evidence that weight gain slowed more in the high cell density group than the other surgery groups. This greater overall reduction in weight in the last week in the high density (200 K) tumour group, and over the last 3 days in the 20 K group resulted in a significant 'Group×Time' interaction ($F(2,12) = 4$, $p = 0.045$).

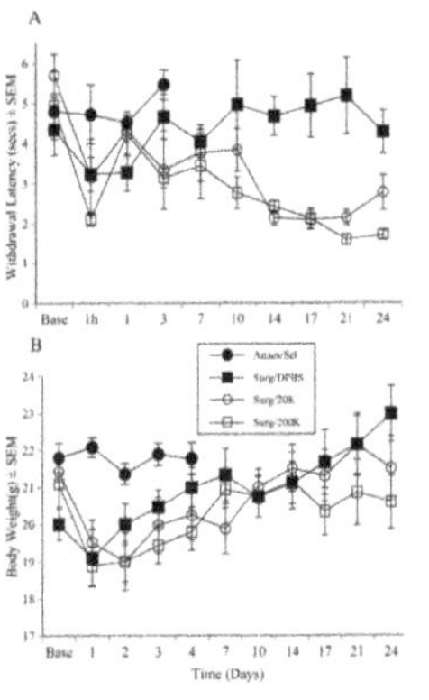

**Figure 2. Hargreaves study results.** The results of nociceptive testing (A) and recording weight changes (B) (mean±SEM) in mice that underwent anaesthesia only (Anaes), or anaesthesia followed by laparotomy for orthotopic implantation of DPBS (100 µl) or MBT-2 bladder tumour cells ($2\times10^4$ or $2\times10^5$; 20 K or 200 K, respectively) (n = 5 per group)). (A) Hargreaves recordings were at baseline (Base), 1 hour (1 h), and then on the days indicated by the *abscissa.* Mice implanted with the highest cell concentration showed lower Hargreaves response thresholds ($p = 0.02$) than the anaesthesia only controls over the first 3 days (indicating hyperalgesia). Also, beginning on day 14, mice with tumours developed significant hyperalgesia compared to surgery/saline controls ($p = 0.019$, 0.001 ($2\times10^4$ or $2\times10^5$ groups respectively)). (B) Tumour groups lost significantly more weight over the first 3 days than either the anaesthesia only or surgery controls ($p \leq 0.04$), but mean baseline body weight was recovered in these mice by post-operative day 4.

## Behaviour Study

Of the 20 mice implanted for the behaviour study (non-surgically) 12 (60%) developed tumours. The implant procedure caused only marginal weight loss (0.8±0.1 g), and all mice fully recovered their starting weights by day 2. The time to detect a solid tumour mass was relatively uniform (28±1.7 days), but subsequent tumour development was considerably more varied. The time from tumour detection to reaching end-point criteria ranged from 10 to 23 days (mean 13.6±3.5). The first mouse was euthanased on day 37 following implantation and 2 mice survived without obvious concerns for 50 days (when the study ended). An inverse relationship was predicted between *ex-vivo* tumour wet weights and survival time (days from detection to euthanasia), but no such relationship was found; average tumour mass was 1.1±0.17 g, range 0.4 to 2 g. The net effect of the varied tumour growth rate was that numbers in the tumour groups were progressively depleted, so aside from immediately following implantation, plotting results on a conventional ascending timescale was not helpful. For both the behaviour and body weight data we therefore examined the results in reverse of the time (day) mice were euthanased; predicting this would be the time when the tumour and control groups would be most distinct. The data were first standardised by matching those from the tumour group to equivalent control data (in terms of elapsed study time). Figure 3 shows the behaviour results from the last 15 days before each mouse was euthanased, with data from an equivalent elapsed study time in controls mice. Panels 3a–d respectively show distance travelled, active, rearing and grooming behaviour frequency. The ANOVA showed tumour bearing mice travelled significantly less overall (Figure 3a; $F(1,22) = 6.65$, $p = 0.017$), and the group difference widened as time progressed. This was especially obvious from 7 days prior to euthanasia when the tumour mice began a marked decline in activity, whereas the opposite effect was observed in controls, leading to a significant 'Group×Time' interaction ($F(14, 308) = 4.1$, $p = 0.001$). There were less obvious group differences in active behaviour (Figure 3b). The groups were not significantly different overall, but the pattern of increasing activity in controls versus a decline in tumour mice was maintained, but was only marginally significant ('Group×Time'; $F(14,308) = 2.3$, $p = 0.04$). The last 7 days was again the time when group differences were most apparent, however, there was a noticeable spike in active behaviour in tumour mice 3 days prior to euthanasia that partially impacted on the distance measure. Rearing behaviour showed the most obvious group separation, with the tumour mice rearing less during the entire 2 weeks prior to euthanasia (Figure 3c; $F(1,22) = 14.3$, $p = 0.001$). There was no particularly obvious decline in tumour versus control mice over the terminal 7 days, but rearing was maintained at a markedly greater

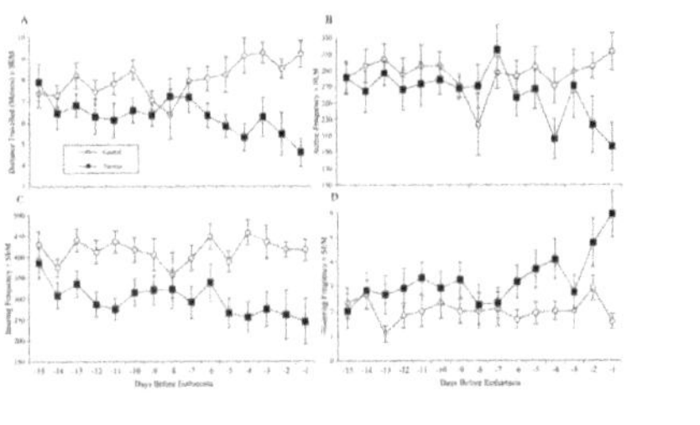

**Figure 3. Behaviour study results - Changes preceding euthanasia.** Results of automated behaviour analysis (HCS) during the period 15 to 1 day prior to euthanasia in the Hargreaves study (mean±SEM). (A) Tumour mice travelled significantly less distance overall ('Group', $p = 0.017$) and showed a pronounced decline over the 8 days before euthanasia ('Group×Time', $p = 0.001$). (B) Active behaviour showed a decline during the days preceding euthanasia (−3 to −1). (C) Tumour mice reared less over the entire 2 weeks prior to euthanasia than controls ('Group', $p = 0.001$) and (D) groomed more overall ('Group', $p = 0.038$), but more intensively so over the final 7 study days ('Group×Time', $p = 0.048$).

frequency in controls (416±90 vs. 245±189). Grooming showed a slight overall increase in both groups over time ('Time' factor significant; F(14,308) = 2.1, p = 0.05; Figure 3d). The tumour mice also groomed more frequently overall (F1,22) = 4.9, p = 0.038), but again, the major effect in tumour mice was an increase in grooming frequency over the final 7 days (significant 'Group x Time' interaction; F(14,308) = 2.1, p = 0.048). This result was rendered only modestly significant due to another incongruous effect 3 days prior to euthanasia when grooming frequency fell in tumour mice. Rest periods (inactive behaviour) were no more frequent in control or tumour mice until the final 3 days when tumour mice tended to show a reduction compared to only a very slight increase in controls (not shown).

The body weight data on the day each mouse was euthanased were matched as previously described: with results in tumour mice matched to data from an equivalent elapsed study time in a randomly chosen non-tumour control. This was repeated for each day prior to euthanasia. Figure 4 shows the mean body weights of the control and tumour groups from 37 days prior to euthanasia. The pre-study weights of the 2 groups were not significantly different. Both groups were gaining weight 37 days prior to the eventual study end, however, the tumour group stopped gaining weight 2 weeks later (22 days before euthanasia). ANOVA showed a significant 'Group×Time' interaction 12 days prior to euthanasia (F(1,23) = 8.55, p = 0.008). *Post-hoc* analyses (independent samples t-tests) showed that by this time the mean weight of tumour bearing mice was 25±1.1 g, compared to 26±1.3 g in controls (p = 0.015). The control mice then steadily increased in weight whereas the reverse occurred in the tumour group (or at least they continued to fail to gain weight). By the end of the study (on day −1) the mean weight of control mice was 27±1.8 g compared to 24.5±2.5 g in the tumour group (p = 0.009). In the tumour mice this amounted to a proportional weight loss of 4.6% compared to the time when they were heaviest (Day 24 prior to euthanasia). We tried to minimise any masking effect of underlying tumour burden on this weight estimate by subtracting *ex-vivo* tumour wet weights, but did not find mice with larger tumours lost significantly more weight.

## Conditioned Place Preference Studies

The results of the CPP pilot study are shown in Figure 5 according to mean S+ preference scores of the groups given saline and each morphine dose. ANOVA indicated a significant overall 'Group' difference (F(1,2) = 5.6, p = 0.013). The *post-hoc* analysis showed mice given 5 mg/kg morphine had significantly elevated S+ scores over tests 2 to 4 compared to the saline controls (p = 0.005) or the mice given the lower morphine dose (p = 0.041). Saline was predictably ineffective, but as 1 mg/kg morphine was also not different from saline an intermediate morphine dose of 2 mg/kg was chosen for the main CPP study.

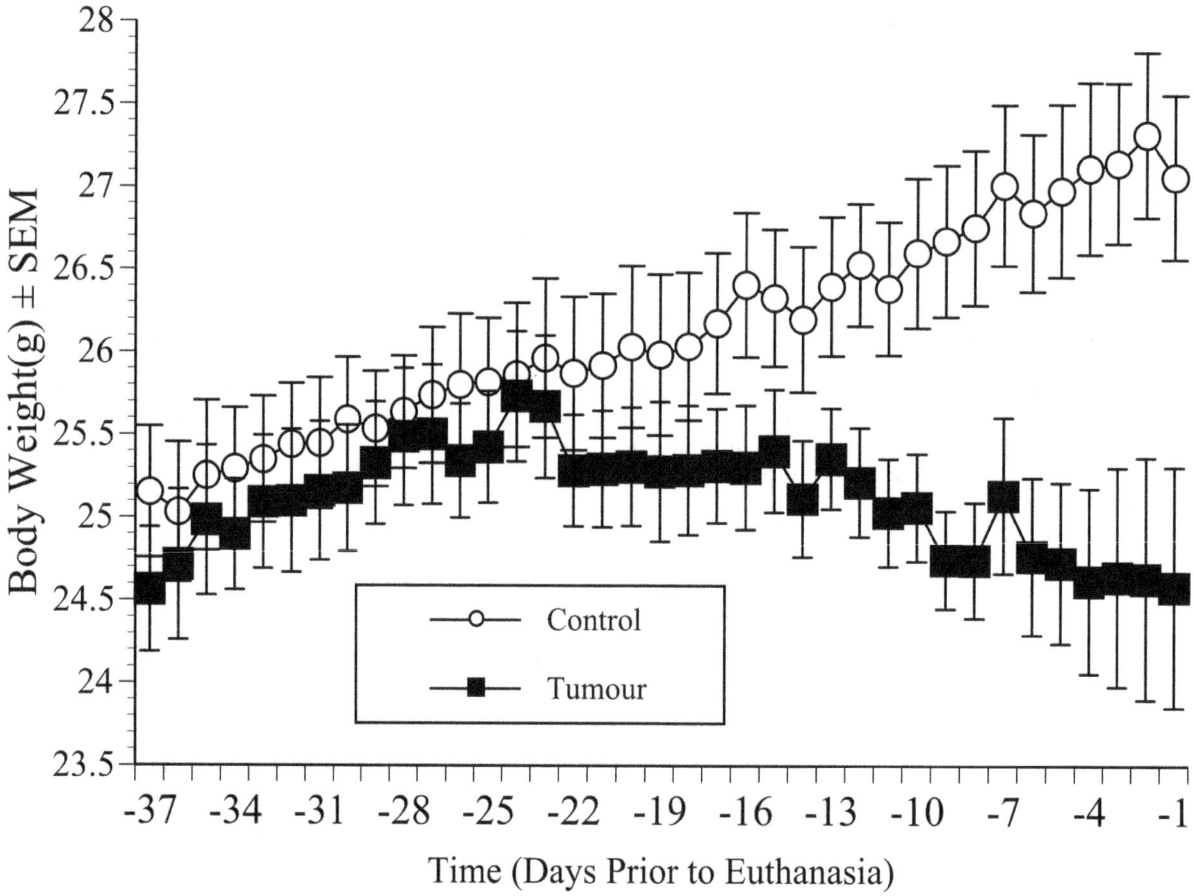


**Figure 4. Body weight in catheterised mice (implanted non-surgically).** The mean (±SEM) body weight of groups of mice implanted orthotopically with either MBT-2 tumours ($5\times10^6$ cells/mouse; 50 µl) or an equal volume of saline, and used to collect behaviour data (n = 12 per group; graft successes only). As in Figure 3, data on days prior to euthanasia are shown following time matching (equivalent elapsed study time). Tumour-bearing mice were significantly lighter than controls from day 12 ('Group'; p = 0.008) and progressively lost more weight until the study end.

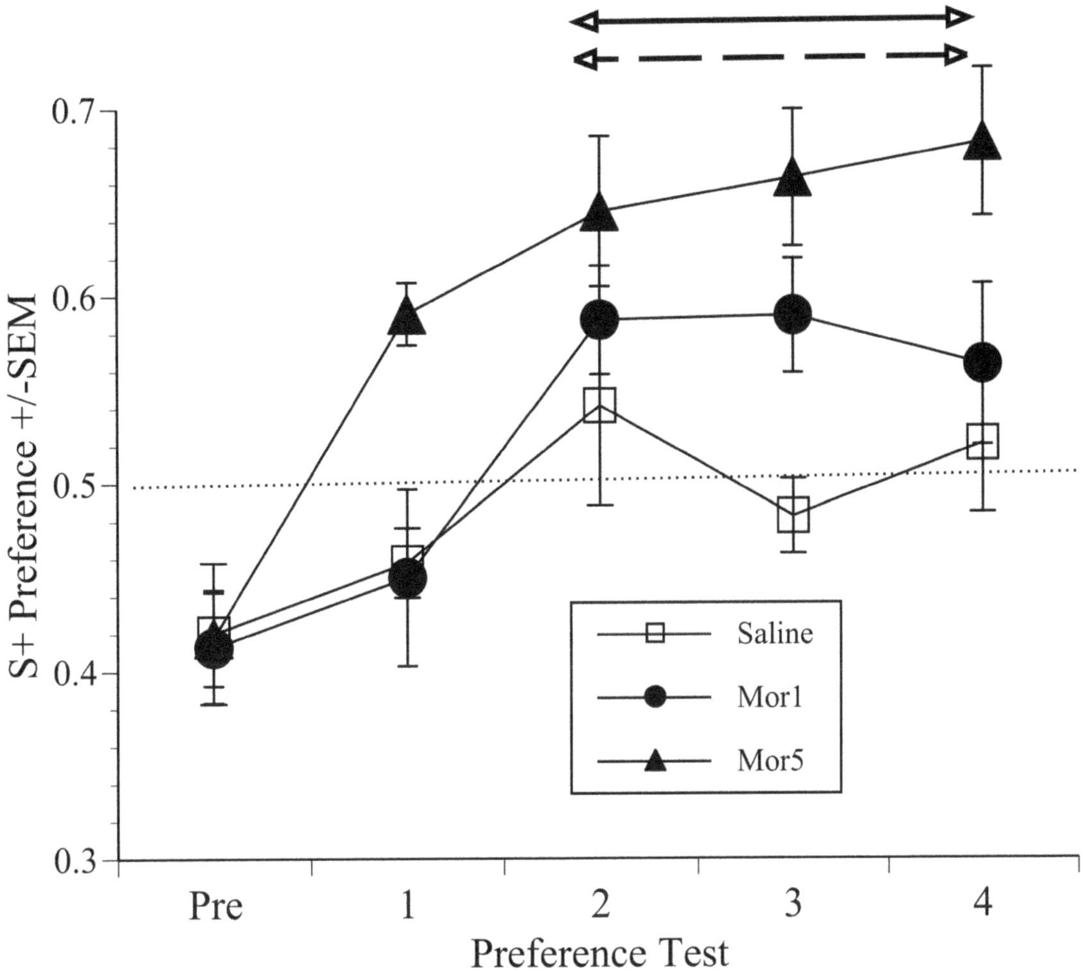


**Figure 5. CPP pilot study results.** Mean S+ chamber preference scores (±SEM) across 4 successive tests in mice conditioned to saline (0.03 mls; n = 4) or morphine (Mor) at 1 or 5 mg/kg (n = 8/group). Mice were conditioned in their initially non-preferred chamber (Pre). Scores above 0.5 (dotted line) indicate enhanced S+ (morphine or saline) chamber preference. Arrowed lines at the top of the chart denote the time period over which the preference for 5 mg/kg morphine exceeded 1 mg/kg ($p<0.05$; dashed arrowed line) or saline ($p<0.01$; solid arrowed line).

Implant success in the main CPP study was 70% with 21 of the 30 implanted mice developing tumours. As planned, four non-growth mice were randomly assigned to control groups, one of which subsequently developed a tumour (so data were rejected). Although overall engraftment was improved from that seen in the behaviour study, the time from implantation to detection of a solid tumour mass over the bladder was more varied. Of the mice where grafts were successful, 75% presented tumours within 14–21 days. Subsequent rates of tumour development were also varied, leading to a broad range of times from tumour detection to the time that mice were euthanased (13–46 days). This meant the number of tests conducted in tumour mice before they reached the endpoint criteria ranged from only 4 to 15 CPP trials (mean ± SD; 8.4±2.73). To minimise the impact of this variation we re-applied the selection procedure to focus on the times likely to reveal group differences; where tumour-bearing mice should show an enhanced morphine preference if they were experiencing pain. As the minimum number of tests was four, the results of the last 4 tests prior to euthanasia were examined (i.e. CPP tests −4, −3, −2 & −1); equivalent to days 10, 7, 4 and 1 day before the study ended. As in the behaviour analysis, data from the non-tumour control (saline or morphine) groups were time-matched as far as was possible to the total number of cycles of conditioning/preference testing undergone by individuals in the equivalent tumour groups.

There were no significant differences in S+ scores between the morphine and saline treated mice on the 3 test days after tumour detection, and both the normal and tumour bearing mice trained only to saline displayed essentially equal preference to the S+ and S− chambers over these trials (i.e. preference scores close to 0.5; data not shown). This illustrated that the apparatus and study design were unbiased. As predicted, the responses to morphine were clearer over the last 4 preference trials (Figure 6). From 10 to 4 days before euthanasia (preference tests −4 to −1) there was little change in morphine preference in controls, but the morphine-treated tumour mice displayed the highest S+ place preference scores of all four groups; the combined effect being an overall significant effect of drug treatment ($F(1,29) = 4.9$, $p = 0.035$). The morphine preference in the tumour group increased over the final 3 preference tests (7 days). Mean S+ preference over this time was calculated and results compared between groups using ANOVA. This also showed a significant overall treatment effect ($F(3,29) = 6.74$, $p = 0.001$). *Post-hoc* tests showed tumour mice conditioned to morphine had significantly elevated S+ scores in comparison to both the saline controls

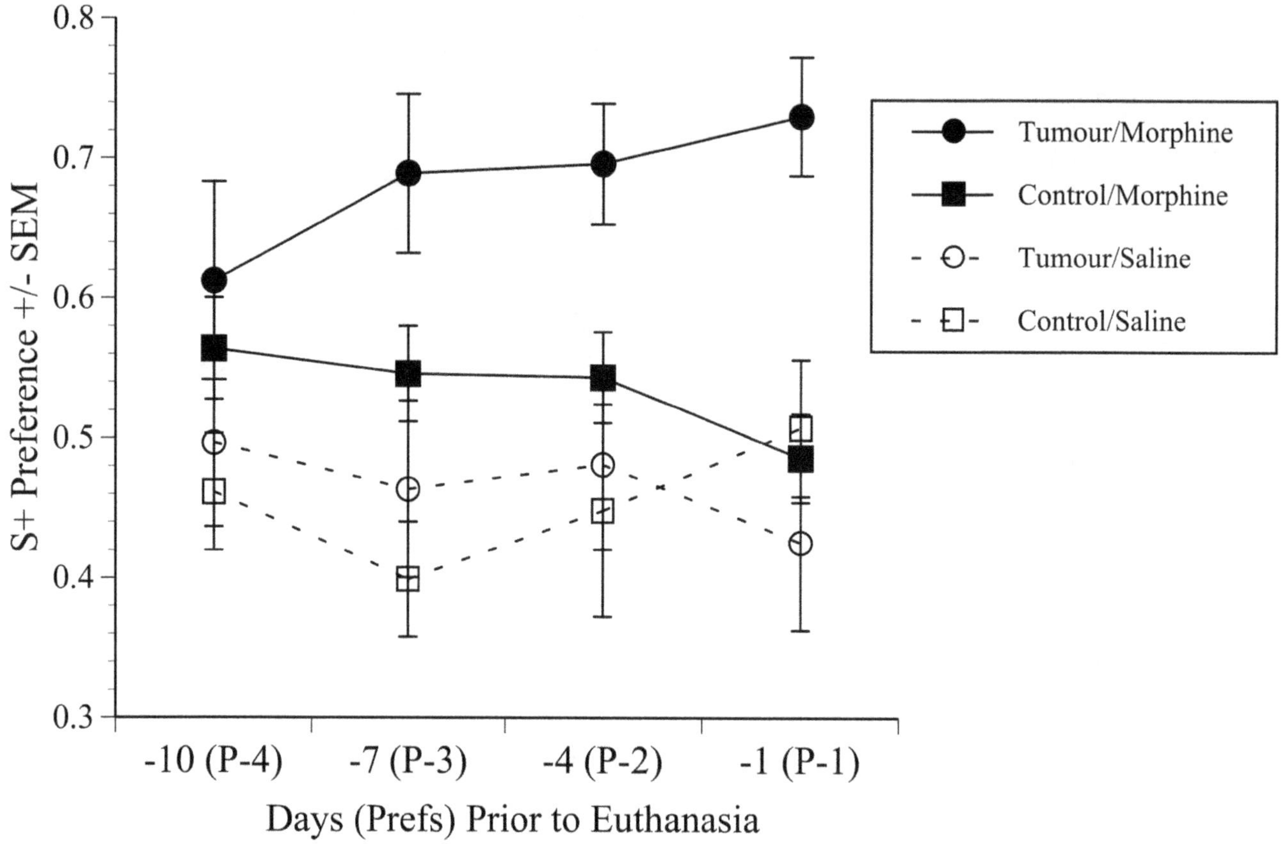


**Figure 6. CPP morphine preference scores preceding euthanasia.** Mean S+ chamber preference scores (±SEM) during the last 4 preference tests (actual days in brackets) prior to euthanasia (Day −1(1)) in normal (Control) and tumour bearing (Cancer) groups conditioned to Saline or Morphine (2 mg/kg; s/c). Scores above 0.5 indicate an enhanced S+ chamber preference. Note especially the cancer mice conditioned to morphine show enhanced morphine seeking (higher CPP S+ score) than either the saline or tumour control groups ($p = 0.005$; $p < 0.001$, respectively), but from days −7 to −1 prior to euthanasia their morphine chamber preference also significantly exceeded the morphine preference of controls conditioned to morphine ($p = 0.02$).

($p = 0.005$) and the saline tumour mice ($p < 0.001$). The key comparison, however, was between the morphine preference scores of the tumour and control mice. Mice with tumours had a significantly greater preference for the morphine paired chamber than the morphine controls ($p = 0.02$). These findings were consistent with the notion that mice in pain will show a place preference to a compartment paired with an analgesic drug over one paired with only saline, but crucially, more so than the drug preference shown by normal mice.

Analysis of the body weight data indicated there were no significant group differences at baseline (before cell implantation). Body weights from the time period over which the CPP results indicated was the most important phase of the study were then assessed; the final 4 preferences tests (Figure 7). We used calculations of change in weight from before the previous test day (14 days prior to euthanasia). Repeated measures ANOVA was used with 'Time' (4 levels) as a within-subjects factor, and both 'Drug' (morphine or saline) and 'Treatment' (cancer or control) as between subject's factors. Over the final 10 days of the study the tumour bearing mice showed a small but nevertheless significant reduction in weight (1.6±0.8) compared to non-cancer mice. The non-cancer groups either maintained body weight or showed a marginal weight increase during this period (0.6±1 g) (significant 'Time×Treatment' interaction; $F(2,50) = 11$, $p < 0.001$). Morphine had no significant effects on body weight.

There was only a marginal difference in mean tumour burden between the saline and morphine groups; tumour wet-weight at *post-mortem* was 1.04±0.75 in the saline group versus 0.83±0.45 g in mice conditioned to morphine. An independent samples t-test showed morphine was unlikely to be responsible for this very slight difference ($t(16) = 0.91$, $p = 0.4$). We initially explored whether tumour burden was a significant contributor to morphine chamber preference on the last CPP test (Preference test P-1). Pearson's correlation showed no significant relationship between S+ preference scores and tumour burden in the saline group ($r = -0.19$; $p = 0.64$; Figure 8a), however, tumour burden was significantly positively correlated with preference for the morphine paired chamber ($r = 0.70$; $p = 0.034$; Figure 8b). The same relationship between tumour burden and morphine seeking was also apparent at 4 days (Preference test P-2) before euthanasia ($r = 0.72$; $p = 0.029$ (not shown)). However, the same comparison at the P-2 time point in mice conditioned to saline was not significant ($r = 0.22$; $p = 0.59$) (P-2 data not drawn)). These results therefore showed that increasing tumour burden made a positive contribution to morphine chamber preference.

The final phase of data collection in the CPP study was to determine whether we could recognise any behaviour-based evidence of reduced pain following terminal morphine treatment. We assessed the effect of the training dose of morphine given on the last study day on grooming, rearing and inactive behaviour

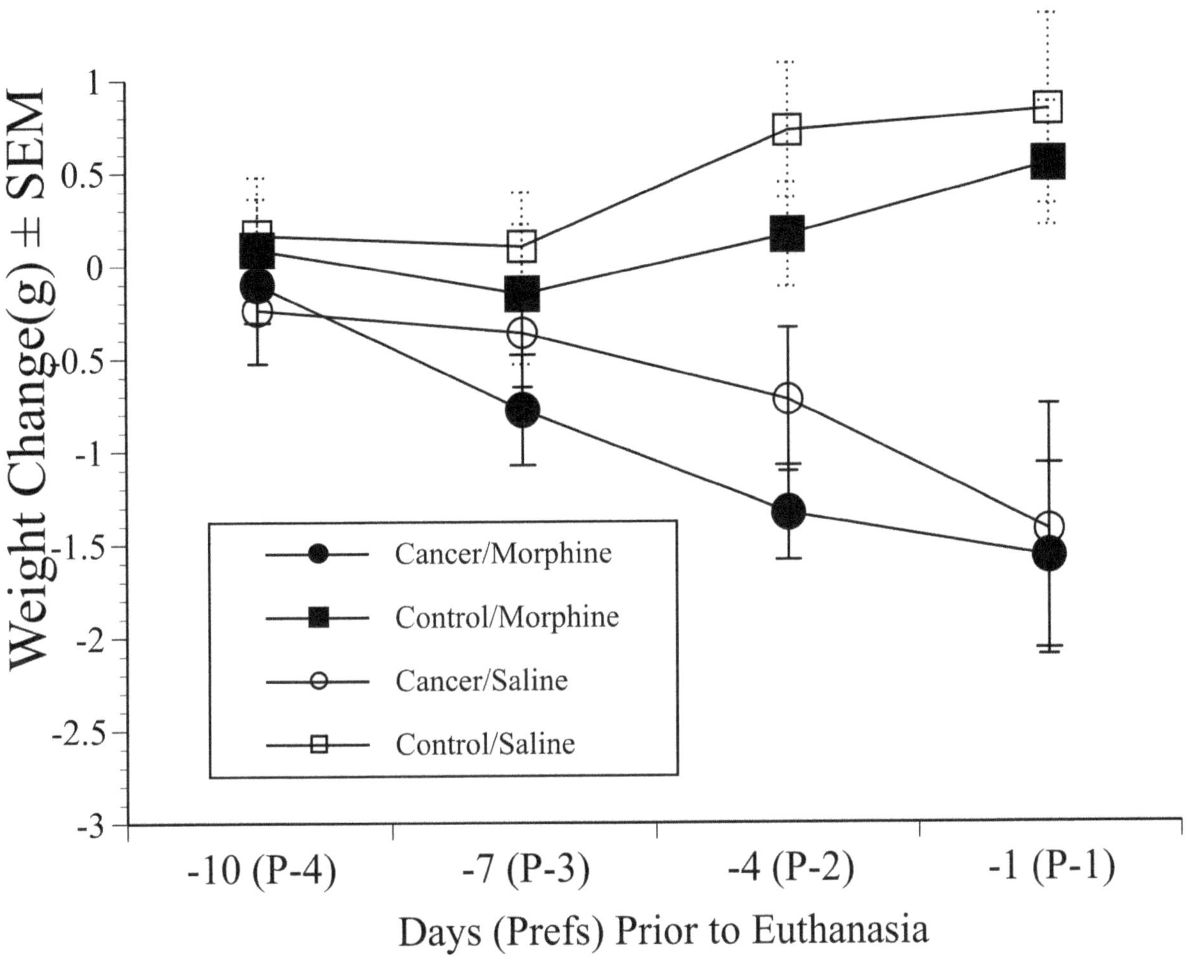


**Figure 7. Body weight change in mice used in CPP testing.** Mean weight (±SEM) on days −10 to −1 prior to euthanasia relative to weight observed on day −14 in mice in the main CPP study. Weights in tumour-bearing mice significantly declined over the final 7 study days compared to control groups ('Group (Cancer vs Control)×Time', p = 0.001), with no apparent effect of morphine.

frequency (Figure 9). For reasons previously given, total distance travelled was the only measure needed to evaluate changes in active behaviour. The analysis used 'Time' (pre and post-morphine) and 'Group' (tumour vs. non-tumour) as within and between subject's factors, and *post-hoc* analyses (Bonferroni) identified individual group differences. Prior to morphine the tumour-bearing mice travelled significantly less distance than controls (F(1.28) = 6.4, p = 0.017; Figure 9a). This increased in all mice following morphine ('Time' factor significant; F(1, 28) = 9.2, p = 0.005). Rearing frequency was similar across all groups initially, and all groups showed significantly reduced rearing behaviour following morphine ('Time' factor significant; F(1,27) = 83, p<0.001; Figure 9b). The mice with tumours initially groomed more than controls (F(1,28) = 104, p = 0.001), and morphine had no significant effect on this in either control group, and no significantly greater effect in tumour mice irrespective of whether they had previously been exposed to morphine (Figure 9c). Inactive behaviour was significantly more frequent in the controls versus the tumour groups prior to morphine (F(1,28) = 11.2, p = 0.002; Figure 9d), but all mice rested more frequently following drug treatment (F(1,28) = 36.7, p<0.001).

## Discussion

The work had two main aims. The first was to determine whether a relatively common mouse bladder cancer model had negative impacts on welfare, including effects caused by *malaise*, anxiety and ultimately pain. If there were any such effects we hoped to highlight these and provide information on potential refinements to prevent possible suffering in similar studies in the future. A second aim was to determine whether the Conditioned Place Preference (CPP) test provides a potentially more relevant alternative to testing analgesics against cancer pain than other presently available methods. The work consisted of a series of studies where in addition to CPP testing, we investigated the development of hyperalgesia, behaviour changes and potential prophylactic effects of morphine in terminal-stage cancer-bearing mice.

In the first study the Hargreaves method was used to evaluate any development of thermal hyperalgesia over a 24 day period following surgical implantation of bladder tumour cells. We found withdrawal thresholds reduced between 10 to 14 days prior to euthanasia, and this hyperalgesic effect was maintained until the end of the study. This increase in peripheral sensitisation provided our first evidence that this type of cancer might progressively impact negatively on welfare. A subsequent investigation exam-

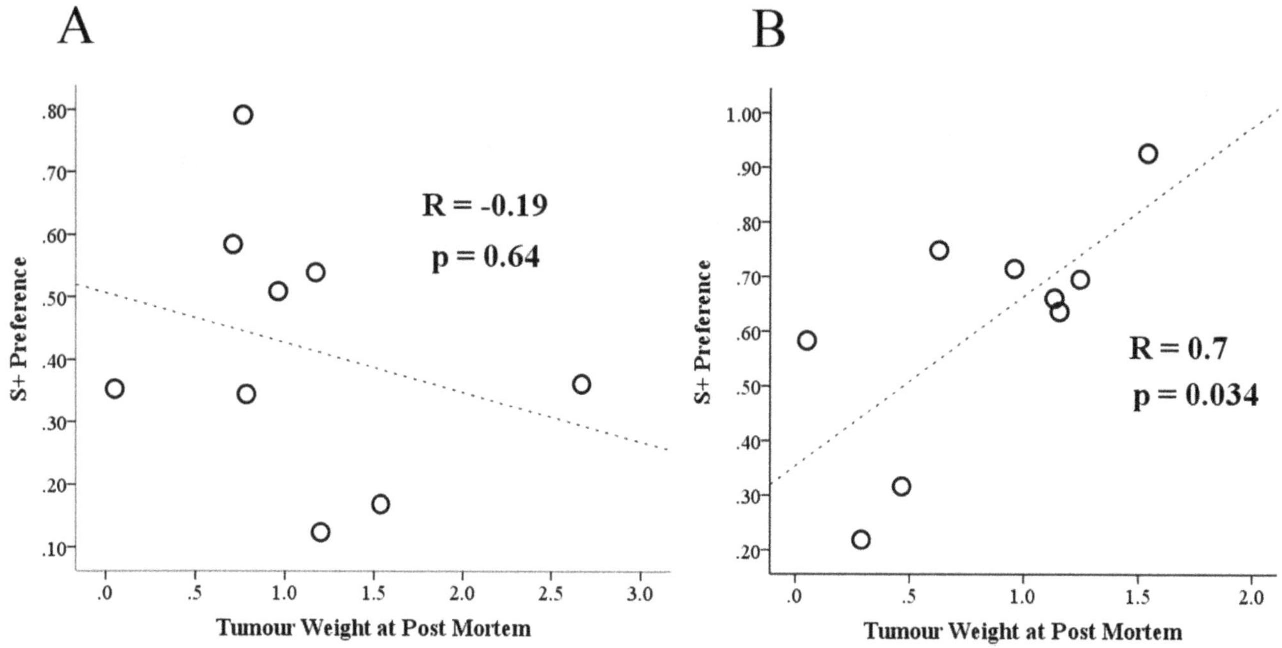


**Figure 8. Relationship between morphine seeking (CPP score) and tumour burden.** Scatterplots showing: (A) the relationship between relative S+ preference scores for saline on the day immediately prior to euthanasia versus post-mortem (wet) tumour weights (day P-1; Pearson's Correlation); and (B) the same relationship between tumour weight and S+ chamber preference on day P-1 for mice exposed to morphine. Tumour mass bore no significant relationship with saline chamber preference, but as panel B shows, morphine seeking significantly increased with increasing tumour burden.

ined changes in the behaviour of mice implanted with tumours via a potentially more refined non-surgical approach. Recordings of behaviour were processed using an automated system. This showed abnormal behaviour changes began between 7 and 10 days before the study ended, with the most notable effects being reduced distance travelled, reduced active and rearing behaviour and increased abdominal grooming. Changes to behaviours such as these have previously been attributed to abdominal pain in mice [30,31,56] and are similar to those that occur post-operatively in rats [21]. However, the most conclusive evidence that the mice

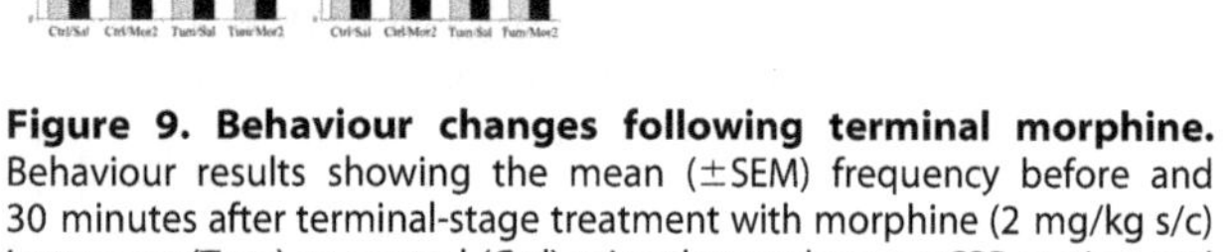

**Figure 9. Behaviour changes following terminal morphine.** Behaviour results showing the mean (±SEM) frequency before and 30 minutes after terminal-stage treatment with morphine (2 mg/kg s/c) in tumour (Tum) or control (Ctrl) mice that underwent CPP testing and were conditioned to morphine (Mor2) or saline (Sal). (A) Distance travelled; (B) Rearing; (C) Grooming; (D) Inactive periods (Pre) and following (Post) morphine treatment (2 mg/kg s/c). Morphine significantly increased overall activity, indicated by increased distance travelled and reduced rearing ('Time'; $p = 0.005$; $p = 0.001$, Distance and Rearing respectively). Grooming was reduced by morphine but not significantly, and inactive frequency increased ('Time', $p < 0.001$, respectively).

actually experienced pain came from the CPP study. Morphine seeking was found to be significantly positively linked to tumour burden, but most importantly, tumour bearing mice developed a greater preference for the morphine-paired chamber than any other group. They may also have found the placebo-paired chamber aversive, but the pattern of drug seeking strongly indicated the change in compartment preference was due to the negatively reinforcing (pain relieving) properties of morphine. As with the nociceptive and behaviour changes, the changes in morphine-seeking primarily emerged during the last 10 days of the study (4 preference tests). This not only indicated the presence of pain, but showed CPP testing could be a potentially effective and relevant means of evaluating analgesics against cancer and other types of pain.

Our findings were obtained despite a number of challenges, mainly the variable success of implanting tumours and the subsequent rates of cancer growth. Although engraftment was 100% using the surgical approach, it dropped to only 60% on our first attempt to implant via the urethra, then improved to 70% in the CPP study. There were several reasons why we persisted with non-surgical implantation of tumours despite the lower graft success. This method initially offered the possibility of being less costly, both financially and in terms of welfare. Conditioning of the bladder epithelium using a mild acid rinse and subsequent buffering was meant to maintain graft success but be less invasive. Non-surgical implantation also meant there was a reduced likelihood of needing to provide peri-operative analgesics; an issue that often concerns researchers who wish to rule out non-specific influences on tumour development. Potential welfare benefits were indicated by an absence of post-procedural weight loss compared to the effects of surgery. Mice that underwent surgical implantation also showed reduced thermal response thresholds, both immediately following surgery and during the latter stage of cancer growth; albeit unfortunate that we had no comparable nociceptive data from the catheterised mice. Finally, stress such as caused by surgery is a known tumour growth promoter [33,57], and any more rapid development could have been detrimental to the eventual timescale for CPP testing. Although tumour seeding was lower and subsequent growth slower via the urethral route, a positive aspect was that this allowed more time for CPP conditioning and also accommodated our preferred approach of only recruiting mice once tumours were detected. Establishing the most appropriate time to begin CPP testing was important since conditioning disease/pain-free mice to morphine could have had other unwanted consequences; e.g. tolerance issues or opioid-induced hyperalgesia. Avoiding these may have been important in our eventual ability to illustrate greater morphine seeking in tumour mice. Directly incorporating nociceptive testing was initially considered in determining when to begin conditioning (i.e. when thresholds reduced), but would have added a further unknown and potentially confounding variable; effectively a third compartment/place to which mice would have been exposed for relatively long periods. From an oncology perspective, however, implanting mice via the urethra may not have been the best option. This is because there are also valid welfare arguments in favour of surgical implantation, especially when tumour growth is more varied. Such variation could increase the number of animals needed to achieve adequate statistical power; making it even more challenging to determine an appropriate study end-point. The longer study duration would also increase facility (housing/husbandry) costs; an obviously important factor in overall cost-benefit analyses.

The behaviour study was meant to establish if bladder cancer impacted on aspects of behaviour in a similar way to other sources of abdominal pain in mice (e.g. vasectomy [31]), and thus required extensive collection of video footage for automated analysis using HCS software. We have previously used this system to assess the behaviour of mice, and shown it can provide precision equivalent to manual scoring [27,28]. However, this was where the varied tumour growth had its first major impact; forcing us to apply the data matching procedure to meaningfully analyse the results. We evaluated responses across 5 behaviour categories during the 2 weeks before euthanasia. This was the period of tumour growth considered most likely to encompass the time of development of any tumour-related pain. Abdominal grooming was more frequent in tumour-bearing mice, whereas distance travelled was reduced, and active behaviour and rearing all occurred substantially less frequently than in controls, especially over the final 7 days prior to euthanasia (Figure 3). There were, however, some unexpected findings. There was an increase in active behaviour and reduced grooming in tumour mice 3 days before euthanasia (Figures 3b and d), and another decline in active behaviour in controls on day −8. We looked for some unplanned event as a possible explanation (e.g. unscheduled husbandry), but the laboratory records held no clues. An adverse reaction to palpation was also unlikely as this was repeated on each of the 2 days that followed without any apparent impact. The effects were also unlikely to have been due to the data manipulation procedure as the period over which matching was conducted spanned 2 weeks and 7 separate dates. Indeed, we cannot offer a more rational explanation, and can only state that some mice were prone to some unusual activity patterns. Nevertheless, the clear disparity between the control and tumour mice over the period preceding euthanasia highlighted this as a key period for later evaluation in the CPP study.

The morphine doses chosen for the CPP pilot study (1 and 5 mg/kg) was another key decision. This was based on evidence of significant anti-nociceptive effects in both phasic (thermal) and tonic (abdominal writhing) tests in mice [54,55]. The larger dose had also previously been shown to elicit relatively robust CPP in rats, whereas 1 mg/kg was only marginally effective [39]. As non-tumour mice in the pilot study developed CPP to 5.0 or 1.0 mg/kg morphine in as a few as two to four conditioning trials (Figure 5) an intermediate dose of 2 mg/kg was chosen for the main study. However, the apparent speed of development of CPP, even in mice given 1 mg/kg, necessitated extending the amount of time used for later preference trials. Exploration time was increased to 45 minutes in the main study, however, only the first 15 minutes served as the dependent measure of preference. This was done in an attempt to minimise CPP development in non-tumour control mice as drug-free tests of this length can serve to facilitate extinction. The design of the main CPP experiment was informed by the original studies where the potential of CPP for evaluating the negatively reinforcing (i.e. analgesic) properties of drugs. Initially, arthritic rats showed an enhanced choice preference to a morphine paired chamber relative to drug treated controls [39] and it was concluded that this was because morphine was more rewarding in the context of pain. However, this interpretation was somewhat obscured in that non-inflamed rats showed an equivalent chamber time preference, and only the choice measure was significant. Sufka [39] describes some possible reasons; one being that choice testing could be a more relevant measure of response strength, whereas time could be influenced by factors unrelated to reinforcement. The intrinsically rewarding properties of morphine also presented challenges of interpreting unconditioned responding (the animals' subjective state), and why choice was superior to time. Then, however, a series of 6 discrete trials was used over 3 days of testing. Although we could not conduct similar choice trials due to a greater burden of conditioning and testing, we investigated the surrogate measure of entrances to each compartment over the first 60 s of each preference test. This, however, did not prove more informative than time preference so the results were not presented. Sufka's original conclusion regarding the value of the CPP methodology in the context of negative reinforcement was ultimately strengthened when a Bradykinin $B_1$ antagonist was used, which unlike morphine, had no intrinsically rewarding effects but was also preferred by formalin treated versus control rats [40]. This highlighted CPP as a method that could be applied outside of its usual domain for testing the abuse liability of drugs, and it has since been applied in several neuropathic and inflammatory pain models, all of which have successfully used 'time' as the dependent measure of unconditioned responding [41–43,45,46]. These studies, and the results presented here show CPP testing is one of the very few methods with potential for effectively differentiating between the sensory (nociceptive) and affective dimensions of pain. We know of only one previous study where the CPP methodology has been used to assess cancer pain [58], and this failed to show CPP to morphine 24 days after development intra plantar melanoma. Notably, they used a much higher morphine dose than in our study (10 mg/kg), so the lack of effects may have been due to tolerance issues or drug-induced hyperalgesia; both very common effects of repetitive opioid treatment. There was little evidence for either in our study since there were no differential behavioural responses to terminal morphine treatment in pre-exposed or drug naïve mice. Additionally, the morphine preference of controls changed relatively little from 10 to 4 days before euthanasia, whereas drug-seeking significantly increased over the same time period in the tumour mice. Tolerance would presumably have increased drug seeking in controls, and conversely, hyperalgesia should have prevented this in cancer mice. In reality, however, we may actually have underestimated when pain began because the first time that the cancer-bearing morphine group showed significantly elevated morphine seeking was 7 days (3 preference tests) before euthanasia. As learning this association could conceivably have required several conditioning cycles, the actual time when pain (and its relief) became salient cues may have been at some earlier time point.

Since the tumour model described by Betourne et al. [58] should still have caused localised pain, another possible explanation of their negative findings could be that the mice were so incapacitated that they were insufficiently motivated make a chamber choice. However, other design differences could also offer an explanation. As in Sufka's original study [39], all other studies where the CPP paradigm has been applied to pain have used the traditional approach of conditioning (using one or several drug exposures) followed by preference testing. We applied CPP testing where there could be severe, but slowly developing pain, but additionally, we wished not only to assess its presence but capture its onset. This meant applying a radical design change, incorporating repeated sets of conditioning trials interspersed with multiple preference tests (see Figure 1). So far as we are aware this approach has not been used previously and our positive result may, at least in part, have been due to the more frequent conditioning trials consolidating the association between pain and drug treatment. Our method of processing results by matching mice according to the total number of conditioning and test cycles undertaken, though again unconventional, may also have helped clarify the main effects. As in the behaviour study, this was needed to minimise the impact of the variable tumour growth. This variation meant mice were enrolled in the study at different times, with the net consequence that we could not be certain that animals entered the study at equivalent stages of cancer development. Using the data matching procedure we only examined CPP scores during the likely critical study time of the 10 days before euthanasia. Although this method of processing the data was not ideal, it does not detract from our main conclusion that the increased preference for morphine in cancer mice relative to controls indicated the emergence of pain.

Another study objective was to investigate the need for refinements if there was evidence of pain following tumour implantation. To this end we tested if a pre-procedural dose of meloxicam (5 mg/kg) was an appropriate method of controlling post-surgical in the Hargreaves study. Mice seem to require relatively high doses of NSAIDs [26,59] compared to the recommended rates for pain prevention in rats [23]. This was therefore a comparatively low pre-procedural dose, and was based on investigators' concerns over possible later impacts on tumour development. Although a relatively common reason for excluding analgesics from cancer studies [60] there was no such effect here. In agreement with behavioural and other physiological evidence [23,26] 5 mg/kg meloxicam also did not prevent post-surgical hyperalgesia, so switching to an alternative (e.g. buprenorphine) could be a refinement option, and is one that has already been shown to be less likely to interact with cancer study results [33] than other NSAIDs or opioids.

The effects of morphine were also assessed on euthanasia days when tumours were at an advanced stage. This delayed euthanasia by 75 minutes, but was justifiable since any positive effects could establish if the conditioning dose of morphine was analgesic. If so, this would provide further evidence of pain and establish if this was a refinement option in studies with a strong case for prolonging data collection. Although tumour-bearing mice travelled less and groomed more before morphine, our ability to detect any positive effects was confounded by several non-specific effects of drug treatment. Despite the pre-treatment differences, morphine increased the distance travelled and the frequency of bouts of inactivity and rearing in all mice including the controls (Figure 9). Such non-specific effects of opioids on behaviour are well documented [1,61–64], and we continue to find these can subvert attempts to confirm beneficial effects in studies of post-operative pain in rats in mice [31,65,66]. However, morphine had little influence on grooming in normal mice, and there were indications of post-treatment reductions in grooming in the cancer groups (Figure 9c). Grooming behaviour has previously been concluded to be important for assessing effects due to abdominal surgery or other manipulation likely to induce acute visceral discomfort [30,31,56,67], cancer [68], arthritis [69] and also shows pattern alterations during stress [70]. Perhaps consistent with stress, the cancer-bearing mice were less frequently inactive (unable to rest) prior to morphine (Figure 9d), but again, post-treatment effects were similar in all mice so no positive outcomes were detectable.

To maximise the welfare of mice used in cancer studies the refinements resulting from this work would ideally be widely applicable; such as to soft tissue cancers in general. Present results support this, at least for bladder cancer, since we implanted cells via 2 very different approaches (one surgical, one not) yet still found a commonality in pain symptoms over the final 7–10 study days. An obvious general recommendation would be to monitor animals as closely as possible during this time, possibly adding hyperalgesia and/or behaviour assessments to standard end-point determinations. We cannot state the extent to which behaviour or nociceptive changes should necessitate euthanasia, but increased grooming and the highly significant effects on rearing during cancer development indicate both could be useful. Although the effects on rearing could be also have been caused by *malaise* or some associated lethargy, they still indicated compromised welfare. Nociceptive assessments, however, require specialised equipment (e.g. Hargreaves apparatus) and routine CPP testing would obviously be implausible. The simplest alternative is to rely on weight changes, and accordingly, current model-specific guidelines suggest animals with solid internalised tumours and showing 'severe' cachexia (amounting to between 15 to 20% of baseline body weight) should be euthanased [11]. However, all cancer-bearing mice presently remained within these limits, with the greatest weight loss in the behaviour study being in the tumour group (4.6%). In the CPP study we found the greatest loss was 5 g in a tumour bearing mouse during the final 10 study days. We predicted that the repeated morphine treatments might minimise differences between the tumour and control groups, but seemingly not. One possible explanation is that although both the control and tumour groups were palpated daily, those with tumours may have experienced additional discomfort. We have previously shown that palpation adversely affects the behaviour of rats with bladder cancer [71]. Whether this was currently the case is speculative, but it is nevertheless advisable to be cautious in the manner and frequency of palpation. Body weight assessments should also be adjusted for increased mass due to progression of cancer. Although this was attempted it was found to be difficult, as in any model where tumours are internalised. In any event there was no effective relationship between body weight changes, *ex-vivo* tumour burden and survival (measured by study days from detection to euthanasia). Thus, even if palpation was an effective measure of burden, this would not have been useful in forecasting the need for euthanasia. A more likely scenario was that pain severity and survival were more closely governed by the tissues impacted on during cancer growth rather than burden *per se*. A better approach would be to use more sophisticated methods such as imaging tumours. We plan to use this in future studies to investigate relationships between tumour morphology and welfare, and the general applicability of the CPP and other findings where tumours grow in tissues where they are differentially likely to cause pain. As the majority of evidence indicated the mice were painful despite only moderate weight loss, we suggest protocols relying on this as a primary welfare indicator might consider a more conservative end-point; such as *any* consistent weight loss over a 2 to 3 day period in an otherwise healthy mouse. In studies where more consistent tumour growth is achieved and study duration can be estimated more accurately, our results suggest end-points might be brought forward by at least one week. The precise time is obviously still difficult to identify, but experienced care staff can be exceptionally capable in estimating survival.

A fundamental 3Rs principle is to obtain maximum from the least number of animals, but without compromising scientific integrity. By applying several different assessment methods we hoped to detect cancer pain or other negative impacts on welfare as reliably as possible. Using separate study groups, although a possible weakness, had the major advantage of minimising the burden of testing on individual mice. Indeed, the impact of high intensity testing may be the reason that at least one report has emerged where a range of different 'quality of life' assessments failed to demonstrate negative consequences in a rat neuropathic pain model [50]. We believe the present series of experiments achieved a good level of precision due to the consistency of findings despite some substantial methodological variations. Overall, our studies were conducted in a manner that closely complied with the 3Rs principle of reduction; the majority of data being collected in mice already undergoing cancer trials. However, this meant studying the female mice our colleagues routinely use; due to the greater ease of implanting tumours via the urethra. Oestrus stage could therefore have impacted on our results depending on what stage coincided with conditioning, such as by altering the sensitivity of the mice to morphine. The mice were singly housed, but not isolated. They were also fully acclimated and never in contact with male mice, thus over the course of the study the mice would have undergone several oestrus cycles. It was not feasible to attempt to determine the impact of this on results due to the additional sampling that would have been required. We could have implemented measures to disrupt or halt oestrus, however, the relatively frequent morphine treatments may have caused this already. Determining oestrus stage would also have been very time consuming, and could also have been counterproductive to results. There is extensive literature on sex and strain differences in response to pain and to drug treatment [72–76], so ideally we would repeat the work to establish if the CPP findings generalise to male mice also. However, this would necessitate either surgical tumour implantation, or the more invasive approach of catheterising the urethra of males, both of which could render results questionable. Overall, we argue that it is unlikely that only using female mice significantly weakened our main findings. It could also have been advantageous had we been able to apply the mouse grimace scale (MGS) as an adjunct to the various other measurement parameters [59,77,78]. However, the work was completed prior to its development, and the quality of video recording in the behaviour study, together with the method of filming for analysis by HCS meant the data were not suitable for retrospective analysis using this approach.

## Conclusions

The essence of this work was to address a recently highlighted need for more appropriate (systems-based) methods of analgesic drug screening, and the development of more relevant translational pain models. We used a common mouse cancer model and multiple test methods to simultaneously address a second but no less important aim. This was to establish if cancer has a negative impact on the welfare of mice (predictably caused by pain), as this would demand greater effort in refining present end-point guidelines. The work constitutes the most comprehensive series of studies so far undertaken to determine whether bladder cancer is painful to mice. We showed reduced body condition and weight, changes in spontaneous behaviour, and the development of peripheral sensitivity (hyperalgesia) as tumours developed. Added to this we used the CPP paradigm as a means of offering mice the opportunity to self-report on any awareness of pain. Those with cancer spent longer in an environment where they previously experienced the effects of morphine than mice conditioned to morphine alone. Another critical finding was that morphine seeking was closely linked (increased) with tumour burden. However, the validity of our conclusion that these effects indicated pain hinges on whether mice sought morphine as a result of its association with pain relief. It also assumes that the various other changes provide complementary evidence of this. We argue that according to the triangulation principle these results collectively provide convincing evidence of the presence of clinical-type pain in this mouse cancer model. If not pain, there was at least very strong evidence of negative impacts on welfare highlighting a need for a range of possible refinements. Mice in this bladder cancer model could benefit from removal at least 7, and possibly even 10 days prior to the scheduled end-point. Relying only on weight changes or other model-specific signs may not be sufficient to ensure mice do not experience pain before they are euthanased. Rearing deficits may be a useful early indicator of the onset of adverse effects. We found no evidence that provision of morphine was detrimental either to cancer development or to the welfare of mice. In mice implanted surgically there were also no obvious effects of a pre-surgery dose of meloxicam either on post-surgery nociception or tumour development. A more refined surgical protocol might be one using a more appropriate dose of an NSAID for pain prevention, but this would require preliminary work to determine how these or other pharmacological candidates might impact on result validity. However, depending on the sensitivity of required outcomes, future studies of this type might involve buprenorphine; where it has been shown in at least one cancer study to have negligible or even beneficial effects in terms of both welfare refinement and result validity [33]. In light of the numerous other examples where CPP testing has now been applied to assess centralised pain in models other than cancer, we also conclude that CPP testing offers a method of increasing the translational relevance of the results of analgesic screening studies.

## Acknowledgments

We wish to thank our colleagues of Newcastle University's Northern Institute for Cancer Research (NICR) for help with cell culturing, developing the implant methodology and for providing access to their animals. The manuscript was prepared according to the ARRIVE guidelines [79] recommended by the UK NC3Rs and others.

## Author Contributions

Conceived and designed the experiments: JVR CC PAF HT KS. Performed the experiments: JVR CC PAF HT KS. Analyzed the data: JVR CC PAF HT KS. Contributed reagents/materials/analysis tools: JVR CC PAF HT KS. Wrote the paper: JVR CC PAF HT KS.

## References


1. Cowan A, Doxey JC, Harry EJ (1977) The animal pharmacology of buprenorphine, an oripavine analgesic agent. Br J Pharmacol 60: 547–554.
2. Dennis SG, Melzack R (1979) Comparison of phasic and tonic pain in animals. In: Bonica JJ, editor. Advances in pain research and therapy. New York: Raven Press. 747–760.
3. Mogil JS, Crager SE (2004) What should we be measuring in behavioral studies of chronic pain in animals. Pain 112: 12–15.
4. Sufka K (2011) Translational challenges and analgesic screening assays. Pain 152: 1942–1943.
5. Mao J (2012) Current challenges in translational pain research. Trends Pharmacol Sci 33: 568–573.
6. Duncan IJH (1996) Animal welfare defined in terms of feelings. Acta Agriculturae Scandinavica Section A-Animal Science Supplementum 27: 29–35.
7. Flecknell P, Leach M, Bateson M (2011) Affective state and quality of life in mice. Pain 152: 963–964.
8. Mendl M, Burman OHP, Parker RMA, Paul ES (2009) Cognitive bias as an indicator of animal emotion and welfare: Emerging evidence and underlying mechanisms. Appl Anim Behav Sci 118: 161–181.
9. HMSO (2012) Statistics of Scientific Procedures on Living Animals (Great Britain). London: Her Majesty's Stationary Office.
10. UKCCCR (1998) United Kingdom Co-ordinating Committee on Cancer Research (UKCCCR) Guidelines for the Welfare of Animals in Experimental Neoplasia (Second Edition). Br J Cancer 77: 1–10.
11. Workman P, Aboagye EO, Balkwill F, Balmain A, Bruder G, et al. (2010) Guidelines for the welfare and use of animals in cancer research. Br J Cancer 102: 1555–1577.
12. Asai H, Ozaki N, Shinoda M, Nagamine K, Tohnai I, et al. (2005) Heat and mechanical hyperalgesia in mice model of cancer pain. Pain 117: 19–29.
13. Fox A, Medhurst S, Courade JP, Glatt M, Dawson J, et al. (2004) Anti-hyperalgesic activity of the cox-2 inhibitor lumiracoxib in a model of bone cancer pain in the rat. Pain 107: 33–40.
14. Lee BH, Seong J, Kim UJ, Won R, Kim M (2005) Behavioral characteristics of a mouse model of cancer pain. Yonsei Med J 46: 252–259.
15. Zhang HW, Iida Y, Andoh T, Nojima H, Murata J, et al. (2003) Mechanical hypersensitivity and alterations in cutaneous nerve fibers in a mouse model of skin cancer pain. J Pharmacol Sci 91: 167–170.
16. Calixto-Campos C, Zarpelon AC, Correa M, Cardoso RDR, Pinho-Ribeiro FA, et al. (2013) The Ehrlich tumor induces pain-like behavior in mice: a novel model of cancer pain for pathophysiological studies and pharmacological screening. BioMed Res Int 2013: 624815.
17. Hang L-H, Shao D-H, Chen Z, Chen Y-F, Shu W-W, et al. (2013) Involvement of spinal CC chemokine ligand 5 in the development of bone cancer pain in rats. Basic Clin Pharmacol Toxicol 113: 325–328.
18. Liu M, Yang H, Fang D, Yang J-J, Cai J, et al. (2013) Upregulation of P2×3 receptors by neuronal calcium sensor protein VILIP-1 in dorsal root ganglions contributes to the bone cancer pain in rats. Pain 154: 1551–1568.
19. Zhao J, Zhang H, Liu SB, Han P, Hu S, et al. (2013) Spinal interleukin-33 and its receptor ST2 contribute to bone cancer-induced pain in mice. Neurosci 253: 172–182.
20. Leach MC, Allweiler S, Richardson C, Roughan JV, Narbe R, et al. (2009) Behavioural effects of ovariohysterectomy and oral administration of meloxicam in laboratory housed rabbits. Res Vet Sci 87: 336–347.
21. Roughan JV, Flecknell PA (2001) Behavioural effects of laparotomy and analgesic effects of ketoprofen and carprofen in rats. Pain 90: 65–74.
22. Roughan JV, Flecknell PA (2003) Validation of a behaviour-based postoperative pain-scoring system in rats. Proceedings of the Association of Veterinary Anaesthetists Spring Meeting, Dublin 2002. Vet Anaesth Analg 30: 54.
23. Roughan JV, Flecknell PA (2003) Evaluation of a short duration behaviour-based post-operative pain scoring system in rats. Eur J Pain 7: 397–406.
24. Roughan JV, Flecknell PA (2006) Training in behaviour-based post-operative pain scoring in rats - An evaluation based on improved recognition of analgesic requirements. Appl Anim Behav Sci 96: 327–342.
25. Roughan JV, Flecknell PA, Orr HE (2003) Behavioural assessment of post-operative pain and analgesic effects of carprofen in the domestic rabbit. 8th World Congress of Veterinary Anaesthesia. Knoxville, USA. 143.
26. Wright-Williams SL, Courade J-P, Richardson CA, Roughan JV, Flecknell PA (2007) Effects of vasectomy surgery and meloxicam treatment on faecal corticosterone levels and behaviour in two strains of laboratory mouse. Pain 130: 108–118.
27. Roughan JV, Wright-Williams SL, Flecknell PA (2009) Automated analysis of postoperative behaviour: assessment of HomeCageScan as a novel method to rapidly identify pain and analgesic effects in mice. Lab Anim 43: 17–26.
28. Miller AL, Flecknell PA, Leach MC, Roughan JV (2011) A comparison of a manual and an automated behavioural analysis method for assessing post-operative pain in mice. Appl Anim Behav Sci 131: 138–144.
29. Dickinson AL, Leach MC, Flecknell PA (2009) The analgesic effects of oral paracetamol in two strains of mice undergoing vasectomy. Lab Anim 43: 357–361.
30. Miller AL, Wright-Williams SL, Flecknell PA, Roughan JV (2012) A comparison of abdominal and scrotal approach methods of vasectomy and the influence of analgesic treatment in laboratory mice. Lab Anim 46: 304–310.
31. Wright-Williams S, Flecknell PA, Roughan JV (2013) Comparative effects of vasectomy surgery and buprenorphine treatment on faecal corticosterone concentrations and behaviour assessed by manual and automated analysis methods in C57 and C3H mice. PLoS ONE [Electronic Resource] 8: e75948.
32. Vermeirsch H, Nuydens RM, Salmon PL, Meert TF (2004) Bone cancer pain model in mice: evaluation of pain behavior, bone destruction and morphine sensitivity. Pharmacol Biochem Be 79: 243–251.
33. Franchi S, Panerai AE, Sacerdote P (2007) Buprenorphine ameliorates the effect of surgery on hypothalamus-pituitary-adrenal axis, natural killer cell activity and metastatic colonization in rats in comparison with morphine or fentanyl treatment. Brain Behav Immun 21: 767–774.
34. Martucci C, Panerai AE, Sacerdote P (2004) Chronic fentanyl or buprenorphine infusion in the mouse: similar analgesic profile but different effects on immune responses. Pain 110: 385–392.
35. Valeberg BT, Rustoen T, Bjordal K, Hanestad BR, Paul S, et al. (2008) Self-reported prevalence, etiology, and characteristics of pain in oncology outpatients. Eur J Pain 12: 582–590.
36. van den Beuken-van Everdingen MHJ, de Rijke JM, Kessels AG, Schouten HC, van Kleef M, et al. (2007) Prevalence of pain in patients with cancer: a systematic review of the past 40 years. Ann Oncol 18: 1437–1449.
37. Medhurst S, Bowes M, Kidd BL, Glatt M, Muller M, et al. (2001) Antinociceptive effects of the bisphosphonate, zoledronic acid, in a novel rat model of bone cancer pain. Brit J Pharmacol 134.
38. Bardo MT, Bevins RA (2000) Conditioned place preference: what does it add to our preclinical understanding of drug reward? Psychopharmacology 153: 31–43.
39. Sufka KJ (1994) Conditioned place preference paradigm: a novel approach for analgesic drug assessment against chronic pain. Pain 58: 355–366.
40. Sufka KJ, Roach JT (1996) Stimulus properties and antinociceptive effects of selective bradykinin B1 and B2 receptor antagonists in rats. Pain 66: 99–103.
41. King T, Vera-Portocarrero L, Gutierrez T, Vanderah TW, Dussor G, et al. (2009) Unmasking the tonic-aversive state in neuropathic pain.[Erratum appears in Nat Neurosci. 2010 Aug;13(8):1033]. Nat Neurosci 12: 1364–1366.
42. Qu C, King T, Okun A, Lai J, Fields HL, et al. (2011) Lesion of the rostral anterior cingulate cortex eliminates the aversiveness of spontaneous neuropathic pain following partial or complete axotomy. Pain 152: 1641–1648.
43. Rutten K, De Vry J, Robens A, Tzschentke TM, van der Kam EL (2011) Dissociation of rewarding, anti-aversive and anti-nociceptive effects of different classes of anti-nociceptives in the rat. Eur J Pain 15: 299–305.
44. Davoody L, Quiton RL, Lucas JM, Ji Y, Keller A, et al. (2011) Conditioned place preference reveals tonic pain in an animal model of central pain. J Pain 12: 868–874.
45. Okun A, Liu P, Davis P, Ren J, Remeniuk B, et al. (2012) Afferent drive elicits ongoing pain in a model of advanced osteoarthritis. Pain 153: 924–933.
46. Park HJ, Stokes JA, Pirie E, Skahen J, Shtaerman Y, et al. (2013) Persistent hyperalgesia in the cisplatin-treated mouse as defined by threshold measures, the conditioned place preference paradigm, and changes in dorsal root ganglia activated transcription factor 3: the effects of gabapentin, ketorolac, and etanercept. Anesth Analg 116: 224–231.
47. Bateson PP, Rose SP, Horn G (1973) Imprinting: lasting effects on uracil incorporation into chick brain. Science 181: 576–578.
48. Bateson P (1991) Assessment of pain in animals. Anim Behav 42: 827–839.
49. McNabb CT, Uhelski ML, Fuchs PN (2012) A direct comparison of affective pain processing underlying two traditional pain modalities in rodents. Neurosci Lett 507: 57–61.
50. Urban R, Scherrer G, Goulding EH, Tecott LH, Basbaum AI (2011) Behavioral indices of ongoing pain are largely unchanged in male mice with tissue or nerve injury-induced mechanical hypersensitivity. Pain 152: 990–1000.
51. Hargreaves K, Dubner,R, Brown F, Flores C, Joris J (1988) Basic Section - A new and sensitive method for measuring thermal nociception in cutaneous hyperalgesia. Pain 32, 77–88.
52. Chin J, Kadhim S, Garcia B, Kim YS, Karlik S (1991) Magnetic resonance imaging for detecting and treatment monitoring of orthotopic murine bladder tumor implants. J Urology 145: 1297–1301.
53. Suzuki T, Tsuji M, Mori T, Misawa M, Endoh T, et al. (1996) Effect of the highly selective and nonpeptide delta opioid receptor agonist TAN-67 on the morphine-induced place preference in mice. J Pharmacol Exp Ther 279: 177–185.
54. Dashti-Rahmatababi MH, Hejazian SH, Morshedi A, Rafati A (2007) The analgesic effect of Carum copticum extract and morphine on phasic pain in mice. J Ethnopharmacol 109: 226–228.
55. Stevenson GW, Bilsky EJ, Negus SS (2006) Targeting pain-suppressed behaviours in preclinical assays of pain and analgesia: Effects of morphine on acetic acid-suppressed feeding in C57BL/6J mice. J Pain 7: 408–416.
56. Cesarovic N, Arras M, Jirkof P (2014) Impact of inhalation anaesthesia, surgery and analgesic treatment on home cage behaviour in laboratory mice. Appl Anim Behav Sci.
57. Hasegawa H, Saiki I (2002) Psychosocial stress augments tumor development through beta-adrenergic activation in mice. Jpn J Cancer Res 93: 729–735.
58. Betourne A, Familiades J, Lacassagne L, Halley H, Cazales M, et al. (2008) Decreased motivational properties of morphine in mouse models of cancerous-

or inflammatory-chronic pain: implication of supraspinal neuropeptide FF2 receptors. Neuroscience 157: 12–21.
59. Matsumiya LC, Sorge RE, Sotocinal SG, Tabaka JM, Wieskopf JS, et al. (2012) Using the Mouse Grimace Scale to reevaluate the efficacy of postoperative analgesics in laboratory mice. J Am Assoc Lab Anim 51: 42–49.
60. Sasamura T, Nakamura S, Iida Y, Fujii H, Murata J, et al. (2002) Morphine analgesia suppresses tumor growth and metastasis in a mouse model of cancer pain produced by orthotopic tumor inoculation. Eur J Pharmacol 441: 185–191.
61. Liles JH, Flecknell PA (1993) The effects of surgical stimulus on the rat and the influence of analgesic treatment. Brit Vet J 149: 515–525.
62. Liles JH, Flecknell PA (1993) The influence of buprenorphine or bupivacaine on the post-operative effects of laparotomy and bile-duct ligation in rats. Lab Anim 27: 374–380.
63. Hayes JH, Flecknell PA (1999) A comparison of pre- and post-surgical administration of bupivacaine or buprenorphine following laparotomy in the rat. Lab Anim 33: 16–23.
64. Hayes KE, Raucci JA, Jr., Gades NM, Toth LA (2000) An evaluation of analgesic regimens for abdominal surgery in mice. Contemp Top Lab Anim 39: 18–23.
65. Roughan JV, Flecknell PA (2000) Effects of surgery and analgesic administration on spontaneous behaviour in singly housed rats. Res Vet Sci 69: 283–288.
66. Roughan JV, Flecknell RA (2004) Behaviour-based assessment of the duration of laparotomy-induced abdominal pain and the analgesic effects of carprofen and buprenorphine in rats. Behav Pharmacol 15: 461–472.
67. Craft RM, Henley SR, Haaseth RC, Hruby VJ, Porreca F (1995) Opioid antinociception in a rat model of visceral pain: systemic versus local drug administration. J Pharmacol Exp Ther 275: 1535–1542.
68. Nagahata S, Harano N, Ono K, Seta Y, Shiiba S, et al. (2007) A rat model for cancer pain in the trigemina nerve area. Eur J Pain 11: 69–69.
69. Dimitrijevic M, Laban O, Djuric VJ, Stanojevic S, Miletic T, et al. (2001) Behavior and Severity of Adjuvant Arthritis in Four Rat Strains. Brain Behav Immun 15: 255–265.
70. Kalueff AV, Tuohimaa P (2004) Grooming analysis algorithm for neurobehavioural stress research. Brain Res Protoc 13: 151–158.
71. Roughan JV, Flecknell PA, Davies BR (2004) Behavioural assessment of the effects of tumour growth in rats and the influence of the analgesics carprofen and meloxicam. Lab Anim 38: 286–296.
72. Mogil JS (2006) Sex, gender and pain. In: Cervero F, Jensen TS, editors. Handbook of Clinical Neurology. Amsterdam: Elsevier. 325–341.
73. Mogil JS (2012) Sex differences in pain and pain inhibition: multiple explanations of a controversial phenomenon. Nat Rev Neurosci 13: 859–866.
74. Sorge RE, LaCroix-Fralish ML, Tuttle AH, Sotocinal SG, Austin J-S, et al. (2011) Spinal cord Toll-like receptor 4 mediates inflammatory and neuropathic hypersensitivity in male but not female mice. J Neurosci 31: 15450–15454.
75. Mogil JS, Chesler EJ, Wilson SG, Juraska JM, Sternberg WF (2000) Sex differences in thermal nociception and morphine antinociception in rodents depend on genotype. Neurosci Biobehav R 24: 375–389.
76. Mogil JS, Wilson SG, Bon K, Lee SE, Kyungsoon C, et al. (1999) Heritaility of nociception I: Responses of 11 inbred mouse strains on 12 measures of nociception. Pain 80: 67–82.
77. Leach MC, Klaus K, Miller AL, Scotto di Perrotolo M, Sotocinal SG, et al. (2012) The assessment of post-vasectomy pain in mice using behaviour and the Mouse Grimace Scale. PLoS ONE [Electronic Resource] 7: e35656.
78. Langford DJ, Bailey AL, Chanda ML, Clarke SE, Drummond TE, et al. (2010) Coding of facial expressions of pain in the laboratory mouse. Nat Methods 7: 447–449.
79. Kilkenny C, Browne WJ, Cuthill IC, Emerson M, Altman DG (2010) Improving bioscience research reporting: The ARRIVE guidelines for reporting animal research. J Pharmacol Pharmacother 1: 94–99.

14

# Periaortic Brown Adipose Tissue as a Major Determinant of [$^{18}$F]-Fluorodeoxyglucose Vascular Uptake in Atherosclerosis-Prone, ApoE$^{-/-}$ Mice

**Jakub Toczek*[9], Alexis Broisat[9], Pascale Perret, Marie-Dominique Desruet, Daniel Fagret, Laurent M. Riou, Catherine Ghezzi**

INSERM, UMR 1039, Radiopharmaceutiques Biocliniques; Université Grenoble I, La Tronche, France

## Abstract

***Background:*** [$^{18}$F]-fluorodeoxyglucose (FDG) has been suggested for the clinical and experimental imaging of inflammatory atherosclerotic lesions. Significant FDG uptake in brown adipose tissue (BAT) has been observed both in humans and mice. The objective of the present study was to investigate the influence of periaortic BAT on apolipoprotein E-deficient (apoE$^{-/-}$) mouse atherosclerotic lesion imaging with FDG.

***Methods:*** ApoE$^{-/-}$ mice (36±2 weeks-old) were injected with FDG (12±2 MBq). Control animals (Group A, n = 7) were injected conscious and kept awake at room temperature (24°C) throughout the accumulation period. In order to minimize tracer activity in periaortic BAT, Group B (n = 7) and C (n = 6) animals were injected under anaesthesia at 37°C and Group C animals were additionally pre-treated with propranolol. PET/CT acquisitions were performed prior to animal euthanasia and ex vivo analysis of FDG biodistribution.

***Results:*** Autoradiographic imaging indicated higher FDG uptake in atherosclerotic lesions than in the normal aortic wall (all groups, $P<0.05$) and the blood (all groups, $P<0.01$) which correlated with macrophage infiltration ($R = 0.47$; $P<0.001$). However, periaortic BAT uptake was either significantly higher (Group A, $P<0.05$) or similar (Group B and C, P = NS) to that observed in atherosclerotic lesions and was shown to correlate with in vivo quantified aortic FDG activity.

***Conclusion:*** Periaortic BAT FDG uptake was identified as a confounding factor while using FDG for the non-invasive imaging of mouse atherosclerotic lesions.

**Editor:** Carmine Pizzi, University of Bologna, Italy

**Funding:** The study was funded by grants from the Agence Nationale de la Recherche (ANR, http://www.agence-nationale-recherche.fr/): ANR grant PLAQUIMAG #ANR-09-TECS-017-01 and Institut National de la Santé et de la Recherche Médicale (INSERM, http://www.inserm.fr/). The funders had no role in study design, data collection and analysis, decision to publish, or preparation of the manuscript.

**Competing Interests:** The authors have declared that no competing interests exist.

* Email: jakub.toczek@gmail.com

[9] These authors contributed equally to this work.

## Introduction

Coronary artery disease leads to myocardial infarction mostly through rupture of undetected coronary vulnerable plaques [1]. The non-invasive detection of vulnerable atherosclerotic lesions therefore represents a great yet unmet clinical challenge in the field of nuclear cardiology. Active inflammation, including monocyte/macrophage infiltration is a major criterion in the definition of vulnerable atherosclerotic lesions [2]. Plaque inflammation might be visualized with positron emission tomography (PET) using [$^{18}$F]-fluorodeoxyglucose (FDG) through increased tracer uptake by inflammatory cells with high metabolic activity as initially shown in patients with symptomatic carotid artery disease [3]. While clinical investigation of FDG PET imaging of atherosclerosis has been an active field of research for over a decade, additional studies are still needed to establish the role of FDG–PET in atherosclerosis imaging [4,5]. Moreover, preclinical imaging of atherosclerosis *per se* remains of great interest for preclinical and basic research. However, the potential of FDG for the non-invasive experimental assessment of atherosclerosis in the widely used apolipoprotein E-deficient (apoE$^{-/-}$) mouse model of atherosclerosis has not been clearly defined [6–11].

The brown adipose tissue (BAT) is involved in nonshivering thermogenesis under sympathetic nervous system control and display varying and potentially high levels of metabolic activity depending upon the energetic metabolic status, anaesthetic conditions, pharmacological interventions and external temperature [12]. Accordingly, FDG uptake in brown adipose tissue has been reported to reach significant levels in humans as well as in mice [7,13,14]. A periaortic adipose tissue with virtually identical features to those of brown adipose tissue has been identified and studied [15]. Periaortic BAT is located in the immediate vicinity of aortic atherosclerotic lesions and has recently been assigned an atheroprotective role through adaptive thermogenesis [16]. Despite its anatomical proximity with atherosclerotic lesions, the potential impact of periaortic BAT on noninvasive FDG vascular imaging of atherosclerotic plaques has not been evaluated yet. Therefore, the objective of the present study was to investigate the potential confounding effect of periaortic BAT on apoE$^{-/-}$ mouse aortic atherosclerotic lesion imaging with FDG under experimental conditions affecting BAT metabolic activity. FDG aortic uptake in apoE$^{-/-}$ mice was studied *in vivo* using a state-of-the-art, small-animal dedicated PET/CT camera and *ex vivo* using autoradiographic imaging of the aortic arch in order to discriminate atherosclerotic lesion from periaortic BAT tracer uptake.

## Materials and Methods

### Ethical statement

All animal procedures were conducted under the approval of the animal experimentation ethics committee ComEth Grenoble (authorization # 151_LER-U1039-LR-01). All efforts were made to minimize suffering.

### Animal study

The experimental procedure is summarized in Figure 1. Twenty (20) female apoE$^{-/-}$ mice aged 36±2 weeks and fed a high-fat western type chow containing 0.05% cholesterol (Safe, Augy, France) for 24±6 weeks were used. The mice were housed under controlled humidity, temperature, and light cycle conditions. All animals were kept at 24°C and fasted for 14 h before the imaging protocol. After 13 h of fasting and 1 h before FDG injection, the animals were randomly assigned to 1 of 3 experimental groups, namely Group A, B and C. Animals from Group A (n = 7) were not anesthetized while Group B (n = 7) and Group C (n = 6) animals were anesthetized using intraperitoneal (i.p.) sodium pentobarbital (0.055 mg·kg$^{-1}$) and kept under anesthesia with an i.p. infusion of 0.020 mg·kg$^{-1}$·h$^{-1}$ sodium pentobarbital for 4 h while kept in a 37°C warmed bed with oxygen supplementation. In addition, Group C animals were injected with DL-propranolol (Sigma-Aldrich) 10 mg·kg$^{-1}$ i.p. following anesthesia induction. FDG (12±2 MBq) was injected in the tail vein 1 h after the induction of anesthesia in Group B and C animals whereas Group A animals were injected conscious at the same time point. Animal weight and blood glucose (Accu-check performa, Roche Diagnostics) were assessed before the fasting period as well as before FDG injection in all 3 experimental groups while an additional assessment of glycemia was performed immediately prior to anesthesia induction in Groups B and C. Group A animals were anesthetized for the purpose of image acquisition at 2.25 h following FDG injection (i.e. 0.25 h prior to PET image acquisition, see below) using isoflurane 2% in an oxygen-supplemented gas mixture. FDG image acquisition was started 2.5 h following tracer injection and lasted for 0.5 h in all animals from groups A, B, and C (see details below). All animals were euthanized 3 h following FDG injection through cervical dislocation while still under deep anesthesia.

### PET/CT imaging

Dual modality PET/CT acquisitions were performed using a small animal dedicated system (nanoPET/CT, Bioscan) and proprietary software (Nucline 1.07, Bioscan). A thirty (30) min-long PET acquisition was performed from 2.5 to 3 h p.i. with 1-3 coincidence mode and image reconstruction was performed using constructor's OSEM algorithm. A CT acquisition was then performed using 180 projections (600 ms each) at 45 kVp and reconstructed using dedicated software (Nucline 1.07, Bioscan). PET images were quantified using InVivoScope 2.0 software (Bioscan) and 2 volumes of interest (VOIs) were drawn. A first spherical volume of interest (radius: 0.5 mm) was centered on aortic arch lesions as identified by CT signal enhancement [17] and a second VOI matched the prevertebral course of the thoracic aorta above the diaphragm muscle. Activity concentration in the VOI was expressed as mean standardized uptake value ($SUV_{mean}$), i.e. tissue activity concentration (MBq·mL$^{-1}$)/injected dose (MBq) · body weight (g).

### *Ex vivo* protocol

After euthanasia, multiple tissues samples were harvested, weighed and their activity was measured (Cobra II Auto-Gamma counter, Packard). Tissue activities from gamma-well counting were corrected for decay and tissue activity concentrations were then expressed as a differential uptake ratios (DUR) corresponding to tissue activity concentration (MBq·g$^{-1}$)/injected dose (MBq) · body weight (g). The proximal thoracic aorta was harvested and deep-frozen in −40°C cooled 2-methylbutane along with other tissues samples of known activity concentration. Twenty (20) µm-thick sections were obtained (HM505E, Microm), exposed on an autoradiographic film (08SR2025, Fujifilm) and read using a phosphorimager (BAS-5000, Fujifilm). Exposed tissues sections were stained with HES trichrome coloration (Haematoxylin, Erythrosine, Saffron) while adjacent 8 µm-thick tissue sections were used for immunohistochemistry.

### Immunohistochemistry

Macrophage and BAT immunostainings were performed on 8 µm-thick frozen sections using anti-F4/80 and anti-UCP-1 antibodies, respectively. Briefly, endogenous peroxidases were blocked with hydrogen peroxide on −20°C acetone fixed slices. Following a blocking step at room temperature, the primary antibody was applied on the tissue sections overnight at 4°C (anti-F4/80, 1:200, 14-4801-85 (BM8), eBioscience; and anti-UCP-1, 1:500, sc-6528 (C17), Santa Cruz Biotechnology). The appropriate biotinylated secondary antibody (Jackson ImmunoResearch) was incubated (1 h at RT) prior to revelation with serial incubation of ABC and DAB (Vector Labs) for UCP-1 staining and Simple Stain Mouse MAX PO (rat) kit (N-Histofine) for macrophage staining and counterstaining with hematoxylin was then performed.

### *Ex vivo* image analysis

Regions of interest (ROIs) corresponding to the atherosclerotic lesion, the periaortic BAT and the lesion-free aortic wall were drawn on the digitized HES-stained sections (Discovery.V8, Zeiss). The histological relevance of the ROIs was assessed by means of comparison with an adjacent section immunostained for macrophages and BAT. Following semi-automated landmark-based coregistration, ROIs were used to quantify tracer activity on the autoradiographic image (Gimp 2.6.8 and ImageJ 1.46). The same process was used to quantify activity of reference tissues samples with known amounts of radioactivity, which allowed the conversion of intensity values into MBq.g$^{-1}$. Tissue sections stained for macrophages were digitized (Discovery.V8, Zeiss) and used to assess macrophage infiltration in individual lesions through the evaluation of the F4/80 positive-to-total lesion area ratio (Gimp 2.6.8 and ImageJ 1.46).

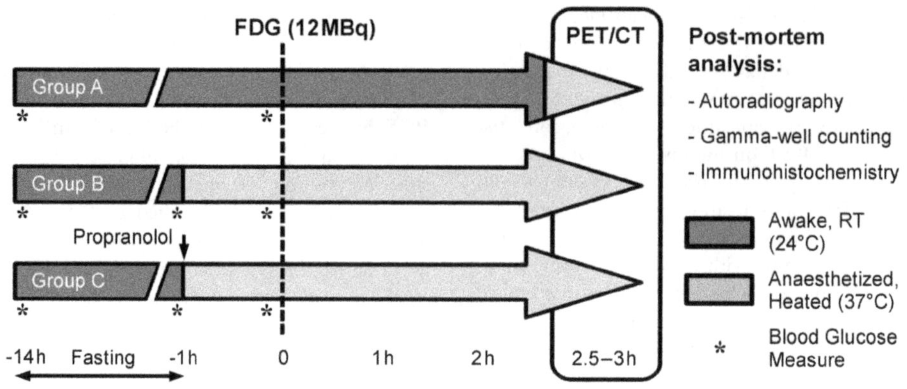


**Figure 1. Experimental protocol.** RT, room temperature.

## Statistical analysis

Numeric parameters were expressed as mean ± SD. Data were tested for homogeneity of variance using Fisher's F-test. Mann and Whitney's U test or Student's t-test were performed to compare data sets. Pearson's product-moment correlation was calculated to assess the significance of linear regressions (R 3.0/R Commander 2.0 and LibreOffice 4.0). A $P$ value of less than 0.05 was considered statistically significant.

# Results

## Blood glucose and body weight

The results are presented in Table 1. Overnight fasting resulted in a significant decrease in blood glucose in all experimental groups (% decrease, 45±12, 45±12, and 41±16 for Group A, B, and C, respectively, $P =$ NS between Groups) while body weight decreased by 7±1%, 7±2%, and 9±2% in Group A, B, and C, respectively ($P =$ NS between Groups). In addition, 1 h of anesthesia did not modify significantly blood glucose in group B animals (4.9±0.4 vs. 4.5±0.9 mmol·L$^{-1}$, $P =$ NS), whereas propranolol injection in anesthetized animals from Group C resulted in a significant increase from 4.8±0.3 mmol·L$^{-1}$ to 6.3±0.8 mmol·L$^{-1}$ ($P<0.01$).

## *Ex vivo* determination of FDG biodistribution

The *ex vivo*-determined FDG biodistibution in the thoracic aorta and surrounding tissues is presented in Table 2. Blood activity was significantly lower in Group A as compared with Group B ($P<0.01$), but not with Group C ($P = 0.15$), with Group B and Group C blood activities being comparable ($P = 0.22$). Heart uptake on one hand and atherosclerotic lesion uptake on the other hand were comparable in Group A and B animals, ($P =$ NS for both) while Group C animals displayed increased cardiac FDG uptake (DUR: 4.61±2.62, $P<0.05$ vs. lesion and Group A and $P = 0.07$ vs. Group B). Diaphragm muscle uptake was higher or tended to be higher in Group A than in Groups B and C ($P = 0.07$ vs. Group B and $P<0.05$ vs. Group C). Interscapular BAT FDG uptake was higher in group A compared to groups B and C ($P<$ 0.05 for both). A positive correlation was observed in FDG uptake between interscapular and periaortic BAT ($R = 0.90$, $P<0.001$).

**FDG uptake in the thoracic aorta.** The adipose tissue surrounding the superior and posterior mediastinum large arteries was identified as periaortic brown adipose tissue (BAT) as indicated by positive anti-UCP-1 immunohistochemical staining (Figure 2A). Macrophage infiltration in aortic atherosclerotic lesions was also demonstrated by F4/80 immunostaining (Figure 2B) and represented approximately 30% of lesion area with no statistical difference between experimental groups. Shown in Figure 3 are representative histological stainings of longitudinal sections of the aortic arch and surrounding tissues together with the corresponding autoradiographic images of FDG activity from Group A, B, and C animals and allowing the distinction between atherosclerotic lesion, normal wall, and periaortic BAT FDG uptake. Quantification of autoradiographic images is provided in Table 2 (see above). The results first indicated that macrophage infiltration in atherosclerotic lesions correlated positively with lesional FDG uptake ($R = 0.47$; $P<0.001$) (Figure 2C). In addition, overall FDG atherosclerotic lesion uptake was not statistically different between experimental groups. Tracer activity in the lesion-free, normal aortic wall was also comparable between experimental groups ($P =$ NS), whereas periaortic BAT tracer

**Table 1.** Blood glucose levels.

| | Fed | Fasting | |
|---|---|---|---|
| | | Anesthesia | FDG injection |
| **Group A** | 8.5±0.6 | N/A | 4.6±0.9† |
| **Group B** | 8.3±1.4 | 4.5±0.9† | 4.9±0.4* † |
| **Group C** | 8.5±0.6 | 4.8±0.3† | 6.3±0.8† ‡ |

Data are mmol·L$^{-1}$.
*, $P<0.05$ vs. Group C;
†, $P<0.05$ vs. Fed;
‡, $P<0.05$ vs. Fasting/Anesthesia.

**Table 2.** *Ex vivo* assessment of FDG biodistribution.

| | Group A | Group B | Group C |
|---|---|---|---|
| **Autoradiography** | | | |
| Atheroscleroctic lesion | 1.57±0.79§ | 1.50±0.74 | 1.39±0.28 |
| Lesion-free aortic wall | 0.54±0.24‡ § | 0.53±0.25‡ § | 0.62±0.26‡ |
| Periaortic BAT | 4.88±2.85‡ | 1.57±1.05* | 1.44±0.99* |
| **Tissues samples** | | | |
| Blood | 0.18±0.04‡ § | 0.34±0.132* ‡ § | 0.22±0.07‡ § |
| Heart | 1.89 ±0.62§ | 1.96±1.33 | 4.64±2.87† ‡ § |
| Thymus | 1.08±0.27§ | 1.32±0.68 | 1.88±1.20 |
| Lymph nodes | 0.84±0.34§ | 1.75±0.94* | 1.36±0.31* |
| Lungs | 0.85±0.20‡ § | 1.47±0.40* | 1.28±0.36* |
| Liver | 0.29±0.06‡ § | 0.59±0.13* ‡ § | 0.50±0.07* ‡ § |
| Diaphragm muscle | 2.97±1.62 | 0.94±1.03* | 0.79±0.30* ‡ |
| Interscapular BAT | 10.32±7.04‡ | 1.74±0.97* | 1.69±0.81* |

Data are DUR.
*, $P<0.05$ vs. Group A;
†, $P<0.05$ vs. Group B;
‡, $P<0.05$ vs. Atheroscleroctic lesion;
§, $P<0.05$ vs. Periaortic BAT.

activity was significantly lower in Groups B and C in comparison with Group A. FDG uptake in atherosclerotic lesions was not statistically different from that observed in the periaortic BAT in Groups B and C ($P = 0.90$ and $P = 0.91$, respectively) whereas accumulation at room temperature in Group A animals resulted in higher uptake in periaortic BAT than in the atherosclerotic lesion ($P<0.05$). Lesion-to-blood and lesion-to-control aorta ratios were comparable between Groups A, B and C ($P=$ NS). Lesion-to-periaortic BAT uptake ratios were of 0.3±0.1, 1.1±0.4 and 1.5±1.0 for Groups A, B, and C respectively, with the higher periaortic BAT FDG activity in Group A resulting in a significantly lower lesion-to-periaortic BAT ratio than in Group B and Group C ($P<0.05$) (Figure 4).

## PET/CT imaging

Representative PET/CT images of FDG uptake in apo$E^{-/-}$ mice are presented in Figure 5, with sagittal, coronal, and transverse views encompassing the aortic arch area as identified using anatomical landmarks from the CT image. Results from image quantification are presented in Table 3. FDG uptake by interscapular BAT was readily observable on images (Figure 5, white arrowheads), with significantly higher mean tracer activity in Group A than in Group B and Group C. Tracer uptake was also noticed at the site of diaphragm aortic insertion (grey arrowheads), with significantly higher activity in Group A than in Groups B and C. FDG activity was observed in the aortic arch (arrows) and thoracic aorta in all experimental groups. Image quantification indicated that significantly higher activity was observed in the aortic arch and thoracic aorta of Group A than in those of Group

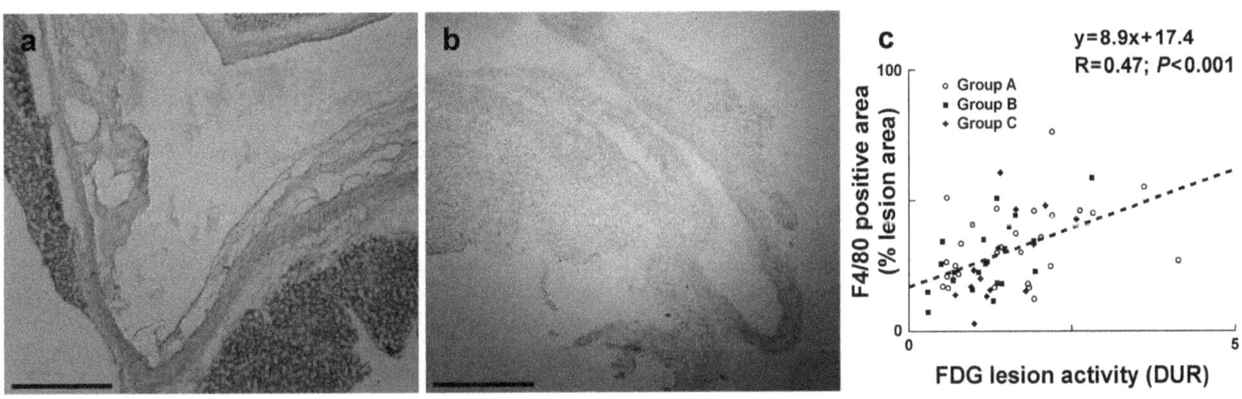


**Figure 2. Immunohistochemical analysis of the aortic arch.** Immunohistochemical stainings of UCP-1 (a) and F4/80 (b) were performed on tissue sections from the aortic arch of apo$E^{-/-}$ mice. UCP-1 staining was used to control the identity of the periaortic adipose tissue. F4/80 macrophage staining was used to quantify atheromatous lesions macrophage infiltration. Scale bar: 200 μm. A positive correlation was observed between macrophage infiltration and FDG uptake assessed through autoradiographic images quantification performed on adjacent tissue sections (c).

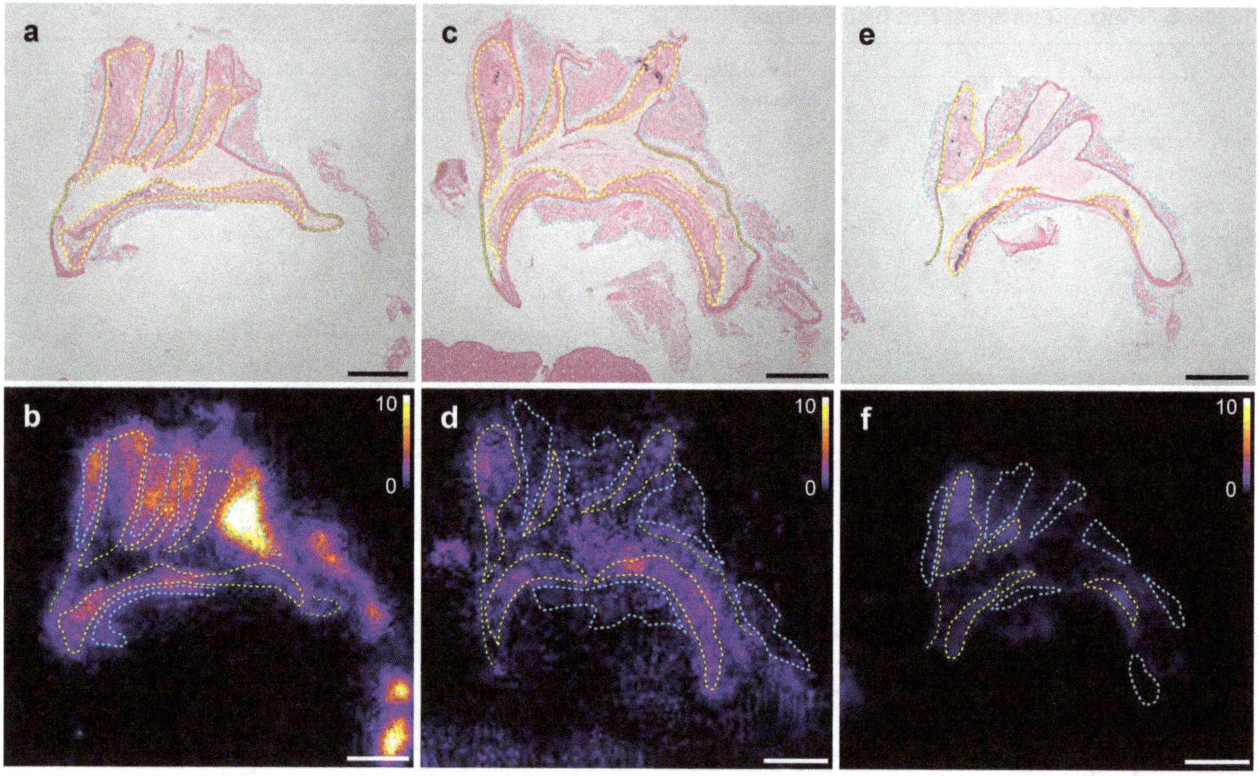


**Figure 3. Autoradiographic analysis of FDG uptake in the aortic arch.** Autoradiographic analysis of FDG uptake in aortic arch from apoE$^{-/-}$ mice from Group A (a, b), B (c, d) and C (e, f). The exposed section were stained with HES trichrome staining (a, c, e), regions of interest were defined (yellow: lesion; green: lesion-free aortic wall; teal: perioartic BAT) and used to quantify the autoradiographic acquisition (b, d, f). Scale bar: 500 μm; autoradiographic images intensity is expressed as DUR.

B animals. Although not significant, a strong trend towards lower activity in Group C, anesthetized and propranolol-treated animals maintained at 37°C was also observed in comparison with Group A ($P = 0.09$ and 0.07 for the aortic arch and thoracic aorta, respectively). Finally, myocardial FDG uptake was significantly higher in Group C animals than in Groups A and B.

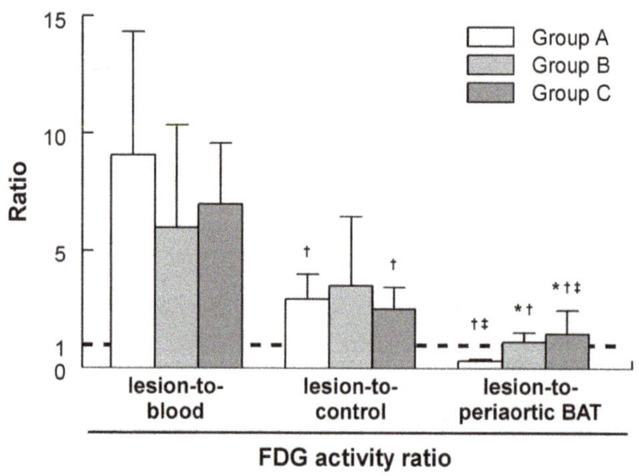


**Figure 4.** ***Ex vivo*****-determined FDG activity ratios.** FDG lesion-to-blood, lesion-to-control and lesion-to periaortic BAT activity ratios from *ex vivo* imaging and biodistribution experiments. *, $P<0.05$ vs. Group A; †, $P<0.05$ vs. lesion-to-blood; ‡, $P<0.05$ vs. lesion-to-control.

Correlation between *in vivo* PET/CT imaging and *ex vivo* biodistribution data are presented in Figure 6. Periaortic BAT uptake positively correlated to $SUV_{mean}$ from *in vivo* PET images at the level of the aortic arch ($R = 0.86$, $P<0.001$) while atherosclerotic lesion, normal wall, and blood tracer activities were not significantly correlated with values from *in vivo* image quantification ($P =$ NS).

## Discussion

The main result from the present study was that quantification of *in vivo* high resolution, small animal-dedicated PET/CT images of aortic FDG uptake in the apoE$^{-/-}$ murine model of atherosclerosis was dependent upon periaortic brown adipose tissue FDG uptake despite favorable, >>1 lesion-to-blood and lesion-to-lesion-free aortic wall tracer activity ratios as assessed by *ex vivo* analysis. In our experimental conditions, including the use of temperatures exceeding thermal neutrality and propranolol, the significant FDG uptake in periaortic BAT represents a confounding factor for the non invasive imaging of FDG uptake in murine aortic atherosclerotic lesions.

### Metabolic conditions and FDG biodistribution

The metabolic status can greatly influence FDG biodistribution. Animal handling was therefore optimized in order to maximize FDG atherosclerotic lesion uptake in contrast with surrounding tissues. All animals were fasted overnight in order to minimize blood glucose level before the experimentation. Anesthesia induction prior to the injection of FDG and maintenance

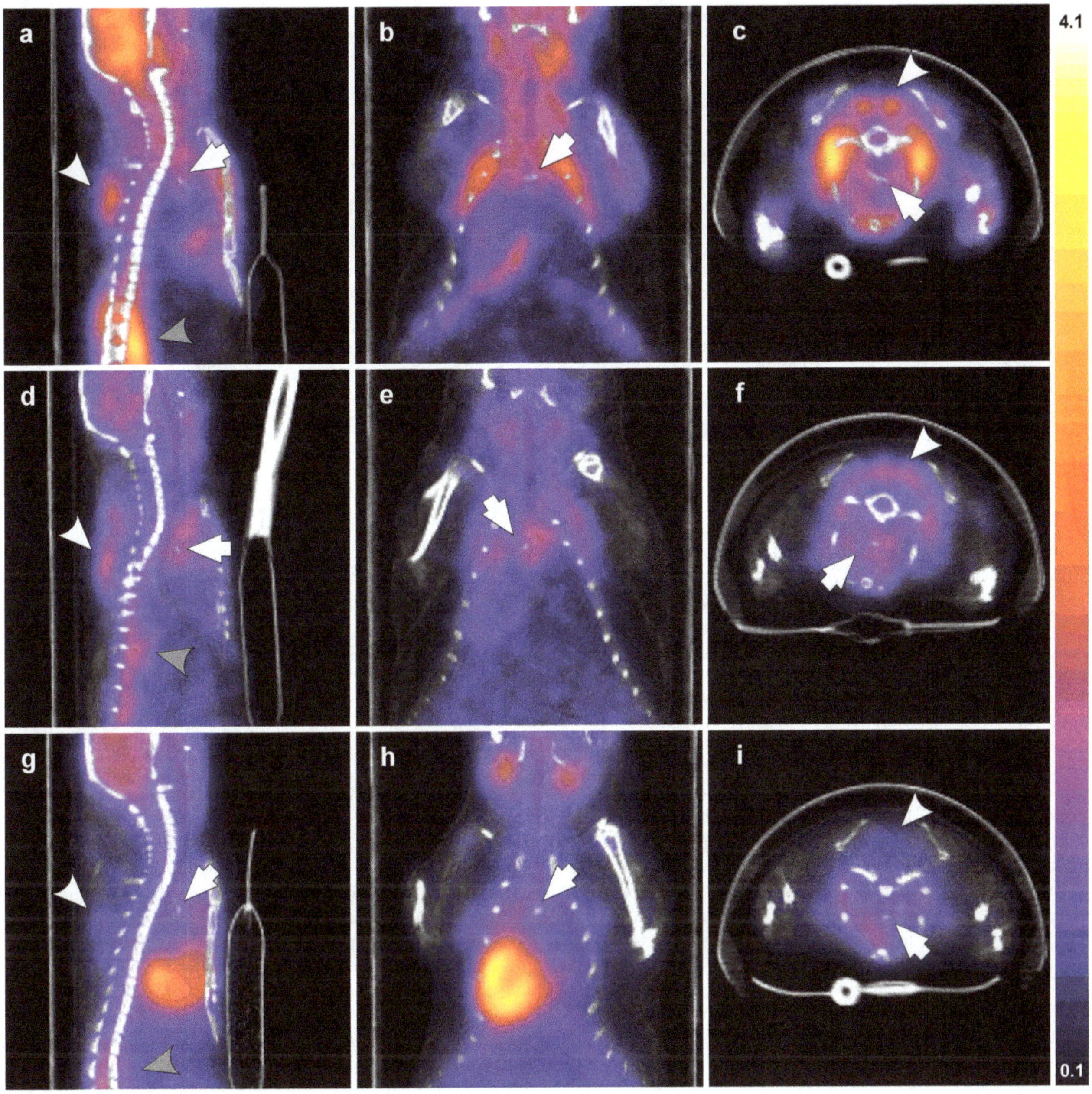


**Figure 5. PET/CT Imaging.** Fusion PET/CT images acquired 2.5 to 3 h after the injection of FDG in apoE$^{-/-}$ mice from Group A (a, b, c), B (d, e, f) and C (g, h, i) groups in sagittal (a, d, g), coronal (b, e, h) and transverse (c, f, i) views centered on the aortic arch (arrows). The interscapular BAT (white arrowheads) and the diaphragm muscle (gray arrowheads) were identified on those views. Scale set at 0.1 to 4.1 SUV for all images.

**Table 3.** In vivo image quantification.

| | Group A | Group B | Group C |
|---|---|---|---|
| Aortic arch | 1.4±0.5 | 0.9±0.2* | 1.0±0.2 ($P$=0.09) |
| Thoracic aorta | 1.2±0.3 | 0.8±0.1† | 0.9±0.1 ($P$=0.07) |
| Interscapular BAT | 5.2±2.4 | 1.1±0.8† | 1.1±0.4† |
| Diaphragm muscle | 2.7±0.7 | 1.0±0.3† | 0.9±0.2† |

Data are $SUV_{mean}$.
*, $P$<0.05 vs. Group A;
†, $P$<0.01 vs. Group A. Given in parentheses are $P$ values for the comparison of Group C vs. Group A.

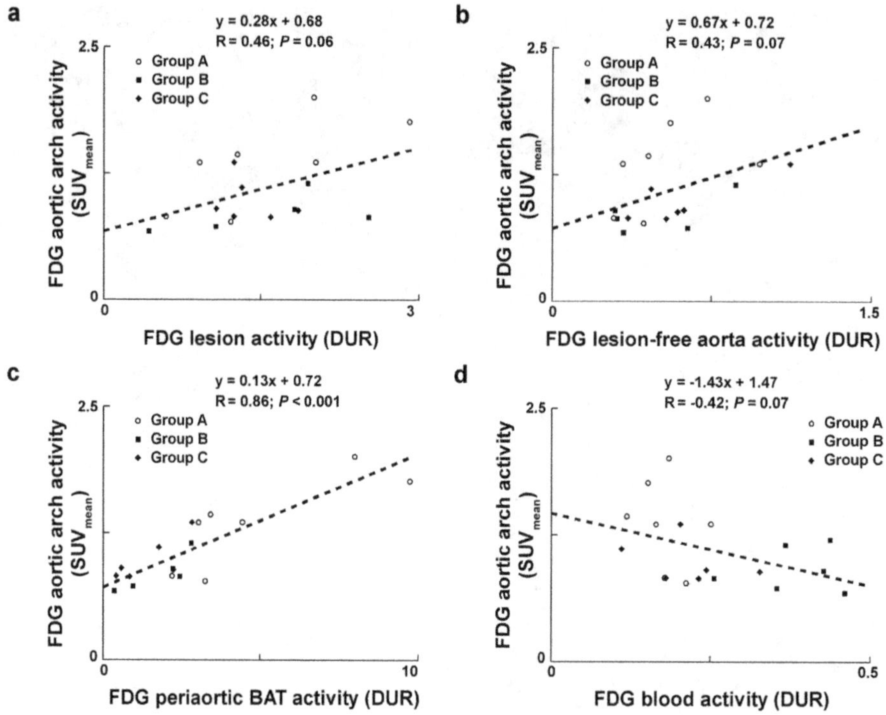


**Figure 6. Correlation between *in vivo* PET/CT imaging and *ex vivo* biodistribution data.** Correlations between FDG activity from *in vivo* PET image quantification using a VOI centered on the aortic arch and *ex vivo*-determined FDG atherosclerotic lesion activity (a), FDG lesion-free aortic activity (b), FDG periaortic BAT activity (c) and FDG blood activity (d).

throughout the accumulation period allowed the lowering of FDG uptake in tissues minimally stimulated in unconscious animals such as the brain and muscles. Sodium pentobarbital anesthesia was chosen over ketamine/xylazine since marked hyperglycemia has been observed with the latter [18]. Isoflurane was also discarded during the FDG accumulation period since it has been shown to increase FDG myocardial uptake [19]. Overall, sodium pentobarbital was expected to have minimal effects on FDG kinetics [20].

As expected from BAT physiology [12], heating the animal over its thermoneutral zone reduced FDG uptake in both the interscapular and periaortic BAT. BAT metabolism is mainly driven through β3-adrenergic activation [21]. An attempt to further reduce BAT FDG uptake was therefore performed using the non-selective β-blocker propranolol using previously described experimental conditions [22]. However, BAT FDG uptake was not further reduced when compared to animals not injected with propranolol, probably due to the fact that warming by itself almost completely inhibited BAT metabolism. In addition, an increase in blood glucose level in the presence of propranolol was observed at the time of tracer injection, which was likely due to the worsening of glycemic control induced by the β-blocker [23] in association with the transient hyperglycemia induced by sodium pentobarbital anesthesia [20]. The anesthesia and propranolol-induced increase in blood glucose level might in turn have caused the observed increase in myocardial FDG uptake reflective of increased myocardial glucose metabolism in animals injected with propranolol.

## Autoradiographic imaging for the distinction between lesion, normal wall, and periaortic BAT FDG uptake

**Atherosclerotic lesion uptake.** FDG lesion-to-lesion-free aortic wall uptake ratio was similar to previously reported values from autoradiographic studies performed in murine models, either on tissues sections [24] or on aorta en face [6]. FDG uptake in lesions positively correlated with macrophage infiltration. Using a similar methodology, such a correlation was already reported in apoE$^{-/-}$ mice when the evaluation was performed at 2 h p.i. [25], while no correlation was found at an earlier time point of 20 min p.i. [6]. Such a correlation is in accordance with the hypothesis of macrophages representing the main source of FDG uptake within plaques, while not excluding that others parameters such as hypoxia [26] or macrophages differentiation [27] might significantly influence FDG uptake within lesions.

**Periaortic BAT uptake.** Similarly to the above mentioned results on interscapular BAT FDG activity from biodistribution and *in vivo* imaging studies, autoradiographic imaging readily showed that periaortic BAT FDG uptake could be lowered using appropriate animal handling. Anesthesia and animal heating allowed a significant reduction of FDG uptake in periaortic BAT which was not further decreased with the use of propranolol. However, qualitative and quantitative autoradiographic image analysis indicated that the lowest achievable periaortic BAT tracer activity remained at a similar level to that measured in adjacent atherosclerotic lesions.

## *In vivo* imaging

Rudd *et al.* have suggested that a potential reason accounting for the initial failure to identify atherosclerotic lesions by FDG PET imaging of apoE$^{-/-}$ mouse might be that the 1 h time point chosen for image acquisition did not allow tracer accumulation into atherosclerotic lesions [8]. Tracer accumulation was therefore allowed for 3 h in the present study, in accordance with the experimental conditions described in recent studies [10]. The effect of animal handling on BAT metabolism was confirmed by *in vivo* imaging indicating varying interscapular BAT FDG uptake, with significantly lower interscapular BAT activity in anesthetized, thermoregulated animals.

The use of a state-of-the-art, small-animal dedicated PET/CT camera prevents the accumulation of FDG in the interscapular region from representing a confounding factor for atherosclerotic lesion imaging as previously suggested [7]. On the other hand, given the moderate size of mouse atherosclerotic lesions in comparison with the spatial resolution of state-of-the-art small-animal dedicated PET systems, partial volume effect is necessarily involved while performing mouse atherosclerotic lesion imaging. This implies that while evaluating FDG uptake of lesions from the aortic sinus, the elevated myocardial FDG uptake represents a major confounding factor; the lesions being present at this anatomical location are therefore not used in studies specifically using FDG [28]. Similarly, the observed activity quantified from a VOI drawn on *in vivo* PET images and centered on atherosclerotic lesions of the aortic arch as identified by signal enhancement on non-contrast CT acquisitions [17] therefore represents FDG uptake in atherosclerotic lesions as well as in tissues immediately adjacent to the atherosclerotic lesions, i.e. the blood, lesion-free aortic wall and periaortic BAT. The results of the present study indicated that $SUV_{mean}$ values measured in the aortic arch on *in vivo* PET images positively correlated with the *ex vivo* determined FDG uptake in periaortic BAT using high resolution *ex vivo* autoradiographic imaging. More precisely, the modulation of periaortic BAT FDG uptake in thermoregulated Group B animals in comparison with control Group A animals as assessed by *ex vivo* analysis resulted in a significantly lower *in vivo* FDG uptake in the VOI encompassing the aortic atherosclerotic lesions. Although lower FDG aortic activity was also observed in Group C than in Group A, the difference did not reach statistical significance most likely due to the fact that propranolol treatment in Group C animals induced a transient increase in glycemia that might have favored FDG uptake by glucose utilizing tissues (see Metabolic condition and FDG biodistribution above).

### Experimental and clinical implications

The present study indicated that the findings from *ex vivo* autoradiographic image analysis indicating higher or similar FDG activity in periaortic BAT than in atherosclerotic lesions translated into significant differences in tracer activity upon *in vivo* image quantification. Periaortic BAT therefore represents a confounding factor for the *in vivo* assessment of FDG atherosclerotic lesion activity in the aorta of $apoE^{-/-}$ mice. Such a limitation to the use of FDG for aortic atherosclerosis imaging should be expected in all mouse models of atherosclerosis. However, recently published data suggested that perivascular adipose tissue around the murine common carotid artery did not significantly participate to overall vascular tracer uptake [11]. Mouse carotid lesions might therefore be more suitable than aortic lesions for mouse atherosclerosis imaging with FDG even though initial experiments of total carotid ligation in $apoE^{-/-}$ mice did not allow to identify FDG uptake in the corresponding lesions [7].

Clinically, BAT activation was initially identified using FDG PET/CT imaging in the supraclavicular area of human adults [29]. BAT activation depends on multiple factors including subject age, adiposity and outdoor temperature [14,30]. Of note, mediastinal BAT activation was also observed in human adults, including in the periaortic and pericardial regions, the latter being in the continuity of pericoronary adipose tissue [31]. Adipose tissue in the vicinity of carotid arteries was also identified as a potential source of FDG uptake [32]. In addition to mouse, perivascular BAT activation could therefore represent a potential confounding factor for atherosclerosis imaging using FDG in humans. However, the retrospective incidence of BAT detection with FDG was shown to be modest since it ranged from 1.7 to 9.3% [30]. In addition, human perivascular coronary adipocytes are white rather than brown adipocytes [33]. Overall, FDG uptake by human adipose tissue should therefore represent a lower bias than that demonstrated in the present study in a preclinical mouse model of atherosclerosis focused on aortic lesions imaging. FDG PET/CT imaging of carotid arteries in the clinical settings is a relatively well-established methodology with good short-term reproducibility [34] which is now used in clinical trials as an end-point to evaluate the effect of therapeutic interventions [35,36]. On the other hand, the elevated FDG myocardial uptake represents a major pitfall for coronary atherosclerosis imaging, despite the use of fasting, low-carbohydrate/high fat meals, or heparin to minimize myocardial activity [37,38].

## Conclusion

In our experimental conditions, FDG uptake in the periaortic BAT of $apoE^{-/-}$ mice was either higher or similar to that observed in the immediately adjacent atherosclerotic lesion depending upon the metabolic status of the animals. These differences in periaortic BAT FDG activity as assessed from *ex vivo* high resolution autoradiographic images translated into corresponding variations in tracer activity as assessed from *in vivo* PET image quantification. Periaortic BAT uptake therefore represents a confounding factor while using FDG imaging for the non-invasive assessment of mouse atherosclerotic lesions, thereby emphasizing the need to carefully design preclinical studies using FDG for the evaluation of lesion inflammation in this animal model.

## Supporting Information

**Data S1 Study Data.*** All study data, including animals age, weight, blood glucose level, FDG injected dose and FDG biodistribution determined *ex vivo *in tissue samples and using autoradiographic analysis and *in vivo *using PET image quantification, are presented in the supporting file.

## Author Contributions

Conceived and designed the experiments: JT AB DF LMR CG. Performed the experiments: JT AB. Analyzed the data: JT AB PP DF LMR CG. Contributed reagents/materials/analysis tools: JT AB PP MDD DF LMR CG. Contributed to the writing of the manuscript: JT AB PP DF LMR CG.

## References


1. Falk E, Nakano M, Bentzon JF, Finn AV, Virmani R (2013) Update on acute coronary syndromes: the pathologists' view. Eur Heart J 34: 719–728. doi:10.1093/eurheartj/ehs411.
2. Naghavi M, Libby P, Falk E, Casscells SW, Litovsky S, et al. (2003) From vulnerable plaque to vulnerable patient: a call for new definitions and risk assessment strategies: Part I. Circulation 108: 1664–1672. doi:10.1161/01.CIR.0000087480.94275.97.
3. Rudd JHF, Warburton EA, Fryer TD, Jones HA, Clark JC, et al. (2002) Imaging atherosclerotic plaque inflammation with [18F]-fluorodeoxyglucose positron emission tomography. Circulation 105: 2708–2711.
4. Sheikine Y, Akram K (2010) FDG-PET imaging of atherosclerosis: Do we know what we see? Atherosclerosis 211: 371–380. doi:10.1016/j.atherosclerosis.2010.01.002.

5. Rosenbaum D, Millon A, Fayad ZA (2012) Molecular imaging in atherosclerosis: FDG PET. Curr Atheroscler Rep 14: 429–437. doi:10.1007/s11883-012-0264-x.
6. Matter CM, Wyss MT, Meier P, Späth N, von Lukowicz T, et al. (2006) 18F-choline images murine atherosclerotic plaques ex vivo. Arterioscler Thromb Vasc Biol 26: 584–589. doi:10.1161/01.ATV.0000200106.34016.18.
7. Laurberg JM, Olsen AK, Hansen SB, Bottcher M, Morrison M, et al. (2007) Imaging of vulnerable atherosclerotic plaques with FDG-microPET: no FDG accumulation. Atherosclerosis 192: 275–282. doi:10.1016/j.atherosclerosis.2006.07.019.
8. Rudd JHF, Fayad ZA, Machac J, Weissberg PL, Davies JR, et al. (2007) Response to "Laurberg JM, Olsen AK, Hansen SB, et al. Imaging of vulnerable atherosclerotic plaques with FDG-microPET: no FDG accumulation" [Atherosclerosis 2006]. Atherosclerosis 192: 453–454; author reply 451–452. doi:10.1016/j.atherosclerosis.2006.10.027.
9. Nahrendorf M, Zhang H, Hembrador S, Panizzi P, Sosnovik DE, et al. (2008) Nanoparticle PET-CT imaging of macrophages in inflammatory atherosclerosis. Circulation 117: 379–387. doi:10.1161/CIRCULATIONAHA.107.741181.
10. Hag AMF, Pedersen SF, Christoffersen C, Binderup T, Jensen MM, et al. (2012) (18)F-FDG PET imaging of murine atherosclerosis: association with gene expression of key molecular markers. PLoS ONE 7: e50908. doi:10.1371/journal.pone.0050908.
11. Wenning C, Kloth C, Kuhlmann MT, Jacobs AH, Schober O, et al. (2014) Serial F-18-FDG PET/CT distinguishes inflamed from stable plaque phenotypes in shear-stress induced murine atherosclerosis. Atherosclerosis 234: 276–282. doi:10.1016/j.atherosclerosis.2014.03.008.
12. Cannon B, Nedergaard J (2004) Brown adipose tissue: function and physiological significance. Physiol Rev 84: 277–359. doi:10.1152/physrev.00015.2003.
13. Nedergaard J, Bengtsson T, Cannon B (2007) Unexpected evidence for active brown adipose tissue in adult humans. Am J Physiol Endocrinol Metab 293: E444–E452. doi:10.1152/ajpendo.00691.2006.
14. Cypess AM, Lehman S, Williams G, Tal I, Rodman D, et al. (2009) Identification and Importance of Brown Adipose Tissue in Adult Humans. New England Journal of Medicine 360: 1509–1517. doi:10.1056/NEJMoa0810780.
15. Fitzgibbons TP, Kogan S, Aouadi M, Hendricks GM, Straubhaar J, et al. (2011) Similarity of mouse perivascular and brown adipose tissues and their resistance to diet-induced inflammation. Am J Physiol Heart Circ Physiol 301: H1425–H1437. doi:10.1152/ajpheart.00376.2011.
16. Chang L, Villacorta L, Li R, Hamblin M, Xu W, et al. (2012) Loss of Perivascular Adipose Tissue on Peroxisome Proliferator–Activated Receptor-γ Deletion in Smooth Muscle Cells Impairs Intravascular Thermoregulation and Enhances Atherosclerosis. Circulation 126: 1067–1078. doi:10.1161/CIRCULATIONAHA.112.104489.
17. Wait JMS, Tomita H, Burk LM, Lu J, Zhou OZ, et al. (2013) Detection of Aortic Arch Calcification in Apolipoprotein E-Null Mice Using Carbon Nanotube–Based Micro-CT System. J Am Heart Assoc 2: e003358. doi:10.1161/JAHA.112.003358.
18. Fueger BJ, Czernin J, Hildebrandt I, Tran C, Halpern BS, et al. (2006) Impact of animal handling on the results of 18F-FDG PET studies in mice. J Nucl Med 47: 999–1006.
19. Toyama H, Ichise M, Liow J-S, Vines DC, Seneca NM, et al. (2004) Evaluation of anesthesia effects on [18F]FDG uptake in mouse brain and heart using small animal PET. Nucl Med Biol 31: 251–256. doi:10.1016/S0969-8051(03)00124-0.
20. Lee K-H, Ko B-H, Paik J-Y, Jung K-H, Choe YS, et al. (2005) Effects of anesthetic agents and fasting duration on 18F-FDG biodistribution and insulin levels in tumor-bearing mice. J Nucl Med 46: 1531–1536.
21. Arch JR, Ainsworth AT, Cawthorne MA, Piercy V, Sennitt MV, et al. (1984) Atypical beta-adrenoceptor on brown adipocytes as target for anti-obesity drugs. Nature 309: 163–165.
22. Tatsumi M, Engles JM, Ishimori T, Nicely O, Cohade C, et al. (2004) Intense (18)F-FDG uptake in brown fat can be reduced pharmacologically. J Nucl Med 45: 1189–1193.
23. Fonseca VA (2010) Effects of beta-blockers on glucose and lipid metabolism. Curr Med Res Opin 26: 615–629. doi:10.1185/03007990903533681.
24. Silvola JMU, Saraste A, Laitinen I, Savisto N, Laine VJO, et al. (2011) Effects of age, diet, and type 2 diabetes on the development and FDG uptake of atherosclerotic plaques. JACC Cardiovasc Imaging 4: 1294–1301. doi:10.1016/j.jcmg.2011.07.009.
25. Zhao Y, Zhao S, Kuge Y, Strauss WH, Blankenberg FG, et al. (2011) Localization of deoxyglucose and annexin A5 in experimental atheroma correlates with macrophage infiltration but not lipid deposition in the lesion. Mol Imaging Biol 13: 712–720. doi:10.1007/s11307-010-0389-7.
26. Folco EJ, Sheikine Y, Rocha VZ, Christen T, Shvartz E, et al. (2011) Hypoxia but not inflammation augments glucose uptake in human macrophages: Implications for imaging atherosclerosis with 18fluorine-labeled 2-deoxy-D-glucose positron emission tomography. J Am Coll Cardiol 58: 603–614. doi:10.1016/j.jacc.2011.03.044.
27. Ogawa M, Nakamura S, Saito Y, Kosugi M, Magata Y (2012) What can be seen by 18F-FDG PET in atherosclerosis imaging? The effect of foam cell formation on 18F-FDG uptake to macrophages in vitro. J Nucl Med 53: 55–58. doi:10.2967/jnumed.111.092866.
28. Camici PG, Rimoldi OE, Gaemperli O, Libby P (2012) Non-invasive anatomic and functional imaging of vascular inflammation and unstable plaque. Eur Heart J 33: 1309–1317. doi:10.1093/eurheartj/ehs067.
29. Cohade C, Osman M, Pannu HK, Wahl RL (2003) Uptake in Supraclavicular Area Fat ("USA-Fat"): Description on 18F-FDG PET/CT. J Nucl Med 44: 170–176.
30. Bauwens M, Wierts R, van Royen B, Bucerius J, Backes W, et al. (2014) Molecular imaging of brown adipose tissue in health and disease. Eur J Nucl Med Mol Imaging 41: 776–791. doi:10.1007/s00259-013-2611-8.
31. Vosselman MJ, van Marken Lichtenbelt WD, Schrauwen P (2013) Energy dissipation in brown adipose tissue: From mice to men. Molecular and Cellular Endocrinology 379: 43–50. doi:10.1016/j.mce.2013.04.017.
32. Falk E, Thim T, Kristensen IB (2009) Atherosclerotic Plaque, Adventitia, Perivascular Fat, and Carotid Imaging. J Am Coll Cardiol Img 2: 183–186. doi:10.1016/j.jcmg.2008.11.005.
33. Chatterjee TK, Stoll LL, Denning GM, Harrelson A, Blomkalns AL, et al. (2009) Proinflammatory phenotype of perivascular adipocytes influence of high-fat feeding. Circulation research 104: 541–549.
34. Rudd JHF, Myers KS, Bansilal S, Machac J, Pinto CA, et al. (2008) Atherosclerosis Inflammation Imaging with 18F-FDG PET: Carotid, Iliac, and Femoral Uptake Reproducibility, Quantification Methods, and Recommendations. J Nucl Med 49: 871–878. doi:10.2967/jnumed.107.050294.
35. Fayad ZA, Mani V, Woodward M, Kallend D, Abt M, et al. (2011) Safety and efficacy of dalcetrapib on atherosclerotic disease using novel non-invasive multimodality imaging (dal-PLAQUE): a randomised clinical trial. The Lancet 378: 1547–1559. doi:10.1016/S0140-6736(11)61383-4.
36. Tawakol A, Fayad ZA, Mogg R, Alon A, Klimas MT, et al. (2013) Intensification of statin therapy results in a rapid reduction in atherosclerotic inflammation: results of a multicenter fluorodeoxyglucose-positron emission tomography/computed tomography feasibility study. J Am Coll Cardiol 62: 909–917. doi:10.1016/j.jacc.2013.04.066.
37. Cheng VY, Slomka PJ, Meunier LL, Tamarappoo BK, Nakazato R, et al. (2012) Coronary Arterial 18F-FDG Uptake by Fusion of PET and Coronary CT Angiography at Sites of Percutaneous Stenting for Acute Myocardial Infarction and Stable Coronary Artery Disease. J Nucl Med 53: 575–583. doi:10.2967/jnumed.111.097550.
38. Joshi NV, Vesey AT, Williams MC, Shah ASV, Calvert PA, et al. (2014) 18F-fluoride positron emission tomography for identification of ruptured and high-risk coronary atherosclerotic plaques: a prospective clinical trial. The Lancet 383: 705–713. doi:10.1016/S0140-6736(13)61754-7.

# 15

# Early Exposure to Volatile Anesthetics Impairs Long-Term Associative Learning and Recognition Memory

**Bradley H. Lee[1], John Thomas Chan[1], Obhi Hazarika[1], Laszlo Vutskits[2], Jeffrey W. Sall[1]***

1 Department of Anesthesia and Perioperative Care, University of California San Francisco, San Francisco, California, Unites States of America, 2 Department of Anesthesiology, Pharmacology and Intensive Care, University Hospital of Geneva, Geneva, Switzerland

## Abstract

***Background:*** Anesthetic exposure early in life affects neural development and long-term cognitive function, but our understanding of the types of memory that are altered is incomplete. Specific cognitive tests in rodents that isolate different memory processes provide a useful approach for gaining insight into this issue.

***Methods:*** Postnatal day 7 (P7) rats were exposed to either desflurane or isoflurane at 1 Minimum Alveolar Concentration for 4 h. Acute neuronal death was assessed 12 h later in the thalamus, CA1-3 regions of hippocampus, and dentate gyrus. In separate behavioral experiments, beginning at P48, subjects were evaluated in a series of object recognition tests relying on associative learning, as well as social recognition.

***Results:*** Exposure to either anesthetic led to a significant increase in neuroapoptosis in each brain region. The extent of neuronal death did not differ between groups. Subjects were unaffected in simple tasks of novel object and object-location recognition. However, anesthetized animals from both groups were impaired in allocentric object-location memory and a more complex task requiring subjects to associate an object with its location and contextual setting. Isoflurane exposure led to additional impairment in object-context association and social memory.

***Conclusion:*** Isoflurane and desflurane exposure during development result in deficits in tasks relying on associative learning and recognition memory. Isoflurane may potentially cause worse impairment than desflurane.

**Editor:** Yael Abreu-Villaça, Universidade do Estado do Rio de Janeiro, Brazil

**Funding:** Funding for the study was provided through National Institutes of Health Grant GM086511 to JWS, the University of California San Francisco Department of Anesthesia and Perioperative Care Hamilton Award to JWS, and by Swiss National Science Foundation Grant 31003A_130625 to LV. The funders had no role in study design, data collection and analysis, decision to publish, or preparation of the manuscript.

**Competing Interests:** The authors have declared that no competing interests exist.

* Email: sallj@anesthesia.ucsf.edu

## Introduction

Every day, anesthetics are used around the world in newborns and infants who undergo medical procedures. There is growing concern that anesthetics can significantly alter the developing brain, and animal models have shown that exposure to anesthetics at an early age lead to neuronal death and long-term cognitive dysfunction [1–3]. Epidemiologic studies suggest that humans are also susceptible to long-term cognitive effects after anesthesia [4,5].

Our knowledge of cognitive effects in humans has been, until recently [6], limited to retrospective studies that typically assess global tests of learning and behavior [4,5,7,8]. For instance, most of these epidemiologic studies identify cognitive or learning disabilities by evaluating databases for individuals with diagnostic codes for unspecified delays, behavioral disorders, language or speech problems [7,8], or through IQ and achievement tests [4,5]. Because these studies examine generalized learning problems, they contribute minimally to our understanding of the memory processes that underlie the cognitive impairment.

An important challenge in the study of anesthetic neurotoxicity is developing a model by which cognitive effects in animals can be translated to humans. Memory processing is highly conserved across rodent and human species [9]. In particular, hippocampal memory functions are very similar between rats and humans [9], and the hippocampus is crucial in spatial encoding, associative learning, and recognition memory in both rats and humans [9–12].

Rodent models therefore provide valuable insight into the types of memory that may be affected in humans. However, behavioral studies are prone to using overlapping models for evaluating learning and memory. Many studies use similar tests, such as the Morris water maze [2,13–15], because they have consistently identified a cognitive deficit. Identifying impairment in specific memory processes, such as recognition and associative memory, in animal models will provide insight into effects in humans and may help guide future assessments of learning and memory in children, as has recently been reported [6].

Recognition memory, which is a subtype of declarative memory, is crucial in humans for recalling different events, objects, and people [16,17]. It has been shown that animals also have episodic-like memory that can be demonstrated through tests involving memory for "what," "where," and "when" details of an event. This was first described in birds [18] and more recently in rodents [12,19–22], and models have since been developed to examine recognition memory in various ways [20,23–25]. Furthermore, many studies find that recognition memory processes rely on the hippocampus and thalamus [19,26], which are areas of neuronal degeneration following anesthesia [2,14].

The present study was designed to evaluate the effects of two commonly used volatile anesthetics – isoflurane and desflurane – on specific learning and memory processes following neonatal exposure. After delivering 1 Minimum Alveolar Concentration [27] of either anesthetic for 4 hours at postnatal day 7 (P7), subjects were evaluated in a set of recognition tasks involving associative memory, as well as social memory, that have been shown to be sensitive to lesions in hippocampal and thalamic circuits [19,28,29].

## Methods

### Subjects

All experiments were conducted with approval from the Institutional Animal Care and Use Committee at the University of California, San Francisco. Five Sprague-Dawley dams with litters of postnatal day 6 (P6) pups from were obtained from Charles River Laboratories (Gilroy, CA). Each litter contained only males and was culled to ten pups. In total, the males were taken from at least ten different litters. On P7, animals from each litter were randomly assigned to control and treatment groups. They were weaned at P23 and housed three per cage under standard lab housing with 12 h light/dark cycle. Animals were food restricted (access to food only during light cycle) for tasks involving object recognition to increase activity and object exploration.

### Anesthesia

Anesthesia was delivered as described previously [14,30,31]. Briefly, animals in the treatment groups received either isoflurane or desflurane as a single agent in air and oxygen ($FiO_2$50%) at 1 Minimum Alveolar Concentration [27] for four hours. MAC was determined by tail clamping every 15 minutes, and anesthetic concentration was adjusted accordingly, so that on average 50% of animals would move in response to clamping (Fig. 1). 12 out of 18 animals anesthetized with isoflurane survived to undergo behavioral testing, and 13 out of 18 animals anesthetized with desflurane survived and underwent behavioral testing. Control animals were concurrently placed in an anesthesia glove box of the same material and conditions without being exposed to anesthesia or tail clamping. Animals were kept on a warming blanket, and temperatures were measured using an infrared laser thermometer and maintained with a goal of 35°C.

### Histology

Brains from the two anesthetized groups and the control group (n = 10 per group) were assessed for acute neuronal death. Twelve hours after anesthesia, animals were transcardially perfused with cold 4% paraformaldehyde in phosphate-buffered saline and brains were removed, postfixed, and sunk in sucrose solution. They were then sliced into 60 micron-thick slices and every other slice was mounted and stained with FluoroJade C, a marker specific for neurodegeneration [32,33] (FJC, 0.001%, Millipore, Billerica, MA). FJ-positive cells were counted using Nikon Eclipse *80i* microscope under 20X magnification in each slice containing the structure of interest. Structures included in analysis were the anterodorsal (AD), anteroventral (AV), laterodorsal (LD), and anteromedial (AM) thalamic nuclei, as well as CA1-3 regions of the hippocampus and the dentate gyrus.

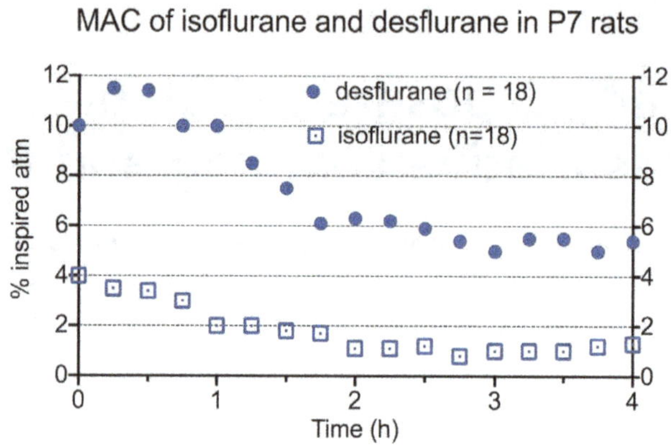


**Figure 1. MAC of isoflurane and desflurane.** Anesthetics were separately delivered to P7 rats in air and oxygen ($FiO_2$ 50%) as previously described[6, 9]. Tail-clamping occurred every 15 minutes, and anesthetic concentration was adjusted to 1 MAC. As before[6, 9], MAC decreases with increasing duration of anesthesia for both agents.

### Object Recognition Tasks

Object recognition was assessed using similar arrangements as others [19,28]. Behavior testing occurred during the light phase of the circadian cycle between 0800 and 1700 hrs in two separate arenas, hereafter referred to as contexts, of identical size (61 cm square base, walls 50 cm high). Context 1 had yellow walls with a base covered in wood-effect vinyl lining, and context 2 had black walls with a black plastic base. Different visual cues were placed on the walls of each context. A video camera (SONY HDR-CX190) was mounted 2 meters above the testing area for recording and observing subjects. For each task, except the allocentric object-location task, subjects were placed into contexts in the same location and facing the south wall (away from the objects). Beginning at P42, subjects were habituated to the two contexts prior to testing by being placed individually into the context for 5 min per day for 4 consecutive days. All animals underwent all behavioral tasks. Subjects were tested on the same day for any given task and in the same sequence of tasks. All tasks were performed in the order presented in subsequent weeks, except for the first two (novel object and object-place) which were performed in the same week. The order of testing during the day was counterbalanced among groups.

Investigation of an object was defined as sniffing or placing the nose within 1 cm of and oriented toward the object. Subjects were recorded, and observers blinded to group assignment were used to determine investigation times. Object investigation times during the initial exposure for each task were compared to assess for possible confounding effects of varying investigation times on the ability to recognize objects. All objects and testing arenas were wiped with 70% ethanol between testing.

**Novel Object Recognition.** Testing began at P48 with novel object recognition. A single trial was performed for each animal consisting of "exposure" and "test" phases separated by a two-minute delay (Fig. 2A). During the exposure, subjects were placed into the context and allowed to explore two *identical* objects for four minutes. After the delay, they were placed into the same context for three minutes with one of the objects replaced with a

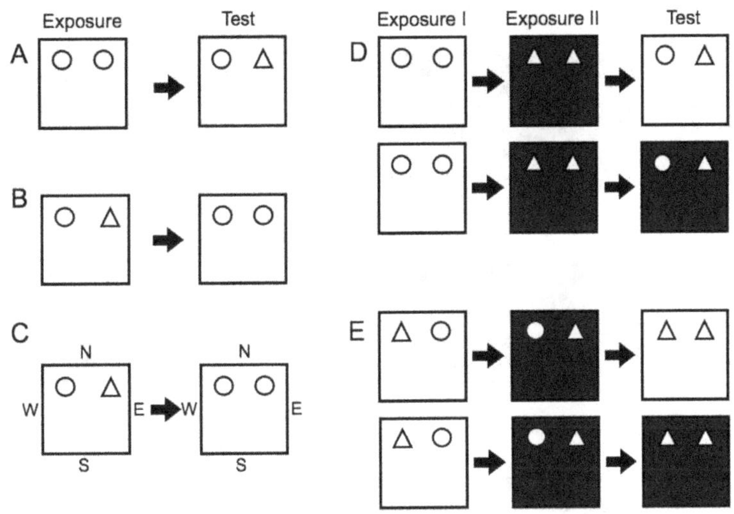


**Figure 2. Object recognition.** For each task, except allocentric object-place recognition, subjects are introduced at and facing the wall away from the objects. (A) *Novel object recognition.* Two identical objects are presented in the exposure, and one (right) is replaced with a novel object in the test phase. (B) *Object-place recognition.* Two different objects are presented, followed by two identical objects. In the test phase, the right object appears in a novel location within the context. (C) In the allocentric version of object-place recognition, subjects are again introduced at and facing the south wall (S) in the exposure. However, for the test phase, subjects are placed at and facing either the east (E) or west (W) wall. (D) *Object-context recognition.* Two different pairs of objects are presented in two different contexts, so each object is associated with a particular context. In the test phase, one object (right object, top row; left object, bottom row) appears within a context in which it has not been explored. (E) *Object-place-context recognition.* Two different objects are first presented in a context. The object locations are then reversed and presented in a different context. Thus, after two exposures, each object is seen in both contexts and both locations (left and right). In the test phase, two objects are presented in either context, so one (right object, top row; left object, bottom row) appears in a novel configuration of place and context.

novel object. Half of the subjects were tested in each context with the location (left or right) of the novel object counterbalanced among subjects.

**Object-Place Recognition.** Subjects were tested in their ability to recognize an object and its location. Two trials were performed, and investigation times were totaled for the two trials. In the exposure, two *different* objects were presented in a context for four minutes. After a two-minute delay, two *identical* copies of one of the previous objects were presented in the same context for three minutes (Fig. 2B). Both objects were equally familiar, but one now occupied a different location within the context.

**Allocentric Object-Place Recognition.** For the previous task, subjects were always introduced into the context facing the wall (south wall) opposite the two objects (Fig. 2C). In the allocentric version of the task, for the initial exposure, subjects were again placed into the context facing the south wall. In the test phase, however, the entry point was varied and half of the subjects were introduced facing either the east or west wall (Fig. 2C). Two trials were performed and the entry point was randomized among subjects.

**Object-Context Recognition.** Subjects were assessed in their ability to recognize an object with a particular context. The task required two separate exposures, each lasting four minutes and separated by a two-minute delay (Fig. 2D). In the first exposure, a pair of *identical* objects was presented in a context. Next, subjects were placed in a *different* context with a *different* pair of objects. In the test phase, lasting three minutes, subjects were placed into a context with one of each previously encountered object. Thus, one object was presented in the same context as before, while the other object appeared within a context in which it had not been explored. Two trials were conducted, and the test phase occurred in opposite contexts for each trial (Fig. 2D).

**Object-Place-Context Recognition.** Subjects were tested in their ability to recognize an object with its location and context (Fig. 2E). In the first exposure, two *different* objects were presented within a context. Next, subjects were placed in the opposite context with the *same* two objects and their locations reversed. Thus, after two exposures, each object was observed in both contexts and locations (left and right). In the test phase, two *identical* copies of either of the previous objects were presented in a context. The location and context associated with one object were familiar, while the other "displaced" object appeared in a location and context in which it had not been observed. Two trials were conducted with the test phase occurring in opposite contexts for each trial (Fig. 2E).

## Social Behavior and Social Recognition

Following object recognition, animals were given unrestricted access to food. Social interaction and recognition were assessed using a discrimination paradigm one week after completing object recognition testing at P80. In the exposure, the subject was presented with a caged stimulus animal and a novel object for five minutes. This arrangement evaluates social behavior by determining whether subjects spend more time investigating the stimulus animal or object[7]. After a sixty-minute delay, subjects were presented simultaneously with the same "familiar" animal and a novel animal for three minutes. Recognition of the previously encountered animal was demonstrated by decreased investigation of the familiar target relative to the novel one.

Same-sex juvenile conspecifics were used as stimulus animals. Male pups five weeks of age were housed individually one week prior to testing. Investigation of the stimulus animal was defined as sniffing or direct contact with the subject's nose or paws. Investigation of the novel object was defined as sniffing or placing the nose within 1 cm of and oriented toward object.

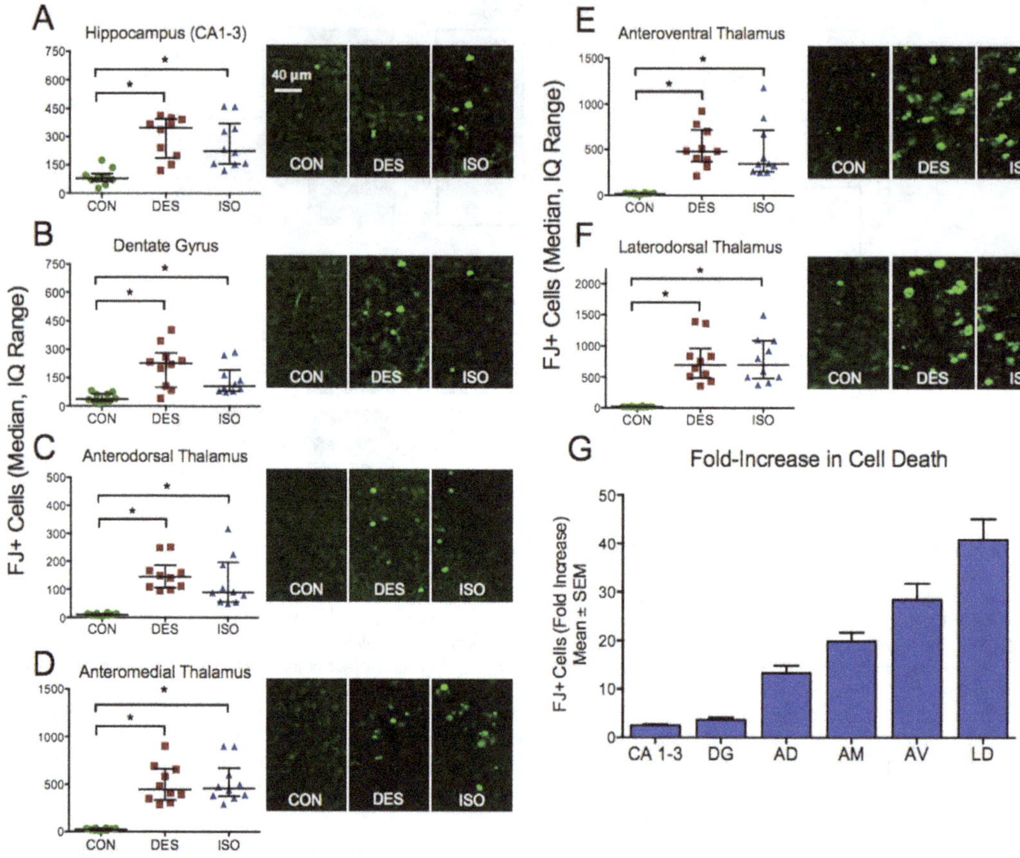


**Figure 3. Neuronal death by group. A to F)** Exposure to either anesthetic - desflurane or isoflurane - led to significantly increased neuronal death in each brain region. The degree of neurodegeneration was similar in desflurane and isoflurane-treated subjects. Sample images from brains at 20X magnification are shown alongside graphs comparing total cell death for each structure. **G)** The average increases in neuronal death relative to controls are shown. *$P<0.05$.

## Statistical Analysis

Data were analyzed using Prism 6 Software for Mac OSX (GraphPad Software Inc., San Diego, CA). Data were assessed for normal distribution using the D'Agostino and Pearson test. Parametric tests were used for normally distributed data; otherwise, nonparametric tests were used for analysis. All comparisons used a two-tail test and a P value less than 0.05 was considered statistically significant.

Total FluoroJade-positive cells for each brain region were compared among the groups – control, desflurane, isoflurane – using one-way ANOVA for parametric data or the Kruskal-Wallis test for nonparametric data. Bonferroni's post-test with multiple comparisons was used following one-way ANOVA, and Dunn's post-test was used with the Kruskal-Wallis test. The fold-increase in neuronal death was determined for each structure by dividing the total FJ-positive cells for all anesthetized animals ($n = 20$) by the average number of FJ-positive cells per structure for control animals ($n = 10$).

Recognition tasks were first assessed by comparing the investigation times of each target using paired tests for each group. Paired t-test was used for normally distributed data, and nonparametric data were analyzed with the Wilcoxon matched-pairs rank test. Also, to identify possible confounding effects of varying investigation times on subsequent object/animal recognition, the times during the exposure phase were compared between the groups using either one-way ANOVA with Bonferroni's post-test or the Kruskal-Wallis test with Dunn's post-test.

In addition, a "discrimination index" (DI) was calculated and represents the relative time spent exploring each target (eg. Familiar versus Novel). To calculate DI, the time spent investigating the familiar target was subtracted from the time spent on the novel target, and this was divided by the total time spent investigating the two (eg. DI = (Novel-Familiar)/(Total Time)). This value was compared to a theoretical value of zero using one sample t-test to assess whether a preference was shown for one of the objects, and a positive DI indicates preference for the novel aspect of the task. For each task, DI of control animals was compared against DI of all anesthetized animals. Also, within the group of anesthetized animals, the DI of desflurane-treated subjects was compared with that of isoflurane-treated subjects. These comparisons were made using either unpaired t-test for parametric data or the Mann Whitney test for nonparametric data.

## Results

### Increased neuronal death occurs similarly in desflurane and isoflurane-treated animals

There was increased neuronal death in each brain region in animals exposed to either desflurane or isoflurane relative to the control animals (Fig. 3). No difference in the extent of cell death was identified between the two anesthetized groups. Anesthetic exposure resulted in significantly increased cell death in the hippocampus (P = 0.0001, one-way ANOVA; control vs. des P = 0.0002, control vs. iso P = 0.0015, des vs. iso P = 0.99, Bonferroni), dentate gyrus (P = 0.0003, one-way ANOVA; control vs. des P = 0.0002, control vs. iso P = 0.03, des vs. iso P = 0.16, Bonferroni), anterodorsal thalamus (P<0.0001, one-way ANOVA; control vs. des P<0.0001, control vs. iso P = 0.0007, des vs. iso P = 0.98, Bonferroni), anteromedial thalamus (P<0.0001, one-way ANOVA; control vs. des P<0.0001, control vs. iso P<0.0001, des vs. iso P = 0.99, Bonferroni), anteroventral thalamus (P<0.0001, Kruskal-Walli test; control vs. des P<0.0001, control vs. iso P = 0.001, des vs. iso P = 0.99, Dunn's), and laterodorsal thalamus (P<0.0001, one-way ANOVA; control vs. des P<0.0001, control vs. iso P<0.0001, des vs. iso P = 0.99, Bonferroni). The relative fold-increase in cell death for each brain region is shown in Figure 3G.

## Novel Object and Object-Place Recognition are Unaffected

Subjects from each group were able to distinguish familiar and novel objects, revealed by increased investigation times of the novel object (control P = 0.006, desflurane P = 0.01, isoflurane P = 0.0003; paired t-test familiar vs. novel, Fig. 4A). Object-place recognition was also intact in each group, and animals spent more time with the object in a novel location (control P = 0.006, desflurane P = 0.001, isoflurane P = 0.0008, paired t-test familiar vs. novel location, Fig. 4C). There was no difference in object exploration times among groups during the exposure for either task (novel object P = 0.5, one-way ANOVA, object-place P = 0.2, Kruskal-Wallis).

Discrimination Indexes [3] for all subjects were greater than zero for both novel object recognition (control P = 0.007, desflurane P = 0.002, isoflurane P = 0.002, one sample t-test, Fig. 4B) and object-place recognition (control P = 0.01, desflurane P = 0.001, isoflurane P = 0.001, one sample t-test, Fig. 4D). No differences in DI were identified between control and anesthetized subjects (novel object P = 0.9, unpaired t-test; object-place P = 0.3, Mann Whitney test) or between desflurane and isoflurane subjects (novel object P = 0.83, unpaired t-test; object-place P = 0.64, Mann Whitney test).

## Isoflurane but not desflurane treated animals are impaired in object-context and social recognition

Only the isoflurane group was impaired in the ability to associate an object with its context and spent similar amounts of time with each object in this task (control P = 0.001, Wilcoxon test familiar vs. novel context; desflurane P = 0.006, isoflurane P = 0.2, paired t-test, Fig. 5A). DIs of control and desflurane subjects were greater than zero but not in isoflurane-treated subjects (control P = 0.004, desflurane P = 0.04, isoflurane P = 0.95, one sample t-test, Fig. 5B). Comparison of DI between control and anesthetized subjects did not reveal a difference (P = 0.094, unpaired t-test, Fig. 5B). Within the anesthetized group, DI did not differ significantly between desflurane and isoflurane-treated subjects (P = 0.32, unpaired t-test). Exploration times in the exposure phases of the object-context task were similar for the three groups (P = 0.6, one-way ANOVA).

Isoflurane animals also had impaired social memory while desflurane animals were unaffected when comparing social target investigation times (control P = 0.0009, desflurane P = 0.002, isoflurane P = 0.08; paired t-test familiar vs. novel animal, Fig. 5C). DIs of control and desflurane subjects were greater than zero (control P = 0.0009, desflurane P = 0.002, one sample t-test, Fig. 5D), although isoflurane DI did not differ significantly from zero (P = 0.064, one sample t-test, Fig. 5D). No difference between DI was identified in control vs. anesthetized groups (P = 0.84, unpaired t-test). In the subset of anesthetized subjects, the isoflurane DI was lower than desflurane DI although it did not reach statistical significance (P = 0.17, unpaired t-test). In the exposure of the social recognition task, animals from all groups displayed normal social behavior and spent significantly greater time investigating the social target relative to the object (all P< 0.0001, paired t-test object vs. social target).

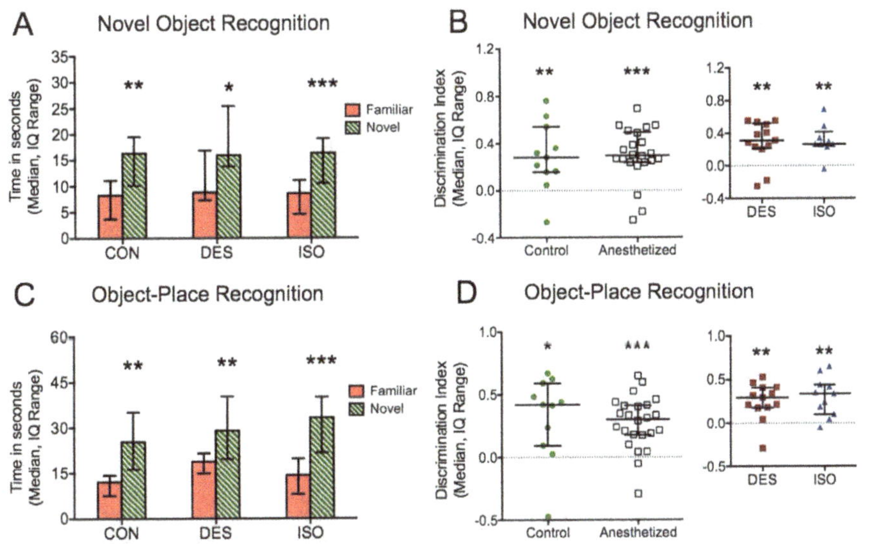


**Figure 4. Novel object and object-place recognition.** A) Subjects all demonstrated successful object recognition and preferentially explored the novel object. B) Each group's DI was significantly greater than zero, and there was no difference in DIs. C) Subjects were also able to identify an object in a novel location, demonstrated by a relative increase in investigation of that object. D) Again, DIs for all subjects were greater than zero with no differences identified. *P<0.05, **P<0.01, ***P<0.001, CON = control, DES = desflurane, ISO = isoflurane.

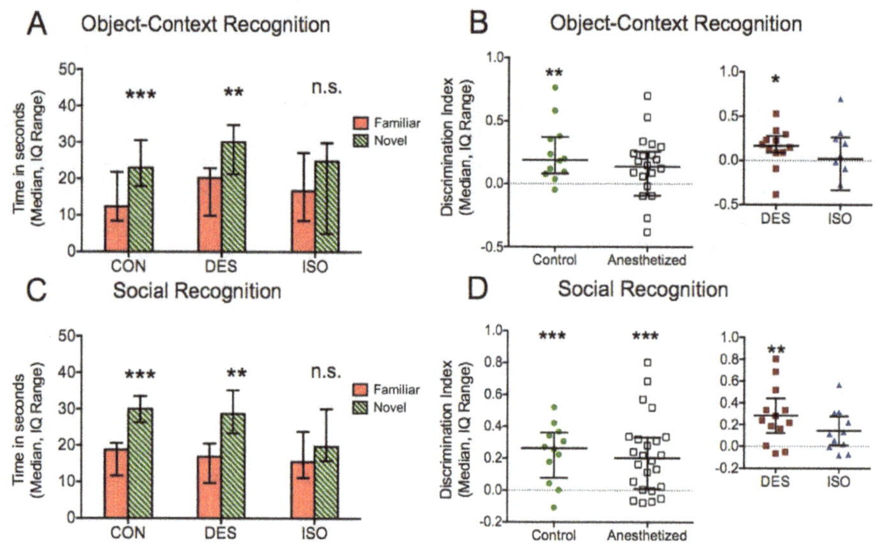


**Figure 5. Object-context and social recognition.** A) Isoflurane-treated animals were impaired in associating an object with a particular context. Animals exposed to desflurane, on the other hand, recognized when an object appeared in a different context and spent more time with that object. B) The DI for anesthetized subjects in this task did not differ from zero, and, within this group, only the desflurane DI significantly exceeded zero. C) Desflurane-treated subjects also had no change in social recognition ability, spending more time with the novel animal, while isoflurane-treated animals had deficient social memory. D) DI for both control and anesthetized animals exceeded zero, although DI for the subset of isoflurane-treated subjects did not. *P<0.05, **P<0.01, ***P<0.001, n.s. = not significant.

## Anesthetized subjects are impaired in allocentric object-place and object-place-context recognition

Animals from both isoflurane and desflurane groups were impaired in object recognition when the entry site was varied in the allocentric version of the object-place task (control P = 0.001, desflurane P = 0.08, paired t-test familiar vs. novel; isoflurane P = 0.2, Wilcoxon test, Fig. 6A). The control DI was greater than zero (P = 0.0004, one sample t-test, Fig. 6B), while neither desflurane nor isoflurane DI differed from zero (desflurane P = 0.094, isoflurane P = 0.31, one sample t-test, Fig. 6B). DI of control animals was also significantly greater than that of anesthetized subjects (P = 0.024, unpaired t-test), although no difference was detected in the subset of desflurane and isoflurane-treated animals (P = 0.95, unpaired t-test).

Anesthetized subjects from both groups were also unable to distinguish objects in the object-place-context task (control P = 0.04, desflurane P = 0.5, paired t-test familiar vs. displaced; isoflurane P = 0.8, Wilcoxon test, Fig. 6C). Only the control DI exceeded zero in this task (control P = 0.021, desflurane P = 0.71, isoflurane P = 0.7, one sample t-test, Fig. 6D). Control DI was again significantly greater than DI for anesthetized subjects (P = 0.04, unpaired t-test), and no difference was found between desflurane and isoflurane DIs (P = 0.59, unpaired t-test). Investigation times during the exposures were similar between groups for each task (allocentric object-place P = 0.1, object-place-context P = 0.7, one-way ANOVA). The summary of all behavioral testing is presented in Table 1, where each group is evaluated whether they demonstrate a preference for the novel portion of the task by recognizing a familiar set of stimuli.

## Discussion

The main finding of this study is that exposure to the volatile anesthetics isoflurane and desflurane causes impairment in tasks relying on specific cognitive processes of associative learning and recognition memory. After exposure to 1 MAC of either anesthetic for 4 hours during the early postnatal period, adult subjects could identify a novel object and recognize changes in an object's spatial location. However, anesthetized animals were unable to recognize an object's location when they entered the testing arena from a different vantage point or perform a complex task requiring the integration of object, place, and context details. In addition, isoflurane-treated subjects were impaired in context-specific object recognition and exhibited deficient social memory.

The behaviors assessed in this study provide valuable insight into the types of learning affected by neonatal anesthesia exposure. The object recognition tasks performed here rely on spatial memory, but they also require associative processing to encode the relationships among distinct elements encountered during a given exposure [28,34,35]. Both control and treatment animals easily recognize a novel object, but animals that were anesthetized on P7 begin to show impairment when presented with objects that were previously in a different location or context, suggesting problems with associative learning. The impairment in the allocentric object-place task may also be related to spatial memory, because the animals are able to identify objects when relying on egocentric cues but struggle when forced to rely on allocentric cues.

Episodic memory is associative in nature, and memory formation relies in large part on our ability to link new experiences and items with closely related ideas, facts, and the environment or context in which we learn them [36]. Clearly, a problem forming associations and relationships would affect memory encoding over time. Furthermore, within the broad domain of episodic memory, recognition memory is a specific type of memory that, according to the dual process model, is comprised of recollection and familiarity [26,36]. It is likely that impairment in the object recognition and associative memory tasks could also result from a deficit in recollection, a process underlying recognition memory [19,28]. We recently reported deficits in recollection in both rodents and children after anesthesia at an early age [6]. Persistent problems with associative and recognition memory in children would have important consequences for learning and development throughout

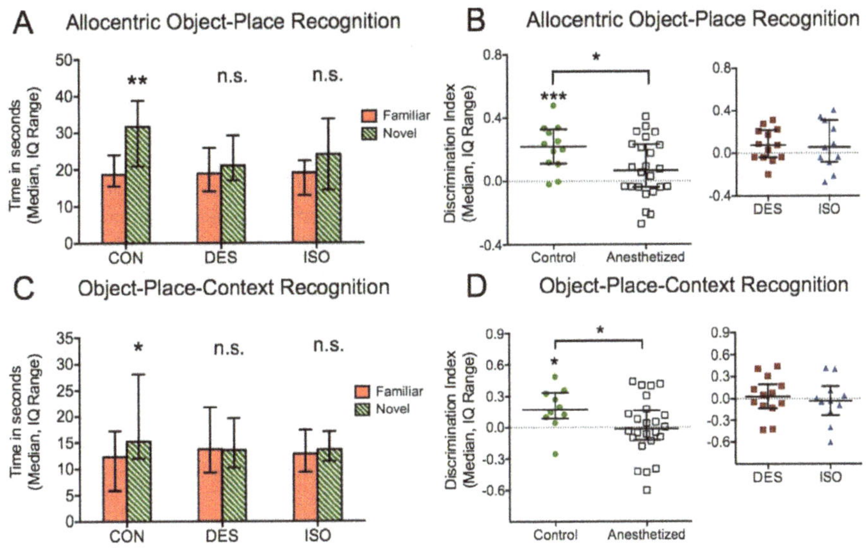


**Figure 6. Allocentric object-place and object-place-context recognition.** A) Exposure to isoflurane or desflurane led to impairment in identifying an object's location when the site of entry into the context was changed. The varied entry points forced subjects to rely on allocentric cues to identify the object's location. B) DI of control animals was significantly greater than that of anesthetized subjects. Neither desflurane nor isoflurane DI significantly exceeded zero. C) Isoflurane and desflurane-treated subjects were also impaired in recognition of an object that required association of its place and context. D) Again, control DI was greater than anesthetized DI. Neither subset of anesthetized subjects - desflurane or isoflurane - had DI greater than zero. *$P<0.05$, **$P<0.01$, n.s. = not significant.

adolescence. The precise cognitive domains that may be impaired in children and how these effects manifest later in life is still unclear, and these are important areas of future investigation.

Isoflurane has been used in numerous studies to investigate the effects of anesthesia and many labs have reported cell death and behavioral changes after isoflurane exposure [1–3,14,30]. The effects associated with desflurane, though, are less well described. Similar to other volatile anesthetics, desflurane in neonates has been shown to induce cell death [37,38]. However, few studies of behavior have been performed, and only one of these has demonstrated cognitive impairment [38]. Kodama and colleagues found that mice exposed to desflurane later developed problems with short-term and long-term memory [38]. In our present study, we demonstrate impairment in desflurane-treated animals using two separate tasks that involve associative learning. Together, these behavioral results show that desflurane, like isoflurane [2,14,30] and sevoflurane [13,30,39], alters long-term cognitive behavior.

Isoflurane-treated animals were impaired in two additional behavioral tasks, suggesting a distinct outcome from those anesthetized with desflurane. Others have also identified distinct outcomes using different anesthetic agents [37,38,40,41], although the reason underlying these behavioral findings is unclear. The types of memory involved in this series of behavioral testing are processed in the medial temporal lobe [19,28], including hippocampus and dentate gyrus, as well as the anterior thalamus and prefrontal cortex [26],[42], and we identified increased neurodegeneration in each of these brain regions. However, the observation of distinct behavioral outcomes occurred in the setting of a similar extent of neuronal injury. The discrepancy between histologic and behavioral findings suggest that, although neuronal death may play a role in determining behavioral phenotype, other effects on neural development likely contribute, as well. In fact, there is evidence that volatile anesthetics can alter synaptogenesis and dendritic spine density even in the absence of cell death [43]. In addition, anesthetics have been shown to result in significant

**Table 1.** Summary of behavioral testing.

| | Discrimination Index for task greater than zero? | | |
|---|---|---|---|
| | **Control** | **DES** | **ISO** |
| Novel Object Recognition | Yes | Yes | Yes |
| Object-Place Recognition | Yes | Yes | Yes |
| Object-Context Recognition | Yes | Yes | *No* |
| Social Recognition | Yes | Yes | *No* |
| Allocentric Object-Place Recognition | Yes | *No* | *No* |
| Object-Place-Context Recognition | Yes | *No* | *No* |

For each test, recognition of a familiar set of stimuli results in preferential exploration of the novel aspect of the task. Discrimination Index (DI) represents the time spent with the novel object or animal relative to the familiar one, and DI significantly greater than zero demonstrates successful recognition in the task.

neuroinflammation [41], changes in cell signaling [44], and stem cell proliferation [45,46]. It is likely that anesthetic effects on these processes of brain development contribute to the ultimate cognitive outcome.

Isoflurane-treated animals also had difficulty with social recognition which is more likely related to long-term memory processes than their capacity for social interaction. Unlike previous reports [39], we found all animals behaved similarly during the exposure portion of the test, spending much more time with a novel animal than an object. In fact, throughout these experiments none of the treatment groups demonstrated a difference in exploration time during the exposure phase. This suggests anesthetic exposure does not alter investigatory or social behavior, motivation, or attention.

## Limitations

The purpose of this study is to evaluate two separate anesthetics using outcomes of cell death and behavior. We cannot make conclusive remarks regarding mechanisms underlying cognitive impairment, and separate studies are needed to better understand these processes. Also, a comprehensive analysis of neuronal death was not undertaken, and it is possible that other brain regions show a difference. The hippocampus and thalamus were chosen, however, because of their underlying role in the investigated behavior.

Social recognition is based on olfaction in rodents [47] and we did not perform a separate experiment to exclude impaired olfaction as the basis for deficient social recognition in our subjects. However, we have previously determined that anesthetic exposure does not impair olfaction [6]. Isoflurane-treated subjects displayed typical social behavior in each part of the test, suggesting impaired recognition was due to effects on memory rather than interest, motivation, or olfaction. Also, although the rats were tested serially, they did not show any signs of decreasing interest with the objects as we used objects that appeared novel to the subjects in each trial. In fact, the exploration times remained very similar across the tests from first to last.

There are numerous studies documenting effects of gestational and early life stress on long-term behavior [48,49]. Because the animals were shipped, rather than bred in the housing facility, it is possible that they were exposed to early life stress that may affect aspects of behavior. Although effects of stress are likely evenly distributed amongst behavior groups, these considerations should be taken into account when interpreting behavioral results.

Finally, the cognitive outcomes from the two anesthetics appear to be different; however, it is possible that the two anesthetics were not entirely equal in depth in spite of being adjusted to 1 MAC. This must be taken into consideration when attempting to make direct comparisons between the two volatile anesthetics.

## Conclusion

Neonatal exposure to isoflurane and desflurane led to impairment in object recognition tasks relying on spatial and associative memory. These findings provide evidence that anesthetics can affect distinct cognitive processes that are fundamental to learning and memory in rodents, as well as humans.

## Author Contributions

Conceived and designed the experiments: BHL JTC OH LV JWS. Performed the experiments: BHL JTC OH LV JWS. Analyzed the data: BHL JTC OH LV JWS. Contributed reagents/materials/analysis tools: BHL JTC OH LV JWS. Contributed to the writing of the manuscript: BHL JTC OH LV JWS.

## References


1. Gentry KR, Steele LM, Sedensky MM, Morgan PG (2013) Early developmental exposure to volatile anesthetics causes behavioral defects in Caenorhabditis elegans. Anesth Analg 116: 185–189.
2. Jevtovic-Todorovic V, Hartman RE, Izumi Y, Benshoff ND, Dikranian K, et al. (2003) Early exposure to common anesthetic agents causes widespread neurodegeneration in the developing rat brain and persistent learning deficits. J Neurosci 23: 876–882.
3. Brambrink AM, Evers AS, Avidan MS, Farber NB, Smith DJ, et al. (2010) Isoflurane-induced neuroapoptosis in the neonatal rhesus macaque brain. Anesthesiology 112: 834–841.
4. Flick RP, Katusic SK, Colligan RC, Wilder RT, Voigt RG, et al. (2011) Cognitive and behavioral outcomes after early exposure to anesthesia and surgery. Pediatrics 128: e1053–1061.
5. Wilder RT, Flick RP, Sprung J, Katusic SK, Barbaresi WJ, et al. (2009) Early exposure to anesthesia and learning disabilities in a population-based birth cohort. Anesthesiology 110: 796–804.
6. Stratmann G, Lee J, Sall JW, Lee B, Alvi BS, et al. (2014) Effect of general anesthesia in infancy on long-term recognition memory in humans and rats. Neuropsychopharmacology 39. EPub ahead of print.
7. DiMaggio C, Sun LS, Kakavouli A, Byrne MW, Li G (2009) A retrospective cohort study of the association of anesthesia and hernia repair surgery with behavioral and developmental disorders in young children. J Neurosurg Anesthesiol 21: 286–291.
8. DiMaggio C, Sun LS, Li G (2011) Early childhood exposure to anesthesia and risk of developmental and behavioral disorders in a sibling birth cohort. Anesth Analg 113: 1143–1151.
9. Bunsey M, Eichenbaum H (1996) Conservation of hippocampal memory function in rats and humans. Nature 379: 255–257.
10. Eichenbaum H, Yonelinas AP, Ranganath C (2007) The medial temporal lobe and recognition memory. Annu Rev Neurosci 30: 123–152.
11. Burgess N, Maguire EA, O'Keefe J (2002) The human hippocampus and spatial and episodic memory. Neuron 35: 625–641.
12. Fortin NJ, Wright SP, Eichenbaum H (2004) Recollection-like memory retrieval in rats is dependent on the hippocampus. Nature 431: 188–191.
13. Shih J, May LD, Gonzalez HE, Lee EW, Alvi RS, et al. (2012) Delayed environmental enrichment reverses sevoflurane-induced memory impairment in rats. Anesthesiology 116: 586–602.
14. Stratmann G, May LD, Sall JW, Alvi RS, Bell JS, et al. (2009) Effect of hypercarbia and isoflurane on brain cell death and neurocognitive dysfunction in 7-day-old rats. Anesthesiology 110: 849–861.
15. Boscolo A, Ori C, Bennett J, Wiltgen B, Jevtovic-Todorovic V (2013) Mitochondrial protectant pramipexole prevents sex-specific long-term cognitive impairment from early anaesthesia exposure in rats. Br J Anaesth.
16. Yonelinas AP (2001) Components of episodic memory: the contribution of recollection and familiarity. Philos Trans R Soc Lond B Biol Sci 356: 1363–1374.
17. Brown MW, Aggleton JP (2001) Recognition memory: what are the roles of the perirhinal cortex and hippocampus? Nat Rev Neurosci 2: 51–61.
18. Clayton NS, Dickinson A (1998) Episodic-like memory during cache recovery by scrub jays. Nature 395: 272–274.
19. Eacott MJ, Norman G (2004) Integrated memory for object, place, and context in rats: a possible model of episodic-like memory? J Neurosci 24: 1948–1953.
20. Eacott MJ, Easton A, Zinkivskay A (2005) Recollection in an episodic-like memory task in the rat. Learn Mem 12: 221–223.
21. Dere E, Huston JP, De Souza Silva MA (2005) Episodic-like memory in mice: simultaneous assessment of object, place and temporal order memory. Brain Res Brain Res Protoc 16: 10–19.
22. Kart-Teke E, De Souza Silva MA, Huston JP, Dere E (2006) Wistar rats show episodic-like memory for unique experiences. Neurobiol Learn Mem 85: 173–182.
23. Eichenbaum H, Fortin N, Sauvage M, Robitsek RJ, Farovik A (2010) An animal model of amnesia that uses Receiver Operating Characteristics (ROC) analysis to distinguish recollection from familiarity deficits in recognition memory. Neuropsychologia 48: 2281–2289.
24. Easton A, Eacott MJ (2010) Recollection of episodic memory within the medial temporal lobe: behavioural dissociations from other types of memory. Behav Brain Res 215: 310–317.
25. Sauvage MM (2010) ROC in animals: uncovering the neural substrates of recollection and familiarity in episodic recognition memory. Conscious Cogn 19: 816–828.
26. Aggleton JP, Dumont JR, Warburton EC (2011) Unraveling the contributions of the diencephalon to recognition memory: a review. Learn Mem 18: 384–400.
27. Macbeth AH, Edds JS, Young WS 3rd (2009) Housing conditions and stimulus females: a robust social discrimination task for studying male rodent social recognition. Nat Protoc 4: 1574–1581.

28. Langston RF, Wood ER (2010) Associative recognition and the hippocampus: differential effects of hippocampal lesions on object-place, object-context and object-place-context memory. Hippocampus 20: 1139–1153.
29. Cross L, Brown MW, Aggleton JP, Warburton EC (2012) The medial dorsal thalamic nucleus and the medial prefrontal cortex of the rat function together to support associative recognition and recency but not item recognition. Learn Mem 20: 41–50.
30. Ramage TM, Chang FL, Shih J, Alvi RS, Quitoriano GR, et al. (2013) Distinct long-term neurocognitive outcomes after equipotent sevoflurane or isoflurane anaesthesia in immature rats. Br J Anaesth.
31. Stratmann G, Sall JW, Eger EI 2nd, Laster MJ, Bell JS, et al. (2009) Increasing the duration of isoflurane anesthesia decreases the minimum alveolar anesthetic concentration in 7-day-old but not in 60-day-old rats. Anesth Analg 109: 801–806.
32. Schmued LC, Stowers CC, Scallet AC, Xu L (2005) Fluoro-Jade C results in ultra high resolution and contrast labeling of degenerating neurons. Brain Res 1035: 24–31.
33. Wang L, Liu YH, Huang YG, Chen LW (2008) Time-course of neuronal death in the mouse pilocarpine model of chronic epilepsy using Fluoro-Jade C staining. Brain Res 1241: 157–167.
34. Aggleton JP, Sanderson DJ, Pearce JM (2007) Structural learning and the hippocampus. Hippocampus 17: 723–734.
35. Mumby DG, Gaskin S, Glenn MJ, Schramek TE, Lehmann H (2002) Hippocampal damage and exploratory preferences in rats: memory for objects, places, and contexts. Learn Mem 9: 49–57.
36. Mayes A, Montaldi D, Migo E (2007) Associative memory and the medial temporal lobes. Trends Cogn Sci 11: 126–135.
37. Istaphanous GK, Howard J, Nan X, Hughes EA, McCann JC, et al. (2011) Comparison of the neuroapoptotic properties of equipotent anesthetic concentrations of desflurane, isoflurane, or sevoflurane in neonatal mice. Anesthesiology 114: 578–587.
38. Kodama M, Satoh Y, Otsubo Y, Araki Y, Yonamine R, et al. (2011) Neonatal desflurane exposure induces more robust neuroapoptosis than do isoflurane and sevoflurane and impairs working memory. Anesthesiology 115: 979–991.
39. Satomoto M, Satoh Y, Terui K, Miyao H, Takishima K, et al. (2009) Neonatal exposure to sevoflurane induces abnormal social behaviors and deficits in fear conditioning in mice. Anesthesiology 110: 628–637.
40. Liang G, Ward C, Peng J, Zhao Y, Huang B, et al. (2010) Isoflurane causes greater neurodegeneration than an equivalent exposure of sevoflurane in the developing brain of neonatal mice. Anesthesiology 112: 1325–1334.
41. Shen X, Dong Y, Xu Z, Wang H, Miao C, et al. (2013) Selective anesthesia-induced neuroinflammation in developing mouse brain and cognitive impairment. Anesthesiology 118: 502–515.
42. Aggleton JP, Hunt PR, Nagle S, Neave N (1996) The effects of selective lesions within the anterior thalamic nuclei on spatial memory in the rat. Behav Brain Res 81: 189–198.
43. Briner A, De Roo M, Dayer A, Muller D, Habre W, et al. (2010) Volatile anesthetics rapidly increase dendritic spine density in the rat medial prefrontal cortex during synaptogenesis. Anesthesiology 112: 546–556.
44. Masaki E, Kawamura M, Kato F (2004) Attenuation of gap-junction-mediated signaling facilitated anesthetic effect of sevoflurane in the central nervous system of rats. Anesth Analg 98: 647–652, table of contents.
45. Sall JW, Stratmann G, Leong J, McKleroy W, Mason D, et al. (2009) Isoflurane inhibits growth but does not cause cell death in hippocampal neural precursor cells grown in culture. Anesthesiology 110: 826–833.
46. Lin N, Moon TS, Stratmann G, Sall JW (2013) Biphasic change of progenitor proliferation in dentate gyrus after single dose of isoflurane in young adult rats. J Neurosurg Anesthesiol 25: 306–310.
47. Tang AC, Reeb BC, Romeo RD, McEwen BS (2003) Modification of social memory, hypothalamic-pituitary-adrenal axis, and brain asymmetry by neonatal novelty exposure. J Neurosci 23: 8254–8260.
48. Koenig JI, Elmer GI, Shepard PD, Lee PR, Mayo C, et al. (2005) Prenatal exposure to a repeated variable stress paradigm elicits behavioral and neuroendocrinological changes in the adult offspring: potential relevance to schizophrenia. Behav Brain Res 156: 251–261.
49. Weinstock M (2001) Alterations induced by gestational stress in brain morphology and behaviour of the offspring. Prog Neurobiol 65: 427–451.

# 16

# Characterization of a Novel *BCHE* "Silent" Allele: Point Mutation (p.Val204Asp) Causes Loss of Activity and Prolonged Apnea with Suxamethonium

**Herve Delacour[1]*, Sofya Lushchekina[2], Isabelle Mabboux[1], Aurore Bousquet[1,3], Franck Ceppa[1,3], Lawrence M. Schopfer[4], Oksana Lockridge[4], Patrick Masson[4,5]**

**1** Bégin Military Teaching Hospital, Department of Biology, Unit of Human Genetics, Saint Mandé, France, **2** Modeling of Biomolecules Lab., N.M. Emanuel Institute of Biochemical Physics, Russian Academy of Sciences, Moscow, Russia, **3** Val de Grace Military Medical School, Paris, France, **4** Eppley Institute, University of Nebraska Medical Center, Omaha, Nebraska, United States of America, **5** DYNAMOP, Institut de Biologie Structurale, Grenoble, France

## Abstract

Butyrylcholinesterase deficiency is characterized by prolonged apnea after the use of muscle relaxants (suxamethonium or mivacurium) in patients who have mutations in the *BCHE* gene. Here, we report a case of prolonged neuromuscular block after administration of suxamethonium leading to the discovery of a novel *BCHE* variant (c.695T>A, p.Val204Asp). Inhibition studies, kinetic analysis and molecular dynamics were undertaken to understand how this mutation disrupts the catalytic triad and determines a "silent" phenotype. Low activity of patient plasma butyrylcholinesterase with butyrylthiocholine (BTC) and benzoylcholine, and values of dibucaine and fluoride numbers fit with heterozygous atypical silent genotype. Electrophoretic analysis of plasma BChE of the proband and his mother showed that patient has a reduced amount of tetrameric enzyme in plasma and that minor fast-moving BChE components: monomer, dimer, and monomer-albumin conjugate are missing. Kinetic analysis showed that the p.Val204Asp/p.Asp70Gly-p.Ala539Thr BChE displays a pure Michaelian behavior with BTC as the substrate. Both catalytic parameters $K_m = 265$ µM for BTC, two times higher than that of the atypical enzyme, and a low $V_{max}$ are consistent with the absence of activity against suxamethonium. Molecular dynamic (MD) simulations showed that the overall effect of the mutation p.Val204Asp is disruption of hydrogen bonding between Gln223 and Glu441, leading Ser198 and His438 to move away from each other with subsequent disruption of the catalytic triad functionality regardless of the type of substrate. MD also showed that the enzyme volume is increased, suggesting a pre-denaturation state. This fits with the reduced concentration of p.Ala204Asp/p.Asp70Gly-p.Ala539Thr tetrameric enzyme in the plasma and non-detectable fast moving-bands on electrophoresis gels.

**Editor:** Fernando Rodrigues-Lima, University Paris Diderot-Paris 7, France

**Funding:** This work was funded by the Val de Grace Military Medical School, and the Russian Foundation for Basic Research (project 13-04-40287-H to S.L.). The funders had no role in study design, data collection and analysis, decision to publish, or preparation of the manuscript.

**Competing Interests:** The authors have declared that no competing interests exist.

* Email: herve.delacour@santarm.fr

## Introduction

Butyrylcholinesterase (EC 3.1.1.8; BChE) also known as pseudocholinesterase, is the sister enzyme of acetylcholinesterase (EC 3.1.1.7; AChE). It is present in most tissues and in human plasma at a concentration about 50 nM. Though BChE lacks obvious physiological functions, it is of toxicological and pharmacological importance in detoxifying or catabolising ester-containing drugs [1]. Furthermore, individuals deficient in BChE appear asymptomatic, apart from a heightened sensitivity to the muscle relaxants suxamethonium and mivacurium, two BChE substrates used as myorelaxant [2]. In patients with usual BChE levels, these drugs are rapidly hydrolysed in plasma and their duration of action is short (<10 min). BChE deficiency results in slower hydrolysis of these drugs and, consequently, a prolonged neuromuscular block, leading to apnea. Prolonged neuromuscular block occurs with BChE deficiencies of marked severity (impairment >70%). Although many acquired conditions may affect BChE activity (liver or renal diseases, malnutrition, pregnancy, malignancy), BChE deficiency is mainly due to mutations in the *BCHE* gene (MIM 177400) [2].

Prolonged apnea following injection of succinylcholine was first described in 1953 [3]. The genetic variation of BChE deficiency was described by Kalow and Genest in 1957 and is said to be a cornerstone in pharmacogenetics/pharmacogenomics [4]. The human *BCHE* gene is located on chromosome *3q26.1*, contains 3 coding exons, and spans approximately 64 kb. Genetically inherited BChE deficiency shows autosomal recessive inheritance. It has been estimated that almost 24% of the human population carries at least one variant *BCHE* allele [5]. Currently, close to 70 natural mutations have been documented in human *BCHE*. Most of them have an adverse effect on BChE activity. This may occur either by deleterious effects of point mutations on catalytic functioning, or by point mutations that affect protein expression, which may result in an absence of BChE altogether [2]. Although the majority of these mutations are rare, two of them, the atypical variant (c.293A>G, p.Asp70Gly, rs1799807) and the K-variant (c.1699G>A, p.Ala539Tyr, rs1803274), are relatively common, homozygotes occurring at 1:3,000 and 1:100 in the Caucasian population respectively.

Here we report a case of prolonged neuromuscular block after administration of suxamethonium leading to the discovery of a novel *BCHE* variant. DNA sequencing showed that this variant results from a point mutation c.695T>A (p.Val204Asp). Inhibition studies, kinetic analysis and molecular dynamics were undertaken to understand how this mutation determines the "silent" phenotype.

## Subjects and Methods

### Patients

The patient is a one-month old infant boy (subject II-1), who presented a prolonged neuromuscular block (16 hours) after administration of a single dose of succinylcholine (2 mg/kg) for pyloric stenosis surgery. His parents have no medical or surgical history. Biological investigations mentioned below were performed on plasma from the patient and his parents. The parents signed an informed consent to participate in the genetic study, which was approved by the Research and Ethics Committee of the Begin Military Teaching Hospital.

### Reference plasma samples

Three reference plasma samples of phenotype UU, UA and AS (DNA sequence for the silent BChE unknown) from O. Lockridge's plasma sample collection were used for control of catalytic and inhibition properties and electrophoresis of plasma BChE samples.

### Chemicals

Butyrylthiocholine iodide (BTC), Benzoylcholine chloride (BzCh) and dibucaine chloride were purchased from Sigma (St Louis, Missouri, United States of America). Succinyldithiocholine was custom synthesized by Molecular Probes Inc. Other chemicals were of biochemical grade.

### BChE activity

Total plasma BChE activity was measured with butyrylthiocholine iodide (BTC) as substrate on a Cobas® 6000 system (Roche Diagnostics) according to the method described by the manufacturer ([BTC] = 7.56 mM at pH = 7.7 and 37°C). Under these conditions the reference interval for BChE activity in healthy individuals was 5,320–12,920 IU/L for men, 4,260–11,250 IU/L for women under 39-years, and 2,260–6,460 IU/L for infants [6].

Activity of BChE in plasma or serum was also measured in the laboratory using a single beam spectrophotometer. Two substrates were used: BTC and BzCh. Activity with BTC was determined using Ellman's method in 0.1 M phosphate buffer pH 7.0 at 25°C [7]. Plasma samples (10 μL) were preincubated for 5 min with the chromogenic reagent 20 mM DTNB (50 μL) in 1,275 μL of the buffer solution prior to assay to neutralize plasma-containing free thiol compounds (under these conditions, free-thiol-containing molecules present in plasma samples were neutralized in less that 3 min). After adding 1 mM BTC, assays were recorded at 412 nm taking $\varepsilon_{412} = 16{,}360\ M^{-1}\,cm^{-1}$. Activity with BzCh was determined according to Kalow and Genest by recording decrease in absorbance at 240 nm ($\Delta\varepsilon = 6{,}700\ M^{-1}.cm^{-1}$) of 50 μM BzCh in 67 mM phosphate buffer pH 7.4 at 25°C [4]. For both assays, one unit (U) of enzyme activity is defined as the amount of enzyme that hydrolyzes one μmol of substrate per minute.

### Genotyping and mutational analysis

Blood samples were collected from the patient and his parents. Genomic DNA was extracted from peripheral blood leucocytes with use of the QIAamp Blood-DNA mini reagent set (Qiagen) according to the manufacturer's instructions. DNA was eluted in 100 μL of water in the final step and stored at −20°C until required. Sequencing of the coding exons and exon-intron boundaries of the *BCHE* gene was performed after PCR amplification of genomic DNA, with specific primers (Table 1). All of the coding exons and the flanking introns of the *BCHE* gene were amplified by PCR using the following conditions: 1 cycle of 95°C for 10 min; 40 cycles of denaturation at 95°C for 30 s, annealing at 56°C for 30 s, and an extension at 72°C for 40 s; 1 cycle of 72°C for 7 min. The reaction mixture of final volume 25 μL contained 100 ng DNA template, 1×PCR Buffer (Invitrogen), 2.0 mmol $MgCl_2$, 0.2 mmol dNTP, 1 μmol of each primer, and 0,625 U Taq Gold DNA polymerase. PCR products were purified with use of the High Pure PCR Product Purification Kit

**Table 1.** Oligonucleotide primers used in PCR for the amplification of the *BCHE* gene.

| Primer name | Sequence (5′-3′) | Tm |
|---|---|---|
| 2-1F | GGCCTTTACAGAAGCAGGTTT | 59.8 |
| 2-1R | TTTTTGGTTTAGGTGCTGGAA | 59.6 |
| 2-2F | CGGTAACAGCCTTTCTTGGA | 60.2 |
| 2-2R | AGCTGCTCCTGCACTTTCTC | 59.9 |
| 2-3F | GGATTCCAGCACCTAAACCA | 59.9 |
| 2-3R | CCCATAGGGGACAACAAATG | 60.0 |
| 2-4F | GGTTGCTCTAGAGAGAATGAGACTG | 60.1 |
| 2-4R | GTTTGGAGGATCGGTGTTCA | 60.9 |
| 2-5F | CCAGGAGTGAGTGAGTTTGGA | 60.3 |
| 2-5R | AAAAATAAAACCAGCTTTGGTACA | 58.3 |
| 3F | TTCTTTAAAGCTCTTGTGAACAGTG | 59.2 |
| 3R | CACCGTGCCTTGGAGAGTAT | 60.1 |
| 4F | GAGAAAATGGCTTTTGTATTCG | 58.0 |
| 4R | CGTTCTAGCCATTTGGGTTT | 59.1 |

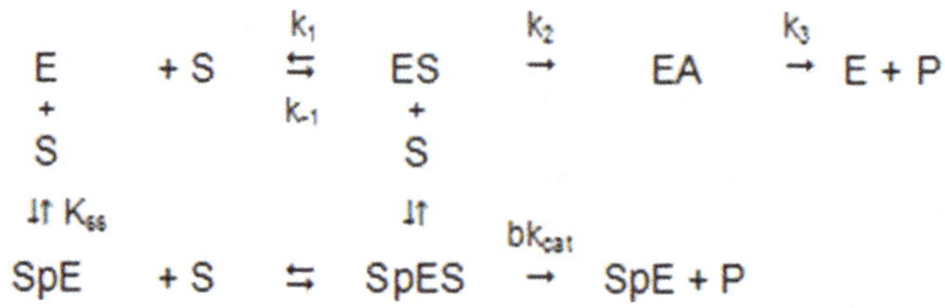


**Figure 1. Model of BChE catalyzed-hydrolysis of substrates.**

(Roche Diagnostics) according to the manufacturer's instructions. Both strands were sequenced using amplification primers as sequencing primers and BigDyeDeoxy terminator cycle sequencing according to the manufacturer's instruction (Beckman Coulter). Purified sequencing fragments were separated by capillary electrophoresis and detected by laser-induced fluorescence on a Beckman Ceq 8000 (Beckman Coulter). Polyphen [8] and Mutation Taster [9] were used to perform *in silico* prediction of the impact of nucleotide changes on the protein structure and function.

## Inhibition studies

Inhibition numbers (i.e. the dibucaine number and the fluoride number) for plasma BChE samples were determined according to classical procedures using BzCh as the substrate in 67 mM phosphate buffer pH 7.4 at 25°C. An inhibition number is defined as the percentage of inhibition of hydrolysis of 50 µM BzCh by a fixed concentration of inhibitor. The dibucaine number (DN) was determined using 10 µM dibucaine according to Kalow and Genest [4]. The fluoride number (FN) was determined using 50 µM sodium fluoride according to Harris and Whittaker [10].

## Determination of catalytic parameters

Catalytic parameters for hydrolysis of BTC were determined in 0.1 M phosphate buffer pH 7.0 at 25°C. Measurements were performed using Ellman's method [7]. Hydrolysis rates were recorded for 2 min after preincubation of plasma samples in the presence of DTNB as mentioned above. Wide ranges of substrate

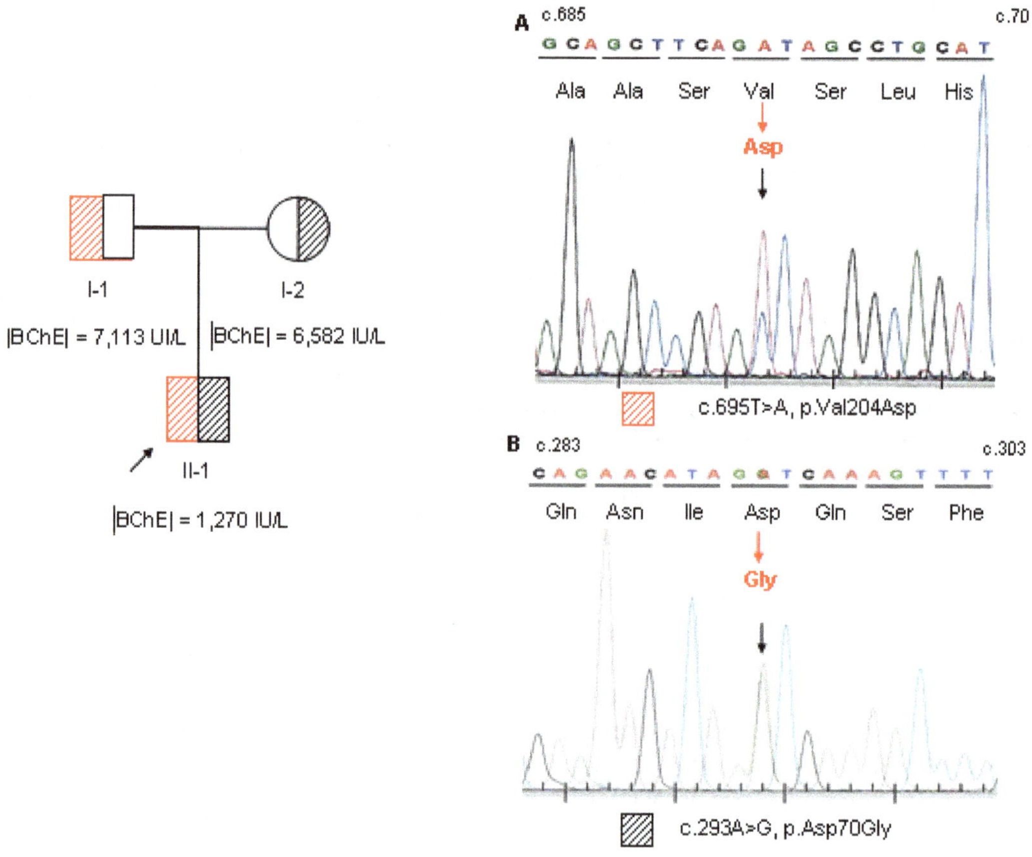


**Figure 2. Pedigree of the family with BChE activities and genotypes.** BChE activities were measured on Cobas® 6000 system. Results of genotyping are given as electropherograms. Sequence analyses reveal (A) an heterozygous mutation c.695T>A (p.Val204Asp). This mutation is observed in the proband and in patient I-1; (B) an heterozygous mutation c.293A>G (p.Asp70Gly, atypical variant). This mutation is observed in the proband and in patient I-2 and (C) an heterozygous mutation c.1699G>A (p.Ala539Thr, Kalow variant, electrophorogram not shown). This mutation is observed in the proband and in patient I-2.

**Table 2.** Evolutionary conservation of the region of BChE including in the variant site p.Val204Asp.

| Class | Species | Sequence | Swissprot accession # |
|---|---|---|---|
| Mammalia | *H. sapiens* | TLFGESAGAAS**V**SLHLLSPG | P06276 |
| | *B. taurus* | TLFGESAGAAS**V**SLHLLSPE | P32749 |
| | *O. cuniculus* | TLFGESAGAAS**V**SLHLLSPR | P21927 |
| | *F. catus* | TLFGESAGAGS**V**SLHLLSPR | O62760 |
| | *C. familiaris* | TLFGESAGAGS**V**GLHLLSPR | F1PEN8 |
| Aves | *G. gallus* | TIFGESAGSAS**V**SYHILSPK | Q90ZK8 |
| Amphibia | *X. tropicalis* | TIFGHSAGAAS**V**GFHLISTK | F7BPW9 |
| Osteichthyes | *G. aculeatus* | TLFGESAGSAS**V**GFHLLSPG | G3NW96 |

concentrations were used: from 10 µM to 50 mM for BTC. Spontaneous hydrolysis of substrates was recorded and subtracted for each enzymatic measurement at corresponding substrate concentrations.

BChE catalyzed-hydrolysis of substrates can be described by the model (Fig. 1) and by Eq 1 [11]:

$$v = \frac{k_{cat}[E]}{1+K_m/[S]}\left(\frac{1+b[S]/K_{ss}}{1+[S]/K_{ss}}\right) \quad (1)$$

At low substrate concentration, hydrolysis kinetics for all substrates follow the simple boxed reaction scheme that corresponds to the simple Michaelis-Menten mechanism in which the Michaelis constant, $K_m$, is described by Eq 2:

$$K_m = \frac{K_s k_3}{(k_2+k_3)} \quad (2)$$

with $K_s = k_{-1}/k_1$, the dissociation of the ES complex, $k_2$ and $k_3$ the rate constant for acylation (EA) and deacylation, respectively. The catalytic constant $k_{cat}$ is:

$$k_{cat} = V_{max}/[E] = \frac{k_2 k_3}{(k_2+k_3)} \quad (3)$$

with $V_{max}$, the maximum velocity, and [E], the enzyme active site concentration.

At high concentration, for positively charged substrates like BTC a second substrate molecule binds to the peripheral anionic site (PAS, p) of wild-type enzyme (Usual): SpE, and the ternary complex $S_PES$ makes products. $K_{ss}$ is the dissociation constant of this ternary complex. As a consequence, the kinetics deviate from the Michaelian model; there is either activation by excess substrate, e.g. with BTC, or inhibition by excess substrate, e.g. with BzCh. In Eq 1, the b factor refers to the effect of the second substrate molecule on the $k_{cat}$. If $b>1$, there is activation; if $b<1$, there is inhibition. If there is no binding on the PAS, $b = 1$, and Eq 1 reduces to the simple Michaelis-Menten equation.

Catalytic parameters were determined by non-linear fitting of substrate-dependent hydrolysis rate curves. Because BChE has a non-Michaelian behavior with BTC as substrate, Eq 1 was used to describe hydrolysis of BTC. On the other hand, owing to the structure of SCdTC which contains 2 thiocholine groups (one binds on the catalytic active center and the other binds to the PAS) the catalytic behavior is Michaelian, and Eq 1 reduces to Eq 3 [12].

## Nondenaturing gradient gel electrophoresis

Nondenaturing gradient gel (4–30%) electrophoresis of plasma samples (5 µL/lane) was carried out as described [13]. BChE active bands were stained using the methods of Karnovsky and Roots [14] with BTC as the substrate as described elsewhere [13].

## Micropurification of plasma BChE and denaturing gel electrophoresis

BChE was immunopurified from 0.5 ml plasma by binding to monoclonal mAb2 immobilized on Sepharose 4B [15]. Activity

**Table 3.** Activity, dibucaine (DN) and fluoride (FN) inhibition numbers of family member's butyrylcholinesterase (average values from triplicate measurements ± standard errors).

| Individual | BChE genotype | Abbreviation | Activity with BTC* (U/mL) | Activity with BzCh° (U/mL) | DN | FN |
|---|---|---|---|---|---|---|
| II-1 | p.Val204Asp/p.Asp70Gly-p.Ala539Thr | AKS | 0.41±0.02 | 0.16±0.002 | 7.2±6.9 | 15.7±3.7 |
| I-1 | p. Val204Asp/Usual | US | 2.26±0.13 | 0.61±0.01 | 75.3±2.3 | 51.6±5.0 |
| I-2 | p.Asp70Gly-p.Ala539Tyr/Usual | AKU | 2.51±0.10 | 0.63±0.01 | 58.3±3.6 | 42.6±4.0 |
| Control #1 | Usual/Usual | UU | 2.93±0.17 | 0.71±0.04 | 78.8±5.9 | 52.1±5.5 |
| Control #2 | p.Asp70Gly/p.Asp70Gly | AA | 1.16±0.001 | 0.39±0.02 | 5.1±7.6 | 13.0±4.1 |
| Control #3 | p.Asp70Gly/Silent | AS | 0.32±0.17 | 0.12±0.001 | 11.1±5.6 | 15.0±2.1 |

*) 1mM; °) 50 µM.
BChE genotype abbreviations are A for atypical (D70G), K for Kalow variant (A539T), U for usual, S for silent. The proband is II-1; his father is I-1; his mother is I-2.

**Table 4.** Catalytic properties of patient and parents's butyrylcholinesterase with BTC as the substrate at pH 7.0 and 25°C (average values from duplicate measurements ± standard deviation).

| | | BTC | | | |
|---|---|---|---|---|---|
| **Individual** | **BChE genotype** | **$V_{max}$ (U/ml)** | **$K_m$ (µM)** | **$K_{ss}$ (mM)** | **b*** |
| II-1 | p.Val204Asp/p.Asp70Gly-p.Ala539Thr | 0.50±0.01 | 265±25 | - | 1.0 |
| I-1 | p. Val204Asp/Usual | 7.51±0.01 | 21±2 | 0.49±0.08 | 2.4±0.2 |
| I-2 | p.Asp70Gly-p.Ala539Tyr/Usual | 6.07±0.01 | 27±2 | 0.51±0.02 | 2.5±0.7 |
| Control #1 | Usual/Usual | −(a) | 18±5(a) | 1.0±0.1(a) | 3.2±0.1(a) |
| Control #2 | p.Asp70Gly/p.Asp70Gly | −(b) | 150±50(b) | 1.1 (b) | 1.2±0.2(b) |

litterature values [12]: a and b) $k_{cat}=V_{max}/[E]=24\ 000\pm10\ 000\ min^{-1}$; b*: substrate activation factor (see Eq 1).

assays showed that 97% of the BChE activity had disappeared from plasma following overnight incubation with mAb2-Sepharose. Beads (0.04 mL) were washed with phosphate buffered saline, and desalted by washing with water. Beads were transferred to 0.45 µm Durapore centrifugal filters. BChE protein was released from the beads with 80 µL of 0.4 M acetic acid pH 2.6. The filtered acid extract was dried in a vacuum centrifuge, dissolved in 35 µL of SDS/dithiothreitol loading buffer, heated in a boiling water bath for 3 min and loaded on an SDS gel. Denaturing gel electrophoresis in SDS in the presence of dithiothreitol was carried out according to Laemli [16] on 4–30% gradient polyacrylamide gels. Protein bands were stained with Coomassie Brilliant Blue.

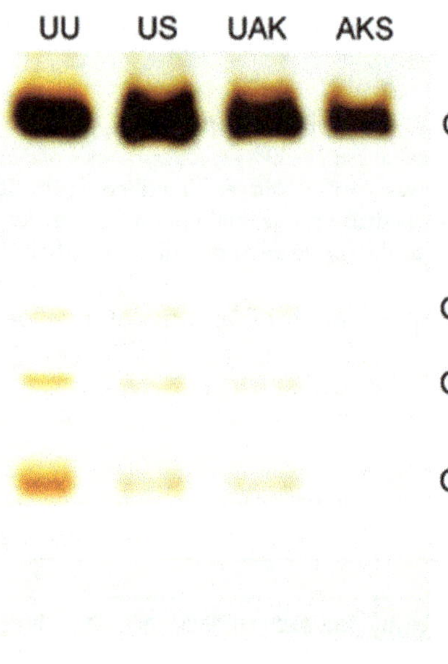


**Figure 3. Activity stained polyacrylamide gels of plasma BChE samples.** Nondenaturing gel stained for BChE activity. Plasma samples (5 µl per lane) were genotype UU, wild-type usual control; genotype US, the father (I-1) heterozygous for the silent variant; genotype UAK, the mother (I-2) heterozygous for the atypical/K variant; and genotype AKS, the son heterozygous (II-1) for the atypical/K variant and silent BChE. The majority of the plasma BChE is a tetramer (C4). Minor activity bands are for monomer (C1), a BChE monomer- albumin dimer (C2), and a BChE dimer (C3). The AKS plasma has weaker staining intensity for tetrameric BChE (C4) and no apparent minor bands of BChE activity.

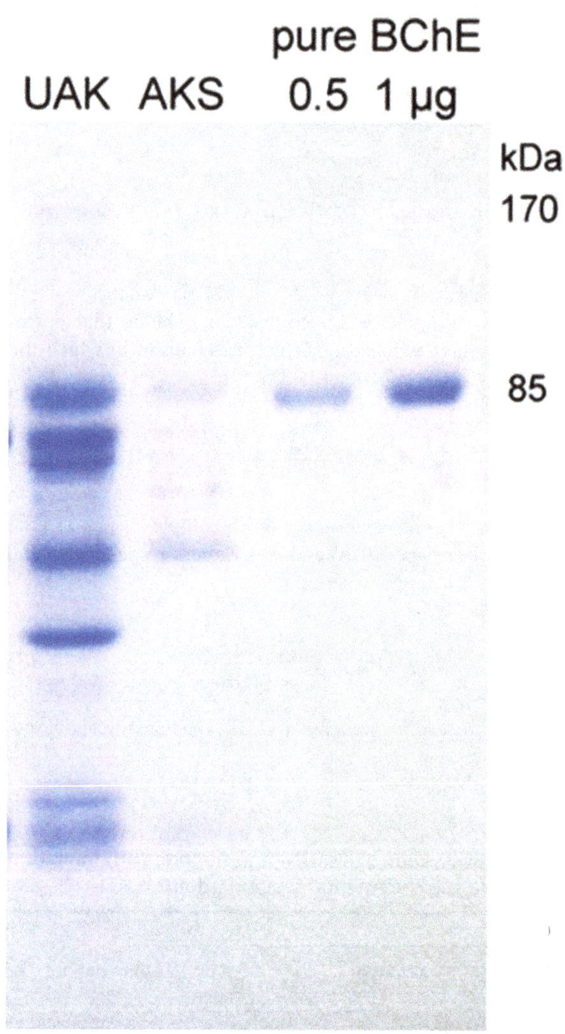


**Figure 4. Coomassie Brilliant Blue stained SDS-electrophoresis gel of immunopurified plasma BChE of patient (p.Val204Asp/ p.Asp70Gly. Ala539Thr; designated AKS) and his mother (p.Asp70Gly-Ala539Thr; designated UAK).** Pure human BChE has a monomer band at 85 kDa and a dimer band at 170 kDa. Comparison to pure BChE standards shows that about 1 µg BChE protein was immunopurified from 0.5 ml plasma of genotype UAK, but only 0.2 µg BChE protein from 0.5 ml plasma of genotype AKS.

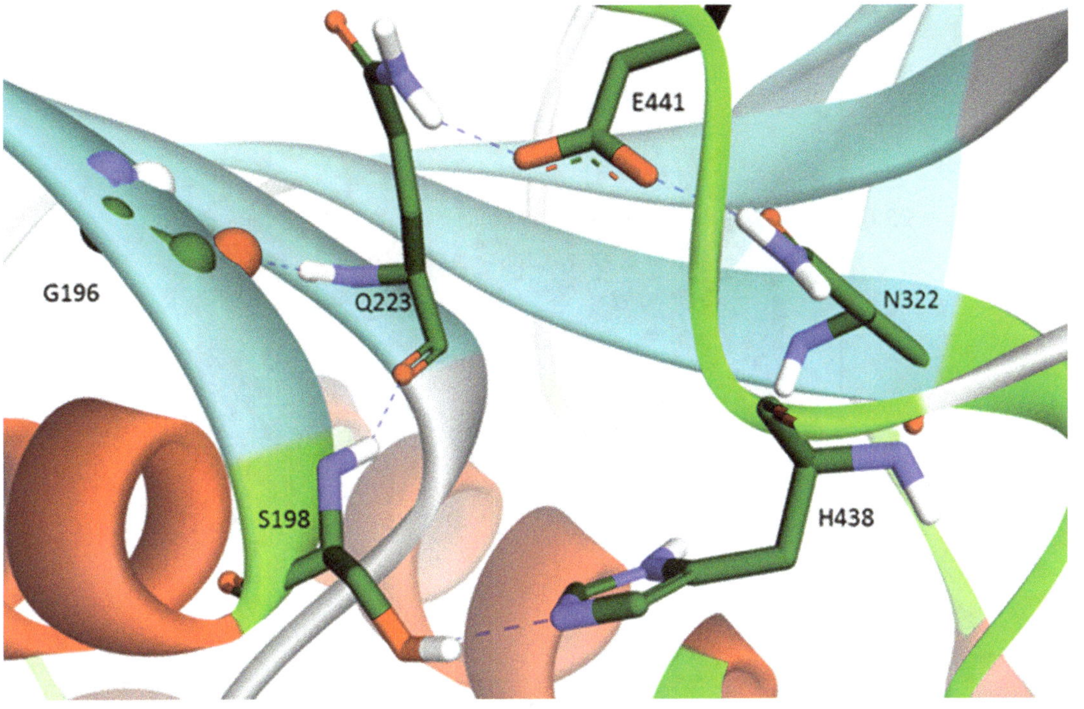


**Figure 5. Hydrogen bonding network in usual BChE keeps the α/β-unit turn carrying the catalytic Ser198 close to the loop carrying the catalytic His438.** Strands of the β-sheet are fixed together among other hydrogen bonds by ones formed by backbone atoms of Gln223 on one strand, and Gly196 and Ser198 on the other. Side chain of Gln223 forms hydrogen bond with Glu441, this hydrogen bond is maintained during the MD trajectory for usual BChE. As Glu441 is located on the same loop with the catalytic His438, this hydrogen bond is essential for keeping Ser198 and His438 close enough to form functional catalytic triad.

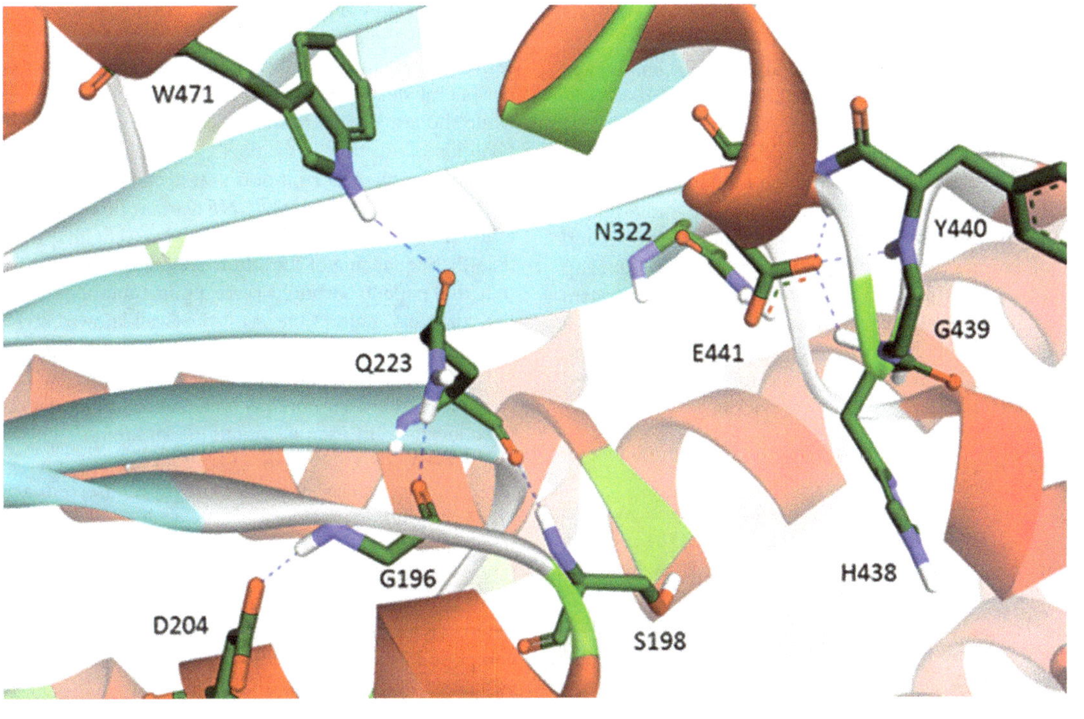


**Figure 6. Hydrogen bonding network in p.Val204Asp BChE formed during MD simulation.** Histidine 438 faces away from Serine 198, thus disrupting the function of the catalytic triad. This conformational change explains why mutation V204D causes the BChE enzyme to lose activity.

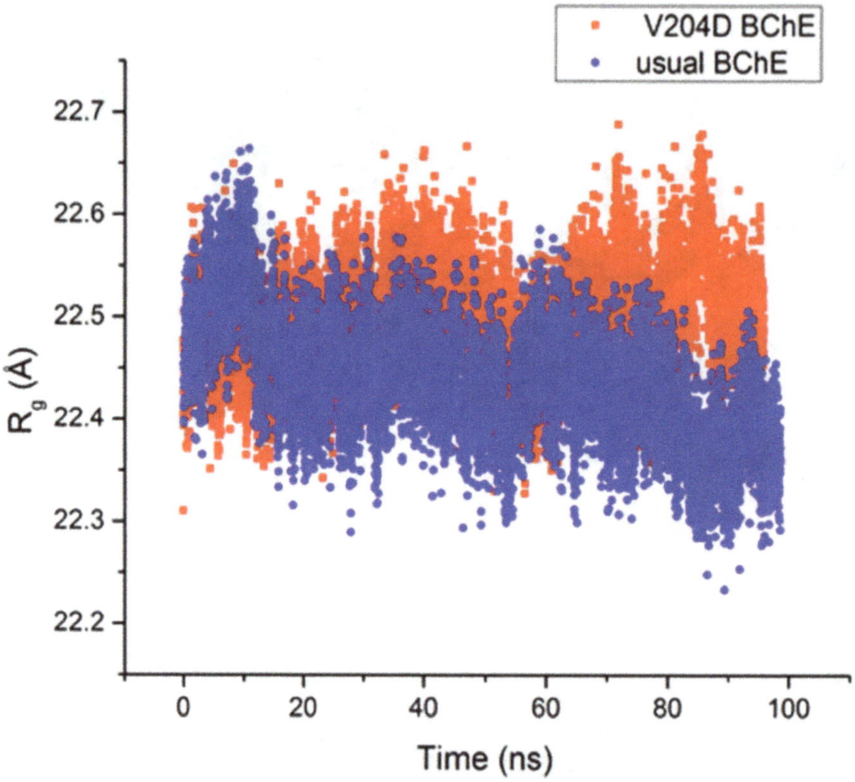


**Figure 7. Radius of gyration of BChE in p.Val204Asp mutant and the usual enzyme.** Along the MD trajectory size of usual BChE is maintained at the same level while for the mutant it gradually increases what indicates transition to a molten globule state.

### Molecular dynamics study

Model structures for wild type (usual BChE) and p.Val204Asp mutant were prepared from the X-ray coordinates of PDB ID 1P0I [17] as described in our previous studies [18,19]. For p.Val204Asp mutant of BChE, the Val204 side chain was manually converted to aspartic acid and its side chain was minimized with other protein atoms fixed. Minimization and MD simulations were performed with the NAMD 2.9 program [20] and the CHARMM36 force field [21] on the Lomonosov Moscow State University supercomputer [22]. After solvation and addition of ions, protein structures were saturated with water molecules and water box equilibrating runs were performed as described in [18]. This was followed by a full dynamic simulation of each system performed for 100 ns under periodic boundary conditions at a constant temperature of 298 K and constant pressure 1 atm. Structural analysis of the obtained MD trajectories was performed with ProDy [23] and VMD [24] software packages.

## Results and Discussion

The crystal structure of human BChE was described in 2003 [17]. The active, or acylation site (Ser198...His438...Glu325 triad) lies near the base of a gorge, approximately 20 Å from the surface. An adjacent site, the choline-binding site, also called the anionic site (Trp82...Tyr128...Phe329), is responsible for binding the choline moiety of the substrate, and positioning the ester bond for nucleophilic attack by the serine of the active site. Two additional structures, also located near the base of the gorge, are the oxyanion hole (Gly116...Gly117...Ala199) and the acyl pocket (Trp231...Leu286...Val288), which stabilize the substrate during hydrolysis. A peripheral anionic site (Asp70...Tyr332) is involved in the initial binding of the substrate and in activation control.

Various mutations affect BChE activity. In some cases, residues involved in the catalytic process are mutated: e.g. Ser198 of the active site, Tyr128 of the choline binding site, or Asp70 of the peripheral site. The first two mutations result in a silent enzyme, while the last one causes a reduction in substrate affinity and an abolition of substrate activation. Other mutated residues fall within conserved sequences or motifs that are distant from the active site.

Here we report a novel *BCHE* variant in a patient presenting a marked deficiency in BChE activity (|BChE| = 1,270 IU/L) (Fig. 2). Sequencing of the whole coding region of *BCHE* revealed that this patient harbored three point mutations in a compound heterozygous state. One was the well-known atypical variant (c.293A>G, p.Asp70Gly). The second one was the Kalow-variant (c.1699G>A, p.Ala539Thr). The last one, which was not previously described nor was included in any mutation databases, introduced a mis-sense mutation at amino acid residue 204 (c.695T>A, p.Val204Asp, GenBank Accession #KJ513459) (Fig. 2). It involves a residue highly conserved across species (Table 2). *In silico* predictions identified this mutation as potentially deleterious: i.e. PolyPhen-2 score of 1.0 (sensitivity: 0.00, specificity: 1.00), and Mutation Taster score of 152. This mutation was observed in the patient's father (patient I-1) at heterozygous state, whereas the mother (patient I-2) was compound heterozygote for the atypical variant and the Kalow variant.

Mutations near residue Val204 have previously been described: p.Ala199Val [25], p.Ala201Thr [26] and p.Ser203Pro [27]. These mutations result in a silent enzyme. However, the mechanisms by which these mutations determine the silent phenotype were not established.

In the present work kinetic analysis, inhibition studies and molecular dynamics studies have led to an understanding of how mutation p.Val204Asp disrupts the catalytic triad and determines the "silent" phenotype.

Results of phenotyping are in Table 3. Results are consistent with reported values of activity, DN and FN for heterozygous human BChE of genotype Silent (p.Val204Asp)/p.Asp70Gly-p.Ala539Thr (Proband), Silent (p.Val204Asp)/Usual (father) and Usual/p.Asp70Gly-p.Ala539Thr (mother).

Hydrolysis kinetics of BTC were performed under steady-state conditions. The catalytic behavior of the patient's BChE (p.Val204Asp/p.Asp70Gly-p.Ala539Thr) follows the Michaelis-Menten model (boxed reactions in Scheme 1). $K_m$ was about 10 times higher than that of the Usual enzyme (18±5 μM) and two times that of the atypical enzyme (150±50 μM) (Control #2 in Table 4). The catalytic behavior of the parent's BChE fits with expected values for heterozygous enzyme tetramers containing half of usual (U) subunits. The low $K_{ss}$ of the patient's mother can be explained by the reduced affinity of BTC for the PAS in K-subunits ($K_{ss}$ value of K-BChE was reported to be two-fold lower than Kss of the usual enzyme) [28]. According to Eq 1, the two-fold reduced $K_{ss}$ did not significantly affect kinetic measurements at BTC concentrations lower than 10 mM, i.e. performed at 1mM and 7.56 mM.

Kinetic analysis of the patient's BChE with BTC as the substrate showed that there was no substrate activation (b = 1), see Individual II-1 in Table 4. This fact indicates that the PAS is not functional in p.Val204Asp subunits or that subunits carrying the p.Val204Asp mutation are totally inactive at all BTC concentrations. Because the tetrameric enzyme is a hybrid of silent subunits carrying the mutation p.Val204Asp and subunits carrying the two mutations p.Gly70Asp and p.Ala539Thr, $V_{max}$ was expected to be reduced compared to parent's BChE (I-1, I-2) and control BChEs (#1,2). However, $V_{max}$ in the patient's BChE was unexpectedly low (Tables 3 and 4). This result, was corroborated by electrophoresis data on both activity stained gels and Coomassie Brilliant Blue stained gels of highly purified BChE (Figs. 3 and 4), which indicated that the concentration of BChE in the patient's plasma is lower than the average BChE concentration of 50 nM. This suggests that mutation p.Val204Asp may either reduce the biosynthesis of enzyme or more likely destabilizes the enzyme and accelerates its clearance from the bloodstream. If the latter possibility is correct this would suggest that mutation p.Val204Asp alters the 3D structure of silent subunits. The MD study on p.Val204Asp mutant protein sheds light on this issue.

An additional cause for the low enzyme concentration could be the p.Ala539Thr mutation. Residue Ala539 is involved in the tetramerization domain of BChE [29]. Mutation p.Ala539Thr (K variant) was found to destabilize the enzyme structure [30]. Therefore the presence of the K variant in subunits carrying the p.Asp70Gly mutation may have also contributed to the low enzyme concentration in the patient's plasma.

Comparison of MD trajectories for usual BChE and p.Val204Asp mutant showed that in the mutant, shortly after the beginning of simulation, the catalytic triad is disrupted. The side chains of Ser198 and His438 move too far from each other to perform catalysis. By contrast, the catalytic triadstays operative during the whole MD trajectory for usual BChE. In usual BChE these catalytic residues are maintained in close proximity by a network of hydrogen bonds involving Gln223, Glu441 and Asn322, which bring the α/β-unit turn carrying the catalytic Ser198 close to the loop carrying the catalytic His438 (Fig. 5). Introduction of a charged amino acid instead of Val204 results in establishment of new hydrogen bonds and disruption of the initial bonds. Asp204 forms a hydrogen bond with Gly196. This causes Gly196 to turn about 90° out of the β-sheet plane (Fig. 6). As a result the Gly196 oxygen backbone forms a hydrogen bond with the Gln223 side chain, instead of with backbone peptide bonds, as for β-sheet strands in usual BChE (Fig. 5). In addition to partial disruption of the β-sheet, this switches hydrogen bonding of the Gln223 side chain from Glu441 to Trp471. In the usual BChE the hydrogen bond between Gln223 and Glu441 links together the β-sheet and the loop carrying the catalytic His438. For Glu441 new hydrogen bonds are formed in the mutant: 3 hydrogen bonds with peptide bond groups of neighboring residues on the His438 loop (Fig. 6). However, Glu441 still interacts with the Asn322 side chain, as in usual BChE. This likely prevents the protein from unfolding. In other words, the overall effect of the mutation p.Val240Asp is disruption of hydrogen bonding between Gln223 and Glu441. This leads the catalytic Ser198 to move away from the loop carrying the catalytic His438 with subsequent disruption of the functional catalytic triad. Therefore, BChE subunits carrying this mutation have no activity regardless of the type of substrate. This mutation also has an impact on the overall protein structure and causes an increase in the radius of gyration along the MD trajectory of p.Val204Asp BChE compared to the usual BChE (Fig. 7). However it does not cause any significant secondary structure change except for that mentioned above (result not shown). The increased gyration radius suggests that the enzyme is in a pre-molten globule state, susceptible to unfolding. This statement would thus explain why the BChE concentration is reduced in plasma.

## Conclusions

In conclusion, this work explains how a point mutation (Val204Asp) far from the active site leads to a "silent" BChE phenotype where the BChE enzyme has no activity regardless of the type of substrate, and has a structure that is not recognized by a monoclonal to native BChE. MD simulations suggest that the enzyme is in a pre-denaturation state.

## Acknowledgments

The authors thank the patient and his family for agreeing to participate in this study. They thank Ms Blandine HARY and Mr Sébastien COURCELLE for their technical help. We thank the Supercomputing Center of Lomonosov Moscow State University for supercomputing time.

## Author Contributions

Conceived and designed the experiments: HD SL OL PM. Performed the experiments: SL IM AB OL PM. Analyzed the data: HD SL FC OL LS PM. Contributed reagents/materials/analysis tools: HD SL OL PM. Wrote the paper: HD SL PM.

## References

1. Masson P, Lockridge O (2010) Butyrylcholinesterase for protection from organophosphorus poisons: catalytic complexities and hysteretic behavior. Arch Biochem Biophys 494: 107–120.

2. Johnson G, Moore SW (2012) Why has butyrylcholinesterase been retained? Structural and functional diversification in a duplicated gene. Neurochem Int 61: 783–797.

3. Forbat A, Lehmann H, Silk E (1953) Prolonged apnoea following injection of succinylcholine. Lancet 265: 1067–1068.
4. Kalow W, Genest K (1957) A method for the detection of atypical forms of human serum cholinesterase; determination of dicucaine number. Can J Biochem Physiol 35: 339–346.
5. Souza RL, Mikami LR, Maegawa RO, Chautard-Freire-Maia EA (2005) Four new mutations in the BCHE gene of human butyrylcholinesterase in a Brazilian blood donor sample. Mol Genet Metab 84: 349–353.
6. Zsigmond EK, Downs JR (1971) Plasma cholinesterase activity in newborns and infants. Canad Anaest Soc J 18: 278–285.
7. Ellman GL, Courtney KD, Andres V, Featherstone RM (1961) A new and rapid colorimetric determination of acetylcholinesterase activity. Biochem Pharmacol 7: 88–95.
8. Adzhubei IA, Schmidt S, Peshkin L, Ramensky VE, Gerasimova A, et al. (2010) A method and server for predicting damaging missense mutations. Nat Methods 7: 248–249.
9. Schwarz JM, Rödelsperger C, Schuelke M, Seelow D (2010) MutationTaster evaluates disease-causing potential of sequence alterations. Nat Methods 7: 575–576.
10. Harris H, Whittaker M (1961) Differential inhibition of human serum cholinesterase with fluoride: recognition of two new phenotypes. Nature 191: 556–562.
11. Radić Z, Pickering NA, Vellom DC, Camp S, Taylor P (1993) Three distinct domains in the cholinesterase molecule confer selectivity for acetyl- and butyrylcholinesterase inhibitors. Biochemistry 32: 12074–12084.
12. Masson P, Legrand P, Bartels CF, Froment MT, Schopfer LM, et al. (1997) Role of aspartate 70 and tryptophane 82 in binding of succinydithiocholine to human butyrylcholinesterase. Biochemistry 36: 2266–2277.
13. Li B, Sedlacek M, Manoharan I, Boopathy R, Duysen EG, et al. (2005) Butyrylcholinesterase, paraoxonase, and albumin esterase, but not carboxylesterase, are present in human plasma. Biochem Pharmacol 70: 1673–16784.
14. Karnovsky MJ, Roots LA (1964) A "direct-coloring" thiocholine method for cholinesterases. J Histochem Cytochem 12: 219–221.
15. Checler F, Grassi J, Masson P, Vincent JP (1990) Monoclonal antibodies allow precipitation of esterasic but not peptidasic activities associated with butyrylcholinesterase. J Neurochem 55: 750–5.
16. Laemmli UK (1970) Cleavage of structural proteins during the assembly of the head of bacteriophage T4. Nature 227: 680–685.
17. Nicolet Y, Lockridge O, Masson P, Fontecilla-Camps JC, Nachon F (2003) Crystal structure of human butyrylcholinesterase and of its complexes with substrate and products. J Biol Chem 278: 41141–41147.
18. Masson P, Lushchekina S, Schopfer LM, Lockridge O (2013) Effects of viscosity and osmotic stress on the reaction of human butyrylcholinesterase with cresyl saligenin phosphate, a toxicant related to the aerotoxic syndrome: Kinetic and molecular dynamics studies. Biochem J 454: 387–399.
19. Lushchekina SV, Nemukhin AV, Varfolomeev SD, Masson P (2014) Molecular modeling evidence for His 438 flip in the mechanism of BuChE hysteretic behavior. J Mol Neurosci 52: 434–445.
20. Phillips JC, Braun R, Wang W, Gumbart J, Tajkhorshid E, et al. (2005) Scalable molecular dynamics with NAMD. J Comput Chem 26: 1781–1802.
21. Best RB, Zhu X, Shim J, Lopes PEM, Mittal J, et al. (2012) Optimization of the Additive CHARMM All-Atom Protein Force Field Targeting Improved Sampling of the Backbone φ, ψ and Side-Chain χ1 and χ2 Dihedral Angles. J Chem Theor Comput 8: 3257–3273.
22. Sadovnichy V, Tikhonravov A, Voevodin V, Opanasenko V (2013) "Lomonosov": Supercomputing at Moscow State University. In Contemporary High Performance Computing: From Petascale toward Exascale, J.S. Vetter, ed. (Boca Raton, USA, CRC Press), pp 283–307.
23. Bakan A, Meireles LM, Bahar I (2011) ProDy: Protein Dynamics Inferred from Theory and Experiments. Bioinformatics 27: 1575–1577.
24. Humphrey W, Dalke A, Schulten K (1996) VMD: visual molecular dynamics. J Mol Graph 14: 33–38.
25. Sakamoto N, Hidaka K, Fujisawa T, Maeda M, Iuchi I (1998) Identification of a point mutation associated with a silent phenotype of human serum butyrylcholinesterase-a case of familial cholinesterasemia. Clin Chim Acta 274: 159–166.
26. Primo-Parmo SL, Bartels CF, Wiersema B, van der Spek AFL, Innis JW, et al. (1996) Characterization of 12 silent alleles of the human butyrylcholinesterase (BCHE) gene. Am J Hum Genet 58: 52–64.
27. Hidaka K, Watanabe Y, Tomita M, Ueda N, Higashi M, et al. (2001) Gene analysis of genomic DNA from stored serum by polymerase chain reaction: identification of three missense mutations in patients with cholinesterasemia and ABO genotyping. Clin Chim Acta 303: 61–67.
28. Varkey Altamirano C, Bartels CF, Lockridge O (2000) The butyrylcholinesterase K-variant shows similar protein turnover and quaternary interaction to the wild-type enzyme. J Neurochem 74: 869–877.
29. Varkey Altamirano C, Lockridge O (1999) Conserved aromatic residue of the C-terminus of human butyrylcholinesterase mediate the association of tetramers. Biochemistry 38: 13414–13412.
30. Podoly E, Hanin G, Soreq H (2010) Alanine-to-threonine substitutions and amyloid disease: butyrylcholinesterase as a case study. Chem Biol Interact 187: 64–71.

# 17

# Allopregnanolone and Its Precursor Progesterone Do Not Reduce Injury after Experimental Stroke in Hypertensive Rats – Role of Postoperative Temperature Regulation?

**Neil J. Spratt[1,2]*, Amelia J. Tomkins[1], Debbie Pepperall[1], Damian D. McLeod[1], Mike B. Calford[1,3]**

1 School of Biomedical Sciences, University of Newcastle, and Hunter Medical Research Institute, Newcastle, Australia, 2 Hunter New England Local Health District, Newcastle, Australia, 3 School of Medicine, The University of Tasmania, Hobart, Australia

**Abstract**

Allopregnanolone is a neurosteroid synthesized from progesterone in brain. It increases inhibition through modulation of the gamma-aminobutyric acid type A (GABA-A) receptor. Both agents are putative neuroprotectants after ischemic stroke. We sought to confirm their effectiveness in a hypertensive rat stroke model, with intra- and post-operative temperature regulation. The primary study compared allopregnanolone, progesterone or vehicle control treatments, administered 105 minutes after induction of temporary middle cerebral artery occlusion in spontaneously hypertensive rats. Temperature was controlled intraoperatively and a heat mat used in the 6 hours postoperatively to permit animal temperature self-regulation. The primary outcome was infarct volume and secondary outcomes were tests of sensory and motor function. There was no significant effect of treatment on any outcome measure. Given prior reports of GABA-A receptor agonists causing hypothermia, follow-up experiments were conducted to examine postoperative temperature regulation. These did not reveal a difference in postoperative temperature in neurosteroid-treated animals compared to control. However, in all rats maintained postoperatively in ambient temperature, moderate hypothermia was observed. This was in contrast to rats maintained over a heat mat. The lowest mean postoperative temperature was between 34.4–34.9°C in all 3 groups. These data do not support a neuroprotective effect of allopregnanolone or progesterone in ischemic stroke in hypertensives in the setting of normothermia. Given previous evidence of synergy between neuroprotective agents and hypothermia, demonstration of neuroprotective effect of these agents in the absence of postoperative hypothermia would be prudent before consideration of these agents for further clinical investigation.

**Editor:** Shaida A. Andrabi, Johns Hopkins University, United States of America

**Funding:** This work was supported by grants from the Greater Building Society/Hunter Medical Research Institute, the Sylvia and Charles Viertel charitable foundation, the Royal Australian College of Physicans / High Blood Pressure Foundation and by the NHMRC (program grant 454417). Dr. Spratt was supported by a NHMRC Career Development Fellowship, APP1035465. The funders had no role in study design, data collection and analysis, decision to publish, or preparation of the manuscript.

**Competing Interests:** The authors have declared that no competing interests exist.

* Email: neil.spratt@newcastle.edu.au

## Introduction

The neurosteroid allopregnanolone is synthesized *de novo* or from systemic progesterone in neurons [1,2]. It is the most potent known endogenous positive modulator of the inhibitory GABA-A receptor. Both allopregnanolone and its parent compound, progesterone, have been shown to reduce injury following experimental brain injury including traumatic brain injury, and stroke [3,4,5,6]. Two previous studies of allopregnanolone in experimental stroke have shown a trend to greater neuroprotective efficacy than progesterone using young, healthy rats [4]. Similar or greater effect sizes have also been seen in mice. Neuroprotection was shown not to be influenced by the presence or absence of the progesterone receptor, thereby supporting the interpretation that the effect is GABA-A mediated [6]. In both of these studies, as well as in studies of other conditions, temperature was measured and regulated in the intraoperative, but not the postoperative phase. However previous investigations with another GABA-A agonist showed that this agent resulted in hypothermia postoperatively [7].

According to the recommendations of the Stroke Therapy Academic Industry Roundtable (STAIR) [8] for preclinical development of potential neuroprotectives, it is also important to confirm neuroprotection in a disease model. Therefore, the primary aim of this study was to evaluate the putative neuroprotective effect of allopregnanolone and progesterone in experimental stroke in spontaneously hypertensive rats (SHR), measuring the effect of these agents on infarct volume with secondary outcomes of neurobehavioral scores. A randomized, blinded placebo-controlled study was undertaken comparing treatment with allopregnanolone, progesterone or vehicle control after 90 minute temporary middle cerebral artery occlusion (MCAo). This methodologically rigorous design was used in accordance with good laboratory practice recommendations [9]. Particular attention was paid to body temperature. Observation of post-stroke body temperature alterations in some animals in the treatment groups led to the hypothesis that hypothermia may account for some of the neuroprotective benefits of these agents reported in previous studies, in which post-operative temperature was not recorded. A second series of experiments was therefore conducted to monitor postoperative temperature continuously with the aim of determining the effects of neurosteroids on post-stroke thermoregulation. Both aims were achieved.

## Methods

### Animals

All animal experimentation was undertaken with the approval of the animal care and ethics committee of the University of Newcastle (Approval No. 1025) and in compliance with the requirements of the Australian Code of Practice for the Care and Use of Animals for Scientific Purposes. A total of 62 male spontaneously hypertensive rats (SHR) (290–350 g) were used (Animal Resource Centre (ARC), Perth, Australia). For stroke experiments, 46 animals were used. For follow up experiments of body temperature during anesthetic recovery 16 animals were used. Animals were housed 2–3 per cage in a temperature and humidity controlled environment on a 12 hour light-dark cycle and were fed a standard laboratory rat chow.

### Surgery and administration of study compounds

MCAo was performed under isoflurane anesthesia using silicone tipped intraluminal filaments (silicone tip external diameter and length 0.35 & 2.5 mm respectively) as reported previously [10]. A simple test of forelimb flexion was performed immediately prior to re-induction of anesthesia for reperfusion at 90 minutes. Animals without evidence of neurological deficit were excluded from further study. At 105 minutes post-MCAo (while still anesthetized post-reperfusion), rats were randomized to receive 1.5 mL i.p. from a coded syringe containing allopregnanolone, progesterone (both 8 mg/kg), or vehicle (30% cyclodextran) mixed by sonication and warmed to body temperature. Six hours post-MCAo a second identical injection was given subcutaneously. Animals were only randomized to treatment following reperfusion of the MCA. Treatment was contained in identical syringes labeled with randomly generated 3 digit numbers. The allocation code was prepared by a non-randomising investigator, and kept in a sealed envelope in a locked cabinet until the completion of all analyses. Hence all investigators were blind to treatment allocation until completion of all analyses. Sample sizes were calculated to enable detection of a 30% difference between treatment groups with a power of 80% at alpha 0.05.

### Temperature regulation

During surgery, animals were maintained at 37°C on a rectal temperature regulated homeothermic heating mat (Physitemp Instruments). Heart and respiratory rates, oxygen saturations and tail-cuff systolic blood pressure (NIBP-R controller, ADInstruments) were monitored throughout surgery. Following MCAo, animals were woken from anesthetic and housed individually in cages placed ½ over a heating mat maintained at 37°C for the first 6 hours postoperatively, after which they were returned to the animal house. Rectal temperature was taken at 2, 6 and 24 hours post-stroke.

### Outcome analyses

The prespecified primary outcome was infarct volume at 24 hours, and secondary outcomes were a composite behavioral score and performance on the "sticky-dot removal test". Neurological scoring was performed at 2 and 24 hours. This consisted of a composite score of forelimb flexion, torso twisting and lateral push [11]. At 24 hours the sticky-dot (adhesive removal) test was performed [12,13]. In the 4 weeks prior to stroke induction, animals received at least 3 training sessions with 3 repetitions per session or until they consistently removed the adhesive label from the forepaws immediately after it was applied. For outcome analysis, speed of removal of an adhesive label from the distal forepaw was recorded for each side, and speed relative to contralateral and to pre-stroke baseline were calculated. Following final behavioral testing, animals were perfused intracardially with 4% paraformaldehyde under deep anesthesia [10]. Brains were post-fixed in 10% neutral buffered formalin, processed and paraffin embedded. Five micron thick sections at 1 mm intervals were stained with hematoxylin and eosin. Photographed areas of infarction and hemispheric areas were measured using Image J software (NIH, Bethesda). If there were any areas where there was any uncertainty regarding the presence of infarction based on the photomicrograph alone, the sections were correlated with high power microscopic evaluation of the region in question. Volumes were calculated as a percentage of the ipsilateral hemisphere.

### Effect on body temperature of recovery at ambient temperature

A secondary study was performed to investigate the possibility that allopregnanolone and/or progesterone may disrupt normal thermoregulation in the immediate postoperative phase. Animals were subjected to isoflurane anesthesia for 1 hour, during which they had a temperature datalogger (SubCue, Calgary, Canada) inserted in the extraperitoneal potential space, under the abdominal musculature. Core body temperature was logged every 5 minutes for the following 24 hours. Immediately prior to recovery from anesthesia animals received an intraperitoneal injection of allopregnanolone ($n=6$), progesterone ($n=4$) or vehicle ($n = 6$), with a follow up subcutaneous dose 6 hours later, following the same regime as for the stroke experiments, including concealment of treatment allocation. Intraoperative temperature was maintained on a homeothermic heating mat, however after waking from anesthesia animals were placed back in standard cages with bedding materials, without the use of a hot water heat mat. Ambient temperature adjacent to the cages was recorded.

Temperature data from a third cohort of animals are presented for comparison of temperature regulation after MCAo with the use of a heat mat postoperatively.. These animals were normothermic control animals from a separate study of the use of hypothermia post stroke. They had stroke surgery, data logger implantation and were then placed in cages ½ over heating mats for 6 hours postoperatively, exactly as was done for the initial cohort.

### Statistics

Comparisons of infarct volumes and other continuous variables were performed using one-way ANOVA with Tukey's multiple comparisons test. Categorical variables such as behavioral scores were analysed using a Kruskal-Wallis test with post hoc Dunn's test for significant results. Temperature data in part 2 was analysed using 2-way ANOVA with repeated measures and Bonferroni post-hoc tests. Infarct volumes are presented as mean ±95% confidence intervals. Physiological and other data are presented as mean± standard deviations, unless otherwise specified.

### Exclusions

In total, 8 animals were excluded from analysis. Three had no stroke deficit prior to reperfusion, 2 had the occluding suture inadvertently completely withdrawn at reperfusion (leaving a potential silicone embolus intravascularly). Two animals were excluded due to inadvertent administration of (concealed) treatment at the incorrect time interval and 1 animal was excluded due to death at 4 hours postoperatively, rendering both infarct and behavioural outcomes unobtainable. This animal did not have a large deficit on neurological score 2 hours previously, and the death remained unexplained after post-mortem examination (this animal received allopregnanolone). A further animal (allopregnanolone) had unquantifiable infarct volume due to damage to the brain during the fixation process. Therefore for the allopregnanolone group infarct volume data n = 11, and behavioral data n = 12. Progesterone and vehicle groups had n = 13 for all data.

## Results

### Stroke Outcomes

No significant differences were detected in physiological data at baseline or during the intra- and postoperative periods between any groups (allopregnanolone, progesterone and vehicle) (Table 1).

Infarct volumes were 34±15%, 39±15% and 36±9% (means ±95% confidence interval) of the hemispheric volume in the allopregnanolone, progesterone and vehicle treatment groups respectively (Figure. 1). There were no significant differences between groups. Similarly, there were no significant differences between groups on any individual or composite behavioral scores (Table 2). Despite no significant differences at any time point of the group means of postoperative temperature, at 24 hours there were three outlier animals with core temperature below 35°C. This was the only time point at which cages were not ½ over a heat mat, and all the outliers were from the allopregnanolone group. This observation prompted the second series of experiments to evaluate body temperature changes during the early postoperative recovery period.

### Postoperative temperature changes

In the second series of experiments (body temperature during recovery), there were no significant differences in ambient air temperature adjacent to the recovery cages. Ambient temperatures were 21.2±0.3, 21.3±0.7 and 21.1±0.4°C next to the allopregnanolone, progesterone and vehicle group cages, respectively. In all animals, core body temperatures dropped by 5–7% of baseline to, 34.9±0.4°C, 34.4±0.8°C, and 34.4±0.4°C for allopregnanolone, progesterone and vehicle groups respectively. These low temperatures occurred at a mean time of 44±20 minutes, 45±14 minutes, and 48±10 minutes post recovery from anesthesia for allopregnanolone, progesterone and vehicle groups respectively. There were no significant temperature differences between treatment groups at any time. The mean temperatures of all groups at each time point are presented at Figure. 2 (note these are somewhat higher than the numbers presented above, due to pooling of groups and the resultant variability in timing of the lowest temperature in each animal). Datalogger insertion had no significant effect on body temperature, since the mean rectal temperatures obtained in the initial experiments (stroke + treatment) at 2, 6 and 24 hours were not significantly different to the datalogger temperatures at the same times in the separate post-stroke comparison group. Temperatures at 2 h were 37.3±0.6 and 36.9±0.6°C, at 6 h were 37.6±0.7 and 37.7±0.3°C, and at 24 h were 36.9±1.1 and 37.5±0.6°C for rectal and datalogger temperatures, respectively.

## Discussion

We found that allopregnanolone and progesterone had no neuroprotective effect in hypertensive animals when body temperature was carefully maintained during and after surgery (Figure 1). Neither drug had an independent effect on body temperature (Figure 2). These randomized, blinded and appropriately powered data suggest that neither drug is likely to be of major benefit to hypertensive patients, which comprise >50% of the stroke population.

This data is in stark contrast to previously published studies of the use of allopregnanolone in experimental stroke in rats and mice [4,6]. The dosage of the steroids used in the present study

**Table 1.** Physiological data in the three treatment groups.

| | Vehicle | Progesterone | Allopregnanolone |
|---|---|---|---|
| Preoperative Weight (g) | 349 (±36) | 338 (±25) | 357(±27) |
| **Intraoperative** | | | |
| Temperature (°C) | 37.2(±0.4) | 37.4(±0.2) | 37.4(±0.3) |
| Heart Rate | 348(±24) | 342(±28) | 356(±20) |
| Systolic Blood Pressure (mmHg) | 106(±19) | 124(±33) | 115(±24) |
| Respiratory Rate | 44.4(±3.8) | 46.1(±4.7) | 48.2(±7.0) |
| Oxygen Saturations (%) | 97.2(±1.6) | 96.5(±1.5) | 95.5(±1.2) |
| **Reperfusion** | | | |
| Temperature (°C) | 37.3(±0.6) | 37.2(±0.6) | 37.5(±0.9) |
| Heart Rate | 348(±54) | 356(±18) | 384(±28) |
| Respiratory Rate | 37.9(±4.7) | 38.0(±6.8) | 43.2(±11.0) |
| Oxygen Saturations (%) | 96.6(±1.7) | 96.4(±2.2) | 97.2(±1.2) |
| **Postoperative** | | | |
| 24 h weight loss (g) | 22(±8.5) | 16(±6.8) | 17(±6.8) |
| 2 h Temperature (°C) | 37.3(±0.6) | 37.2(±0.6) | 37.3(±0.6) |
| 6 h Temperature (°C) | 37.8(±0.4) | 37.5(±0.7) | 37.7(±1.1) |
| 24 h Temperature (°C) | 37.2(±1.1) | 36.9(±0.7) | 36.6(±1.5) |

Data are presented as mean ±sd.

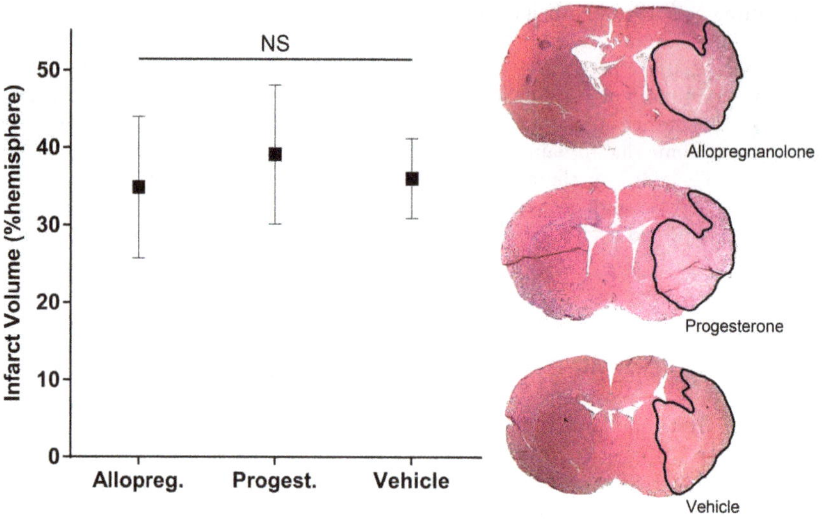


**Figure 1. Infarct volume after administration of allopregnanolone, progesterone or vehicle control, expressed as a percentage of the ipsilateral hemisphere (mean +95% confidence intervals, allopregnanolone n = 11, progesterone n = 13, vehicle n = 13).** There was no significant difference between any group. Representative H&E stained sections of each treatment group are displayed with the area of infarct outlined in black.

match those found effective in the earlier studies. Results are also in contrast to multiple studies of the use of progesterone in experimental stroke [4,14,15,16,17,18,19], as well as the use of both agents in other models of brain injury [3,5,20,21,22,23,24,25,26,27,28]. However, there have been other similarly negative studies in ovariectomised female rats treated with either allopregnanolone or progesterone [29,30]. Additionally, a recent single animal data meta-analysis of progesterone neuroprotection after stroke presented evidence of significant publication bias – i.e. that negative studies may not have been published [29]. What might account for the difference of the current study from those showing neuroprotection?

One significant difference between this study and previous neuroprotection studies using these agents (in stroke and other models of neural injury), is the provision of warming during the postoperative period (6 hours), and the measurement of body temperature during this interval. All mammals including humans are prone to development of postoperative hypothermia if warming is not provided [31]. This can be profoundly neuroprotective and has led to false positive detection of neuroprotection, a phenomenon reported for other GABAergic agents such as clomethiazole [7]. Neither allopregnanolone nor progesterone altered body temperature beyond the moderate hypothermia induced by anesthesia for several hours in all non-stroked animals (Figure 2). However, some other neuroprotective agents have been shown to have a synergistic effect with mild hypothermia [32,33]. Such synergy could be exploited for treatment, however inducing even mild hypothermia in patients is far more difficult than in postoperative small animals.

Another important difference was the use of spontaneously hypertensive rats. Few stroke neuroprotection studies examine efficacy in the face of the co-morbidities common in patients, however this was a key recommendation of the STAIR committee update [34]. While the benefits of hypothermia are maintained in the face of hypertension [35], this does not appear to always be the case for neuroprotective agents in experimental models. The degree of neuroprotection produced by the spin-trap agent NXY-059 in SHRs was significantly less than that in normotensive strains [36]. This agent was not shown to have any benefit in the subsequent large-scale clinical trial [37]. While neuroprotection by progesterone has been reported after MCAo in SHRs [18], those experiments were not temperature controlled in the postoperative phase.

Timing of stroke treatment with neuroprotectants is also critical. Reports on the importance of reperfusion injury [38] also suggest that treatment administration prior to reperfusion [4], rather than after, may be important in the neuroprotective activity of these agents. However, such a hypothesis is not consistent with reported neuroprotection by progesterone following permanent MCAo [19].

**Table 2.** 24 hour behavioral score and sticky dot removal test scores.

| Test | Allopregnanolone | Progesterone | Vehicle | P |
|---|---|---|---|---|
| Forelimb flexion | 0.40±0.32 | 0.92± 0.52 | 1.23± 0.39 | 0.06 |
| Torso twisting | 0.60± 0.32 | 0.69± 0.47 | 0.77± 0.39 | 0.90 |
| Lateral push | 0.60± 0.32 | 0.31± 0.26 | 0.54± 0.28 | 0.33 |
| Total | 1.60± 0.67 | 1.92± 0.98 | 2.62± 0.79 | 0.23 |
| Sticky dot removal (s) | 283± 182 | 138± 117 | 174± 31 | 0.35 |

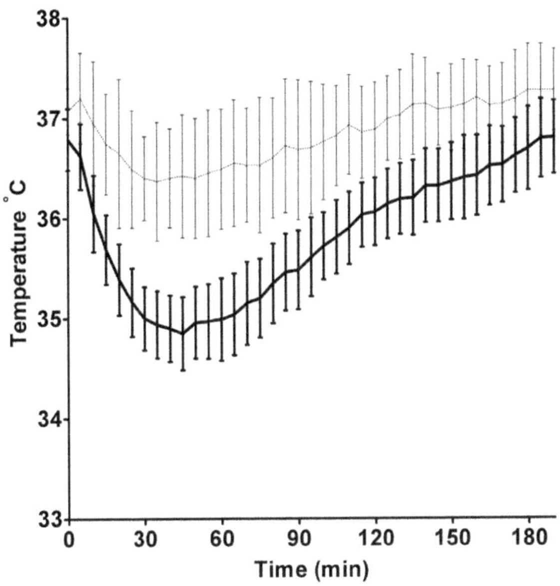


**Figure 2. Core body temperatures during the first 3 hours of recovery following a 1 hour anesthetic.** Data are presented as mean ±95% C.I. Animal temperatures were recorded by extraperitoneal datalogger. Dark lines are pooled data from the 3 treatment groups (non-stroke surgery animals, n = 16) that recovered from anesthesia in regular cages at ambient laboratory temperature (21.2±0.5°C). There was no statistically significant difference in postoperative temperatures between these 3 groups. For comparison, lighter lines are data from 9 animals that were recovered in cages ½ over a heat mat. These animals formed the normothermic control group for a separate study of hypothermia, and received stroke surgery +3 hours anesthesia before recovery. Temperatures in both groups were regulated during anesthesia. There was a statistically significant difference between animals warmed postoperatively to those kept at room temperature ($p<0.0001$).

Potential limitations of this study are that we used an early sacrifice time (24 h) and that we only investigated one dose of the neurosteroids. Had there been benefit of treatment at 24 h, confirmation of neuroprotection would have been required with longer survival studies to exclude the possibility of treatment merely delaying rather than preventing infarct progression The dose of progesterone used was that previously found effective in both SHR and other strains [18], and the allopregnanolone dose chosen was based on that shown to be successful in other strains of rat in studies of occlusion and neurotrauma [4,27,28]. The lack of treatment effect in this study may suggest a need for further dose studies to determine the full limitations of neuroprotection of these neurosteroids, and whether higher doses are effective in hypertensives.

This study was designed in order to avoid some of the experimental factors that have been identified as being of importance in previous failures of translation of successful neuroprotectants from the laboratory into clinical practice [36]. The use of *a priori* sample size calculations, randomization, concealment of treatment allocation and blinded outcome assessment have been shown to be important aspects of trial design, preventing overestimate of efficacy of the intervention [9,39,40]. An important corollary is that implementation of such good laboratory practice is expected to reduce the number of 'false positive' results, and will therefore increase the number of negative results.

In contrast to prior studies, the current data demonstrate no difference in infarct volume or functional outcome measures compared to vehicle control in animals receiving either allopregnanolone or progesterone at standard doses. The use of postoperative temperature maintenance in this study, in contrast to previous investigations, raises the possibility that these agents are not effective at normal body temperatures or in the setting of hypertension – both of which are most commonly present in stroke patients. These findings suggest a need for further experimental study to determine the suitability of allopregnanolone or its precursors for clinical trial.

## Acknowledgments

We would like to acknowledge the assistance of Dr Seth Tarrant, who conducted preliminary experimental work, and A. Prof David Howells for advice on preparation of the manuscript and editorial contributions.

## Author Contributions

Conceived and designed the experiments: NS MC. Performed the experiments: NS AT DP DM. Analyzed the data: NS AT DP DM. Wrote the paper: NS AT DM MC.

## References


1. Agis-Balboa RC, Pinna G, Zhubi A, Maloku E, Veldic M, et al. (2006) Characterization of brain neurons that express enzymes mediating neurosteroid biosynthesis. Proc Natl Acad Sci U S A 103: 14602–14607.
2. Saalmann YB, Kirkcaldie MT, Waldron S, Calford MB (2007) Cellular distribution of the GABAA receptor-modulating 3alpha-hydroxy, 5alpha-reduced pregnane steroids in the adult rat brain. J Neuroendocrinol 19: 272–284.
3. He J, Hoffman SW, Stein DG (2004) Allopregnanolone, a progesterone metabolite, enhances behavioral recovery and decreases neuronal loss after traumatic brain injury. Restorative Neurology & Neuroscience 22: 19–31.
4. Sayeed I, Guo Q, Hoffman SW, Stein DG (2006) Allopregnanolone, a progesterone metabolite, is more effective than progesterone in reducing cortical infarct volume after transient middle cerebral artery occlusion. Ann Emerg Med 47: 381–389.
5. Stein DG, Wright DW, Kellermann AL (2008) Does progesterone have neuroprotective properties?. Annals of Emergency Medicine 51: 164–172.
6. Liu A, Margaill I, Zhang S, Labombarda F, Coqueran B, et al. (2012) Progesterone receptors: a key for neuroprotection in experimental stroke. Endocrinology 153: 3747–3757.
7. Chaulk D, Wells J, Evans S, Jackson D, Corbett D (2003) Long-term effects of clomethiazole in a model of global ischemia. Exp Neurol 182: 476–482.
8. Stroke Therapy Academic Industry Roundtable (STAIR) (1999) Recommendations for standards regarding preclinical neuroprotective and restorative drug development. Stroke 30: 2752–2758.
9. Macleod MM, Fisher M, O'Collins V, Sena ES, Dirnagl U, et al. (2008) Good Laboratory Practice. Preventing Introduction of Bias at the Bench. Stroke: Published online before print August 14, 2008.
10. Spratt NJ, Fernandez J, Chen M, Rewell S, Cox S, et al. (2006) Modification of the method of thread manufacture improves stroke induction rate and reduces mortality after thread-occlusion of the middle cerebral artery in young or aged rats. J Neurosci Methods 155: 285–290.
11. Petullo D, Masonic K, Lincoln C, Wibberley L, Teliska M, et al. (1999) Model development and behavioral assessment of focal cerebral ischemia in rats. Life Sci 64: 1099–1108.
12. Aronowski J, Samways E, Strong R, Rhoades HM, Grotta JC (1996) An Alternative Method for the Quantitation of Neuronal Damage After Experimental Middle Cerebral Artery Occlusion in Rats: Analysis of Behavioral Deficit. J Cereb Blood Flow Metab 16: 705–713.
13. Schallert T, Whishaw IQ (1984) Bilateral cutaneous stimulation of the somatosensory system in hemidecorticate rats. Behav Neurosci 98: 518–540.
14. Jiang N, Chopp M, Stein D, Feit H (1996) Progesterone is neuroprotective after transient middle cerebral artery occlusion in male rats. Brain Res 735: 101–107.
15. Murphy SJ, Littleton-Kearney MT, Hurn PD (2002) Progesterone Administration During Reperfusion, But Not Preischemia Alone, Reduces Injury in Ovariectomized Rats. J Cereb Blood Flow Metab 22: 1181–1188.
16. Alkayed NJ, Murphy SJ, Traystman RJ, Hurn PD, Miller VM (2000) Neuroprotective Effects of Female Gonadal Steroids in Reproductively Senescent Female Rats. Stroke 31: 161–168.

17. Chen J, Chopp M, Li Y (1999) Neuroprotective effects of progesterone after transient middle cerebral artery occlusion in rat. Journal of the Neurological Sciences 171: 24–30.
18. Kumon Y, Kim SC, Tompkins P, Stevens A, Sakaki S, et al. (2000) Neuroprotective effect of postischemic administration of progesterone in spontaneously hypertensive rats with focal cerebral ischemia. Journal of Neurosurgery 92: 848–852.
19. Sayeed I, Wali B, Stein DG (2007) Progesterone inhibits ischemic brain injury in a rat model of permanent middle cerebral artery occlusion. Restorative Neurology & Neuroscience 25: 151–159.
20. Azcoitia I, Fernandez-Galaz C, Sierra A, Garcia-Segura LM (1999) Gonadal hormones affect neuronal vulnerability to excitotoxin-induced degeneration. Journal of Neurocytology 28: 699–710.
21. Callier S, Morissette M, Grandbois M, Pelaprat D, Di Paolo T (2001) Neuroprotective properties of 17beta-estradiol, progesterone, and raloxifene in MPTP C57Bl/6 mice. Synapse 41: 131–138.
22. Garcia-Estrada J, Del Rio JA, Luquin S, Soriano E, Garcia-Segura LM (1993) Gonadal hormones down-regulate reactive gliosis and astrocyte proliferation after a penetrating brain injury. Brain Research 628: 271–278.
23. O'Connor CA, Cernak I, Johnson F, Vink R (2007) Effects of progesterone on neurologic and morphologic outcome following diffuse traumatic brain injury in rats. Experimental Neurology 205: 145–153.
24. O'Connor CA, Cernak I, Vink R (2003) Interaction between Anesthesia, Gender, and Functional Outcome Task following Diffuse Traumatic Brain Injury in Rats. Journal of Neurotrauma 20: 533–541.
25. O'Connor CA, Cernak I, Vink R (2005) Both estrogen and progesterone attenuate edema formation following diffuse traumatic brain injury in rats. Brain Research 1062: 171–174.
26. VanLandingham JW, Cutler SM, Virmani S, Hoffman SW, Covey DF, et al. (2006) The enantiomer of progesterone acts as a molecular neuroprotectant after traumatic brain injury. Neuropharmacology 51: 1078–1085.
27. Djebaili M, Hoffman SW, Stein DG (2004) Allopregnanolone and progesterone decrease cell death and cognitive deficits after a contusion of the rat pre-frontal cortex. Neuroscience 123: 349–359.
28. Djebaili M, Guo Q, Pettus EH, Hoffman SW, Stein DG (2005) The Neurosteroids Progesterone and Allopregnanolone Reduce Cell Death, Gliosis, and Functional Deficits after Traumatic Brain Injury in Rats. Journal of Neurotrauma 22: 106–118.
29. Wong R, Renton C, Gibson CL, Murphy SJ, Kendall DA, et al. (2013) Progesterone treatment for experimental stroke: an individual animal meta-analysis. J Cereb Blood Flow Metab 33: 1362–1372.
30. Parker SM, Hurn PD, Murphy SJ (2005) Progesterone and allopregnanolone as neuroprotectants in ischemic ovariectomized mouse brain. J Cereb Blood Flow Metab 25: S21–S21.
31. Armstrong SR, Roberts BK, Aronsohn M (2005) Perioperative hypothermia. Journal of Veterinary Emergency and Critical Care 15: 32–37.
32. Campbell K, Meloni BP, Zhu H, Knuckey NW (2008) Magnesium treatment and spontaneous mild hypothermia after transient focal cerebral ischemia in the rat. Brain Res Bull.
33. Berger C, Schabitz W-R, Wolf M, Mueller H, Sommer C, et al. (2004) Hypothermia and brain-derived neurotrophic factor reduce glutamate synergistically in acute stroke. Experimental Neurology 185: 305–312.
34. Fisher M, Feuerstein G, Howells DW, Hurn PD, Kent TA, et al. (2009) Update of the stroke therapy academic industry roundtable preclinical recommendations. Stroke 40: 2244–2250.
35. van der Worp HB, Sena ES, Donnan GA, Howells DW, Macleod MR (2007) Hypothermia in animal models of acute ischaemic stroke: a systematic review and meta-analysis. Brain 130: 3063–3074.
36. Macleod MR, van der Worp HB, Sena ES, Howells DW, Dirnagl U, et al. (2008) Evidence for the Efficacy of NXY-059 in Experimental Focal Cerebral Ischaemia Is Confounded by Study Quality. Stroke 39: 2824–2829.
37. Shuaib A, Lees KR, Lyden P, Grotta J, Davalos A, et al. (2007) NXY-059 for the treatment of acute ischemic stroke. N Engl J Med 357: 562–571.
38. Lust WD, Taylor C, Pundik S, Selman WR, Ratcheson RA (2002) Ischemic cell death: dynamics of delayed secondary energy failure during reperfusion following focal ischemia. Metabolic Brain Disease 17: 113–121.
39. Zivin JA (2008) Identifying Low-Quality Preclinical Studies. Stroke 39: 2697–2698.
40. Kilkenny C, Browne WJ, Cuthill IC, Emerson M, Altman DG (2010) Improving bioscience research reporting: the ARRIVE guidelines for reporting animal research. PLoS Biol 8: e1000412.

18

# Multiple Interacting Factors Influence Adherence, and Outcomes Associated with Surgical Safety Checklists: A Qualitative Study

**Anna R. Gagliardi[1]*, Sharon E. Straus[2], Kaveh G. Shojania[3], David R. Urbach[4]**

**1** University Health Network, Toronto, Ontario, Canada, **2** St. Michael's Hospital, Toronto, Ontario, Canada, **3** Sunnybrook Health Sciences Centre, Toronto, Ontario, Canada, **4** University Health Network, Toronto, Ontario, Canada

## Abstract

***Objectives:*** The surgical safety checklist (SSC) is meant to enhance patient safety but studies of its impact conflict. This study explored factors that influenced SSC adherence to suggest how its impact could be optimized.

***Methods:*** Participants were recruited purposively by profession, region, hospital type and time using the SSC. They were asked to describe how the SSC was adopted, associated challenges, perceived impact, and suggestions for improving its use. Grounded theory and thematic analysis were used to collect and analyse data. Findings were interpreted using an implementation fidelity conceptual framework.

***Results:*** Fifty-one participants were interviewed (29 nurses, 13 surgeons, 9 anaesthetists; 18 small, 14 large and 19 teaching hospitals; 8 regions; 31 had used the SC for ≤12 months, 20 for 13+ months). The SSC was inconsistently reviewed, and often inaccurately documented as complete. Adherence was influenced by multiple issues. Extensive modification to accommodate existing practice patterns eliminated essential interaction at key time points to discuss patient management. Staff were often absent or not paying attention. They did not feel it was relevant to their work given limited evidence of its effectiveness, and because they were not engaged in its implementation. Organizations provided little support for implementation, training, monitoring and feedback, which are needed to overcome these, and other individual and team factors that challenged SSC adherence. Responses were similar across participants with different characteristics.

***Conclusions:*** Multiple processes and factors influenced SSC adherence. This may explain why, in studies evaluating SSC impact, outcomes were variable. Recommendations included continuing education, time for pilot-testing, and engaging all staff in SSC review. Others may use the implementation fidelity framework to plan SSC implementation or evaluate SSC adherence. Further research is needed to establish which SSC components can be modified without compromising its effectiveness.

**Editor:** Delphine Sophie Courvoisier, University of Geneva, Switzerland

**Funding:** Research funding that supported this work was awarded to SES and KGS by the Canadian Health Services Research Foundation (now called Canadian Foundation for Healthcare Improvement) which took no part in study design, data collection and analysis, decision to publish, or preparation of the manuscript.

**Competing Interests:** The authors have declared that no competing interests exist.

* Email: anna.gagliardi@uhnresearch.ca

## Introduction

Checklists have become a commonly used tool to facilitate the delivery of high quality health care [1]. They are meant to improve patient outcomes by specifying care recommendations and health professional roles to standardize and coordinate care delivery, and enhance inter-professional communication [2,3]. Checklists have been widely implemented in operating rooms to address preventable adverse events that arise during, or as a result of surgical procedures following publication of an international study sponsored by the World Health Organization (WHO) that showed it reduced surgical mortality and complications [4–6]. The surgical safety checklist (SSC) prompts oral confirmation by surgical team members of key processes at three time points – before anesthesia administration (i.e. patient identity confirmed, site marked, anesthesia safety check completed, other patient risks such as allergy, aspiration risk, and anticipated blood loss), immediately prior to incision (i.e. team member introductions, confirmation of patient, site, side and procedure being performed, discussion of any other concerns), and before the patient is taken out of the operating room (i.e. procedure recorded, instrument count, key recovery or management concerns) [6].

While the findings of several observational studies and systematic reviews support its effectiveness [7–9], other studies have reported inconsistent, or little to no impact of the SSC compared with usual care [10–12]. Variable adherence with the SSC may account for its inconsistent impact. A systematic review of 20 studies that examined the impact of the SSC on teamwork in the operating room found that hospitals which achieved higher adherence with SSC use were more likely to significantly reduce postoperative complications [13]. However, multiple studies demonstrated that recorded adherence is unreliable and significantly higher than observed adherence [14–16].

Several processes and factors may influence adherence with the SSC and, hence it's capacity to improve surgical outcomes. Adaptation, either modification or removal of one or more of the processes at any of the three time points specified in the SSC, may limit team interaction, the completion of crucial tasks, or the delivery of essential components of care [17]. Implementation may not be successful if no interventions are used to promote use of the SSC, or if those strategies are less than effective. For example, some research suggests that SSC use must be aligned with institutional values, enabled with training and coaching, and encouraged by local champions and real-time feedback of performance data [7,8]. Poor or incomplete integration of the SSC into operating room processes may limit adherence if staff are not aware of it, or can easily bypass its use in favour of usual practices [7,8,18]. Monitoring may be necessary to identify and address adherence issues and ensure sustained SSC use [17,19]. Adherence may also be influenced by individual (beliefs about SSC effectiveness, uncertainty about when and how to use it, perceived interruption of workflow and redundancy with other checklists or processes, resistance to change) and team-related factors (professional hierarchy in the operating room where individual physicians rather than multidisciplinary teams make decisions) [8,9,13,20–23].

A large proportion of in-hospital adverse events are surgery-related and preventable [24]. The SSC may prevent such adverse events but its impact has been inconsistent due to variable adherence. Research to date has not revealed how to promote and support SSC adherence. One, few qualitative studies explored SSC introduction and use so we have little insight on whether and how various processes and factors such as those described above may influence adherence. Two, most of those studies involved one or a few participating hospitals so findings may be setting-specific. Three, adoption of an innovation is not a discrete event and must be evaluated longitudinally [25]. Most studies assessed adherence or clinical impact from one week to three months after the SSC was introduced so adoption may not yet have occurred, and issues influencing adherence may not yet have arisen. The overall objective of this study was to understand and compare the processes and factors influencing SSC adherence in multiple hospitals of different types that had been exposed to the SSC for various lengths of time. In particular, we interviewed nurses, surgeons and anaesthetists from community and academic hospitals in several jurisdictions that had used the SSC for one year or less, or longer than one year to learn how various processes and factors influenced SSC adherence. This may reveal approaches for optimizing SSC adherence, which could be tested in future research and, if widely adopted, lead to more consistent SSC use, and improved outcomes among surgical patients.

## Methods

### Approach

Qualitative interviews were conducted to explore how adaptation, implementation, integration and monitoring or other process, and individual, team or other factors influenced SSC adherence. Qualitative research elicits detailed information about beliefs and experiences, and the factors that shape them to create a thorough understanding of an issue. A grounded theory approach was used to collect and analyze data such that views, experiences, needs and suggestions emerged freely during interviews and inductively during data analysis rather than being restricted to the components of established theory [26]. Rigour was optimized by sampling participants with various characteristics that could influence their views and experiences; exploring responses inductively for emerging ideas; demonstrating responses from an array of participants by anonymously identifying exemplary quotes; comparison of independently-derived analysis across two individuals, and thorough, high-level interpretation of the findings [27]. It was further ensured by complying with Relevance, Appropriateness, Transparency and Soundness (RATS) principles for reporting of qualitative research [28]. This research was based in Canada which features ten provinces and three territories, and where the health care system is largely publicly funded. This research was approved by the University Health Network Research Ethics Board (10-0659-AE) and all participants signed a consent form prior to interviews.

### Sampling and recruitment

Purposive sampling was used to identify practicing clinicians with differing characteristics including role (nurses, surgeons, anaesthetists), geographic region (provinces), type of hospital (teaching, large community, small community less than 100 beds) and time using the SSC (≤12 months, 13+ months). Hospitals that had adopted the surgical checklist were identified by the Canadian Patient Safety Institute (http://www.patientsafetyinstitute.ca/) which advocated for SSC adoption in Canada. The list of hospitals they provided included the name and contact information for a front line nurse or nurse leader who was most familiar with implementation of the SSC at each hospital. Contact information for surgeons and anesthetists at those hospitals was acquired through random sampling of publicly available directories from the College of Physicians and Surgeons for respective provinces. All individuals were invited to participate by regular mail or email with an invitation letter and consent form. A reminder was sent to non-respondents at two and four weeks from initial contact. The intent was to recruit, from among those who consented, 10 of each professional role from across Canada who differed in non-mutually exclusive fashion by type of hospital and time using the SSC for a minimum total of 30 participants.

### Data collection

Interviews were conducted in English language with all consenting participants via telephone by a trained research assistant. Participants were asked about perceived benefits of, and adherence with the SSC; how the SSC was adapted, implemented, integrated and monitored; factors influencing these processes; and suggestions for improving SSC adherence. Interviews of approximately 45 minutes were audio-recorded, then transcribed verbatim. Interviews were conducted over eight months from January 6, 2011 to August 14, 2011. Detailed information from representative, rather than a large number of cases is needed in qualitative research [26]. Sampling was concurrent with data collection and analysis, and proceeded until unique themes no longer emerged from successive interviews (saturation). This was determined by discussion of emerging themes between two independent reviewers, the principal investigator and research assistant.

### Data analysis

Unique themes were identified in an inductive manner through iterative stages [29,30]. First, interview transcripts were read to identify, define and organize themes in participant responses relevant to each of the main interview questions (first level coding).

Second, a codebook was developed to organize codes reflecting emerging themes, their definition, sample quotes illustrating application of that code, and an account of decisions related to that code. Third, transcripts were reviewed (constant comparative technique) to assess whether and how to expand or merge themes (second level coding). Interview transcripts and the codebook were analyzed independently by the research analyst and principal investigator. The two met to compare findings and achieve consensus by discussion. Data (quotes labeled with an anonymous identifier reflecting profession, province, type of hospital and time using the SSC) were tabulated for each main interview question by theme and profession to identify trends.

Once data were analyzed and organized in this manner, the findings were further interpreted according to a conceptual framework of implementation fidelity, defined as the degree to which programs are implemented as intended [31]. Implementation fidelity must be evaluated to assess whether lack of impact of a program is due to poor implementation or inadequacies in the program. This framework proposes that program Adherence (program is delivered or used as intended) is influenced by several inter-related factors including program Differentiation (core elements essential for success are known and maintained), Facilitation (training, tools, interventions to promote and support adherence), Quality of delivery (whether and how participants undertake or use the program in an ideal manner), participant Responsiveness (participants are engaged in, and view the program as relevant) and Complexity (number and type of issues challenging adherence). To do this, themes and exemplary quotes from interview findings were matched with domains of the framework. For example, themes related to adherence and adaptation corresponded directly with Adherence and Differentiation, respectively. The framework domain Responsiveness was populated with themes about perceived benefits of the SSC, and themes about engagement and relevance within interview findings related to SSC implementation. The framework domain of Quality was populated with themes within interview findings related to SSC integration. The framework domains of Facilitation and Complexity were populated with themes reflecting organizational, team and individual factors from within findings relevant to implementation, integration and monitoring.

## Results

### Participants

Of 607 physicians invited to participate, 551 either declined or did not respond, 56 consented and 22 were interviewed. Of 306 nurses invited to participate, 226 either declined or did not respond, 80 consented and 29 were interviewed. Participants included 29 nurses, 13 surgeons and 9 anaesthetists from 18, 14 and 29 small community, large community and teaching hospitals, respectively (Table 1). Thirty-one had used the SSC for 12 months or less, and 20 had used the SSC for 13 or more months. Participants represented the provinces of British Columbia (10), Alberta (10), Saskatchewan (1), Ontario (17), Quebec (3), New Brunswick (6), Prince Edward Island (1), and Nova Scotia (3).

### SSC adherence

Study findings organized by main interview question, then theme and type of health professional are available in Table S1 (Adherence with Surgical Safety Checklists: Summary of study findings). When asked about adherence, most participants said that the SSC was incompletely and inconsistently reviewed and documented for each patient. Several mentioned that review of the SSC was marked as complete even when this was not the case. Experiences or views were similar across participants from different geographic regions, and from different health professional groups. Some differences by hospital type and length of time using the SSC were apparent. They are noted in the following interpretation of study findings according to the domains of the implementation fidelity conceptual framework, which was used to organize the multiple processes and factors that influenced adherence. The interpretation is summarized in Table 2 with select participant quotes.

### Factors influencing SSC adherence

**Differentiation.** Most participants said that they modified the SSC considerably. In several cases one or more versions were blended to create an entirely new SSC. The SSC was often modified to make it easier to use and accommodate existing local practices or processes, for example, who should be present for completion of each component, and where components were completed if not in the operating room. Therefore multidisciplinary interaction at key time points may not have occurred. Participants who had used the SSC for longer periods of time were more likely to say that they had added dimensions to the checklist (i.e. handoffs, anesthesia relevant items, patient positioning and destination following surgery), changed the order of items, and had adapted it over an extended period of time. Participants from small hospitals were more likely to remove items relevant to surgical procedures that they did not perform, and waive the need for team introductions. Rapid turnovers, call backs and emergency cases also challenged SSC adherence. Modification was viewed as necessary, so maintaining the integrity of the SSC was not a concern. In fact, a few physicians recommended that the SSC should be more easily modifiable to suit different procedures.

**Responsiveness.** Most participants viewed the SSC as relevant and cited numerous benefits associated with its use. This included better use of time in the operating room; improved communication, teamwork and staff satisfaction; and patients and families were comforted knowing that the SSC was used. Several said that, due to the SSC, they were better prepared including having the proper equipment and antibiotics available, consistent site marking, correct labelling of specimens, and informed consent for all procedures. In general this enabled the right surgery on the right patient on the right side. A few noted that incidents had been averted. Despite these positive remarks, engagement was viewed as less than ideal. For example, many participants said that staff should have been involved in adapting and implementing the SSC as a means of fostering ownership. Instead they felt it had been imposed on them by management, which hurt morale and caused tension in the operating room. They also questioned why it was necessary and doubted that it improved efficiency, therefore it was not perceived as highly relevant.

**Quality.** The SSC was available in operating rooms as a laminated card or sheet, or wall poster, and verbally reviewed as was the intent. However, the intended multidisciplinary interaction among staff was frequently not achieved. Staff were often absent at one or more of the three key time points. Some were even obstructive by refusing to participate in SSC review. Even when SSC items were being reviewed, staff were talking or not paying attention, and this was described as "going through the motions", which diminished the impact of the SSC to "just another tick box". Therefore the quality of inter-professional communication was limited, and items pertinent to patient safety may not have been reviewed in a mindful manner. Processes in place to document that the SSC had been reviewed were variable across hospitals. In some sites this was done verbally only. Other hospitals used either paper forms or electronic medical records to

**Table 1.** Participant characteristics by profession, type of hospital and time using the surgical checklist.

| Type of Hospital | Profession | | | Subtotal |
|---|---|---|---|---|
| | Nurse | Surgeon | Anesthetist | |
| Small community (<100 beds) | 14 | 3 | 1 | 18 |
| ≤12 mo | 11 | 3 | – | 14 |
| 13+ mo | 3 | – | 1 | 4 |
| Large community | 7 | 3 | 4 | 14 |
| ≤12 mo | 4 | 2 | 4 | 10 |
| 13+ mo | 3 | 1 | – | 4 |
| Teaching | 8 | 7 | 4 | 19 |
| ≤12 mo | 3 | 3 | 1 | 7 |
| 13+ mo | 5 | 4 | 3 | 12 |
| Subtotal | 29 | 13 | 9 | 51 |

document completion of either the entire SSC or each of its three components. Those using the SSC for a shorter period of time were not aware if completion was documented for each patient.

**Facilitation.** Little organizational support was available to promote and facilitate SSC use. Staff were informed by email or memo that they were to use the SSC. Nurses, who were largely responsible for planning SSC implementation, said that there was little time to prepare or pilot-test the SSC prior to full launch, and that no resources were provided by hospital management for more thorough or robust implementation efforts. Furthermore, hospital leadership was not seen as involved in either promoting or actively implementing the SSC. Many participants said that they did not receive information or training on how to use the SSC, and that identifying facilitators, in particular physician champions, would have improved SSC uptake.

Monitoring of SSC use was variable. Some participants, largely from hospitals using it for a shorter length of time, said that audit reports based on nursing documentation of SSC use were shared with staff and hospital managers but this was weekly at some sites and yearly at others. A few sites monitored SSC use with observational spot checks. There appeared to be no incentives to prompt SSC use or consequences associated with non-adherence. Some nurse managers held discussions with non-compliant individuals. Those using the SSC for a longer period of time were more likely to say that adherence issues resulted in an incident report and/or discussion among the operating room team or surgical services committee. Rarely was non-adherence reported to those in leadership roles. Several participants recommended regular local audits of SSC use, or random audits conducted by groups independent of the operating room team or external to the organization, and consequences associated with non-compliance. In contrast, others said that SSC use would be promoted if local data were more routinely collected, analyzed and shared to demonstrate its impact, necessitating additional clerical support to alleviate the nursing workload.

**Complexity.** Multiple individual and team factors interacted to influence adherence. All participants noted that the nursing workload had increased, in large part due to the need for SSC documentation. Many participants said that staff were uncertain about how to use the SSC and who was responsible for leading it. Participants said that SSC use was limited by the traditionally physician-dominated hierarchical culture of the operating room and lack of confidence among nurses leading SSC review, particularly when faced with resistance from staff who were most often surgeons, leading to tension and avoidance of SSC review. Physician resistance to change was attributed to individual beliefs about relevance given the lack of strong evidence on SSC effectiveness, physician age, perceived redundancy with other checklists or processes, and concerns about surgical delays as a result of taking time to review the SSC. To rectify these issues, participants recommended that surgeons lead review of the SSC, continuing education be offered on how to use the SSC, and networking take place with other hospitals to share strategies for promoting SSC compliance.

**Interpretation Summary.** Use of the implementation fidelity conceptual framework to analyze study findings confirms that multiple processes and factors influence SSC adherence, including issues that were proposed in other research and several unique factors that emerged from this research. Staff did not adhere to the technical and qualitative manner in which the SSC was meant to be used. In part this was because they did not feel it was relevant to their work, and had not been engaged in its adaptation and implementation, so did not fully or meaningfully take part in reviewing the SSC for each patient (Responsiveness, Quality - qualitative manner). In part this was due to the fact that extensive modification of the SSC to accommodate existing, preferred practice patterns eliminated essential interaction to discuss patient management issues at key time points (Differentiation - technical manner). Complexity of the SSC was high given the many individual and team factors that further challenged SSC adherence. Organizations provided few resources and supports for thorough implementation, training, monitoring and feedback (Facilitation), which are clearly needed to overcome challenges associated with Responsiveness, Differentiation, Quality and Complexity. It is notable that, overall, responses were similar across different types of health professionals and hospitals, and among those exposed to the SSC for different periods of time.

## Discussion

This study found that SSC adherence was poor though often documented as complete, as was identified in other studies [7,14–16]. This was at odds with many positive views articulated about its benefits. Analysis of findings using an implementation fidelity conceptual framework revealed that multiple processes and factors influenced SSC adherence. This may explain why, in studies evaluating SSC impact, outcomes were variable despite

**Table 2.** Key findings according to a conceptual framework of implementation fidelity.

| Framework Domain | Themes from Study Findings | Exemplary Quotes from Study Findings |
|---|---|---|
| Adherence (SSC used - all items reviewed by team at key times and documented) | Portions not completed for every patient | No one goes through the whole list of every single item (Sx01ON-T-short); Consistent application of the checklist in every case (Ax09NB-T-long); They trickle out with the debriefing (Nx05ON-S-short); Getting the surgeons to be in the room for the briefing (Nx03AB-L-long) |
| | Documentation incomplete or inaccurate | If some part of the checklist were done then it's considered complete (Sx04BC-T-long); Nurses are biased to mark it complete otherwise the manager will say how come this case went ahead (Sx11ON-T-long); There is no recording that each component was asked or that each individual was present (Sx09ON-T-long) |
| Differentiation (Core elements essential for success are maintained) | Adapted other versions or newly developed | We came up with our own (Nx06NS-L-short); As issues came up there would be discussions about what should or should not be in the checklist (Sx09ON-T-long) |
| | Modification viewed as necessary | It needs to be easily modifiable (Sx11ON-T-long); Flexibility in modification of the checklist (Sx07AB-L-short) |
| Responsiveness(Participants are engaged and view the program as relevant) | Numerous perceived benefits were noted | It builds and fosters a team mentality (Sx04BC-T-long); It reassures the family (Sx06AB-T-short); We've improved the use of appropriate peri-operative antibiotics (Ax06NB-T-long); Mislabeling of specimens is really improved (Nx15BC-S-short) |
| | In contrast, use was imposed so staff did not feel engaged, and SSC relevance was questioned | It's been forced on us. It's hurt morale and caused tension in the OR (Ax05BC-L-short); Involve the people who're gonna be using it in its development so you feel ownership (Sx05BC-S-short); It's an additional layer that doesn't improve efficiency (Ax07BC-L-short); Lingering beliefs in why it is necessary (Sx07AB-L-short) |
| Quality (Participants use the SSC in an ideal manner) | Staff absent at key times, not paying attention or obstructive | Surgeons were refusing to do it (Sx04BC-T-long); Some days it doesn't seem like a team effort (Ax09NB-T-long); Everybody being in the room at the same time was one of our biggest challenges (Nx09ON-S-short) |
| | SSC reviewed but not in a mindful manner | There are a lot of people that are just going through the motions (Sx12BC-T-long); People who aren't listening, aren't participating, rolling their eyes (Nx01NB-L-short) |
| | Available in OR as card or wall poster | Small cards were placed in every OR (Ax07BC-L-short); We have a large poster in each of the ORs (Sx08BC-T-short) |
| | Documentation processes variable | Nurses in the OR have a booklet where they mark off for every case if the surgical checklist was used (Nx10AB-S-short); Nurses have three check boxes on the electronic patient record (Ax01ON-T-long) |
| Facilitation (Resources, training, interventions or other strategies provided or enabled by the organization that promoted and supported adherence) | Implemented by alerting staff to impending use | We were informed by letters (Ax08NB-L-short); A memo went out to everybody that it was gonna be starting (Nx05NS-L-short) |
| | Little time to prepare or pilot-test | We would probably start one service at a time because it was extremely overwhelming to implement it all at the same time in five services (Nx20SK-S-long) |
| | Little training on SC use | We don't know how to do it, we're not trained (Sx12BC-T-long); They could have done a better job of educating people (Ax04NB-T-short) |
| | Little support from facilitators | Identify surgeon champions (Sx04BC-T-long); Need leaders in the physician group to sell it (Nx23ON-T-long) |
| | Little support from hospital leadership (resources or visible involvement) | Needs to be supported by the medical quality committee of the hospital (Ax02ON-L-short); I just didn't get the support that I would have needed to be able to implement that fully (Nx02ON-L-long) |
| | Monitoring and feedback varied | We do audits quarterly (Nx01NB-L-short); Feedback that was accurate and meaningful (Ax07BC-L-short) |
| | Non-adherence addressed at few sites | I follow up with them individually (Nx12ON-S-short); We try to review it in the OR committee monthly meeting (Sx06AB-T-short) |
| | No incentives or accountability | There are no consequences (Nx02ON-L-long); There's no punishment (Sx07AB-L-short); If it was mandatory people might be more diligent (Nx05NS-L-short) |
| Complexity (Number and type of issues challenging adherence - team and individual factors) | Beliefs about effectiveness | Ongoing data demonstrating its impact on patient care (Sx09ON-T-long); People like to know this is evidence-based (Nx29AB-T-long); There was little evidence that it has been proven to make any difference in patient outcome (Ax05BC-L-short) |
| | Resistance to change | Getting acceptance from surgeons and anaesthesiologists (Ax07BC-L-short); Older practitioners are very set in their ways and it's hard to change them (Sx11ON-T-long) |
| | Concerns about delays | It does delay getting the case started (Sx04BC-T-long); Cause of inefficiency in our operating room (Ax05BC-L-short) |

**Table 2.** Cont.

| Framework Domain | Themes from Study Findings | Exemplary Quotes from Study Findings |
|---|---|---|
| | Lack of knowledge about how to use it | People were not fully understanding what the components of the checklist were (Nx25ON-T-long); I'm still unclear as to who it is that's supposed to lead the discussion (Sx04BC-T-long) |
| | Increased workload for nurses | It's one more job for the nurse to do (Nx02ON-L-long); Layering on further administrative burden (Ax07BC-L-short); Documentation has dramatically increased, and it has taken away from patient care (Sx09ON-T-long) |
| | Hierarchical OR culture is a barrier to team interaction | Nurses were intimidated so there was friction between team members (Ax02ON-L-short); Flatten the hierarchy (Sx12BC-T-long); Some nurses are really shy to speak up (Nx26ON-T-short) |

Profession (Nx = nurse, Sx = surgeon, Ax = anesthetist), Province (two-letter identifier), Hospital type (S = small, L = large, T = teaching), Time using the surgical checklist (short = ≤12 months, long = 13+ months).

documentation of high adherence. This study confirms the assertion by Carroll et al. that any evaluation of adherence with a quality improvement intervention such as the SSC must measure not only adherence, but all of the implementation fidelity domains which influence it, and that evaluation must be longitudinal since issues may not emerge immediately upon introduction of the intervention [31]. This would also suggest that those planning to introduce the SSC or other quality improvement intervention could use the implementation fidelity conceptual framework as a means of planning how to promote, support and sustain its use.

The SSC was adapted to accommodate existing practice patterns. Therefore the intended timing and quality of team interaction at key intervals was not achieved. No one questioned SSC integrity, likely because tailoring was encouraged by national and international SSC advocates [6]. Further research is needed on the extent to which SSC modification influences adherence and associated clinical outcomes. This would establish which elements must remain in the SSC, and which can be modified and how without compromising effectiveness. This too is recommended by Carroll et al. who state that an evaluation of outcomes "...may identify those components that are essential to the intervention, and must be implemented if the intervention is to have its intended effects. This evaluation may in turn inform the content of the intervention by determining the minimum requirements for high implementation fidelity" [31].

Use of the SSC was mandated by government and hospital management, and email, sometimes supplemented with meetings, was widely used to notify staff about the SSC. Educational material and meetings are known to have minimal impact on the uptake of innovations [32]. Participants recommended staff engagement, multidisciplinary interaction, use of champions and facilitators, and more time to thoughtfully plan, develop, pilot-test and implement the SSC. Those using the SSC for a longer period of time reflected on the lack of resources provided by management to support SSC implementation, and of advocacy from professional societies. Leadership promotion of, and involvement in strategic initiatives are recognized as determinants of success and organizational performance [33–35]. Participants also recommended ongoing networking with other hospitals to learn from each other's experiences. Knowledge networks, quality improvement collaboratives and communities of practice are known to support collaboration and the exchange of knowledge to achieve a common goal in both the management and health care sectors [36–38]. Tools exist for diagnosing barriers or organizational quality improvement culture [39–41]. This would establish baseline levels of acceptance and capacity to inform the selection of one or more implementation strategies appropriate for overcoming identified challenges.

The SSC was widely available in operating rooms in the form of a laminated card or wall poster. However portions were often not completed, and staff were absent or not paying attention. Those using the SSC for a shorter time noted uncertainty about how to use it. Even among those who used it for a longer period of time, physician resistance was evident and, given traditional operating room hierarchy, nurses were reluctant to direct physicians. In many cases it was marked as having been completed despite these circumstances. These issues were also revealed in other research [8,9,20–23]. To address resistance participants recommended that physicians assume the responsibility for leading SSC review. This was evaluated in a study where each team member was required to lead the review of the SSC component most relevant to their role [42]. Completion of all items increased from 54% when previously surgeon-led to 97% after the intervention, and the improvement was sustained at 18 months. Social identity theory refers to shared knowledge, values and practices in members of social or professional groups, however social identity can be threatened when individuals are forced to collaborate with members of other groups, therefore continuing education on SSC use must be multidisciplinary in nature [43]. Such an educational program could also include conflict management training that describes, and provides alternatives for negative behaviour [44].

Sharing of audit data with staff appeared more common among those using the SSC for a shorter period of time. Those using the SSC for a longer period of time were more likely to have team conversations about adherence. Otherwise there were no repercussions for non-compliance. Perhaps this was due to resolution through discussion, or perhaps because no accountability mechanisms were in place to address non-compliance. Some participants recommended that SSC use should be mandatory; monitored with regular or random audits by an arms-length group; and that consequences be applied for non-compliance. Monitoring and sharing of performance data with staff, and consequences such as reprimanding and penalizing were found to improve SSC compliance in other research [17,19]. However, evidence on the impact of punitive, top-down strategies to motivate performance is mixed, and conflicts with theories of adult learning [45,46]. In contrast, others said that external research or local data demonstrating impact would promote SSC use. While this would require clerical support to alleviate the nursing workload, audit and feedback can improve professional practice, particularly when the source is a supervisor or colleague, it is provided more than once, it is delivered in both verbal and written formats, and when it includes both explicit targets and an action plan [47].

Transferrability of our finding to other settings may be limited. We attempted to mitigate this through purposive sampling of participants based on a range of characteristics that may have influenced their views. Those using the SSC for a longer period of time noted that they had adapted it over an extended period of time, and non-compliance was addressed through team discussion. This suggests that the process of adoption is not linear, and time may be needed to use the SSC, experience challenges, work out solutions, develop teamwork, monitor adherence, and address ongoing non-compliance. However, most challenges and recommendations were remarkably similar across participants representing different regions, professions, types of hospitals and length of exposure to the SSC, and confirm previous research. Therefore these findings may be broadly relevant. Applicability of the findings may be limited because data were collected in 2011. However, impact of the surgical checklist remains topical given inconsistent findings across studies, and the findings offer insight on how to enhance SSC adherence. Some researchers favor in-person interviews to collect non-verbal cues that can be used to further interpret meaning while others prefer telephone interviews because participants may often be more forthcoming when not faced by the interviewer [26]. We chose the latter approach, in part because telephone interviews can be easily accommodated in busy professional schedules, and minimize research costs when participants are geographically dispersed as in this study. Data suggest that participants were quite frank about their experiences thus having conducted telephone interviews may not have limited our data collection.

Overall, this study supports the assertion that variability in SSC impact across previous studies may be attributed to multiple processes related to adapting, implementing, integrating and monitoring SSC use, and interacting organizational, team and individual factors that influenced SSC adherence. Views were mixed about accountability, so further research is needed to identify the approaches that best incentivize SSC adherence. Some participants noted that evidence of SSC impact is needed to convince clinicians of its importance and motivate adherence. Concerns about effectiveness were also identified in other studies of SSC use [8,9]. The need for longitudinal evaluation of outcomes is also evident. It would be interesting to repeat interviews among the same population to explore whether adherence had improved and why, or whether it was challenged by the same or different factors. Future studies to demonstrate SSC impact should aim to better implement and integrate the SSC, and assess its impact only after a sufficient period of adjustment. Planning and evaluation could be guided by the domains of the implementation fidelity conceptual framework, which proved to be very useful in analyzing the myriad of contextual factors influencing SSC adherence.

## Supporting Information

**Table S1** Adherence with Surgical Safety Checklists: Summary of study findings.

## Author Contributions

Conceived and designed the experiments: ARG SES KGS DRU. Performed the experiments: ARG. Analyzed the data: ARG SES KGS DRU. Contributed reagents/materials/analysis tools: ARG SES KGS DRU. Contributed to the writing of the manuscript: ARG SES KGS DRU.

## References


1. Hales B, Terblanche M, Fowler R, Sibbald W (2008) Development of medical checklists for improved quality of patient care. Int J Qual Health Care; 20: 22–30.
2. Lemieux-Charles L, McGuire W (2006) What do we know about health care team effectiveness? A review of the literature. Med Care Res Rev 63: 263–300.
3. Lingard L, Regehr G, Orser B, Reznick R, Baker GR, et al. (2008) Evaluation of a preoperative checklist and team briefing among surgeons, nurses and anesthesiologists to reduce failures in communication. Arch Surg 143: 12–17.
4. Gawande AA, Thomas EJ, Zinner MJ, Brennan TA (1999) The incidence and nature of surgical adverse events in Colorado and Utah in 1992. Surgery 126: 66–75.
5. Kable AK, Gibbert RW, Spigelman AD (2002) Adverse events in surgical patients in Australia. Int J Qual Health Care 14: 269–276.
6. Haynes AB, Weiser TG, Berry WR, Lipsitz SR, Breizat AH, et al. (2009) A surgical safety checklist to reduce morbidity and mortality in a global population. NEJM 360: 491–499.
7. Borchard A, Schwappach DLB, Barbir A, Bezzola P (2012) A systematic review of the effectiveness, compliance and critical factors for implementation of safety checklists in surgery. Ann Surg 256: 925–933.
8. Treadwell JR, Lucas S, Tsou AY (2014) Surgical checklists: a systematic review of impacts and implementation. BMJ Qual Saf 23: 299–318.
9. Tang R, Ranmuthugala G, Cunningham F (2014) Surgical safety checklists. ANZ J Surg 84: 148–154.
10. Lubbeke A, Hovaguimian F, Wickboldt N, Barea C, Clergue F, et al. (2013) Effectiveness of the Surgical Safety Checklist in a High Standard Care Environment. Med Care 51: 425–429.
11. Tillman M, Wehbe-Janek H, Hodges B, Smythe WR, Papaconstantinou HT (2013) Surgical care improvement project and surgical site infections: can integration in the surgical safety checklist improve quality performance and clinical outcomes? J Surg Res 184: 150–156.
12. Urbach DR, Govindarajan A, Saskin R, Wilton AS, Baxter NN (2014) Introduction of surgical safety checklists in Ontario, Canada. NEJM 370: 1029–1038.
13. Russ S, Rout S, Sevdalis N, Moorthy K, Darzi A, et al. (2013) Do safety checklists improve teamwork and communication in the operating room? Ann Surg 258: 856–871.
14. Saturno PJ, Soria-Aledo V, Da Silva Gama ZA, Lorca-Parra F, Grau-Polan M (2014) Understanding WHO surgical checklist implementation. World J Surg 38: 287–295.
15. Aveling EL, McCulloch P, Dixon-Woods M (2013) A qualitative study comparing experiences of the surgical safety checklist in hospitals in high-income and low-income countries. BMJ Open 3: e0003039.
16. Bergs J, Hellings J, Cleemput I, Zurel O, De Troyer V, et al. (2014) Systematic review and meta-analysis of the effect of the World Health Organization surgical safety checklist on postoperative complications. BJS 101: 150–158.
17. Hannam JA, Glass L, Kwon J, Windsor J, Stapelberg F, et al. (2013) A prospective, observational study of the effects of implementation strategy on compliance with a surgical safety checklist. BMJ Qual Saf 22: 940–947.
18. Vats A, Vincent CA, Nagpal K, Davies RW, DArzi A, et al. (2010) Practical challenges of introducing WHO surgical checklist: UK pilot experience. BMJ 340: 133–135.
19. Healy JM (2012) How hospital leaders implemented a safe surgery protocol in Australian hospitals. Int J Qual Health Care 24: 88–94.
20. Waehle HV, Haugen AS, Softeland E, Hjalmhult E (2012) Adjusting team involvement: a grounded theory study of challenges in utilizing a surgical safety checklist as experienced by nurses in the operating room. BMC Nursing 11: 16.
21. Fourcade A, Blache JL, Grenier C, Bourgain JL, Minvielle E (2012) Barriers to staff adoption of a surgical safety checklist. BMJ Qual Saf 21: 191–197.
22. O'Connor P, Reddin C, O'Sullivan M, O'Duffy F, Keogh I (2013) Surgical checklists: the human factor. Pat Saf Surg 7: 14.
23. Pickering SP, Robertson ER, Griffin D, Hadi M, Morgan LJ, et al. (2013) Compliance and use of the World Health Organization checklist in U.K. operating theatres. BJS 100: 1664–1670.
24. De Vries EN, Ramrattan MA, Smorenburg SM, Gouma DJ, Boermeester MA (2008) The incidence and nature of in-hospital adverse events: a systematic review. Qual Saf Health Care 17: 216–223.
25. Dopson S (2007) A view from organizational studies. Nurs Res 56): S72–77.
26. Strauss AL (2003) Qualitative analysis for social scientists. Cambridge: Cambridge University Press.
27. Barbour RS (2011) Checklists for improving rigour in qualitative research: a case of the tail wagging the dog? BMJ 322: 1157–1117.
28. Clark JP (2003) How to peer review a qualitative manuscript. In Peer Review in Health Sciences. Second edition. Edited by Godlee F, Jefferson T. London, UK: BMJ Books.
29. Miles MB, Huberman AM (1994) Qualitative analysis: an expanded sourcebook. Thousand Oaks, CA: Sage Publications.
30. Pope C, Ziebland S, Mays N (2000) Analysing qualitative data. BMJ 320: 114–116.

31. Carroll C, Patterson M, Wood S, Booth A, Rick J, et al. (2007) A conceptual framework for implementation fidelity. Implement Sci 2: 40.
32. Forsetlund L, Bjorndal A, Rashidian A, Jamtvedt G, O'Brien MA, et al. (2009) Continuing education meetings and workshops: effects on professional practice and health care outcomes. Cochrane Database Syst Rev 2: CD003030.
33. Kash BA, Spaulding A, Johnson CE, Gamm L (2014) Success factors for strategic change initiatives: A qualitative study of healthcare administrators' perspectives. J Healthc Manag 59: 65–81.
34. Mannion R, Davies HTO, Marshall MN (2005) Cultural characteristics of "high" and "low" performing hospitals. J Health Organ Manage 19: 431–439.
35. Davies HT, Mannion R, Jacobs R, Powell AE, Marshall MN (2007) Exploring the relationship between senior management team culture and hospital performance. Med Care Res Rev 64: 46–65.
36. Li LC, Grimshaw JM, Nielsen C, Judd M, Coyte PC, et al. (2009) Use of communities of practice in business and health care sectors: A systematic review. Implement Sci 4: 27.
37. Siriwardena AN, Shaw D, Essam N, Togher FJ, Davy Z et al. (2014) The effect of a national quality improvement collaborative on prehospital care for acute myocardial infarction and stroke in England. Implement Sci 9: 17.
38. Wales A, Graham S, Rooney K, Crawford A (2012) Scotland's Knowledge Network: translating knowledge into action to improve quality of care. Scott Med J 57: 221–224.
39. Huijg JM, Gebhardt WA, Dusseldorp E, Verheijden MW, van der Zouwe N, et al. (2014) Measuring determinants of implementation behaviour: psychometric properties of a questionnaire based on the theoretical domains framework. Implement Sci 9: 33.
40. Simpson KM, Porter K, McConnell ES, Colon-Emeric C, Daily KA, et al. (2013) Tool for evaluating research implementation challenges: A sense-making protocol for addressing implementation challenges in complex research settings. Implement Sci 8: 2.
41. Hagedorn HJ (2010) The relationship between baseline organizational readiness to change assessment subscale scores and implementation of hepatitis prevention services in substance use disorders treatment clinics. Implement Sci 5: 46.
42. Porter AJ, Narimasu JY, Mulroy MF, Koehler RP (2014) Sustainable, effective implementation of a surgical preprocedural checklist: an "attestation" format for all operating team members. Jt Comm J Qual Patient Saf 40: 3–9.
43. Owen JA, Brashers VL, Littlewood KE, Wright E, Childress RM, et al. (2014) Designing and evaluating an effective theory-based continuing interprofessional development program to improve sepsis care by enhancing healthcare team collaboration. J Interprof Care 28: 212–217.
44. Rogers D, Lingard L, Boehler ML, Espin S, Klingensmith M, et al. (2011) Teaching operating room conflict management to surgeons: clarifying the optimal approach. Med Educ 45: 939–945.
45. Scott A, Sivey P, Ait Ouakrim D, Willenberg L, Naccarella L et al. (2011) The effect of financial incentives on the quality of health care provided by primary care physicians. Cochrane Database Syst Rev 9: CD008451.
46. Kaufman DM (2003) Applying educational theory in practice. BMJ 326: 213–216.
47. Ivers N, Jamtvedt G, Flottorp S, Young JM, Odgaard-Jensen J, et al. (2012) Audit and feedback: Effects on professional practice and healthcare outcomes. Cochrane Database Syst Rev 6: CD000259.

# 19

# Investigation of Cross-Species Translatability of Pharmacological MRI in Awake Nonhuman Primate - A Buprenorphine Challenge Study

**Stephanie Seah[1,2]*, Abu Bakar Ali Asad[1,2], Richard Baumgartner[3], Dai Feng[3], Donald S. Williams[1], Elaine Manigbas[4], John D. Beaver[4¤a], Torsten Reese[2¤b], Brian Henry[2], Jeffrey L. Evelhoch[1], Chih-Liang Chin[1,2]**

**1** Imaging, Merck & Co. Inc., West Point, Pennsylvania, United States of America, **2** Translational Medicine Research Centre, MSD, Singapore, Singapore, **3** Biostatistics and Research Decision Sciences, Merck & Co. Inc., Rahway, New Jersey, United States of America, **4** Imaging, Maccine Pte Ltd, Singapore, Singapore

## Abstract

***Background:*** Pharmacological MRI (phMRI) is a neuroimaging technique where drug-induced hemodynamic responses can represent a pharmacodynamic biomarker to delineate underlying biological consequences of drug actions. In most preclinical studies, animals are anesthetized during image acquisition to minimize movement. However, it has been demonstrated anesthesia could attenuate basal neuronal activity, which can confound interpretation of drug-induced brain activation patterns. Significant efforts have been made to establish awake imaging in rodents and nonhuman primates (NHP). Whilst various platforms have been developed for imaging awake NHP, comparison and validation of phMRI data as translational biomarkers across species remain to be explored.

***Methodology:*** We have established an awake NHP imaging model that encompasses comprehensive acclimation procedures with a dedicated animal restrainer. Using a cerebral blood volume (CBV)-based phMRI approach, we have determined differential responses of brain activation elicited by the systemic administration of buprenorphine (0.03 mg/kg i.v.), a partial μ-opioid receptor agonist, in the same animal under awake and anesthetized conditions. Additionally, region-of-interest analyses were performed to determine regional drug-induced CBV time-course data and corresponding area-under-curve (AUC) values from brain areas with high density of μ-opioid receptors.

***Principal Findings:*** In awake NHPs, group-level analyses revealed buprenorphine significantly activated brain regions including, thalamus, striatum, frontal and cingulate cortices (paired *t*-test, versus saline vehicle, $p<0.05$, $n=4$). This observation is strikingly consistent with μ-opioid receptor distribution depicted by [6-O-[$^{11}$C]methyl]buprenorphine ([$^{11}$C]BPN) positron emission tomography imaging study in baboons. Furthermore, our findings are consistent with previous buprenorphine phMRI studies in humans and conscious rats which collectively demonstrate the cross-species translatability of awake imaging. Conversely, no significant change in activated brain regions was found in the same animals imaged under the anesthetized condition.

***Conclusions:*** Our data highlight the utility and importance of awake NHP imaging as a translational imaging biomarker for drug research.

**Editor:** Alessandro Gozzi, Italian Institute of Technology, Italy

**Funding:** This research was funded by Merck & Co. The authors would like to declare that the following individuals are current or former employees of the funder - Stephanie Seah, Abu Bakar Ali Asad, Richard Baumgartner, Dai Feng, Don Williams, Torsten Reese, Brian Henry, Jeff Evelhoch and Chih-Liang Chin. Their roles include study design, data collection and analysis, decision to publish and preparation of the manuscript.

**Competing Interests:** Merck provided all funds for this work. As mentioned in the financial disclosures, some authors are current or former employees of Merck and may own stock or hold stock options in Merck. Co authors Elaine Manigbas and John Beaver were employees of Maccine Pte. Ltd.

* Email: stephanie.seah@merck.com

¤a Current address: Translational Imaging, Global Pharmaceutical Research and Development, Abbott Park, Illonois, United States of America
¤b Current address: MR Imaging, CIC biomaGUNE, San Sebastián, Gipuzkoa, Spain

## Introduction

Pharmacological MRI (phMRI) is a neuroimaging technique that allows characterization of changes in neural activity following drug challenge. Drug-induced pharmacodynamic responses detected from alterations in blood oxygenation level dependence (BOLD) signals or relative cerebral blood volume/flow (rCBV/rCBF) can provide as imaging biomarkers to delineate the central effect of drug actions [1,2,3,4]. As a result, significant effort has been devoted to implement phMRI as a translational research tool to develop novel CNS compounds, considering that this *in vivo* imaging technique can be performed in both animals [5,6,7,8] and humans [9,10,11,12]. To date, phMRI has been adopted to interrogate several key neurotransmitter systems, and these findings collectively have highlighted the value of phMRI to elucidate neurobiological mechanisms of drug actions and to gain better understanding of human diseases. In most preclinical imaging studies, animals were anesthetized during image acquisition to minimize movements; however, several lines of evidence have shown that the use of anesthesia could attenuate basal neuronal activity and likely confound drug-induced brain activation patterns [13,14,15,16,17,18,19,20]. Therefore, it is critical to establish translational platforms that permit investigation of pharmacological responses of experimental therapeutics in preclinical species, healthy volunteers and eventually in patients. To this end, phMRI in awake animals has been extensively pursued across various species, such as rodents [19,21,22,23] and nonhuman primates (NHPs) [17,18,24,25,26,27,28].

Awake NHP models are particularly attractive for neuroscience research, in light of greater similarities with humans in clinical and pathological characteristics [29]. It has been demonstrated that NHP and human brains share features in neuronal cytoarchitecture [30] and functional connections [31]. Additionally, the activity and distribution of neurotransmitter systems [32,33], drug metabolism and pharmacokinetic responses [34] are more comparable to human in NHP than in rodent. Nonetheless, despite the improved cross-species translatability offered by awake NHP imaging, animal movements during image acquisition can pose as a major obstacle, since excessive motion can lead to image blurring or ghosting artifacts, and higher baseline signal fluctuations that could diminish sensitivity to detect changes of drug-induced phMRI signals. Furthermore, the level of resting state stability could vary significantly among imaging sessions, which can attribute to compromised test-retest reliability and hindrance to conducting longitudinal studies. To circumvent this challenge, several groups have attempted to develop awake NHP imaging paradigms, in which extensive acclimation procedures are often required [17,27,35,36,37]. Animals were trained to remain still and gradually habituate to the actual scanning environment while using a dedicated animal restrainer that affords better securing of the animal's head and/or body, such as a head-post model [35] or non-invasive helmet approaches [27,36]. In addition, improved data acquisition methods [37], use of contrast agent [38] and optimized data analysis strategies [39] have also been explored to enhance phMRI sensitivity. Nonetheless, it will be essential to establish a systematic approach to evaluate phMRI baseline signals attributable to animal movements and thus characterize the utility, or limitation, of these awake imaging platforms.

Buprenorphine is an opioid agonist that has a high affinity to various opioid receptors, such as μ, δ, κ subtypes [40], and it has been used clinically to treat opiate addiction or pain [41,42]. The clinical efficacy of buprenorphine for pain and opiate addiction is thought to be due to partial agonism at μ–opioid receptors and/or antagonism at κ–opioid receptors [41,42]. Previous studies performed by Upadhyay et al. have shown that buprenorphine elicited BOLD responses in humans correspond to brain regions with abundant μ–opioid receptors and modulate brain functional connectivity ascribed to pain-processing circuitry [43]. Interestingly, congruency in the spatial pattern of buprenorphine-induced brain activation between humans and conscious rats was also observed [21]. In light of these studies in both humans and awake rats, a phMRI study of buprenorphine in awake NHP can assess the congruency of imaging endpoints across species, and thereby determine the utility of an awake NHP imaging platform for translational research.

In this study, we sought to investigate differential responses in brain activity in NHP produced by the systemic administration of buprenorphine under awake and anesthetized conditions. We hypothesized that buprenorphine-induced brain activation pattern observed from awake NHP should highlight the known μ-opioid receptor distribution [44,45] and afford investigation of cross-species translatability of awake NHP imaging in conjunction with previous phMRI data obtained from humans and awake rats [21,43].

Toward this goal, we first constructed a dedicated animal restrainer based on a design previously reported by Andersen et al. [35] and then developed an awake NHP training protocol. Each animal received comprehensive training, including incremental sessions in a mock MRI scanner and acclimatization to the actual imaging environment. The effectiveness of training was evaluated via measured circulating cortisol levels and behavioral scores (e.g. rated by the trainer). Consequently, these criteria were used to select animals thought to be most habituated to the scanner environment for subsequent imaging studies. During the imaging phase, resting state BOLD signals were acquired under awake (both test and re-test) and anesthetized conditions to determine resting state baseline stability and reliability, which served as a measure of the effectiveness or limitation of our acclimation procedures. To assess the cross-species translatability of our awake NHP platform, we imaged brain activity induced by buprenorphine infusion (0.03 mg/kg i.v.) using a CBV-based phMRI approach, where an ultrasmall superparamagnetic iron oxide (USPIO) contrast agent was applied to increase sensitivity [46]. Imaging experiments were conducted following a within-subject study design to differentiate the central effect of buprenorphine and saline vehicle in NHPs imaged under both awake and isoflurane-anesthetized conditions. To characterize the regional specificity of drug effect, a group-level and region-of-interest (ROI) data analysis pipeline was implemented based on a standard monkey brain atlas [47], where drug-induced CBV-based signal change time-course data and corresponding area-under-curve (AUC) were derived from selected brain regions with high density of μ–opioid receptors.

## Materials and Methods

### Ethics Statement

The following experiments were conducted in accordance with the Institutional Animal Care and Use Committee at Merck & Co. The current study, in addition to its protocol, was approved by the Institutional Animal Care and Use Committee at Merck & Co (Permit Number: 11102130610016). No animals were sacrificed for the purpose of this experiment. Trained veterinarians and animal technicians were involved in the care of the animals as well as all the animal procedures performed during this study.

### Animals

Adult female cynomolgus monkeys (Macaca fascicularis, PT Prestasi Fauna Nusantara, Indonesia; $n = 12$, age $= 4$ years - 6 years, body weight $= 2$ kg~4 kg) were allocated for this study. Animals were pair housed at the Maccine facility in temperature- (18 °C–26 °C) and humidity-controlled (30%–70%) rooms maintained on a 12:12 light/dark cycle with lights on at 7:00 AM. Mirrors were placed outside the home cage, and cage toys/ manipulative enrichment, such as Kong toys, Flexi keys, were provided and rotated every week. Radios and televisions were also used as supplementary enrichments. Animals were fed with a diet of monkey chow free of animal protein, as well as a controlled amount of fruits or vegetables, offered twice daily. Aside from daily fruit rations, frozen homemade treats (i.e. fruits, raisins, cereals, etc.) were provided once a week. Tap water was offered ad libitum. Prior to the commencement of the study, a complete physical examination, including hematological/blood chemistry analysis, was performed and reviewed by the attending veterinarian.

## Awake Training Protocol

Based on previous work done by Andersen et al. [35], a dedicated animal restrainer was constructed, and the animals were habituated to the restrainer and MRI scanner environment for awake imaging. To alleviate stress and minimize movement during awake imaging, each animal was blindfolded and trained in a phased manner, gradually habituated through different training procedures over several months (see Fig. 1; Phase 1a–c). As shown in Figure 1, our training protocol includes *restrainer training*, *mock scanner training* and *head-post surgery and head-restraint tethering training* phases. During each training session, animal's behavioral gestures (e.g. vocalization, excessive movement, head/body turn) were monitored and scored by a trainer. A low cumulative behavioral score at the end of the training was indicative of a well-behaved animal, suitable for the imaging study. Briefly, during Phase 1a: *restrainer training*, animals were trained to remain still in a primate restraining chair for a period of 30 minutes which was gradually prolonged to a steady state of 120 minutes. Upon achieving this requirement, animals were placed in a prone position in a confinement apparatus for 120 minutes to acclimatize to the restrainer environment. Next, animals were gradually exposed to an MRI-compatible restrainer and the duration of the training period increased by 15 minutes weekly until a steady state of 120 minutes was reached. Additionally, to assess the stress level associated with training procedures, cortisol concentrations were also measured using an electrochemiluminescence immunoassay toolkit (ECLIA, Roche Diagnostics, Singapore), in which blood samples (2 mL) were collected prior to placing the animals inside the restrainer tube and 90-minute-post training. Based on the measured cortisol levels and cumulative behavioral scores over the course of Phase 1a, eight animals were selected and progressed to Phase 1b (*mock scanner training*).

In the *mock scanner training* phase, animals were placed in the restrainer in a mock scanner for a 2-hour time period every other day, in order to habituate them to the scanner environment. At the last training session of this phase, cortisol measurements were repeated (pre- and post-training, $n = 8$) to evaluate the effectiveness of acclimation, and the results were compared with a non-trained control cohort ($n = 6$). Finally, in the *head-post surgery and head-restraint tethering* phase for the selected animals, the head-post component of the restrainer was surgically attached to the skull of each subject [35]. Head tethering restraint training started after animals had fully recovered from the surgery and occurred twice a week until the actual imaging study.

## Animal Preparation for the Imaging Study

Animals progressed from the training procedures to imaging studies (see Fig. 1), where they were imaged under both awake and anesthetized conditions for the stability and test-retest reliability study of resting state BOLD signal and subsequently the phMRI experiments. For the anesthetized imaging study, animals were sedated with ketamine (10 mg/kg IM) for induction, while ear plugs and eye lubricant were applied to all the animals, prior to bringing them into the scanner room. The animal was then placed on the patient bed of the MRI scanner in a prone position and ventilated by an MRI-compatible ventilator and bellows system (SurgiVet, Dublin, OH). Anesthesia was maintained through inhalation of a mixture of isoflurane (2%) in medical air. Physiological parameters of each animal, including heart rate, $SpO_2$, $EtCO_2$, and respiration rate were monitored and recorded throughout the imaging session using an MR-compatible Datex-Ohmeda physiological monitoring system (GE Healthcare, WI). The temperature of the animal was measured via a fiber-optic temperature sensor system (OpSens, Quebec, Canada) and recorded periodically throughout the experiment. For the awake imaging study, animals were blindfolded and placed in a sphinx position within the restrainer used during the training procedures.

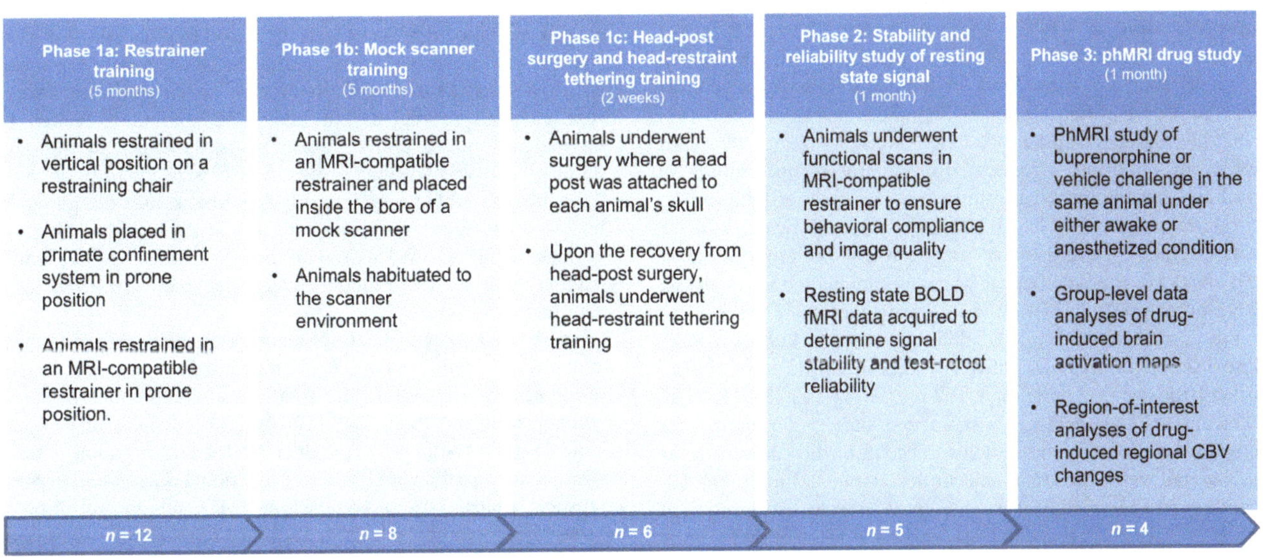


**Figure 1. Study protocol of awake imaging in non-human primates.** Initial Phase 1a–c focus on the training procedures to reduce animal movement/stress during awake imaging; Phase 2 was the assessment of the stability of resting state signal and its test-retest reliability; Phase 3 was the within-subject pharmacological challenge study, where buprenorphine (0.03 mg/kg i.v.) and vehicle were given to the same animals under awake and anesthetized conditions.

A customized head radiofrequency (RF) coil was securely attached to the head-post of the animal. Also, during each awake imaging session, at least one animal trainer would be assigned to visually monitor the animals.

## Evaluation of the Effectiveness or Limitation of Awake Training Protocol

All imaging experiments were conducted on a 3 Tesla TIM Trio MRI scanner (Siemens Medical Solutions, Erlangen, Germany) using a dedicated 8-channel phased-array head coil (RAPID Biomedical GmbH, Germany). Resting state BOLD signal was collected by a single-shot gradient-echo EPI pulse sequence (TR/TE = 3 s/21 ms, in-plane pixel size = 1 mm ×1 mm, slice thickness = 2 mm, and 24 slices with no gap), and 810 imaging volumes (40 minutes in total) were acquired. High resolution brain anatomical images (TR/TE = 700 ms/13 ms, in-plane pixel size = 0.67 mm ×0.67 mm) of individual animals were also acquired in order to co-register with a standard monkey brain atlas [47] for further group-level and ROI analyses. Resting state BOLD signals were acquired from the same animals imaged under anesthetized and awake conditions separately ($n = 5$). Further, to examine the test-retest reliability of resting state BOLD signal during awake imaging, experiments were repeated on a different day. As a result, each animal was imaged three times in total.

## Assessment of Cross-species Translatability of Awake NHP

For the phMRI study, selected animals ($n = 4$) underwent four separate sessions (1-week apart to ensure drug washout) on different days (16 scans in total), where a counterbalanced measures design was used to ensure each animal was imaged under different drug challenge (vehicle or buprenorphine) or imaging condition (awake or anesthetized). For each imaging experiment, brain anatomical image and functional datasets were acquired using the same imaging pulse sequences and parameters described above (see *Evaluation of the Effectiveness or Limitation of Awake Training Protocol* section).

To increase the sensitivity of phMRI signals [46], a CBV-based approach using a USPIO contrast agent, 7.5 mg/kg i.v. of Ferumoxytol (AMAG Pharmaceutical, Cambridge MA), was used. A tail vein line was cannulated for the administration of contrast agent and drug, while the indwelling catheter was attached to a saline-filled syringe placed on an infusion pump (Harvard Apparatus, Holliston, MA) located outside the scanner room. All animals were administered intravenously with either 0.03 mg/kg of buprenorphine (Reckitt Benckiser Pharmaceuticals, UK) or saline vehicle. Intramuscular injection of buprenorphine at 0.01 mg/kg or 0.03 mg/kg has been commonly used for analgesia in nonhuman primates [48] and we have adopted the higher dose in the current study. Notably, different doses of buprenorphine were selected in previous phMRI studies in rodent (0.04 mg/kg and 0.1 mg/kg i.v.) or human (0.2 mg/70 kg i.v.) [21,43]. The following imaging protocol was carried out: (i) 5-minute pre-contrast data acquisition, (ii) bolus injection of the contrast agent via the tail vein line (total injection volume = 2 mL), (iii) 10-minute pre-drug baseline acquisition (post-contrast), (iv) infusion of either buprenorphine at 0.03 mg/kg i.v. or saline vehicle (total injection volume = 3 mL) was split into three infusion periods (30 s each) separated by a 1.5-minute interval, in order to minimize potential respiratory suppression related to the buprenorphine injection [43]. Finally, (v) 20-minute period of post-drug imaging acquisition.

## Data Analysis

Data analyses were conducted using the FMRIB Software Library (FSL) (http://www.fmrib.ox.au.ul/fls) and in-house Matlab (MathWorks, Natick, MA). First, voxels of the brain were extracted using a brain extraction tool (FSL BET). To characterize the fluctuation of resting state BOLD signals obtained from awake and anesthetized imaging experiments, time-course data of each voxel was derived and expressed as a percentage change relative to the average signal intensity over the entire imaging time period. Then, for each voxel the mean percentage change was calculated by averaging the absolute value of percentage change over time. Consequently, the mean value and standard deviation over the entire brain volume were calculated and reported. Finally, a Bland-Altman plot was used to assess test-retest reliability of awake resting state BOLD signal.

For the phMRI data analysis, FSL was used. Specifically, our data analysis pipeline included the following steps: motion correction (FSL MCFLIRT), brain extraction, spatial smoothing (FWHM = 2 mm) and co-registration to a standard monkey brain atlas [47]. To depict activated brain regions, time-course relative CBV change, ΔrCBV($t$), was first calculated from the raw data using a known relationship [46,49],

$$\Delta rCBV(t) = \ln[S_{POST}/S(t)]/\ln[S_{PRE}/S_{POST}] \qquad (1)$$

where $t$ is time after drug injection, $S(t)$ is the signal intensity after the drug infusion, $S_{POST}$ is the mean pre-drug baseline signal intensity over the 10-minute period, post contrast agent administration, and $S_{PRE}$ is the mean signal intensity over the 5-minute period, prior to the administration of contrast agent. Then, a general linear model (GLM) was used for the subject-level analysis, where a linear ramp model was used to mimic the infusion response, while the elimination of buprenorphine was based on the known plasma pharmacokinetic of buprenorphine in dogs (brain half-life ~4.5 hr) [50]. Due to the relatively long onset of the ramp function compared to the hemodynamic response function (HRF), the ramp stimulus function in our GLM was not convolved with HRF [43]. To perform unbiased univariate linear regression analysis, nuisance regressors were prepared that account for most of the confounding explanatory variables (EVs), where the mean time-course signals extracted from the ventricles and white matter were included to regress out additional confounds related to physiological noises and/or linear drifts. Further, an in-house Matlab script was written to identify excessive intensity changes (head movement) between imaging time-points, as a de-spiking in the EV. Spike detection was implemented using a median absolute residual variation (MARV) score-based approach [51], while imaging volumes with motion greater than half of a voxel were identified as spikes.

For the group-level and ROI analyses, functional data of each animal was first co-registered to the individual's anatomical images by rigid body translations and rotations and subsequently into a template monkey brain atlas [47] using 12 degrees of freedom affine transformation. These calculated transformation matrix parameters were then applied to the functional dataset and derived statistical maps. Group comparisons were conducted using a mixed-effects paired $t$-test (FSL FLAME) to determine the group means of the differential effect of vehicle and buprenorphine in both anesthetized and awake animals, threshold at $p<0.05$, in order to identify brain regions affected by the drug or vehicle challenge under awake and anesthetized imaging. In addition, to illustrate the temporal dynamics of rCBV change, time-course data for each imaging condition from selected brain regions were

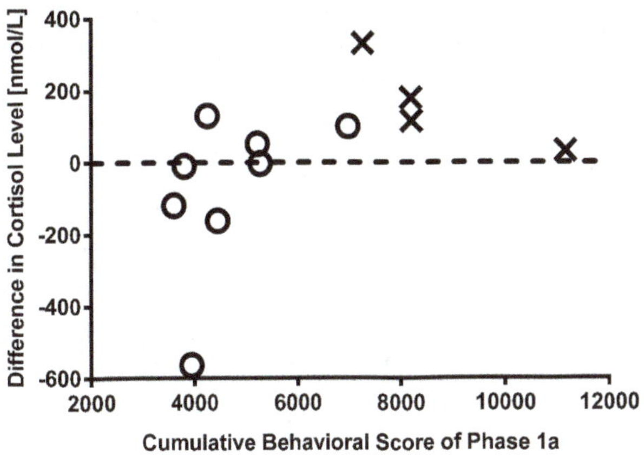


**Figure 2. Differences in plasma cortisol concentration and cumulative behavioral scores during Phase 1a used to select animals for Phase 1b.** Cumulative behavioral scores over the Phase 1a training obtained from all animals ($n=12$), in which animals with lower behavioral scores ($n=8$, 'O') were selected to transition into the Phase 1b study and ones with higher scores were deselected ($n=4$, '×'). In addition, to assess the stress level during the awake training, plasma cortisol concentrations were measured from these animals at two separate time points (~ one month apart) during this phase, and results indicated that the reduction in cortical level is likely associated with better habituation (i.e. lower behavioral scores).

extracted, detrended and plotted. Regional time-course data was calculated by averaging the rCBV change over all the supra-threshold voxels within specific brain regions. Results obtained from the vehicle infusion were exploited to detrend buprenorphine data on a region-by-region basis. Also, ROI analyses of drug-induced ΔrCBV time-course data were performed, in which AUC were obtained from brain regions with high density of μ-opioid receptor such as putamen, caudate, thalamus, cingulate cortex and frontal cortex, where regional AUC values (mean ± SEM) were

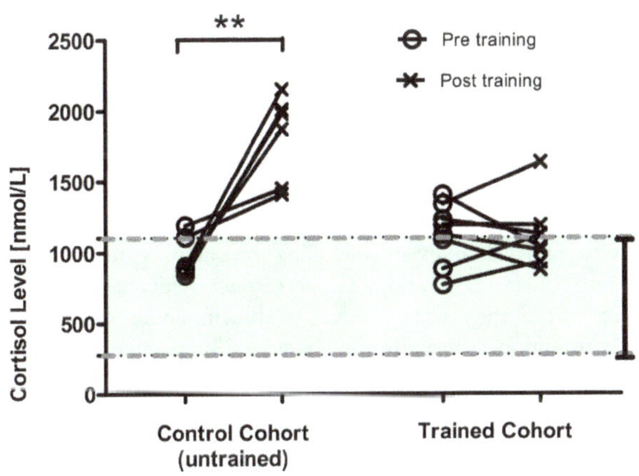


**Figure 3. Awake training increased plasma cortisol concentrations in untrained animals, but not in trained animals.** Plasma cortisol concentrations measured from the animals ($n=8$) at prior- and post-90-minute training session during the Phase 1b period. Results indicate that, at the end of training session cortisol levels are significantly elevated in untrained/control animals ($n=6$), while no significant change was observed in habituated animals (paired $t$-test, **$p<0.01$). The dash lines highlight the range of normal cortisol concentration observed in cynomolgus monkeys (276 nmol/L to 1104 nmol/L) [52].

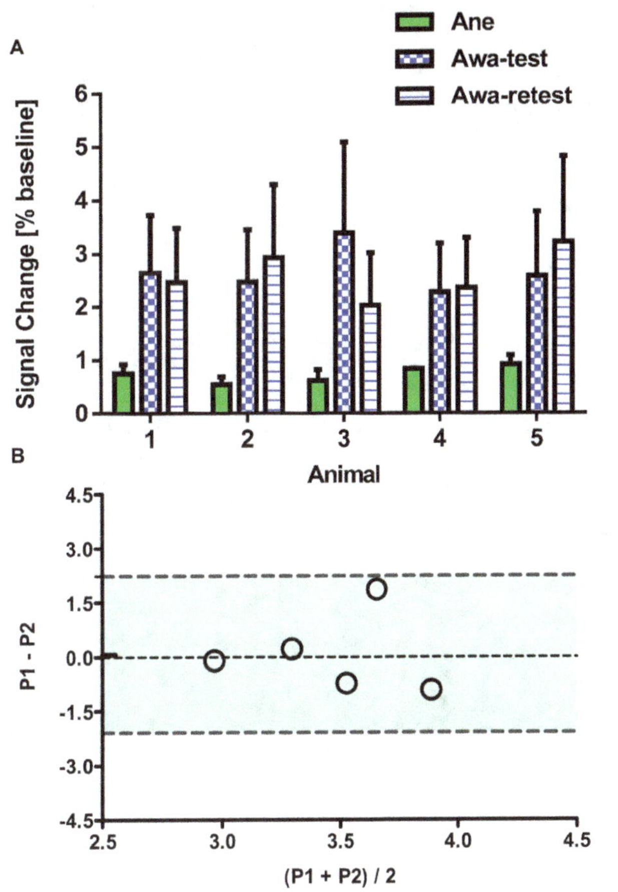


**Figure 4. Comparison of resting state stability between anesthetized and awake imaging and test-retest reliability of awake baseline signal.** (**A**) Resting state variation of BOLD signal (mean ± SD) obtained from each non-human primate (NHP) imaged under either awake (Awa, test and retest) or anesthetized (Ane) condition. (**B**) Bland-Altman plot for awake imaging data and the dash lines highlight the 95% limits of agreement (P1: represents the first test, P2 represents the retest).

calculated from all animals treated with either buprenorphine or vehicle and imaged under both anesthetized and awake conditions. Finally, calculated AUC data were subjected to a paired $t$-test (JMP 7.0.1, SAS Institute, Cary NC), with differences considered statistically significant at $p<0.05$.

## Results

### Behavioral Scores and Cortisol Levels for Animal Selection

Cumulative behavioral scores obtained from all the animals ($n=12$) over the entire Phase 1a period are plotted in Figure 2, in which animals with lower overall behavioral scores (better habituated) were selected to transition from Phase 1a to 1b ($n=8$). These results demonstrate that levels of acclimation can vary within the training cohort, and thereby the selection of desired animals is essential. Within this phase, differences in the cortisol levels measured at two time points (separated by a month) are shown in Figure 2, indicating that elevated cortisol levels are likely observed from animals with higher behavioral scores. To assess the effect of training on stress levels, Figure 3 illustrates the cortisol concentrations obtained from untrained/control animals

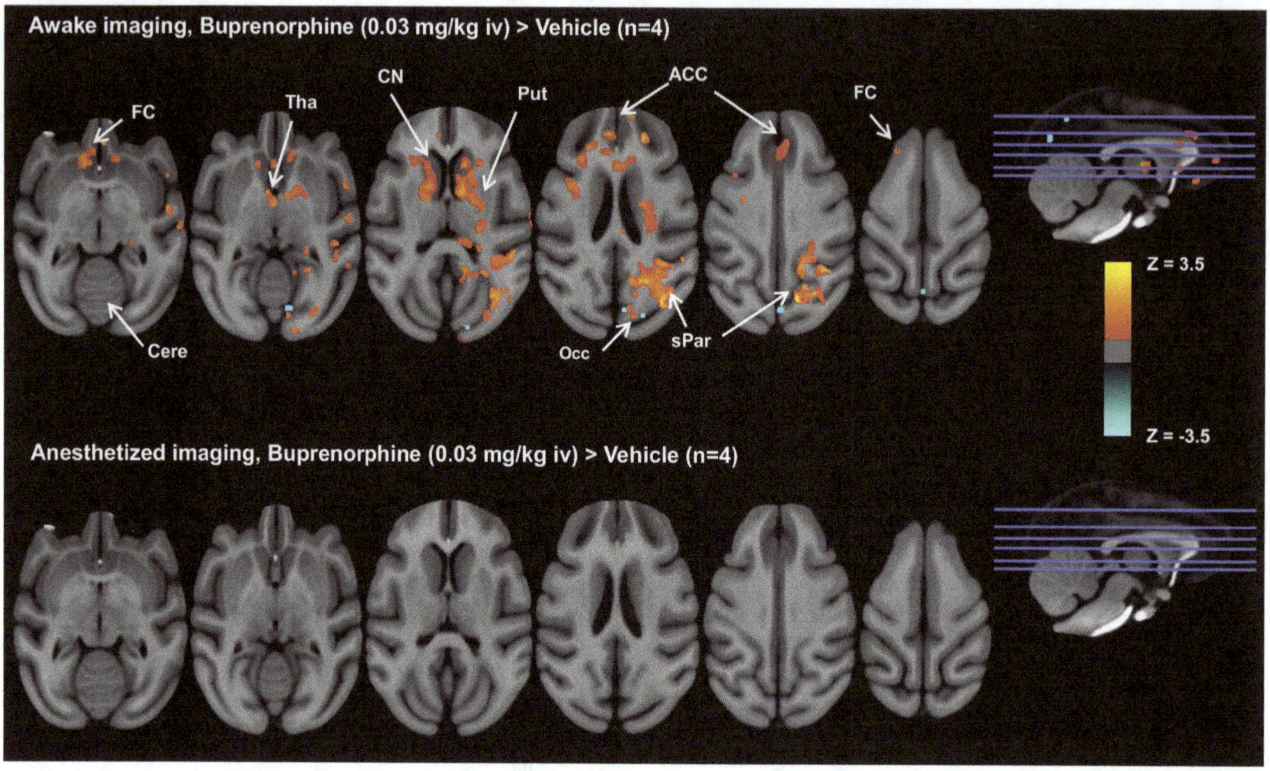


**Figure 5. Group comparisons of brain activation patterns between buprenorphine and vehicle under awake and anesthetized imaging.** Group comparisons of brain activation patterns showing significant effect of buprenorphine versus vehicle (paired *t*-test, $p<0.05$, $n=4$) under awake and anesthetized imaging. In the awake study, buprenorphine activates brain regions with a high density of μ-opioid receptor, including frontal cortex (FC), thalamus (Tha), anterior cingulate cortices (ACC), caudate nucleus (CN), putamen (Put), and superior parietal lobule (sPar), and limited deactivation was found in occipital cortex (Occ). In contrast, no significant difference in brain activation between buprenorphine and vehicle infusion was observed in anesthetized animals.

($n=6$) as well as our imaging cohort ($n=8$) at pre- and 90-minute-post training session (Phase 1b). As shown, cortisol levels were significantly elevated in untrained animals after they underwent the training session (paired *t*-test, $p<0.01$), while no significant difference was observed in habituated animals. Further, only one from the trained imaging cohort had cortisol concentrations substantially above the previously reported normal range (between 276 nmol/L and 1104 nmol/L) [52]. The lower cortisol level found in the trained cohort implies reduced stress levels in these animals and effective habituation to the restrainer and MRI scanner environment. Finally, two animals were deselected from the cohort due to medical conditions (unrelated to the training), while the remaining six animals were moved forward to Phase 1c.

## Effectiveness or Limitation of Awake Training Protocol

Figure 4A shows the percentage variation in resting state baseline signals within the whole brain volume (mean ± SD) from individual animals imaged under awake and anesthetized conditions. Our data indicate that compared to anesthetized imaging, the level of baseline variation was significantly higher (4~5 fold) under the awake condition (paired *t*-test, $p<0.01$). This observation is not unexpected, since there was some animal movement during awake imaging. These findings suggest that a larger change in drug-induced phMRI signals may be needed in order to achieve comparable sensitivity offered by imaging anesthetized animals (i.e. to offset the increased baseline noise). Reasonable test-retest reliability was found from the awake baseline data, considering all the data points were within 95% limits of agreement of the Bland Altman plot (see Fig. 4b). Finally, two animals were deselected from the Phase 3 drug study, due to the increased body weight thus unable to fit into the animal restrainer or the need for repetitive head-post repairs.

## Buprenorphine-induced phMRI response under awake and anaesthetized conditions

Figure 5 illustrates group comparisons of brain activation patterns showing significant effect of buprenorphine versus vehicle on rCBV changes (paired t-test, $p<0.05$, $n=4$), while Table 1 lists the results of ROI analyses, including activated brain regions/coordinates, z-statistics, and total percentage activated volumes calculated from the awake study. As shown, under the awake imaging condition, buprenorphine activated brain regions with a high density of μ-opioid receptor including, frontal cortex, thalamus, cingulate cortex, caudate nucleus, putamen, occipital cortex, and superior parietal lobule. Notably, these findings are strikingly consistent with μ-opioid receptor distribution depicted by [6-O-[$^{11}$C]methyl]buprenorphine ([$^{11}$C]BPN) positron emission tomography (PET) study in baboons, where the highest [$^{11}$C]BPN uptakes was observed in striatum (caudate nucleus and putamen) followed by thalamus, cingulate, frontal, parietal, occipital cortices, and then cerebellum [44]. In accordance with the results obtained from the previous study in conscious rodent and human studies [21], similar region-specificity of activated brain structures are also observed in our awake NHP data. Conversely, no significant activation was observed from anesthetized animals (paired *t*-test, vs. vehicle treatment; see Fig. 5B), despite animal

**Table 1.** Activated brain regions and their volumes induced by buprenorphine infusion derived from the region-of-interest analysis.

| Brain Region | Coordinates (X, Y, Z) [mm] | Z-statistics | Activated Volume (percentage) [mm$^3$] |
|---|---|---|---|
| Cingulate cortex | 29.7, 70.0, 25.2 | 2.52 | 182.52 (10.80%) |
| Gyrus rectus | 29.5, 61.2, 21.0 | 2.61 | 44.39 (11.58%) |
| Orbital gyrus | 26.0, 58.7, 19.5 | 2.39 | 2.83 (0.38%) |
| Caudate Nucleus | 35.5, 57.2, 28.0 | 2.54 | 224.19 (28.51%) |
| Putamen | 24.2, 57.2, 20.7 | 2.43 | 17.84 (2.02%) |
| Superior frontal gyrus | 17.5, 54.5, 35.5 | 2.51 | 77.17 (1.46%) |
| Middle frontal gyrus | 17.2, 54.7, 35.0 | 2.54 | 11.14 (0.86%) |
| Precentral gyrus | 51.5, 50.5, 23.5 | 2.51 | 43.16 (0.79%) |
| Postcentral gyrus | 53.0, 42.0, 25.7 | 2.66 | 34.48 (1.79%) |
| Globus pallidus | 37.0, 50.2, 25.0 | 2.46 | 27.55 (13.42%) |
| Internal capsule | 36.2, 49.7, 24.7 | 2.49 | 23.22 (10.56%) |
| Amygdala | 40.5, 48.2, 12.7 | 2.50 | 13.94 (2.37%) |
| Thalamus | 34.5, 48.2, 27.0 | 2.61 | 34.48 (3.18%) |
| Hippocampus | 43.2, 43.0, 12.7 | 2.61 | 24.06 (4.84%) |
| Insular cortex | 46.7, 42.7, 21.2 | 2.51 | 1.09 (0.28%) |
| Inferior temporal gyrus | 48.0, 40.7, 9.5 | 2.33 | 0.25 (0.03%) |
| Superior temporal gyrus | 50.2, 31.7, 29.5 | 2.53 | 213.33 (6.32%) |
| Middle temporal gyrus | 50.5, 31.0, 29.7 | 2.61 | 43.61 (2.89%) |
| Midbrain | 36.2, 39.7, 18.2 | 2.37 | 3.28 (0.34%) |
| Pulvinar nuclei | 36.5, 36.2, 27.0 | 2.43 | 6.19 (6.14%) |
| Inferior parietal lobe | 38.0, 24.5, 36.7 | 2.63 | 120.39 (4.32%) |
| Superior parietal lobe | 36.2, 21.2, 34.5 | 2.61 | 72.75 (2.56%) |
| Superior occipital | 37.7, 22.5, 35.0 | 2.61 | 87.05 (2.58%) |
| Lateral occipital | 34.2, 12.0, 27.5 | 2.56 | 68.58 (3.16%) |
| Cerebellum | 35.5, 19.0, 22.7 | 2.43 | 5.77 (0.08%) |

Brain regions show differential responses of buprenorphine infusion (0.03 mg/kg i.v.) in awake imaging (vs vehicle, paired *t*-test, $z>2.3$, $n=4$). The *z*-statistic represents the maximum of each brain region with significant difference in rCBV changes between buprenorphine and vehicle treatments, while the coordinates correspond to the location of individual maxima in the standard monkey brain atlas space [47].

physiological parameters (mean ± SEM, $n=4$) being maintained within normal ranges during these experiments (mean heart rate = (119.9±5.1) beats/min, mean $SpO_2$ = 98.8%±0.6%, mean $EtCO_2$ = 22.0%±0.4%, and body temperature = 36.5 °C±0.1 °C). These results exemplify the undesired anesthetic-drug interactions embedded in the anesthetized animal experiments, while highlighting the need for awake imaging for phMRI studies.

Plots of time-course rCBV changes derived from our ROI analyses are shown in Figure 6, in which activated brain regions identified in the group-level brain activation maps (see Fig. 5) showed significant increases in rCBV following buprenorphine infusion. Buprenorphine produced significant increases in rCBV change (mean ± SD) at frontal cortex (7.3%±0.2%), thalamus (6.5%±0.2%), caudate nucleus (6.2%±0.2%), putamen (5.8%±0.2%), and cingulate cortex (5.1%±0.2%). Of note, it appears that rCBV reached the maximum value around 10-minute-post onset of drug infusion and then maintained at steady state that prolonged over the rest of the imaging period. Area-under-curve of the rCBV time-course data over the entire drug infusion period (AUC), or the above-mentioned steady state period ($AUC_{ss}$), were calculated and shown in Figure 7. Results depicted that both AUC and $AUC_{ss}$ calculated from thalamus, caudate nucleus, and putamen are significantly higher in buprenorphine-treated awake animals (paired *t*-test, $p<0.05$, vs vehicle), whilst no significant increases in AUC and $AUC_{ss}$ were found in any brain region from the anesthetized study.

## Discussion

Previous PET studies in baboons with the opioid receptor radioligand, [$^{11}$C]BPN revealed high binding activity in striatum, thalamus, cingulate gyrus, frontal cortex, parietal cortex, occipital cortex and cerebellum (in a descending order) [44] and these findings agree well with the known opioid receptor distribution in post-mortem human brain [53]. In this work, we found that buprenorphine infusion in awake, but not anesthetized, NHP produced significant and persistent increase in rCBV at specific brain regions including frontal and cingulate cortices, caudate nucleus, putamen, thalamus, parietal cortex and occipital cortices (see Fig. 5). These activated brain regions are consistent with the binding sites of μ–opioid receptors highlighted in the PET study [44], reflecting the underlying drug actions and subsequent biological responses. Recently, Becerra et al. demonstrated that brain regions activated by buprenorphine in awake rats paralleled that observed in humans, in which buprenorphine elicited BOLD signals in somatosensory and cingulate cortices, insula, striatum,

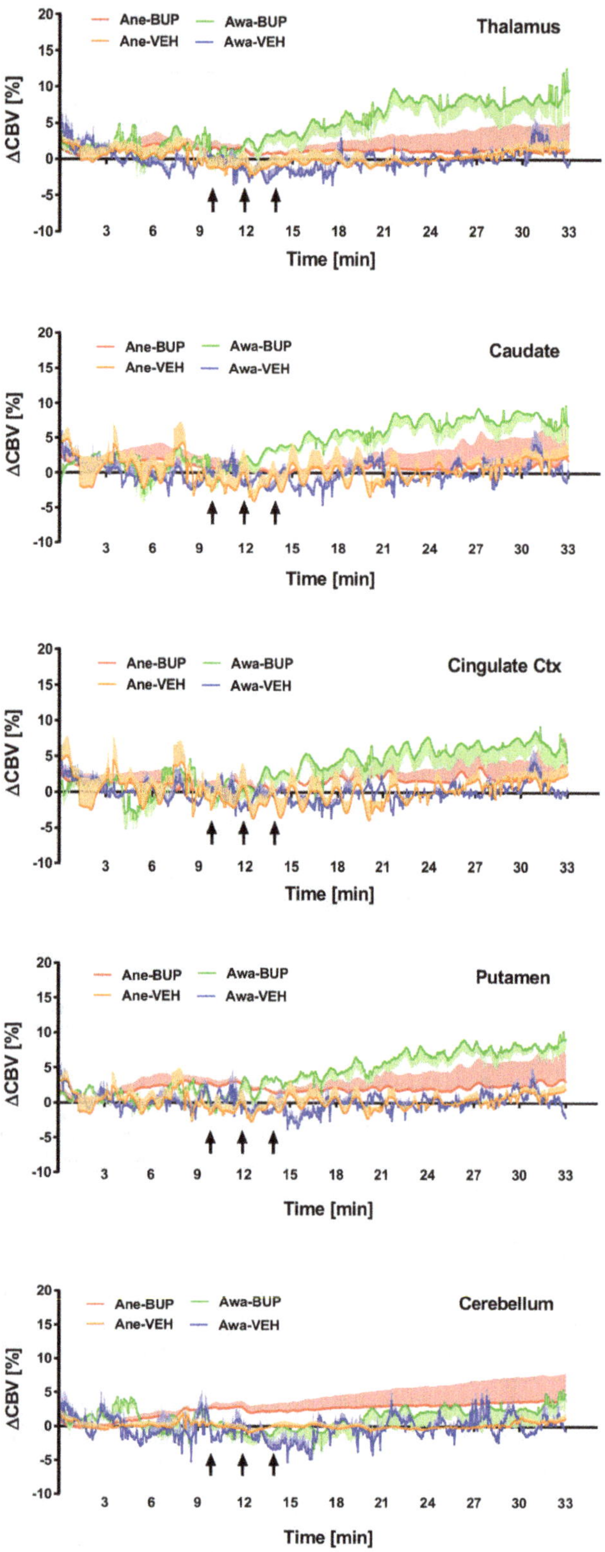


**Figure 6. Regional time-course rCBV changes derived from the region-of-interest analysis.** Plots of regional time-course rCBV change (mean ± SEM) derived from region-of-interest (ROI) analyses of the imaging cohort ($n = 4$) treated with either buprenorphine (BUP at 0.03 mg/kg i.v.) or vehicle (VEH) and imaged under awake (Awa) or anesthetized (Ane) conditions. The black arrows indicate the three individual dosing time periods (30 s drug infusion separated by 1.5-minute intervals), starting at 10-minute after the contrast agent administration. Results indicated that in awake NHP, buprenorphine infusion produces significant increases in rCBV at brain regions with high density of μ-opioid receptors, but not the area with low concentration of μ-opioid receptors (i.e. cerebellum).

thalamus, periaqueductal gray (PAG), and cerebellum in a dose-dependent manner [21]. Further, in contrast to human data, negative BOLD signals were observed in several brain regions in awake rats and this discrepancy was reconciled with the difference in opioid receptor subtypes and binding affinities between these two species [21]. To examine the congruency of phMRI data across rodent, NHP and humans, it appears that the brain activation patterns obtained from our awake NHP study show greater similarity to human data. For example, very limited deactivation, or decreased rCBV, was found in occipital cortex (see Fig. 5). Also, with the exception of activation in the cerebellum, brain regions activated by buprenorphine in awake NHP are depicted in human data. We attributed inconsistency in cerebellar activation to the difference in drug pharmacokinetic or exposure levels, considering that in the baboon PET study [$^{11}$C]BPN uptake at cerebellum peaked within 2-minute post tracer injection and eliminated rapidly [44]. Further, unlike previous rodent and human BOLD fMRI studies [21,43], we used a CBV-based approach in the current work. For the CBV-based approach, changes in MRI signal reflect changes in CBV, rather than the concentration of deoxyhemoglobin as in BOLD imaging [54]. While it could depend on the resting state blood volume at specific brain regions, BOLD and CBV contrasts are known to be spatially [54] and temporally [55] coupled. Overall, our data highlight the importance and utility of awake imaging in NHP.

In anesthetized animals, brain activation patterns induced by buprenorphine challenge differ from the previous PET μ-opioid receptor data. In comparison with the vehicle treatment, buprenorphine challenge did not elicit any significant changes in brain activity (see Fig. 5), possibly due to the effect of anesthesia. Also, ROI analyses indicate that the rank order of regional rCBV changes induced by buprenorphine infusion was different between anesthetized and awake imaging (see Fig, 7). For example, in awake NHP the highest rCBV change was found in frontal cortex and followed by thalamus, caudate, putamen, cingulate cortex, and cerebellum, while the rank order (descending) became frontal cortex, cerebellum, putamen, cingulate cortex, thalamus, and caudate under anesthetized imaging. Anesthetic-drug interactions on brain activity has been investigated by several groups [14,16,18,19], and it was concluded that drug-induced brain activation pattern can vary among the anesthetics used. The extent of anesthesia confounds likely pivots on the particular mechanism of action associated with selected anesthetics and test drugs, which might or might not be an issue, depending on the neurotransmitter system investigated. Considering the observed drug-induced activation can result from drug-receptor down-stream biological effects, the use of anesthesia can modulate both direct and indirect neuronal pathways. As such, it is more desirable to perform imaging in preclinical species without anesthesia that enables qualification of imaging biomarkers which represent a closer scenario to that of clinical investigation.

One of the key challenges for awake imaging is to ensure animals remain still during the data acquisition. Significant efforts have been made to establish comprehensive habituation procedures and specialized animal restrainers in order to minimize head and body motion during data acquisition [16,17,24,27,35, 37,56,57]. For example, Keliris et al. have developed a sophisticated MRI-compatible training chair and head-post restrainer to image alert monkeys in a natural upright sitting position, and they

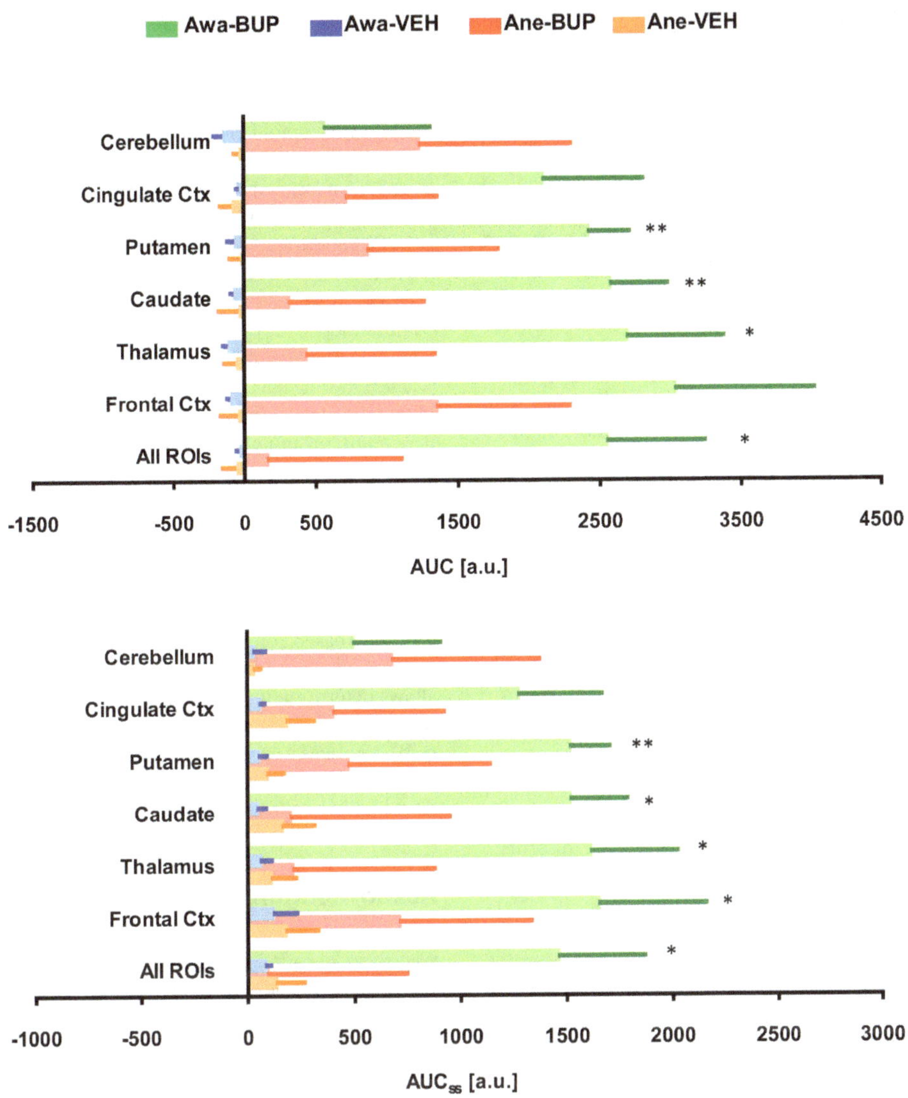


**Figure 7. Area-under-curve of regional time-course rCBV change during post-drug infusion derived from the region-of-interest analysis.** Results obtained from region-of-interest (ROI) analyses of rCBV time-course data showing the area-under-curve (mean ± SEM) of the entire post-drug infusion period (AUC) or only the steady-state time period (AUC$_{ss}$). Animals ($n = 4$) were imaged under awake (Awa) or anesthetized (Ane) conditions and treated with either buprenorphine (BUP at 0.03 mg/kg i.v.) or vehicle (VEH). Our data indicated that in awake animals AUC and AUC$_{ss}$ calculated from thalamus, caudate nucleus, and putamen are significantly higher in buprenorphine-treated animals (paired *t*-test, *$p<0.05$, **$p<0.01$ vs vehicle).

found jaw and body movements are the major causes for the fluctuation of fMRI signals [56]. Alternatively, Chen et al. have proposed another approach of integrating an MRI-compatible chair, head-post holder, and volume coil for awake imaging, where in-plane movements can be limited within 80 µm [37]. We have adopted the awake imaging apparatus developed by Andersen et al. [35] and used a custom-made NHP phased-array head coil that can be attached to the head-post for better signal-to-noise ratio (SNR). Without a dedicated NHP MRI scanner [37,56], we have successfully imaged animals in a sphinx position instead. Improved data acquisition and analysis methods have been also developed to enhance the sensitivity to detect targeted drug responses; for example, USPIO imaging contrast agents have been previously exploited to amplify signal changes [36,38] as well as advanced data analysis pipeline for motion correction [39].

To minimize the amount of stress during awake imaging, our study cohort has been trained over several months to acclimatize to the restrainer and scanner environment (see Fig. 1). Some animals showed signs of gradual adaptation to the training, as indicated by the decreased plasma cortisol concentration and behavioral scores (see Fig. 2). This finding is consistent with the results reported by Lee et al. [58], where a weekly decline in cortisol levels was observed in animals receiving chair training for a month. Cortisol levels were also measured in our study, as animals progressed to Phase 1b. We found no significant difference in cortisol concentrations measured at pre- and post- 90-minute training from the trained cohort, whilst in the untrained animals cortisol concentrations elevated significantly (see Fig 3), suggesting that trained animals have been acclimated to the restrainer.

It is noteworthy that in most awake imaging models, a head-post is surgically implanted for the purpose of head fixation. This invasive procedure is however not ideal since the head-post placement requires surgery and can become loose or even detach over time. While this method might be sub-optimal for a longitudinal study, alternative non-invasive approaches have been recently implemented [27,36]. For example, Shrihasam and his colleagues have developed a non-invasive vacuum helmet technique for imaging alert monkeys, and they found that the degrees of translational and rotational head motion during awake imaging are comparable to the same monkey's movements when restrained by a head-post [36]. Likewise, using the expandable foam in combination with a plastic helmet, Murnane et al. have shown the feasibility of imaging conscious monkeys under cocaine challenge without a head-post [27]. There are also disadvantages for this awake imaging approach. For example, awake training is time-consuming and often requires significant effort and resources to habituate the animal. For the current study, it took more than 10 months to complete the awake training protocol and only a subgroup of animals was suitable for the actual imaging study. Although the stress level can be alleviated by extensive training procedures, this factor cannot be completely eliminated.

To develop novel treatments for neurological diseases or psychiatric disorders, PET or single photon emission computed tomography (SPECT) imaging techniques have proved to be useful tools to confirm blood-brain barrier penetration and drug target engagement in the brain, and derived receptor occupancy–drug concentration curves can guide dose selection in clinical development [59,60]. Conversely, biological consequences of drug actions depicted by awake phMRI can offer complimentary pharmacodynamic biomarkers to PET/SPECT imaging. In light of the low success rate associated with the development of novel compounds to treat neurological diseases or psychiatric disorders, phMRI in alert, behaving NHP can serve as a translational imaging platform that affords pharmacodynamic or safety biomarkers, attributed to targeted mechanisms of action. While animal movement and stress during awake imaging increases the noise associated with this approach, the absence of unwanted anesthetic-drug interactions can outweigh efforts needed to overcome these technical hurdles. For the development of CNS compounds, this requirement can be particularly crucial to assess novel experimental therapeutics.

There are limitations for this current study. First, only four animals progressed to the actual imaging experiments and therefore inter-subject variability cannot be properly evaluated. Second, to fully evaluate the utility of this awake phMRI platform, test-retest study of buprenorphine infusion needs to be explored. Third, in the anesthetized imaging study, buprenorphine did not elicit significant changes in rCBV at brain areas with a high density of μ–opioid receptor (see Figure 5). This observation can be attributed to the level of anesthesia used. Previously, Tinker et al. have reported that the percentage volume of minimum alveolar concentration (MAC) of isoflurane in nonhuman primate is 1.28% and the maintaining dose for most applications is around 1.3× MAC (i.e. ~1.7%) [61], whereas 2% isoflurane in medical air was selected to anesthetize animals in our study. In combination with paralytics (e.g. vercuronium or mivacurium) or fentanyl, the feasibility of using a lower level of isoflurane (0.3%~1%) in fMRI studies has been demonstrated [62,63]. However, anesthesia protocols could vary among different studies, depending on the experimental design.

In summary, we have shown that, in awake NHP buprenorphine activated brain regions ascribed to high density of μ-opioid receptors, including caudate nucleus, putamen, thalamus, and cingulate cortex. More importantly, in conjunction with previous buprenorphine phMRI studies in conscious rats and humans, our results establish utility of buprenorphine phMRI across species. Further, based on a standard monkey brain atlas, we have established robust phMRI data and ROI analysis pipeline that allows determination of group-level brain activation patterns. Our results indicated that in the same animal, buprenorphine-induced rCBV changes in awake animals are significantly higher than those obtained under the anesthetized condition. Taken together, our data highlight the utility and importance of awake NHP imaging platform as a translational imaging biomarker for drug research.

## Acknowledgments

The authors wish to extend our gratitude to Marie A. Holahan and Fuqiang Zhao for insightful discussion. We would also like to thank Htoon Win, Myoe Lynn and Hamzah Isa for their technical support for this work.

## Author Contributions

Conceived and designed the experiments: SS DSW TR BH JLE CLC. Performed the experiments: SS ABMAA EM JDB CLC. Analyzed the data: SS ABMAA RB DF CLC. Wrote the paper: SS ABMAA CLC TR EM.

## References


1. Wise RG, Tracey I (2006) The role of fMRI in drug discovery. J Magn Reson Imaging 23: 862–876.
2. Borsook D, Becerra L, Hargreaves R (2006) A role for fMRI in optimizing CNS drug development. Nat Rev Drug Discov 5: 411–424.
3. Leslie RA, James MF (2000) Pharmacological magnetic resonance imaging: a new application for functional MRI. Trends Pharmacol Sci 21: 314–318.
4. Jenkins BG (2012) Pharmacologic magnetic resonance imaging (phMRI): imaging drug action in the brain. Neuroimage 62: 1072–1085.
5. Gozzi A, Schwarz A, Reese T, Bertani S, Crestan V, et al. (2006) Region-specific effects of nicotine on brain activity: a pharmacological MRI study in the drug-naive rat. Neuropsychopharmacology 31: 1690–1703.
6. Mueggler T, Baumann D, Rausch M, Rudin M (2001) Bicuculline-induced brain activation in mice detected by functional magnetic resonance imaging. Magn Reson Med 46: 292–298.
7. Chin CL, Tovcimak AE, Hradil VP, Seifert TR, Hollingsworth PR, et al. (2008) Differential effects of cannabinoid receptor agonists on regional brain activity using pharmacological MRI. Br J Pharmacol 153: 367–379.
8. Chen YC, Galpern WR, Brownell AL, Matthews RT, Bogdanov M, et al. (1997) Detection of dopaminergic neurotransmitter activity using pharmacologic MRI: correlation with PET, microdialysis, and behavioral data. Magn Reson Med 38: 389–398.
9. Schwarz AJ, Becerra L, Upadhyay J, Anderson J, Baumgartner R, et al. (2011) A procedural framework for good imaging practice in pharmacological fMRI studies applied to drug development #2: protocol optimization and best practices. Drug Discov Today 16: 671–682.
10. De Simoni S, Schwarz AJ, O'Daly OG, Marquand AF, Brittain C, et al. (2013) Test-retest reliability of the BOLD pharmacological MRI response to ketamine in healthy volunteers. Neuroimage 64: 75–90.
11. Wise RG, Williams P, Tracey I (2004) Using fMRI to quantify the time dependence of remifentanil analgesia in the human brain. Neuropsychopharmacology 29: 626–635.
12. Leppa M, Korvenoja A, Carlson S, Timonen P, Martinkauppi S, et al. (2006) Acute opioid effects on human brain as revealed by functional magnetic resonance imaging. NeuroImage 31: 661–669.
13. Austin VC, Blamire AM, Allers KA, Sharp T, Styles P, et al. (2005) Confounding effects of anesthesia on functional activation in rodent brain: a study of halothane and alpha-chloralose anesthesia. Neuroimage 24: 92–100.
14. Gozzi A, Schwarz A, Crestan V, Bifone A (2008) Drug-anaesthetic interaction in phMRI: the case of the psychotomimetic agent phencyclidine. Magn Reson Imaging 26: 999–1006.
15. Hodkinson DJ, de Groote C, McKie S, Deakin JF, Williams SR (2012) Differential Effects of Anaesthesia on the phMRI Response to Acute Ketamine Challenge. Br J Med Med Res 2: 373–385.
16. Ferris CF, Smerkers B, Kulkarni P, Caffrey M, Afacan O, et al. (2011) Functional magnetic resonance imaging in awake animals. Rev Neurosci 22: 665–674.

17. Liu JV, Hirano Y, Nascimento GC, Stefanovic B, Leopold DA, et al. (2013) fMRI in the awake marmoset: Somatosensory-evoked responses, functional connectivity, and comparison with propofol anesthesia. Neuroimage 78: 186–195.
18. Zhang Z, Andersen AH, Avison MJ, Gerhardt GA, Gash DM (2000) Functional MRI of apomorphine activation of the basal ganglia in awake rhesus monkeys. Brain Res 852: 290–296.
19. Chin CL, Pauly JR, Surber BW, Skoubis PD, McGaraughty S, et al. (2008) Pharmacological MRI in awake rats predicts selective binding of alpha4beta2 nicotinic receptors. Synapse 62: 159–168.
20. Lahti KM, Ferris CF, Li F, Sotak CH, King JA (1999) Comparison of evoked cortical activity in conscious and propofol-anesthetized rats using functional MRI. Magn Reson Med 41: 412–416.
21. Becerra L, Upadhyay J, Chang PC, Bishop J, Anderson J, et al. (2013) Parallel Buprenorphine phMRI Responses in Conscious Rodents and Healthy Human Subjects. J Pharmacol Exp Ther 345: 41–51.
22. Febo M, Segarra AC, Nair G, Schmidt K, Duong TQ, et al. (2005) The neural consequences of repeated cocaine exposure revealed by functional MRI in awake rats. Neuropsychopharmacology 30: 936–943.
23. Baker S, Chin CL, Basso AM, Fox GB, Marek GJ, et al. (2012) Xanomeline modulation of the blood oxygenation level-dependent signal in awake rats: development of pharmacological magnetic resonance imaging as a translatable pharmacodynamic biomarker for central activity and dose selection. J Pharmacol Exp Ther 341: 263–273.
24. Vanduffel W, Fize D, Mandeville JB, Nelissen K, Van Hecke P, et al. (2001) Visual motion processing investigated using contrast agent-enhanced fMRI in awake behaving monkeys. Neuron 32: 565–577.
25. Stefanacci L, Reber P, Costanza J, Wong E, Buxton R, et al. (1998) fMRI of monkey visual cortex. Neuron 20: 1051–1057.
26. Dubowitz DJ, Chen DY, Atkinson DJ, Grieve KL, Gillikin B, et al. (1998) Functional magnetic resonance imaging in macaque cortex. Neuroreport 9: 2213–2218.
27. Murnane KS, Howell LL (2010) Development of an apparatus and methodology for conducting functional magnetic resonance imaging (fMRI) with pharmacological stimuli in conscious rhesus monkeys. J Neurosci Methods 191: 11–20.
28. Mandeville JB, Choi JK, Jarraya B, Rosen BR, Jenkins BG, et al. (2011) FMRI of cocaine self-administration in macaques reveals functional inhibition of basal ganglia. Neuropsychopharmacology 36: 1187–1198.
29. McClure HM (1984) Nonhuman primate models for human disease. Adv Vet Sci Comp Med 28: 267–304.
30. Petrides M, Pandya DN (2002) Comparative cytoarchitectonic analysis of the human and the macaque ventrolateral prefrontal cortex and corticocortical connection patterns in the monkey. Eur J Neurosci 16: 291–310.
31. Nakahara K, Adachi Y, Osada T, Miyashita Y (2007) Exploring the neural basis of cognition: multi-modal links between human fMRI and macaque neurophysiology. Trends Cogn Sci 11: 84–92.
32. Mansour A, Khachaturian H, Lewis ME, Akil H, Watson SJ (1988) Anatomy of CNS opioid receptors. Trends Neurosci 11: 308–314.
33. Smith HR, Beveridge TJ, Porrino LJ (2006) Distribution of norepinephrine transporters in the non-human primate brain. Neuroscience 138: 703–714.
34. Reuning RH, Ashcraft SB, Wiley JN, Morrison BE (1989) Disposition and pharmacokinetics of naltrexone after intravenous and oral administration in rhesus monkeys. Drug Metab Dispos 17: 583–589.
35. Andersen AH, Zhang Z, Barber T, Rayens WS, Zhang J, et al. (2002) Functional MRI studies in awake rhesus monkeys: methodological and analytical strategies. J Neurosci Methods 118: 141–152.
36. Srihasam K, Sullivan K, Savage T, Livingstone MS (2010) Noninvasive functional MRI in alert monkeys. Neuroimage 51: 267–273.
37. Chen G, Wang F, Dillenburger BC, Friedman RM, Chen LM, et al. (2012) Functional magnetic resonance imaging of awake monkeys: some approaches for improving imaging quality. Magn Reson Imaging 30: 36–47.
38. Leite FP, Tsao D, Vanduffel W, Fize D, Sasaki Y, et al. (2002) Repeated fMRI using iron oxide contrast agent in awake, behaving macaques at 3 Tesla. NeuroImage 16: 283–294.
39. Stoewer S, Goense JB, Keliris GA, Bartels A, Logothetis NK, et al. (2011) Realignment strategies for awake-monkey fMRI data. Magn Reson Imaging 29: 1390–1400.
40. Sadee W, Rosenbaum JS, Herz A (1982) Buprenorphine: differential interaction with opiate receptor subtypes in vivo. J Pharmacol Exp Ther 223: 157–162.
41. Heel RC, Brogden RN, Speight TM, Avery GS (1979) Buprenorphine: a review of its pharmacological properties and therapeutic efficacy. Drugs 17: 81–110.
42. Lewis JW (1985) Buprenorphine. Drug Alcohol Depend 14: 363–372.
43. Upadhyay J, Anderson J, Schwarz AJ, Coimbra A, Baumgartner R, et al. (2011) Imaging Drugs with and without Clinical Analgesic Efficacy. Neuropsychopharmacology 36: 2659–2673.
44. Galynker I, Schlyer DJ, Dewey SL, Fowler JS, Logan J, et al. (1996) Opioid Receptor Imaging and Displacement Studies with [6-O-[11C]methyl] Buprenorphine in Baboon Brain. Nuclear Medicine & Biology 23: 325–331.
45. Greenwald MK, Johanson CE, Moody DE, Woods JH, Kilbourn MR, et al. (2003) Effects of buprenorphine maintenance dose on mu-opioid receptor availability, plasma concentrations, and antagonist blockade in heroin-dependent volunteers. Neuropsychopharmacology 28: 2000–2009.
46. Mandeville JB, Marota JJ, Kosofsky BE, Keltner JR, Weissleder R, et al. (1998) Dynamic functional imaging of relative cerebral blood volume during rat forepaw stimulation. Magn Reson Med 39: 615–624.
47. Frey S, Pandya DN, Chakravarty MM, Bailey L, Petrides M, et al. (2011) An MRI based average macaque monkey stereotaxic atlas and space (MNI monkey space). Neuroimage 55: 1435–1442.
48. Nunamaker EA, Halliday LC, Moody DE, Fang WB, Lindeblad M, et al. (2013) Pharmacokinetics of 2 formulations of buprenorphine in macaques (Macaca mulatta and Macaca fascicularis). J Am Assoc Lab Anim Sci 52: 48–56.
49. Wu EX, Tang H, Jensen JH (2004) Applications of ultrasmall superparamagnetic iron oxide contrast agents in the MR study of animal models. NMR Biomed 17: 478–483.
50. Andaluz A, Moll X, Abellan R, Ventura R, Carbo M, et al. (2009) Pharmacokinetics of buprenorphine after intravenous administration of clinical doses to dogs. Vet J 181: 299–304.
51. Jenkinson M, Beckmann CF, Behrens TE, Woolrich MW, Smith SM (2011) Fsl. Neuroimage.
52. Thrall M, Weiser G, Allison R, Campbell T, editors (2012) Veterinary hematology and clinical chemistry 2ed: John Wiely & Sons, Inc.
53. Pfeiffer A, Pasi A, Mehraein P, Herz A (1982) Opiate receptor binding sites in human brain. Brain Res 248: 87–96.
54. Mandeville JB, Marota JJ (1999) Vascular filters of functional MRI: spatial localization using BOLD and CBV contrast. Magn Reson Med 42: 591–598.
55. Shen Q, Ren H, Duong TQ (2008) CBF, BOLD, CBV, and CMRO(2) fMRI signal temporal dynamics at 500-msec resolution. J Magn Reson Imaging 27: 599–606.
56. Keliris GA, Shmuel A, Ku SP, Pfeuffer J, Oeltermann A, et al. (2007) Robust controlled functional MRI in alert monkeys at high magnetic field: effects of jaw and body movements. Neuroimage 36: 550–570.
57. Pinsk MA, Moore T, Richter MC, Gross CG, Kastner S (2005) Methods for functional magnetic resonance imaging in normal and lesioned behaving monkeys. J Neurosci Methods 143: 179–195.
58. Lee JI, Shin JS, Lee JE, Jung WY, Lee G, et al. (2012) Changes of N/L ratio and cortisol levels associated with experimental training in untrained rhesus macaques. J Med Primatol 42: 10–14.
59. Wong DF, Tauscher J, Grunder G (2009) The role of imaging in proof of concept for CNS drug discovery and development. Neuropsychopharmacology 34: 187–203.
60. Hargreaves RJ (2008) The role of molecular imaging in drug discovery and development. Clin Pharmacol Ther 83: 349–353.
61. Fish R, Danneman PJ, Brown M, Karas A (2011) Anesthesia and Analgesia in Laboratory Animals. Elsevier Science: 350.
62. Logothetis NK, Pauls J, Augath M, Trinath T, Oeltermann A (2001) Neurophysiological investigation of the basis of the fMRI signal. Nature 412: 150–157.
63. Wey HY, Li J, Szabo CA, Fox PT, Leland MM, et al. (2010) BOLD fMRI of visual and somatosensory-motor stimulations in baboons. Neuroimage 52: 1420–1427.

# 20

# Positive End-Expiratory Pressure and Variable Ventilation in Lung-Healthy Rats under General Anesthesia

**Luciana M. Camilo[1], Mariana B. Ávila[1], Luis Felipe S. Cruz[1], Gabriel C. M. Ribeiro[2], Peter M. Spieth[3], Andreas A. Reske[4], Marcelo Amato[5], Antonio Giannella-Neto[2], Walter A. Zin[1], Alysson R. Carvalho[1,2]***

**1** Laboratory of Respiration Physiology, Carlos Chagas Filho Institute of Biophysics, Universidade Federal do Rio de Janeiro, Rio de Janeiro, Brazil, **2** Laboratory of Pulmonary Engineering, Biomedical Engineering Program, Alberto Luis Coimbra Institute of Post-Graduation and Research in Engineering, Universidade Federal do Rio de Janeiro, Rio de Janeiro, Brazil, **3** Pulmonary Engineering Group, Department of Anesthesiology and Intensive Care Medicine, Technische Universität Dresden, Germany, **4** Department of Anesthesiology and Intensive Care Medicine, University of Leipzig, Leipzig, Germany, **5** Cardio-Pulmonary Department, Pulmonary Division, Hospital das Clínicas, Universidade de São Paulo, São Paulo, Brazil

## Abstract

***Objectives:*** Variable ventilation (VV) seems to improve respiratory function in acute lung injury and may be combined with positive end-expiratory pressure (PEEP) in order to protect the lungs even in healthy subjects. We hypothesized that VV in combination with moderate levels of PEEP reduce the deterioration of pulmonary function related to general anesthesia. Hence, we aimed at evaluating the alveolar stability and lung protection of the combination of VV at different PEEP levels.

***Design:*** Randomized experimental study.

***Setting:*** Animal research facility.

***Subjects:*** Forty-nine male Wistar rats (200–270 g).

***Interventions:*** Animals were ventilated during 2 hours with protective low tidal volume ($V_T$) in volume control ventilation (VCV) or VV and PEEP adjusted at the level of minimum respiratory system elastance (Ers), obtained during a decremental PEEP trial subsequent to a recruitment maneuver, and 2 $cmH_2O$ above or below of this level.

***Measurements and Main Results:*** Ers, gas exchange and hemodynamic variables were measured. Cytokines were determined in lung homogenate and plasma samples and left lung was used for histologic analysis and diffuse alveolar damage scoring. A progressive time-dependent increase in Ers was observed independent on ventilatory mode or PEEP level. Despite of that, the rate of increase of Ers and lung tissue IL-1 beta concentration were significantly lower in VV than in VCV at the level of the PEEP of minimum Ers. A significant increase in lung tissue cytokines (IL-6, IL-1 beta, CINC-1 and TNF-alpha) as well as a ventral to dorsal and cranial to caudal reduction in aeration was observed in all ventilated rats with no significant differences among groups.

***Conclusions:*** VV combined with PEEP adjusted at the level of the PEEP of minimal Ers seemed to better prevent anesthesia-induced atelectasis and might improve lung protection throughout general anesthesia.

**Editor:** Jorge IF Salluh, D'or Institute of Research and Education, Brazil

**Funding:** The work was supported by grants from the Brazilian Council for Scientific and Technological Development (CNPq) and Carlos Chagas Filho Rio de Janeiro State Research Supporting Foundation (FAPERJ). The funders had no role in study design, data collection and analysis, decision to publish, or preparation of the manuscript.

**Competing Interests:** The authors have declared that no competing interests exist.

* Email: acarvalho@biof.ufrj.br

## Introduction

Pulmonary atelectasis is a common complication during general anesthesia [1]. Anesthesia-induced atelectasis causes an increase in intrapulmonary shunt [2] and highly correlates with the progressive reduction in lung compliance and oxygenation impairment throughout surgery [1,3]. Recruitment maneuvers have been used to open up atelectatic areas but their beneficial effects seemed to be just transitory and atelectasis rapidly recurs if no positive end-expiratory pressure (PEEP) is applied [4–8].

High levels of PEEP are often associated with decreased venous return [9,10], increased pulmonary vascular resistance, decreased

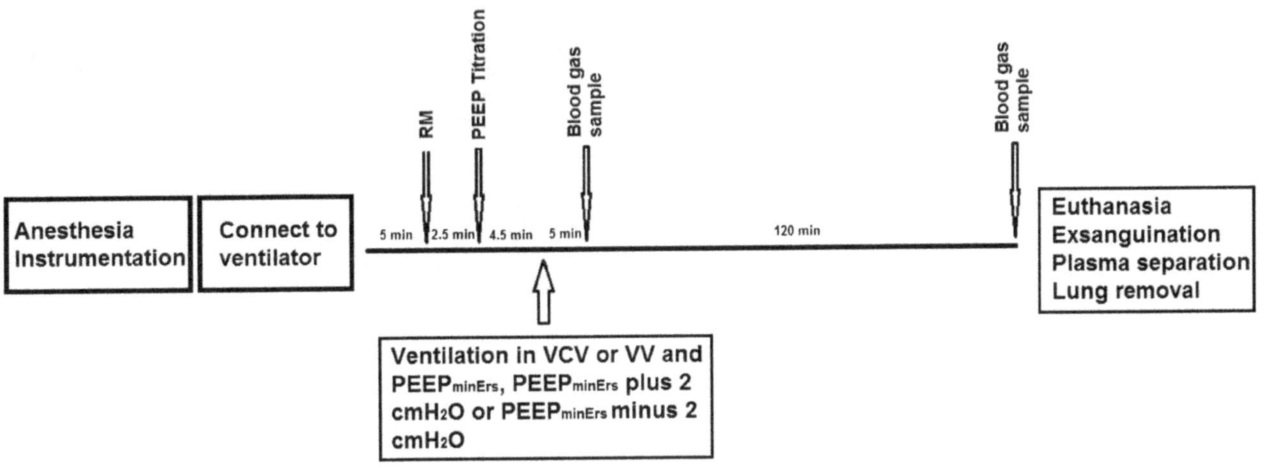


**Figure 1. Time course of respiratory system elastance and slope. A.** Respiratory system elastance (Ers) throughout ventilation protocols. Red points are minute-averaged values of Ers and its fitted line (blue line). **B.** Slope of Ers calculated by angular coefficient of the groups: VCV_E (volume-controlled mode and $PEEP_{minErs}$; n = 6), VCV_E+2 (volume-controlled mode and $PEEP_{minErs}$ plus 2 $cmH_2O$; n = 6), VCV_E-2 (volume-controlled mode and $PEEP_{minErs}$ minus 2 $cmH_2O$; n = 6), VV_E (variable ventilation and $PEEP_{minErs}$; n = 6), VV_E+2 (variable ventilation and $PEEP_{minErs}$ plus 2 $cmH_2O$; n = 5), VV_E-2 (variable ventilation and $PEEP_{minErs}$ minus 2 $cmH_2O$; n = 6). Effect of ventilator mode, PEEP and interaction were tested with two-way ANOVA followed by Tukey post-hoc. Time effect was tested by generalized linear model. Statistical significance was accepted at $p<0.05$. *$p<0.05$.

left ventricular compliance [11,12], cardiac output and systemic oxygen delivery [13,14], and still may result in lung overdistension with increased dead space ventilation and lung rupture [15–18]. In this line, the use of the so called open-lung PEEP [19] is still a challenge at the operating room routine [20,21].

During controlled mechanical ventilation the breathing pattern is monotonous (tidal volume and respiratory rate are constant) and highly different from that observed in spontaneously breathing healthy subjects, which have an important intrinsic variability on tidal volume ($V_T$) and respiratory rate (RR) [22–26]. Indeed, the addition of an extrinsic variability on ventilatory breathing pattern during mechanical ventilation, commonly referred to as variable ventilation (VV) [23,26], appears to contribute to sustained improvement in gas exchange with reduced mechanical stress in several experimental models of acute lung injury [23,27–29] and in lung-healthy patients during general anesthesia [30,31]. Furthermore, the release of pro-inflammatory mediators (IL-6, IL-8, TNF-alpha) is significantly less in VV than in controlled ventilation [26,29,32].

Taking together, the combination of VV and PEEP may yield a better pulmonary function than protective low $V_T$ strategies with comparable PEEP values [26]. We speculate that association VV and PEEP may result in increased alveolar stability, improved pulmonary function and attenuated inflammatory response in mechanically ventilated lung-healthy rats. Hence, we aimed at evaluating the physiological effects of the combination of VV and different levels of PEEP, adjusted after a recruitment maneuver and a decremental PEEP trial, on the improvement of alveolar stability and lung protection.

## Materials and Methods

Forty-nine male Wistar rats (200–270 g) were used in the present study. All animals received humane care in compliance with the "Principles of Laboratory Animal Care" formulated by the National Society for Medical Research and the "Guiding Principles in the Care and Use of Animals" approved by the Council of the American Physiological Society, USA. The experimental protocol was approved by the Ethics Committee on the Use of Animals, Health Sciences Centre, Federal University of Rio de Janeiro (approval number: IBCCF 103).

All animals were sedated (diazepam 5 mg, ip), anesthetized (ketamine, 60 mg/kg, ip), and intubated with a snugly fitting cannula (1.5 mm ID). Animals were placed in supine position on a surgical table and a catheter (18 G, Arrow International, USA) was inserted into the right carotid artery for continuous arterial pressure (AP) monitoring and blood sampling. At the end of surgical instrumentation, animals were paralyzed (pancuronium bromide, 0.3 mg/kg, iv) and mechanically ventilated (Inspira ASV, Harvard Apparatus, Holliston, MA, USA) using a volume controlled ventilation (VCV) mode, with a tidal volume ($V_T$) of 6 mL/kg, respiratory rate (RR) of 90 breaths/min, inspiratory to expiratory time ratio (I:E) of 1:2, positive end-expiratory pressure (PEEP) of 0 $cmH_2O$ and fraction of inspired oxygen of 0.5 (Baseline).

### Ventilation Protocol

After 5 minutes of stabilization period under baseline settings, lungs were recruited by increasing PEEP from 0 to 3, 6, 7 and 8 $cmH_2O$, 30 seconds per step. Just afterwards, PEEP was progressively reduced from 8 to 0 $cmH_2O$, in steps of 1 $cmH_2O$ for 30 s per step and the PEEP of minimum respiratory system elastance ($PEEP_{minErs}$) was determined.

To investigate the physiological effects of each ventilation strategy (VCV or VV) combined with 3 different levels of PEEP, ventilation lasted 2 hours with the same baseline settings but with: 1) VCV or VV with mean $V_T$ of 6 mL/kg and PEEP adjusted at the $PEEP_{minErs}$ (VCV_E or VV_E, respectively n = 7 per group); 2) VCV or VV with PEEP adjusted at the $PEEP_{minErs}$ plus 2 $cmH_2O$ (VCV_E+2 or VV_E+2, respectively n = 7 per group); and 3) VCV or VV with PEEP adjusted at the $PEEP_{minErs}$ minus 2 $cmH_2O$ (VCV_E-2 or VV_E-2, respectively n = 7 per group).

Fig. 1 illustrates the time course of the experimental protocol. Seven animals were surgically instrumented and immediately sacrificed (Fig. 1) to be used as controls for protein assays and histology.

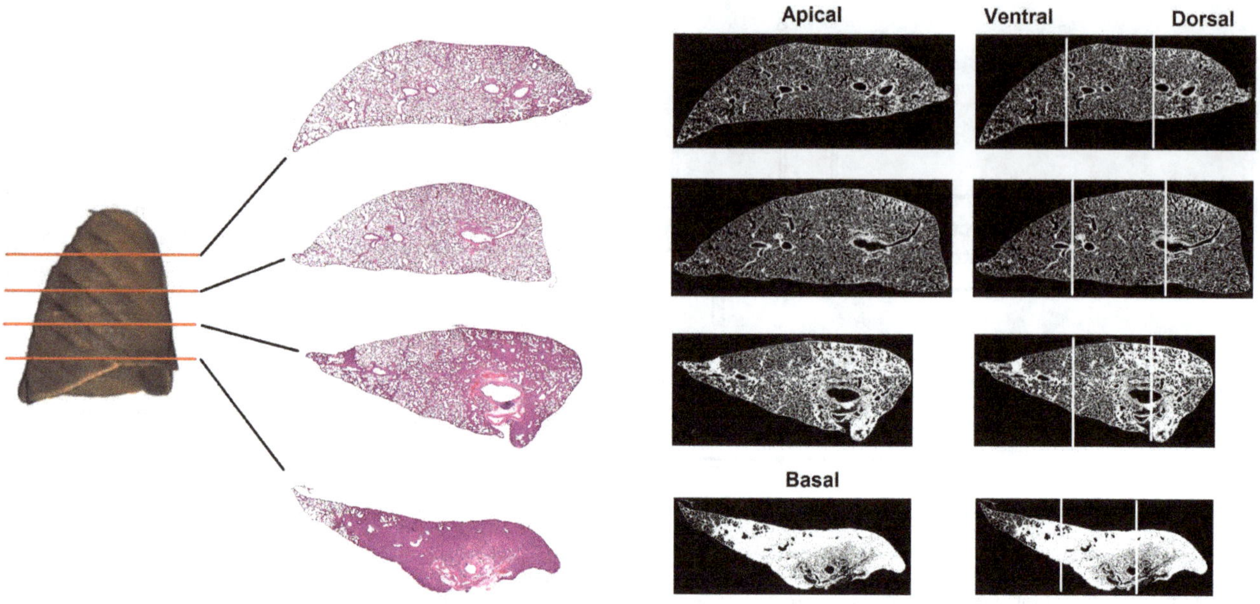


**Figure 2. Air fraction obtained by histology images.** Air fraction analysis of apex and base (A) and ventral and dorsal lung areas (B) in the groups: VCV_E (volume-controlled mode and $PEEP_{minErs}$; n = 6), VCV_E+2 (volume-controlled mode and $PEEP_{minErs}$ plus 2 $cmH_2O$; n = 6), VCV_E-2 (volume-controlled mode and $PEEP_{minErs}$ minus 2 $cmH_2O$; n = 6), VV_E (variable ventilation and $PEEP_{minErs}$; n = 6), VV_E+2 (variable ventilation and $PEEP_{minErs}$ plus 2 $cmH_2O$; n = 5), VV_E-2 (variable ventilation and $PEEP_{minErs}$ minus 2 $cmH_2O$; n = 6). Ventilatory mode and PEEP effects were tested with two-way ANOVA followed by Tukey post hoc. t test was used to detect differences between ventilated and non-ventilated groups and then correction by comparisons ensued. Statistical significance was accepted at $p<0.05$. *$p<0.05$.

## Variable Ventilation Design

VV mode was designed to provide different range of $V_T$ adjusted to achieve a desired target variability level. The widths of the $V_T$ distributions were set by assigning a random sequence of $V_T$ values taken from a Gaussian probability distribution falling between ±10% of the mean $V_T$ (6 mL/kg). A sequence of 5400 values of $V_T$ was applied during the first hour and repeated in the second hour of the protocol. Thus, the measured mean and ± one SD was 5.9±0.8 mL/kg. RR was kept constant throughout the protocol as previously proposed [26].

## Data Acquisition and Processing

Airway pressure (Paw) and flow (F) were continuously recorded using a heated-controlled pneumotachograph (Hans Rudolph model 8430B, Shawnee, KS, USA) connected between the endotracheal tube (ETT) and a Y-piece of the ventilatory circuit. The pneumotachograph was connected to a differential pressure transducer for Paw (105124-9, SCIREQ, Montreal, QC, Canada) and flow (105159-6, SCIREQ, Montreal, QC, Canada) measurements. Arterial blood pressure as well as the electrocardiogram was continuously acquired with a Multi-parameter physiologic monitor (LifeWindow LW6000 Digicare Biomedical Technology, Boynton Beach, FL, USA). Paw and flow signals were low-pass filtered at 30 Hz and all signals were then digitized at 1000 Hz using a 16-bit AD converter (NI-6009, National Instruments, Austin, TX, USA) and recorded with a built-purpose routine (Data Acquisition System, DAS) written in LabVIEW (National Instruments, Austin, TX, USA). Volume was calculated by numerical integration of flow. All transducers were calibrated before the experiments.

During the entire protocol, respiratory system elastance (Ers) was estimated in real-time by means of the recursive least square method (5 s forgetting time constant) considering the linear single-compartment model (Equation 1) in a subroutine of the DAS software.

$$Paw(t) = Rrs \cdot F(t) + Ers \cdot V(t) + EEP \tag{1}$$

Where Rrs and Ers represent the resistance and elastance of the respiratory system, respectively, and EEP is the total end-expiratory pressure at null volume (V) and flow (F).

After the experiments, all mechanical parameters were also calculated offline on a breath-by-breath basis for the whole 120 minutes of ventilation period. For such purpose the least square method was applied to Equation 1 and a routine (Mecanica) written in MATLAB (The Mathworks Inc., Natick, MA, USA) was employed. The mean Ers was calculated for every 1-minute period, and the temporal dynamics of Ers was assessed by the slope (a) of a linear function described by Ers (t) = a.t+b; where t is time in minutes and b is the Ers at the beginning of ventilation protocols.

Mean arterial pressure (MAP) was also calculated offline as the mean value of arterial pressure beat-by-beat throughout the experimental protocols.

Arterial blood samples were anaerobically collected and immediately processed to measured $PaO_2$, $PaCO_2$ and pH (i-STAT, Abbott Laboratories, Abbott Park, IL, USA), at 5 (M5) and 120 minutes (M120) of the ventilation protocols.

## Digital histology image acquire and processing

At the end of the experimental protocol, mechanical ventilation was returned to baseline settings. After heparinization the animals were euthanized by sectioning the abdominal vena cava. The trachea was clamped at end-expiration and the lungs were extracted *en bloc*, the right and left lungs were isolated and fixed

**Table 1.** Ventilatory and hemodynamic variables.

| Group | VCV_E-2 | VV_E-2 | VCV_E | VV_E | VCV_E+2 | VV_E+2 | Mode | PEEP | Interaction |
|---|---|---|---|---|---|---|---|---|---|
| Ppeak ($cmH_2O$) | 11±1.6 | 12±1.3 | 14±0.5 | 13±1.3 | 15±0.8 | 14±1.3 | ns | ** | ns |
| Pmean ($cmH_2O$) | 5±0.8 | 5±0.7 | 6±0.6 | 6±0.7 | 9±0.6 | 8±0.7 | ns | ** | ns |
| PEEP ($cmH_2O$) | [1–2] | [1–2] | [3–4] | [3–4] | [5–7] | [5–6] | ns | ** | ns |
| Mean $V_T$ (mL/kg) | 5.8±0.2 | 6.1±0.7 | 5.5±0.3 | 5.7±0.2 | 5.6±0.4 | 6.0±1.1 | ns | ns | ns |
| RR (bpm) | 84±0.6 | 84±0.6 | 84±1.4 | 84±0.2 | 84±0.4 | 84±0.2 | ns | ns | ns |
| $CVV_T$ (%) | 1±0.2 | 8±1.0 | 2±0.5 | 8±0.4 | 1±0.3 | 10±3.3 | ** | ns | ns |
| MAP (mmHg) | 110±15 | 120±21 | 101±28 | 97±23 | 118±24 | 115±19 | ns | ns | ns |
| HR (bpm) | 410±65 | 389±38 | 383±68 | 406±32 | 402±70 | 393±57 | ns | ns | ns |

Values are mean ± SD from initial 5 minutes of ventilation. PEEP values are given as range (minimum and maximum). Definition of abbreviations: VCV_E = volume-controlled mode and $PEEP_{minErs}$; VCV_E+2 = volume-controlled mode and $PEEP_{minErs}$ plus 2 $cmH_2O$; VCV_E-2 = volume-controlled mode and $PEEP_{minErs}$ minus 2 $cmH_2O$; VV_E = variable ventilation and $PEEP_{minErs}$; VV_E+2 = variable ventilation and $PEEP_{minErs}$ plus 2 $cmH_2O$; VV_E-2 = variable ventilation and $PEEP_{minErs}$ minus 2 $cmH_2O$; BW = body weight; Ppeak = peak airway pressure; Pmean = mean airway pressure; PEEP = positive end-expiratory pressure; $V_T$ = tidal volume; RR = respiratory rate; CVVT = tidal volume coefficient of variation; MAP = mean arterial pressure; HR = heart rate. Differences among groups were tested with two-way ANOVA. Statistical significance was accepted at p<0.05. **p<0.0001, ns: non-significant.

in formaldehyde 10% in Millonig's phosphate buffer (100 ml HCHO, 900 ml H2O, 18.6 g NaH2PO4, and 4.2 NaOH) and subsequently embedded in paraffin. 4-µm thick transversal slices were cut from the apex to the base of the left lung and stained with hematoxylin-eosin.

The histologic lung slices were then digitized (3DHistech Panoramic Scan, Budapest, Hungary) and images were processed using a routine written in MATLAB (MathWorks, Inc., Natick, MA, USA) in order to quantify the fraction of air in each specimen. The specimen images were converted to binary images, the total specimen area was computed and the relative proportion between the amount of parenchyma, edema or infiltration (presented in white color) and air (presented in black) were determined in each specimen (Fig. 2).

Diffuse alveolar damage (DAD) was evaluated using an histopathological scoring system by an expert blinded to the [33]. Briefly, five typical features of DAD were evaluated, according to their extent and severity. Single features, namely alveolar edema, interstitial edema, inflammatory infiltration, hemorrhage and micro-atelectasis were scored ranging from 0–9 and the cumulative DAD score, ranging from 0–45, was calculated by summarizing the single score features.

## Protein assays

The right lung homogenates and plasma samples collected at the end of ventilation protocols were used for the assessment of pro-inflammatory (TNF-α, IL-1β, IL-6, CINC-1) mediators with the ELISA technique, with high sensitivity kits (R&D Systems Inc., Minneapolis, MN, USA) according to the manufacturer's instructions.

## Statistical analysis

Statistical analysis was performed with SigmaPlot 11 (Systat, Chicago, IL, USA). The normality of the data (Kolmogorov-Smirnov test with Lilliefors correction) and the homogeneity of variances (Levene median test) were tested. Then, Two-way ANOVA (mode and PEEP and their interactions as independent factors) was used. For *post-hoc* analyses, we used Tukey pairwise comparison. To compare non-ventilated and ventilated groups, the t-test was performed followed by the Bonferroni multiple comparison correction. A general linear model for repeated measures was used to evaluate the influence of time on deterioration of Ers throughout each ventilation protocol. All tests considered a critical $p<0.05$.

# Results

Ventilatory and hemodynamic data are shown in Table 1. Tidal volume ($V_T$), respiratory rate (RR), mean arterial pressure (MAP) and heart rate (HR) did not differ among groups. $PEEP_{minErs}$, determined during the decremental PEEP trial, did not differ among groups, ranging between 3 to 5 $cmH_2O$. The coefficient of variation of $V_T$ was significantly higher, as expected, in VV groups compared to VCV (8.5±0.5% *vs* 1.6±0.6%, respectively; p<0.001). Mean airway pressure (Pmean), peak airway pressure (Ppeak) and positive end-expiratory pressure (PEEP) were significantly different among PEEP settings (p< 0.0001).

The dynamics of Ers in each animal at each ventilation protocol is represented in Figure 3A. In all groups, Ers depended on time (p<0.0001) and always increased throughout ventilation period. The rate of change of Ers(t) (slope) clearly decreased with PEEP both in VCV or VV (p<0.001). However, Ers(t) slope in the VV mode and $PEEP_{minErs}$ was significantly lower than in VCV

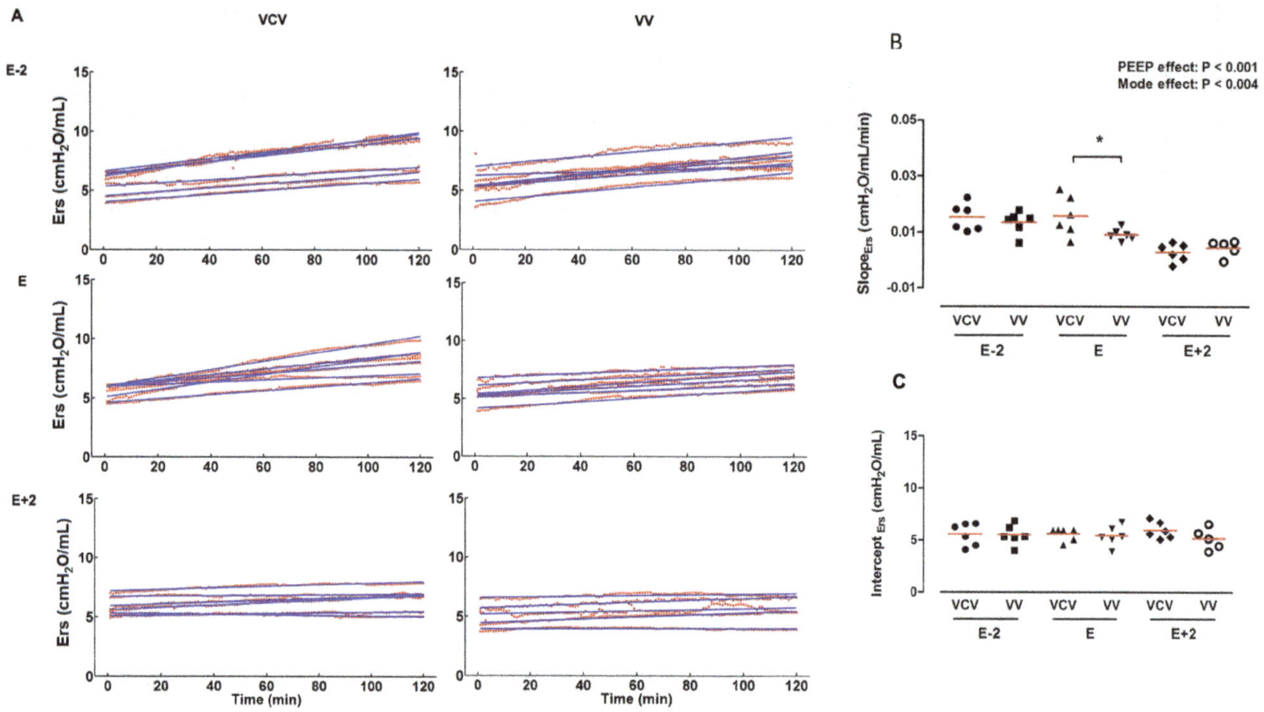

**Figure 3. Lung cytokines.** Lung tissue concentration of TNF-α (A), IL-6 (B), CINC-1(C) and IL-1β(D) in the groups: VCV_E (volume-controlled mode and $PEEP_{minErs}$; n=6), VCV_E+2 (volume-controlled mode and $PEEP_{minErs}$ plus 2 $cmH_2O$; n=6), VCV_E-2 (volume-controlled mode and $PEEP_{minErs}$ minus 2 $cmH_2O$; n=6), VV_E (variable ventilation and $PEEP_{minErs}$; n=6), VV_E+2 (variable ventilation and $PEEP_{minErs}$ plus 2 $cmH_2O$; n=5), VV_E-2 (variable ventilation and $PEEP_{minErs}$ minus 2 $cmH_2O$; n=6). Red lines represent mean values. Ventilatory mode and PEEP effects were tested with two-way ANOVA followed by Tukey post hoc. T-test was used to detect differences between ventilated and non-ventilated groups and then correction by multiple comparison. Statistical significance was accepted at $p<0.05$. *$p<0.05$.

(0.016±0.007 vs 0.009±0.002 $cmH_2O/L/min$, respectively; $p<0.001$), thus suggesting better Ers stability (Fig. 3B).

Oxygenation and gas exchange data are shown in Table 2. $PaO_2/FiO_2$, $PaCO_2$ and pH did not differ either among groups or with PEEP, ventilatory mode and time. All mechanically ventilated animals presented a significant reduction in the air fraction in dorsal and basal regions, which means that collapse, edema or consolidation are concentrated in these areas, independently of ventilatory mode or PEEP level (Fig. 4A). Additionally,

**Table 2.** Gas exchange.

| Group | Time | pH | $PaO_2/FiO_2$ | $PaCO_2$ (mmHg) |
|---|---|---|---|---|
| VCV_E-2 | 5 min | 7.27±0.05 | 345±117 | 58±12 |
| | 120 min | 7.25±0.06 | 395±144 | 56±7 |
| VV_E-2 | 5 min | 7.34±0.03 | 297±64 | 47±6 |
| | 120 min | 7.30±0.05 | 367±53 | 54±10 |
| VCV_E | 5 min | 7.32±0.03 | 270±122 | 49±10 |
| | 120 min | 7.24±0.04 | 276±126 | 55±8 |
| VV_E | 5 min | 7.30±0.02 | 319±52 | 56±5 |
| | 120 min | 7.23±0.06 | 370±68 | 58±10 |
| VCV_E+2 | 5 min | 7.26±0.04 | 348±127 | 60±6 |
| | 120 min | 7.20±0.06 | 420±119 | 58±8 |
| VV_E+2 | 5 min | 7.30±0.04 | 283±63 | 54±8 |
| | 120 min | 7.23±0.07 | 294±127 | 52±20 |

Values are expressed by mean ± SD. Definition of abbreviation: VCV_E: volume-controlled mode and $PEEP_{minEr}$; VCV_E+2: volume-controlled mode and $PEEP_{minErs}$ plus 2 $cmH_2O$; VCV_E-2: volume-controlled mode and $PEEP_{minErs}$ minus 2 $cmH_2O$; VV_E: variable ventilation and $PEEP_{minErs}$; VV_E+2: variable ventilation and $PEEP_{minErs}$ plus 2 $cmH_2O$; VV_E-2: variable ventilation and $PEEP_{minErs}$ minus 2 $cmH_2O$. Differences between groups were tested with Two-way ANOVA. Statistical significance was accepted at $p<0.05$.

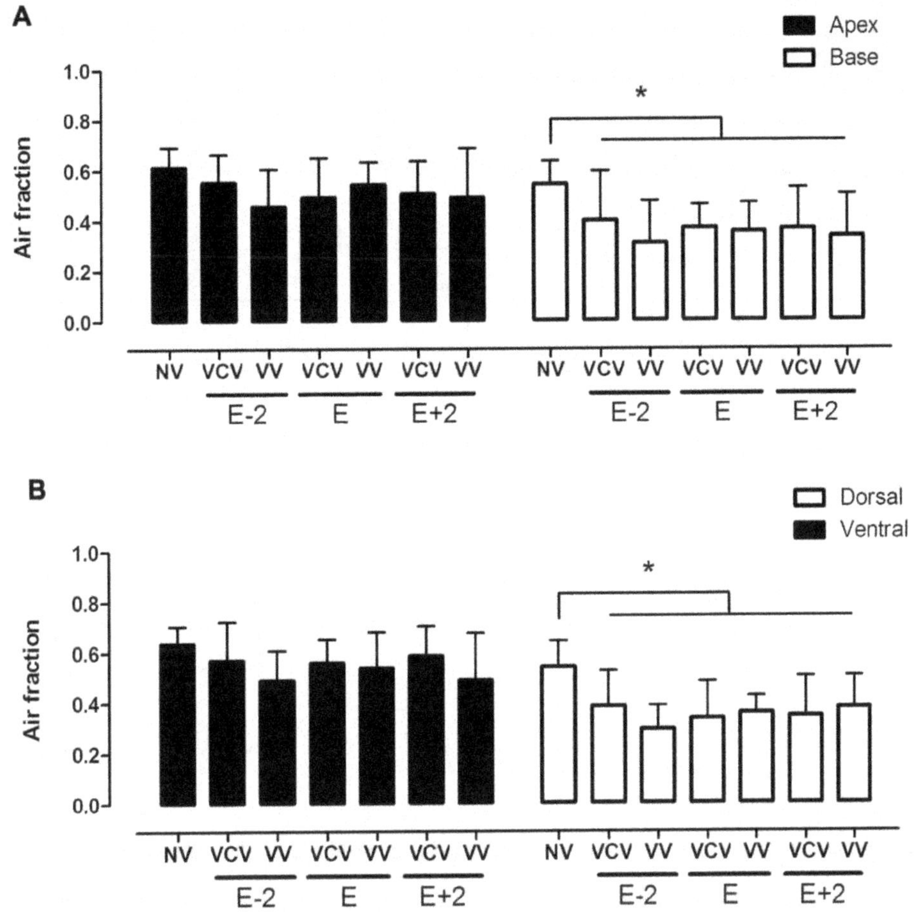


**Figure 4. Plasmatic cytokines.** Plasmatic concentration of TNF-α (A), IL-6 (B), CINC-1(C) and IL-1β (D) ) in the groups: VCV_E (volume-controlled mode and $PEEP_{minErs}$; n = 6), VCV_E+2 (volume-controlled mode and $PEEP_{minErs}$ plus 2 $cmH_2O$; n = 6), VCV_E-2 (volume-controlled mode and $PEEP_{minErs}$ minus 2 $cmH_2O$; n = 6), VV_E (variable ventilation and $PEEP_{minErs}$; n = 6), VV_E+2 (variable ventilation and $PEEP_{minErs}$ plus 2 $cmH_2O$; n = 5), VV_E-2 (variable ventilation and $PEEP_{minErs}$ minus 2 $cmH_2O$; n = 6). Red lines represent mean values. Ventilatory mode and PEEP effects were tested with two-way ANOVA followed by Tukey post hoc. T-test was used to detect differences between ventilated and non-ventilated groups and then correction by multiple comparison. Statistical significance was accepted at $p<0.05$. *$p<0.05$.

no significant differences were observed in the cumulated diffuse alveolar damage score among groups (Fig. 5).

The concentrations of lung tissue pro-inflammatory interleukins were higher in ventilated groups than in non-ventilated controls (Fig. 6). At the level of $PEEP_{minErs}$, VV had significant less IL-1β than VCV (177±96 vs 424±76 pg/mg, respectively; $p<0.001$).

Plasmatic cytokines levels are presented in Figure 7. TNF-α and IL-6 concentration were similar among groups (Figs. 7A to D). We observed that CINC-1 levels were uniformly higher in ventilated groups than in non-ventilated controls (Fig. 7C) and IL-6 was lower in VV than in VCV at E-2 and E+2 PEEPs.

## Discussion

Patients under general anesthesia develop a progressive deterioration of lung function [34], with impaired oxygenation and lung compliance [3,7]. Anesthesia-induced atelectasis might create a hazardous mechanical stress concentration in the neighborhood of atelectatic regions [35]. Such stress can predispose epithelial disruption and loss of function of the alveolar-capillary barrier leading to increased epithelial permeability. As a consequence, alveolar edema that dilutes and/or inactivates surfactant may further aggravate atelectasis [36].

Mechanical ventilation at the operating room has aimed at optimizing gas exchange in spite of lung protection [37]. Protective ventilatory strategies have just recently been applied to general anesthesia in lung-healthy patients [21,38]. Most often, high tidal volumes and low or even no PEEP [39] associated with high inspiratory oxygen fraction are used [7,40]. Even if airway pressure is limited, such ventilatory strategy might generate tidal hyperinflation of previously normally aerated areas (volutrauma), cyclic alveoli and small airways derecruitment (atelectrauma), and increase the levels of local proinflammatory mediators without ultrastructural damage (biotrauma) [41].

Minimization of injurious mechanical forces is the main target of protective ventilatory strategies that help to avoid lung collapse and overdistension by the use of low $V_T$, limitation of the plateau pressure, PEEP, and recruitment maneuvers. However, even during protective low $V_T$ strategies, injurious mechanical stress can derive from concentration of stress in the interface between atelectatic and aerated regions [35], propagation of air/fluid interfaces in the airway producing injury on the bronchiolar epithelium [42], and energy release by the rupture of liquid bridges during airway reopening [43].

In the present study, we hypothesized that the combination of a moderate PEEP [19] and VV can be useful at the scenario of

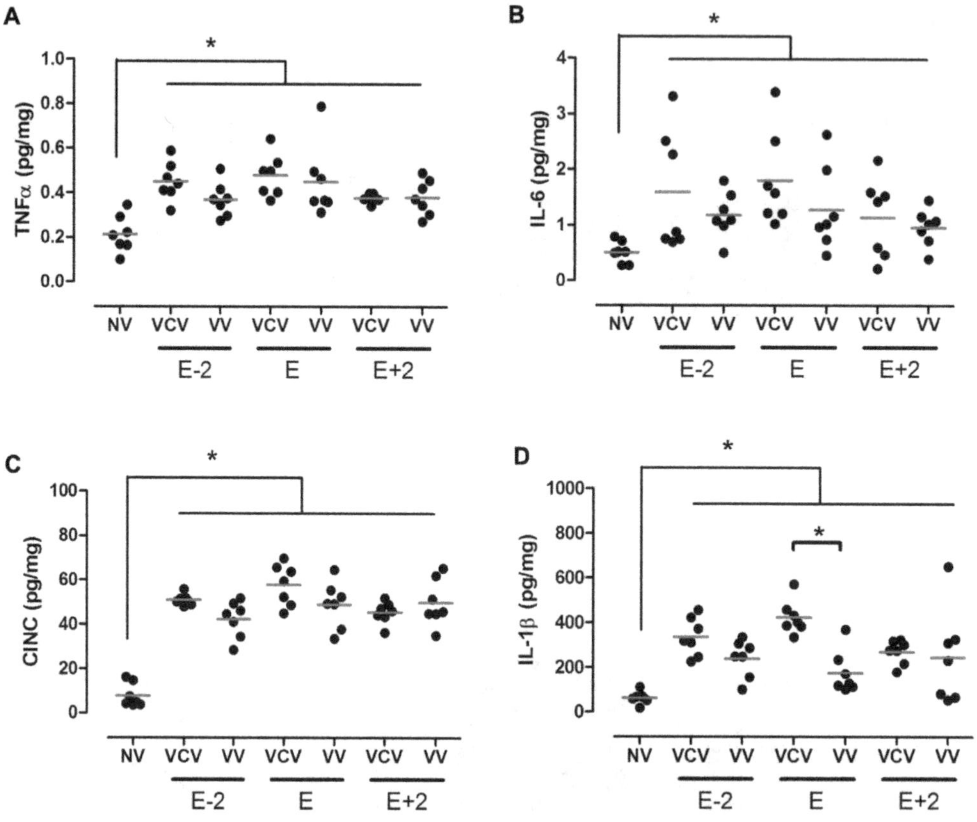


**Figure 5. Diffuse alveolar damage score.** Score of 0–9 to alveolar edema (A), interstitial edema (B), hemorrhage (C), inflammation (D), atelectasis (E) and the cumulative total score in the groups: VCV_E (volume-controlled mode and $PEEP_{minErs}$; n = 6), VCV_E+2 (volume-controlled mode and $PEEP_{minErs}$ plus 2 $cmH_2O$; n = 6), VCV_E-2 (volume-controlled mode and $PEEP_{minErs}$ minus 2 $cmH_2O$; n = 6), VV_E (variable ventilation and $PEEP_{minErs}$; n = 6), VV_E+2 (variable ventilation and $PEEP_{minErs}$ plus 2 $cmH_2O$; n = 5), VV_E-2 (variable ventilation and $PEEP_{minErs}$ minus 2 $cmH_2O$; n = 6). Red lines represent mean values. Ventilatory mode and PEEP effects were tested with two-way ANOVA followed by Tukey post hoc. T-test was used to detect differences between ventilated and non-ventilated groups and then correction by multiple comparison. Statistical significance was accepted at $p < 0.05$. *$p < 0.05$.

general anesthesia as an alternative to ventilatory strategies associated with high PEEP levels.

Our main findings were: 1) a progressive increase in Ers independent of ventilatory mode or PEEP was observed in lung-healthy rats during general anesthesia and muscle paralysis; 2) the rates of rise in Ers as well as lung tissue IL-1β concentration were significantly lower when VV was combined with the PEEP adjusted at the level of minimum Ers; 3) the same rate of increase in Ers observed during VV and PEEP of minimum Ers could only be achieved with higher levels of PEEP in the VCV_E+2 group; 4) even with a protective low-$V_T$ strategy all ventilated animals presented higher levels of pro-inflammatory cytokines in lung tissue samples, independently of ventilatory mode and PEEP level, than non-ventilated animals.

A substantial increase in Ers was observed in all animals, suggesting a progressive alveolar derecruitment induced by anesthesia (Figure 3-A, -B, and -C), as previously suggested [44,45]. Fairly higher levels of PEEP, ranging from 5 to 7 $cmH_2O$, were required to minimize the rate of increase of Ers (Table 1). If we consider that the mean transpulmonary pressure in a rat at functional residual capacity ranges from 2 to 3 $cmH_2O$ [46], a PEEP of 7 $cmH_2O$ represents approximately a 2.3-fold increase. If the mean transpulmonary pressure in humans at functional residual capacity is about 5 $cmH_2O$, our PEEP of 5–7 $cmH_2O$ in rats might correspond to a PEEP ranging from 11 to 16 $cmH_2O$ in humans. Such PEEP levels seem much higher than the standard of care at the operating room for lung-healthy mechanically ventilated patients [21].

Interestingly, the rate of increase in Ers fell when VV was combined with a PEEP at the level of the minimum Ers (ranging from 3 to 4 $cmH_2O$ in the present study, Table 1). If the same aforementioned conversion factor were applied, this PEEP might correspond to 7–9 $cmH_2O$ in lung-healthy patients. Such PEEP levels have been applied as a protective ventilatory strategy in patients undergoing abdominal surgery [21].

Several studies report a better performance of VV than VCV in ARDS experimental models in terms of mechanical function, pro-inflammatory biomarkers [44] and gas exchange [47]. From the mechanistic point of view, the dynamics of recruitment and de-recruitment of some alveolar units are likely to be important determinants of the efficiency of VV [45].

In the anesthesia scenario, VV was applied in a trial with 41 patients undergoing prolonged anesthesia for elective abdominal surgery. A sustained improvement in gas exchange was observed [30]. The benefits of protective low $V_T$ ventilation in patients with ARDS, as well as the use of high levels of PEEP is well studied, but it is still under discussion whether these strategies should also be applied to lung-healthy patients in the anesthesia scenario. Additionally, considering that Ers changes overtime, the PEEP adjusted just after the recruitment maneuver, may not be able to

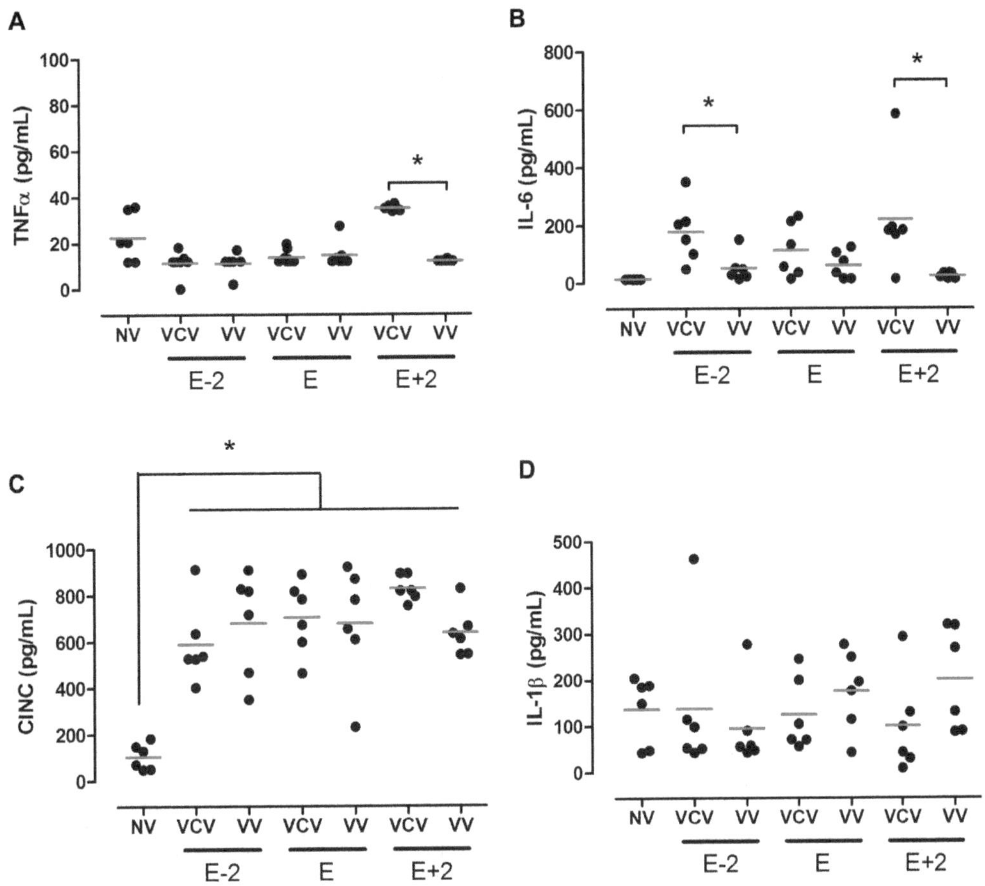


**Figure 6. Lung cytokines.** Lung tissue concentration of TNF-α (A), IL-6 (B), CINC-1(C) and IL-1β(D) in the groups: VCV_E (volume-controlled mode and $PEEP_{minErs}$; n = 6), VCV_E+2 (volume-controlled mode and $PEEP_{minErs}$ plus 2 $cmH_2O$; n = 6), VCV_E-2 (volume-controlled mode and $PEEP_{minErs}$ minus 2 $cmH_2O$; n = 6), VV_E (variable ventilation and $PEEP_{minErs}$; n = 6), VV_E+2 (variable ventilation and $PEEP_{minErs}$ plus 2 $cmH_2O$; n = 5), VV_E-2 (variable ventilation and $PEEP_{minErs}$ minus 2 $cmH_2O$; n = 6). Red lines represent mean values. Ventilatory mode and PEEP effects were tested with two-way ANOVA followed by Tukey post hoc. T-test was used to detect differences between ventilated and non-ventilated groups and then correction by multiple comparison. Statistical significance was accepted at $p<0.05$. *$p<0.05$.

keep lung opened throughout the protocol. In this scenario, VV ventilation can be an aid in lung stabilization.

In our study even though all experimental groups were ventilated with a protective strategy with respect to $V_T$, they presented concentrations of TNF-α, IL-6, CINC-1 and IL-1β in lung homogenate higher than non-ventilated rats, but specifically IL-1β content showed a reduction on VV strategy (Figure 3).

Mechanical ventilation is likely to induce the production and/or secretion of IL-1β in animal models of VILI [48,49]. Since IL-1β is a proinflammatory cytokine and a mediator of sterile inflammation that acts through IL-1R, it may have a role in the mechanism of lung inflammation and injury induced by mechanical stretch [49]. Additionally, activation of the inflammatory response, including increased IL-1β signaling, is a major mechanism of alveolar barrier dysfunction in VILI [48].

Plasmatic concentrations of IL-1β in all groups were compatible with non-ventilated controls. The amount of this protein in the lungs is about four hundred times that in the blood, showing that with 2 hours of ventilation the inflammatory process is mostly confined to the lungs. Our data showed that plasmatic levels of IL-6 were significantly higher in VCV strategies (VCV_E-2 and VCV_ E+2) compared to non-ventilated controls.

Pecchiari et al. recently showed that 4-h mechanical ventilation with different ventilatory modes did not alter lung histology, but exerted distinct effects on pro-inflammatory cytokine concentrations in lung-healthy rats [50]. These results are in agreement with our findings describing differences in cytokine concentration but not in lung histology. A similar behavior was also described by Krebs et al. ventilating lung-healthy rats during 1, 6 or 12 h following the open lung approach [51]. These authors found alterations in pulmonary histology just after 12 h of MV, whereas mRNA expressions of pro-inflammatory and pro-fibrotic cytokines were already elevated at 1 or 6 h of mechanical ventilation. Ventilation with the least injurious volume settings induced biochemical and histological changes consistent with lung impairment in a murine VILI model [52]. It triggered significant gene expression (including those involved in immunity and inflammation such as IL-1β and IL-6) at only 90 min of protective ventilation in the absence of a primary pulmonary insult in rodents [53].

## Limitations

Our findings around the amount of air/non-air expressed by air fraction obtained by histological analysis revealed no differences between VV and VCV, nor in PEEPs. This can be partially attributed to the fact that all lungs were removed under no PEEP. In fact, in absence of PEEP, an immediately collapse takes place

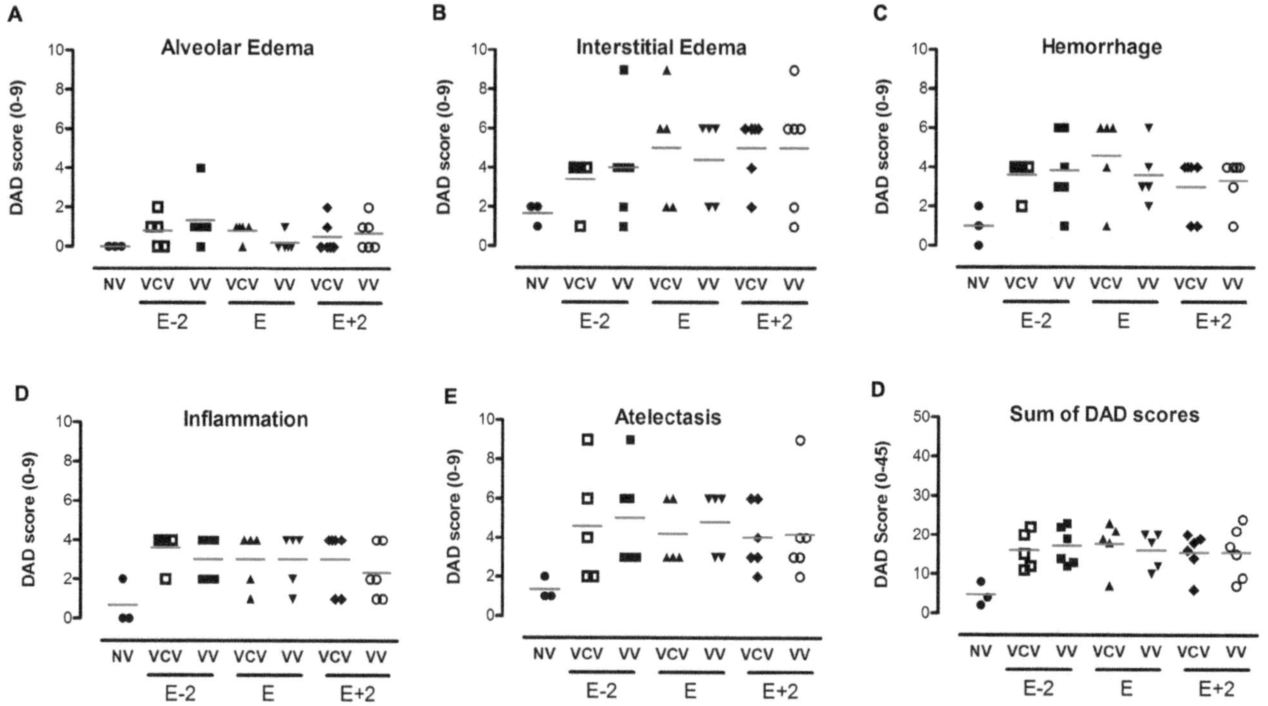


**Figure 7. Plasmatic cytokines.** Plasmatic concentration of TNF-α (A), IL-6 (B), CINC-1(C) and IL-1β (D) ) in the groups: VCV_E (volume-controlled mode and $PEEP_{minErs}$; n = 6), VCV_E+2 (volume-controlled mode and $PEEP_{minErs}$ plus 2 $cmH_2O$; n = 6), VCV_E-2 (volume-controlled mode and $PEEP_{minErs}$ minus 2 $cmH_2O$; n = 6), VV_E (variable ventilation and $PEEP_{minErs}$; n = 6), VV_E+2 (variable ventilation and $PEEP_{minErs}$ plus 2 $cmH_2O$; n = 5), VV_E-2 (variable ventilation and $PEEP_{minErs}$ minus 2 $cmH_2O$; n = 6). Red lines represent mean values. Ventilatory mode and PEEP effects were tested with two-way ANOVA followed by Tukey post hoc. T-test was used to detect differences between ventilated and non-ventilated groups and then correction by multiple comparison. Statistical significance was accepted at $p<0.05$. *$p<0.05$.

and this probably contributed to an increase in the non-air fraction in all groups. However, the decision to excise the lungs with no PEEP was based on the technical difficulty to keep alveolar pressure constant during lung removal.

Another important issue is that in VV we applied a coefficient of variation (CV) of 10% to VT, while most studies use a CV of 30%. This can explain the similar oxygenation or $CO_2$ clearance found in VCV and VV. However, the CV of 30% would generate volumes in the range 2–12 ml/kg, which is not recommended as a protective strategy.

Finally, mechanical ventilation was provided for just 2 h in all ventilated animals. This seems to be a short time period for the observation of any conclusive inflammatory or anti-inflammatory pathway. However, this is the most common period of mechanical ventilation during anesthesia, and only in few cases anesthesia and mechanical ventilations takes longer than this time window [38]. Furthermore, despite no significant differences in terms of oxygenation among ventilatory strategies, the lower concentration of IL-1β in lung tissue in the group of VV and PEEP adjusted at the minimal Ers may suggest a lower biological cost that might impact in a long term ventilation.

## Conclusion

VV with moderate levels of PEEP was associated with improved pulmonary function and alveolar stability in lung-healthy rats under general anesthesia.

## Acknowledgments

The authors thank the Department of Pathology from the University of São Paulo, São Paulo, Brazil for the technical support on the scanning histology specimens.

## Author Contributions

Conceived and designed the experiments: ARC. Performed the experiments: LC MBA. Analyzed the data: LC MBA GCMR LFSC PS ARC MA WAZ AGN AR. Contributed reagents/materials/analysis tools: PS ARC. Contributed to the writing of the manuscript: ARC LC PS WAZ AGN MA AR.

## References

1. Duggan M, Kavanagh BP (2005) Pulmonary atelectasis: a pathogenic perioperative entity. Anesthesiology 102: 838–854.
2. Rusca M, Proietti S, Schnyder P, Frascarolo P, Hedenstierna G, et al. (2003) Prevention of Atelectasis Formation During Induction of General Anesthesia. Anesthesia and analgesia 97: 1835–1839.
3. Duggan M, Kavanagh BP (2007) Atelectasis in the perioperative patient. Current Opinion in Anaesthesiology 20: 37–42.
4. Rothen HU, Sporre B, Engberg G, Wegenius G, Hedenstierna G (1998) Airway closure, atelectasis and gas exchange during general anaesthesia. British Journal of Anaesthesia 81: 681–686.
5. Neumann P, Berglund JE, Fernandez-Mondéjar E, Magnusson A, Hedenstierna G (1998) Dynamics of lung collapse and recruitment during prolonged breathing in porcine lung injury. Journal of Applied Physiology 85: 1533–1543.

6. Rothen HU, Neumann P, Berglund JE, Valtysson J, Magnusson A, et al. (1999) Dynamics of re-expansion of atelectasis during general anaesthesia. British Journal of Anaesthesia 82: 551–556.
7. Hedenstierna G, Rothen HU (2000) Atelectasis formation during anesthesia: causes and measures to prevent it. J Clin Monit Comput 16: 329–335.
8. Hedenstierna G, Rothen HU (2012) Respiratory function during anesthesia: effects on gas exchange. Compr Physiol 2: 69–96. doi:10.1002/cphy.c080111.
9. Lutch Js (1972) Continuous Positive-Pressure Ventilation: Effects on Systemic Oxygen Transport and Tissue Oxygenation. Ann Intern Med 76: 193.
10. Neidhart PP, Suter PM (1988) Changes of right ventricular function with positive end-expiratory pressure (PEEP) in man. Intensive Care Medicine 14 Suppl 2: 471–473.
11. Jardin F, Farcot JC, Boisante L, Curien N, Margairaz A, et al. (1981) Influence of positive end-expiratory pressure on left ventricular performance. The New England journal of medicine 304: 387–392.
12. Huemer G, Kolev N, Kurz A, Zimpfer M (1994) Influence of positive end-expiratory pressure on right and left ventricular performance assessed by Doppler two-dimensional echocardiography. CHEST 106: 67–73.
13. Robotham JL, Lixfeld W, Holland L, MacGregor D, Bromberger-Barnea B, et al. (1980) The effects of positive end-expiratory pressure on right and left ventricular performance. Am Rev Respir Dis 121: 677–683.
14. Wallis TW, Robotham JL, Compean R, Kindred MK (1983) Mechanical heart-lung interaction with positive end-expiratory pressure. J Appl Physiol 54: 1039–1047.
15. Kumar A, Pontoppidan H, Falke Kj, Wilson Rs, Laver Mb (1973) Pulmonary barotrauma during mechanical ventilation. Critical Care Medicine 1: 181.
16. Suter PM, Fairley HB, Isemberg MD (1975) Optimum end-expiratory airway pressure in patients with acute pulmonary failure. The New England journal of medicine 292: 284–289.
17. Carvalho A, Jandre FC, Pino AV, Bozza FA, Salluh JI, et al. (2006) Effects of descending positive end-expiratory pressure on lung mechanics and aeration in healthy anaesthetized piglets. Crit Care 10: R122.
18. Carvalho AR, Pacheco SA, de Souza Rocha PV, Bergamini BC, Paula LF, et al. (2013) Detection of Tidal Recruitment/Overdistension in Lung-Healthy Mechanically Ventilated Patients Under General Anesthesia. Anesthesia and analgesia 116: 677–684.
19. Rouby J-J, Ferrari F, Bouhemad B, Lu Q (2007) Positive end-expiratory pressure in acute respiratory distress syndrome: should the 'open lung strategy' be replaced by a 'protective lung strategy'? Crit Care 11: 180.
20. Imberger G, McIlroy D, Pace NL, Wetterslev J, Brok J, et al. (2010) Positive end-expiratory pressure (PEEP) during anaesthesia for the prevention of mortality and postoperative pulmonary complications. Cochrane Database Syst Rev: CD007922.
21. Severgnini P, Selmo G, Lanza C, Chiesa A, Frigerio A, et al. (2013) Protective mechanical ventilation during general anesthesia for open abdominal surgery improves postoperative pulmonary function. Anesthesiology 118: 1307–1321.
22. Tobin MJ, Chadha TS, Jenouri G, Birch SJ, Gazeroglu HB, et al. (1983) Breathing patterns. 2. Diseased subjects. CHEST 84: 286–294.
23. Suki B, Alencar AM, Sujeer MK, Lutchen KR, Collins JJ, et al. (1998) Life-support system benefits from noise. Nature 393: 127–128.
24. Vassilakopoulos T, Zakynthinos S (2008) When mechanical ventilation mimics nature*. Critical Care Medicine 36: 1009–1011.
25. Shimabukuro DW, Gropper MA (2009) Noisy mechanical ventilation: listen to the melody. Anesthesiology 110: 214–215.
26. Spieth PM, Carvalho AR, Pelosi P, Hoehn C, Meissner C, et al. (2009) Variable tidal volumes improve lung protective ventilation strategies in experimental lung injury. American Journal of Respiratory and Critical Care Medicine 179: 684–693.
27. Wolff G, Eberhard L, Guttmann J, Bertschmann W, Zeravik J, et al. (1992) Polymorphous Ventilation: A New Ventilation Concept for Distributed Time Constants. New Aspects on .... Berlin, Heidelberg: Springer Berlin Heidelberg. 235–252.
28. Mutch WA, Harms S, Lefevre GR, Graham MR, Girling LG, et al. (2000) Biologically variable ventilation increases arterial oxygenation over that seen with positive end-expiratory pressure alone in a porcine model of acute respiratory distress syndrome. Critical Care Medicine 28: 2457–2464.
29. Boker A, Graham MR, Walley KR, McManus BM, Girling LG, et al. (2002) Improved arterial oxygenation with biologically variable or fractal ventilation using low tidal volumes in a porcine model of acute respiratory distress syndrome. American Journal of Respiratory and Critical Care Medicine 165: 456–462.
30. Boker A, Haberman CJ, Girling L, Guzman RP, Louridas G, et al. (2004) Variable ventilation improves perioperative lung function in patients undergoing abdominal aortic aneurysmectomy. Anesthesiology 100: 608–616.
31. Kowalski S, McMullen MC, Girling LG, McCarthy BG (2013) Biologically variable ventilation in patients with acute lung injury: a pilot study. Can J Anesth/J Can Anesth 60: 502–503.
32. Mutch WA, Eschun GM, Kowalski SE, Graham MR, Girling LG, et al. (2000) Biologically variable ventilation prevents deterioration of gas exchange during prolonged anaesthesia. British Journal of Anaesthesia 84: 197–203.
33. Spieth PM, Knels L, Kasper M, Domingues Quelhas A, Wiedemann B, et al. (2007) Effects of vaporized perfluorohexane and partial liquid ventilation on regional distribution of alveolar damage in experimental lung injury. Intensive Care Medicine 33: 308–314.
34. Mead J, Collier C (1959) Relation of volume history of lungs to respiratory mechanics in anesthetized dogs. Journal of Applied Physiology.
35. Mead J, Takishima T, Leith D (1970) Stress distribution in lungs: a model of pulmonary elasticity. Journal of Applied Physiology 28: 596–608.
36. Seeger W, Grube C, Günther A, Schmidt R (1993) Surfactant inhibition by plasma proteins: differential sensitivity of various surfactant preparations. Eur Respir J 6: 971–977.
37. Do Anesthesia H, Affect S (2013) Protect the Lungs during Abdominal Surgery It May Change the Postoperative Outcome. Anesthesiology.
38. Futier E, Constantin J-M, Paugam-Burtz C, Pascal J, Eurin M, et al. (2013) A Trial of Intraoperative Low-Tidal-Volume Ventilation in Abdominal Surgery. The New England journal of medicine 369: 428–437.
39. Jaber S, Coisel Y, Chanques G, Futier E, Constantin J-M, et al. (2012) A multicentre observational study of intra-operative ventilatory management during general anaesthesia: tidal volumes and relation to body weight. Anaesthesia 67: 999–1008.
40. Hedenstierna G, Edmark L, Aherdan KK (2000) Time to reconsider the pre-oxygenation during induction of anaesthesia. Minerva Anestesiol 66: 293–296.
41. Vlahakis NE, Hubmayr RD (2000) Invited review: plasma membrane stress failure in alveolar epithelial cells. Journal of Applied Physiology 89: 2490–6.
42. Bilek AM, Dee KC, Gaver DP (2003) Mechanisms of surface-tension-induced epithelial cell damage in a model of pulmonary airway reopening. Journal of Applied Physiology 94: 770–783.
43. Huh D, Fujioka H, Tung Y-C, Futai N, Paine R, et al. (2007) Acoustically detectable cellular-level lung injury induced by fluid mechanical stresses in microfluidic airway systems. Proc Natl Acad Sci USA 104: 18886–18891.
44. Thammanomai A, Hamakawa H, Bartolák-Suki E, Suki B (2013) Combined Effects of Ventilation Mode and Positive End-Expiratory Pressure on Mechanics, Gas Exchange and the Epithelium in Mice with Acute Lung Injury. PLoS ONE 8: e53934.
45. Ma B, Suki B, Bates JHT (2011) Effects of recruitment/derecruitment dynamics on the efficacy of variable ventilation. Journal of Applied Physiology 110: 1319–1326.
46. Santos RL, Santos MA, Sakae RS, Saldiva PH, Zin WA (1992) Effects of longitudinal laparotomy on respiratory system, lung, and chest wall mechanics. J Appl Physiol 72: 1985–1990.
47. Bellardine CL, Hoffman AM, Tsai L, Ingenito EP, Arold SP, et al. (2006) Comparison of variable and conventional ventilation in a sheep saline lavage lung injury model*. Critical Care Medicine 34: 439–445.
48. Frank JA, Pittet J-F, Wray C, Matthay MA (2008) Protection from experimental ventilator-induced acute lung injury by IL-1 receptor blockade. Thorax 63: 147–153.
49. Wu J, Yan Z, Schwartz DE, Yu J, Malik AB, et al. (2013) Activation of NLRP3 inflammasome in alveolar macrophages contributes to mechanical stretch-induced lung inflammation and injury. J Immunol 190: 3590–3599.
50. Pecchiari M, Monaco A, Koutsoukou A, Valle PD, Gentile G, et al. (2013) Effects of Various Modes of Mechanical Ventilation in Normal Rats. Anesthesiology.
51. Krebs J, Pelosi P, Tsagogiorgas C, Haas J, Yard B, et al. (2011) Time course of lung inflammatory and fibrogenic responses during protective mechanical ventilation in healthy rats. Respir Physiol Neurobiol 178: 323–328.
52. Wolthuis EK, Vlaar APJ, Choi G, Roelofs JJTH, Juffermans NP, et al. (2009) Mechanical ventilation using non-injurious ventilation settings causes lung injury in the absence of pre-existing lung injury in healthy mice. Crit Care 13: R1.
53. Ng CSH, Wan S, Ho AMH, Underwood MJ (2009) Gene expression changes with a "non-injurious" ventilation strategy. Crit Care 13: 403.

21

# Bioimpedance Spectroscopy for Assessment of Volume Status in Patients before and after General Anaesthesia

**Matthäus Ernstbrunner[1], Lisa Kostner[1], Oliver Kimberger[1], Peter Wabel[2], Marcus Säemann[3], Klaus Markstaller[1], Edith Fleischmann[1], Barbara Kabon[1], Manfred Hecking[1,3]***

**1** Medical University of Vienna, Department of Anaesthesiology and Critical Care Medicine, Vienna, Austria, **2** Fresenius Medical Care, Bad Homburg, Germany, **3** Medical University of Vienna, Department of Internal Medicine III, Clinical Division of Nephrology & Dialysis, Vienna, Austria

## Abstract

***Background:*** Technically assisted assessment of volume status before surgery may be useful to direct intraoperative fluid administration. We therefore tested a recently developed whole-body bioimpedance spectroscopy device to determine pre- to postoperative fluid distribution.

***Methods:*** Using a three-compartment physiologic tissue model, the body composition monitor (BCM, Fresenius Medical Care, Germany) measures total body fluid volume, extracellular volume, intracellular volume and fluid overload as surplus or deficit of 'normal' extracellular volume. BCM-measurements were performed before and after standardized general anaesthesia for gynaecological procedures (laparotomies, laparoscopies and vaginal surgeries). BCM results were blinded to the attending anaesthesiologist and data analysed using the 2-sided, paired Student's t-test and multiple linear regression.

***Results:*** In 71 females aged 45±15 years with body weight 67±13 kg and duration of anaesthesia 154±68 min, pre- to postoperative fluid overload increased from −0.7±1.1 L to 0.1±1.0 L, corresponding to −5.1±7.5% and 0.8±6.7% of normal extracellular volume, respectively (both $p<0.001$), after patients had received 1.9±0.9 L intravenous crystalloid fluid. Perioperative urinary excretion was 0.4±0.3 L. The increase in extracellular volume was paralleled by an increase in total body fluid volume, while intracellular volume increased only slightly and without reaching statistical significance ($p = 0.15$). Net perioperative fluid balance (administered fluid volume minus urinary excretion) was significantly associated with change in extracellular volume ($r^2 = 0.65$), but was not associated with change in intracellular volume ($r^2 = 0.01$).

***Conclusions:*** Routine intraoperative fluid administration results in a significant, and clinically meaningful increase in the extracellular compartment. BCM-measurements yielded plausible results and may become useful to guide intraoperative fluid therapy in future studies.

**Editor:** Daniel Schneditz, Medical University of Graz, Austria

**Funding:** The authors have no funding or support to report.

**Competing Interests:** P. Wabel is an employee of Fresenius Medical Care in Germany, which produces the BCM Body Composition Monitor. P. Wabel is holding the following patents in the United States in the field of bioimpedance spectroscopy: 'Method and a device for determining the hydration and/or nutrition status of a patient' (application No. 11/630967, patent reference 035018US01, patent No. 7917202); 'Method and a device for determining the hydration and/or nutrition status of a patient' (application No. 11/630965, patent reference 045010US02, patent No. 8340754).

* Email: manfred.hecking@meduniwien.ac.at

## Introduction

All patients undergoing anaesthesia and surgery routinely receive intravenous (iv) fluid therapy intraoperatively for correction of anaesthesia- and surgery-related hemodynamic disturbances. Timing, amount and the specific type of its administration, however, remain controversial [1]. Based on the assumption of preoperative dehydration and intraoperative 'third space' fluid loss, administering a considerable amount of iv fluid is still a common clinical practice, although positive perioperative fluid balance with postoperative fluid-based weight gain is associated with major complications [2–6]. Cardiac-, pulmonary-, renal- and gastrointestinal function, respectively tissue oxygenation, wound healing and coagulation are all influenced by perioperative fluid therapy [7].

Surgery represents a traumatic insult and initiates an acute stress response leading to secretion of proinflammatory mediators and stress hormones, which control the sympathoadrenal system and the hypothalamic-pituitary-adrenal axis [8,9]. Increased levels of adrenocorticotrophic hormone, antidiuretic hormone, cortisol, aldosterone and catecholamines result in increased catabolism, reduced urinary secretion, disturbed microcirculation and increased vascular permeability leading to salt and fluid retention [10]. Perioperative fluid therapy represents an approach to counteract the incidence and severity of systemic inflammation following surgery [9].

Total body fluid volume (TBV) comprises approximately 50% of the female body mass, i.e. 30 liters in a 60 kg woman. Of this amount, about two-thirds (20 liters) are intracellular volume (ICV) and one-third (10 liters) extracellular volume (ECV) in a healthy, young subject [11–13]. The body composition monitor (BCM, Fresenius Medical Care, Germany) is a novel, whole-body bioimpedance spectroscopy device that measures TBV, ICV and ECV by using a three-compartment physiologic tissue model based on the expected normal volume status with healthy renal function in a normohydrated subject [14]. The BCM was originally developed to calculate fluid overload in patients undergoing renal replacement therapy [15]. Extensive validation of the fluid volumes and body composition obtained with BCM has been performed against reference methods (bromide-, deuterium dilution and total body potassium method) involving healthy volunteers and hemodialysis patients [14,16,17].

To the best of our knowledge, the BCM device has not previously been studied in patients undergoing general anaesthesia, although objective assessment of fluid status before surgery may be useful to optimize intraoperative fluid administration and to prevent postoperative fluid retention. The aim of the present study was to determine the pre- to postoperative fluid distribution using bioimpedance spectroscopy technology, and, by relating changes in volume status to the net administration of iv fluid, to evaluate if BCM-derived measurements yield plausible results.

## Materials and Methods

### Patients

The use of routine BCM-measurements was instituted at the Department of Anaesthesiology of the Medical University of Vienna, as of May 2012, based on the availability of a BCM device provided by the Department of Nephrology. From 12 November 2012 until 31 January 2013, BCM-measurements were consecutively performed directly before general anaesthesia in unselected, conscious females, presenting for various elective gynaecological procedures. Patients with a pacemaker, with a limb amputation or pregnant women were not measured. Patients who had significant blood loss and therefore had received erythrocyte concentrates or colloid solution, and/or all those patients who had not received a urinary catheter were measured, but excluded from the present analysis. All patients fasted overnight for more than 6 hours. All patients received isotonic crystalloid solution (Elo-mel, Fresenius Kabi Austria) continuously, throughout the duration of anaesthesia. The amount and timing of intraoperative fluid administered was at the discretion of the attending anaesthesiologist, who was not informed about the BCM result, thereby reflecting clinical practice, as influenced by cardiovascular signs and fluid losses, without following a fixed fluid regime.

For induction of general anaesthesia propofol, fentanyl and rocuronium were administered intravenously. To secure the airway, an endotracheal tube was inserted as appropriate. Anaesthesia was maintained with sevoflurane in an air/oxygen mixture or with a continuous propofol infusion guided by electroencephalogram (Narcotrend index, MT MonitorTechnik, Bad Bramstedt, Germany). At the discretion of the attending anaesthesiologist, and depending on the anamnesis of the patient, a serotonin antagonist (usually ondansetron), a glucocorticoid (usually dexamethasone) in low dose (4 mg) and/or a total intravenous anaesthesia (TIVA) were administered intraoperatively to prevent postoperative nausea and vomiting (PONV). Urinary catheterization was performed after induction. Body temperature was maintained with temperature controlling devices like Bair Hugger (3 M) and Hotline 2 Fluid Warmer (Smiths Medical). The second BCM-measurement was performed as soon as possible after the end of anaesthesia in the postanaesthesia care unit.

To evaluate the obtained data in the form of the present open, non-interventional, observational cohort study, we obtained approval from the Ethics Committee of the Medical University of Vienna (EK Nr.: 2059/2012) and anonymised all participant information. The study adhered to the Declaration of Helsinki.

### BCM-measurements

BCM-measurements were performed as proposed by the manufacturer. Briefly, four non-recyclable electrode strips were taped to wrist and ankle, respectively hand and foot, on one side of the patient body in supine position. Electrodes were connected to the BCM device using the cable provided by the manufacturer. Body weight and height, patient age and patient gender were entered into the BCM device.

About BCM technology: The measurement itself usually requires <2 minutes; the BCM device measures resistance and reactance at 50 discrete frequencies covering the frequency spectrum from 5 to 1000 kHz. Extracellular and intracellular resistance values are obtained on the basis of a Cole model [18]. Using these resistances values, ECV, ICV and TBV are calculated from a fluid model described by Moissl [17]. Excess extracellular fluid is distinguished from the physiological hydration of lean and adipos tissue, based on a physiological tissue model described by Chamney [14]. This algorithm is built into the BCM device and calculates the normal hydration status for a given weight, i.e. the expected normal values for ECV, which would result with healthy renal function and in a state of normohydration. Specifically, the tissue hydration status is calculated from the difference between the normal ECV expected, and with BCM measured ECV. Excess extracellular fluid (fluid overload: FO) is then indicated as 'overhydration' in liters and in percent above "normal" ECV on the BCM device. In dehydrated patients, the value for 'overhydration' indicated on the BCM device is negative.

Additional information provided by a typical BCM-measurement comprise basic measures of the body composition, such as lean tissue mass, lean tissue index (lean tissue mass/height$^2$), fat mass and fat tissue index (fat tissue mass/height$^2$).

Note that the terms fluid overload, volume overload and overhydration are often used interchangeably. Since 'hydration' refers strictly to water, while 'volume expansion' refers to the accumulation of isotonic fluid (salt and water), we primarily use the term fluid overload and fluid status. Similarly, the term extracellular water used in previous publications [19–22] has here been replaced by extracellular fluid volume (ECV).

### Other measurements and patient characteristics

The patient characteristics recorded for this study included age, height, body weight, body mass index, classification per the American Society of Anaesthesiologists' (ASA) physical status classification system, and New York Heart Association (NYHA) functional classification. All biochemical and hematological analyses (labs) were performed by the Clinical Institute of Laboratory Medicine of the Medical University of Vienna (for methods, see www.kimcl.at). Preoperative measurements of hemoglobin, serum creatinine and gamma glutamyl transferase were available in all patients. Increased vascular permeability might have influenced the BCM results, and is associated with hypoalbuminaemia and inflammation (manifested by high C-reactive protein [CRP] levels). To assess vascular permeability we therefore calculated the capillary leak index as CRP [in milligrams per deciliter] over albumin [in grams per liter], multiplied by 100 [23].

Pre- and postoperative heart rate, blood pressure measurements and fluid balance data were documented in all patients. Measurements of body temperature with single-use oesophageal temperature probes from Dräger were available in 51 patients. Urinary output was recorded in all patients. Net perioperative fluid balance was calculated by subtracting urine output from infused fluid.

### Data analysis: Statistics and sample size considerations

Descriptive statistics (mean ± standard deviation and relative frequency) were used to portray patient characteristics, laboratory values, iv fluid administration and urinary output, as well as all BCM-derived measurements. Changes in BCM-derived measurements from pre- to postoperatively (delta values) were obtained by subtracting the preoperative value from the postoperative value.

The primary parameter of interest was fluid overload (FO in liters and in % ECV). The change in pre- to postoperative FO was evaluated using the paired, two-sided Student's t-test, as proposed in the pre-specified statistical analysis plan of the study protocol. Similar exploratory analyses were conducted for all other parameters obtained before and after anaesthesia. When the distribution of the analyzed variables was tested by Kolmogorov-Smirnov test, fluid therapy was found to be non-normally distributed.

Sample size considerations were based on association analyses using the Pearson correlation test. To detect a moderate, and thereby clinically meaningful correlation ($r = 0.4$) between net perioperative fluid balance and change in FO, a sample of 62 analysable subjects was calculated to provide 90% power to discover that the correlation would be significantly different from there being no correlation (i.e. that the correlation would be near zero) at the 0.05 level.

We used multiple regression analysis to examine the effect of different predictor variables (net perioperative fluid balance, serum albumin, age, body mass index, serum creatinine, preoperative iv fluid therapy, preoperative blood pressure, pre- and postoperative capillary leak index) on the outcome variable (change in ECV).

For calculations we used MS Excel 2011 and IBM SPSS Statistics 22.0.

## Results

### Characteristics of the study population

The study population comprised 71 females, aged 45±15 years, with body weight 67±13 kg (Table 1) after excluding 26 patients without a urinary catheter, 2 patients who had received erythrocyte concentrates intraoperatively without obtaining colloids and 7 patients who had received colloid solution in addition to crystalloid solution. Of these 71 patients, 2 patients had evidence of severe systemic disease, per the ASA physical classification system, and 14 patients were classified as NYHA stage 2 patients. No patient had serum creatinine >1.2 mg/dL, indicating that renal function was not impaired. The gynaecological procedures were 23 laparotomies (32%), 43 laparoscopies (61%) and 5 vaginal operations (7%).

The average preoperative iv fluid volume administered amounted to 0.3 L, with 16 patients having received no fluid at all. The average interval between two BCM-measurements was 189 minutes and the average duration of anaesthesia was 154 minutes. During this period, patients received on average 1.9 L iv crystalloid fluid, 6 patients ≥3 L and 5 patients ≤1 L. During the interval between the two BCM-measurements, the average urinary excretion was 0.3 L, with 3 patients excreting ≥ 1 L. The net perioperative fluid balance amounted to 1.6 L (data shown in Table 1). PONV prophylaxis was administered in 70% of the patients.

### Vital signs, volume status and laboratory tests before and after anaesthesia

Heart rate and blood pressure were lower after anaesthesia than before, while body temperature was the same (Table 2). Before anaesthesia, no patient had fluid overload >15% ECV, and 17 patient were dehydrated <−10% ECV. After anaesthesia, one patient had fluid overload >15% ECV, and 4 patients were dehydrated <−10% ECV. Concomitantly, fluid overload increased significantly by 0.8±0.8 L, from −0.7±1.1 L preoperatively to 0.1±1.0 L postoperatively, equivalent to a 5.9±5.6% rise in ECV. This increase was paralleled by a 1.0±1.4 L rise in TBV. ICV increased only slightly without reaching statistical significance ($p = 0.15$).

Relative to the total body weight, the preoperative TBV was 47.3%, ECV 20.8% and ICV 26.5% (Table 2). The preoperative ECV:ICV ratio was 0.79. Relative TBV, relative ECV and the ECV:ICV ratio increased significantly from pre- to postoperatively, while relative ICV did not increase significantly. Serum protein and serum albumin decreased and CRP increased, from pre- to postoperatively, as manifested by a significant rise in the capillary leak index (Table 2).

### Associations between pre- to postoperative changes in volume status and perioperative fluid volume administration

We evaluated the relationship between perioperative fluid administration and changes in pre- to postoperative fluid status and identified a strong, significant correlation between the net perioperative fluid balance and change in ECV ($r^2 = 0.65$, $p < 0.001$, Figure 1A). We also identified a significant correlation between the net perioperative fluid balance and change in TBV, however, the coefficient of determination was smaller ($r^2 = 0.22$, $p < 0.001$, Figure 1B). Net perioperative fluid balance, respectively change in ECV were not significantly associated with change in ICV (Figure 1C and 1D).

### Association between net perioperative fluid balance and changes in pre- to postoperative ECV with multiple levels of adjustments

Patient-dependent parameters such as age, body mass index and renal function, might alter the relationship between perioperative fluid administration and changes in ECV. We therefore performed a linear regression analysis with net perioperative fluid balance as the predictor and change in ECV as the outcome, consecutively adjusting additionally for serum albumin, age, body mass index, serum creatinine, preoperative blood pressure, preoperative fluid therapy, pre- and postoperative capillary leak index. After stepwise adjustments, the combined effects of the predictors on change in ECV were significant in each model (Models 1–9: $p < 0.001$). The overall model (Model 9) explained 71.3% of variance in change in ECV ($r^2 = 0.713$, $p < 0.001$, Table 3). Only net perioperative fluid balance (Beta = 0.804, $p < 0.001$), preoperative fluid therapy (Beta = −0.152, $p = 0.046$) and postoperative capillary leak index (Beta = 0.202, $p = 0.011$) were significant individual predictors of change in ECV. The addition of all other variables altered the association only slightly. Duration of anaesthesia was not added to the model, because this variable correlated strongly with net perioperative fluid balance.

**Table 1.** Demographic characteristics of the study population.

| | All |
|---|---|
| N Patients | 71 |
| Females | 100% |
| Age [years] | 45±15 (22; 71) |
| Height [cm] | 163±7 (150; 176) |
| Body weight [kg] | 67±13 (49; 87) |
| Body mass index [kg/m$^2$] | 25.1±5.7 (18.2; 33.9) |
| ASA 1 | 40 (56%) |
| ASA 2 | 29 (41%) |
| ASA 3 | 2 (3%) |
| NYHA 1 | 57 (80%) |
| NYHA 2 | 14 (20%) |
| Serum Creatinine [mg/dL] | 0.7±0.1 (0.5; 1.0) |
| Gamma Glutamyl Transferase [U/L] | 19±14 (5; 59) |
| Gynaecological procedure <150 min | 43 (61%) |
| Gynaecological procedure <300 min | 23 (32%) |
| Major gynaecological procedure ≥300 min | 5 (7%) |
| PONV Prophylaxis | 50 (70%) |
| Duration of Anaesthesia [min] | 154±69 (69; 314) |
| Interval between 2 BCM-measurements [min]* | 189±68 (108; 354) |
| Preoperative IV Fluid Volume [mL] | 301±275 (0; 1000) |
| Total Perioperative IV Fluid Volume [mL] | 1929±866 (830; 4160) |
| Urinary Excretion [mL] | 337±209 (100; 1000) |
| Net perioperative fluid balance [mL] | 1600±741 (620; 3316) |

Continuous variables are reported as mean ± standard deviation, (5$^{th}$ and 95$^{th}$ percentile); categorical variables are presented as counts and frequencies. Abbreviations: ASA = American Society of Anaesthesiologists' physical status classification system, NYHA = New York Heart Association functional classification, PONV = postoperative nausea and vomiting, IV = intravenous. Net perioperative fluid balance = total perioperative intravenous fluid volume, corrected for urinary excretion and blood loss. *In 5 cases, the interval between the BCM-measurements was >60 minutes longer than the duration of anaesthesia, due to logistical reasons.

## Discussion

The principal findings of the present study on BCM-derived measurements performed before and after general anaesthesia in gynaecological patients were: [1] 17 of 71 patients (24%) were dehydrated (<−10% ECV), while no patient was volume overloaded (>15% ECV) before anaesthesia; [2] a net perioperative fluid balance of 1.6 L on average, administered perioperatively, led to an average increase of 0.8 L in fluid overload, respectively 0.8 L in ECV from pre- to postoperatively, but not to a significant increase in ICV; [3] concomitantly, we identified a strong, significant correlation between net perioperative fluid balance and change in ECV, which; [4] remained significant after adjustment for serum albumin, age, BMI, serum creatinine, preoperative iv fluid therapy, preoperative blood pressure and capillary leak index. Together, these data indicate that BCM-derived measurements yield plausible results on the perioperative fluid status.

Several methods of body composition analysis based on impedance are available [24,25]. One such method is bioimpedance analysis (BIA) using single-frequency technique (SF-BIA) and another method is BIA at low and high frequency (multi-frequency MF-BIA). TBV and ECV are predicted on the basis of the primary BIA results (reactance and resistance), and ICV is calculated as the difference between TBV and ECV. SF-BIA has previously been used to detect postoperative fluid retention after major thoracic surgery [26], while MF-BIA using 4 frequencies has been employed to monitor fluid shifts after major abdominal surgery [27].

In our study we employed another impedance method, bioimpedance spectroscopy (BIS) using BCM. The BCM device measures at 50 frequencies and employs a unique body composition model for determination of fluid overload, respectively for direct prediction of TBV, ECV and ICV. Recently a study by Raimann at al. compared the precision and accuracy of SF-BIA and BIS to direct estimation methods (DEMs, i.e. deuteriumoxide-diltution, bromide-dilution and total potassium count) for body composition analysis in hemodialysis patients. In comparison to DEMs, SF-BIA and BIS were equally precise in determining TBV and ICV. However BIS-determined ECV was closer to DEM-determined ECV, in comparison to SF-BIA. According to Raimann et al., there is no real "gold standard" method with absolute accuracy for determination of the fluid status due the wide limits of agreement [28].

Another impedance-based method to estimate fluid distribution is bioelectrical impedance vector analysis (BIVA), where a vector of impedance at one frequency is evaluated against an ordinal scale with tolerance interval percentiles from a reference population [24,25]. Body composition is analysed by the patterns of vector distribution independent of body weight. Vector displacement indicates a change in fluid status [29]. BIVA allows a ranking of repeated measurements in the individual subject

**Table 2.** Vital signs, volume status and body composition before and after anaesthesia.

| | Pre | Post | Delta | p-value |
|---|---|---|---|---|
| Body Temperature [°C] | *36.3±0.5* | *36.3±0.4* | *0.0±0.5* | 0.71 |
| Heart Rate [beats/min] | **82±17** | **77±17** | **−5±15** | **0.006** |
| Systolic Blood Pressure [mm Hg] | **135±23** | **124±22** | **−11±25** | **<0.001** |
| Diastolic Blood Pressure [mm Hg] | **82±12** | **70±12** | **−12±15** | **<0.001** |
| Mean Blood Pressure [mm Hg] | **105±17** | **92±15** | **−13±19** | **<0.001** |
| Extracellular Volume [L] | **13.6±1.8** | **14.4±1.9** | **0.8±0.7** | **<0.001** |
| Relative ECV [% body weight] | **20.8±2.3** | **22.0±2.3** | **1.2±1.0** | **<0.001** |
| Intracellular Volume [L] | 17.3±2.4 | 17.5±2.2 | 0.2±1.1 | 0.15 |
| Relative ICV [% body weight] | 26.5±4.2 | 26.8±4.1 | 0.3±1.7 | 0.14 |
| Total Body Volume [L] | **30.9±3.9** | **31.9±3.9** | **1.0±1.4** | **<0.001** |
| Relative TBV [% body weight] | **47.3±6.2** | **48.9±6.1** | **1.6±2.2** | **<0.001** |
| Fluid Overload [L] | **−0.7±1.1** | **0.1±1.0** | **0.8±0.8** | **<0.001** |
| Fluid Overload [% ECV] | **−5.1±7.5** | **0.8±6.7** | **5.9±5.6** | **<0.001** |
| ECV/ICV | **0.79±0.08** | **0.83±0.08** | **0.04±0.06** | **<0.001** |
| Serum Protein [g/L] | *71.4±6.0* | *56.5±8.1* | *−14.2±10.2* | *<0.001* |
| Serum Albumin [g/L] | *43.2±5.5* | *32.4±5.4* | *−12.4±5.9* | *<0.001* |
| C-reactive protein [mg/dL] | *0.6±1.7* | *6.2±5.8* | *5.9±5.8* | *<0.001* |
| Capillary Leak Index [unitless] | *2.8±9.9* | *22.1±18.9* | *25.1±20.3* | *<0.001* |

Delta was calculated by subtracting any patient's preoperative value from the postoperative value. Significance was determined by Student's t-test ($p<0.05$). Italics: Data were incomplete for body temperature (number of missing values: N = 7 [pre], N = 20 [post], N = 20 [delta]), serum protein (number of missing values: N = 15 [pre], N = 39 [post], N = 46 [delta]), serum albumin (number of missing values: N = 42 [pre], N = 40 [post], N = 54 [delta]), C-reactive protein (number of missing values: N = 11 [pre], N = 39 [post], N = 42 [delta]) and Capillary Leak Index (number of missing values: N = 43 [pre], N = 43 [post], N = 55 [delta]), despite significant findings. Note that postoperative laboratory measurements were usually performed on the day after surgery (not simultaneous to the postoperative BCM-measurement). Bold: findings with $p<0.05$. Abbreviations: ECV = Extracellular Volume, ICV = Intracellular Volume, TBV = Total Body Fluid Volume.

compared to the reference population, but no direct prediction of TBV, ECV and ICV, which may limit its use in the clinical setting.

In the present study the values obtained for relative TBV (47.3%), relative ECV (20.8%) and relative ICV (26.5%) are in contrast to the classical textbook knowledge, stating that TBV comprise approximately 50–60% of the body weight in healthy adults [11–13]. Chamney et al. described strikingly similar results in 57 healthy females with a mean BMI of 24.5 kg/m$^2$ measured with DEMs. Specifically, TBV determined by deuterium dilution was equivalent to 46.51% body weight, and ECV determined by bromide dilution was equivalent to 20.71% body weight [14]. Our results therefore seem to perfectly confirm the established validation of BCM-derived volume measurements against DEMs.

Mechanistically, because fluid content of lean tissue is around 73%, while fluid content of adipose tissue is around 10% [30], the proportion of lean to adipose tissue determines the proportion of TBV, ECV and ICV in relation to the body weight [31–33]. As the relative fat content of the whole body increases, the relative TBV decreases and the ECV/ICV ratio increases because the ECV component of adipose tissue becomes more dominant [14]. The difference in fluid content between our gynaecological study population and the average reference female described in the classical textbook seems to reflect differences in body composition and indicates that previous textbook results were generated from subjects, who were generally leaner than the present cohort, as well as those described by Chamney et al. [14].

While the bioimpedance spectroscopy-based BCM is currently used in various nephrological settings, and specifically for the management of fluid withdrawal in patients with end-stage renal disease, it has not previously been studied perioperatively. Roughly a fourth of our patients were dehydrated (ECV <−10%) and 41% of the patients had a calculated fluid deficit >1 L before surgery, although they were allowed to drink clear fluid up to two hours prior to the operation. Using BCM-derived information as a target for initial fluid management could therefore become useful to guide fluid therapy before anaesthesia in order to avoid hypovolaemia and thereby hypotension after induction [34]. On the other hand BCM could potentially assist in preventing postoperative fluid overload after major surgery.

The systemic stress response to anaesthesia and surgery is characterized by secretion of corticotrophin, antidiuretic hormone and cortisol, activation of the renin- angiotensin-aldosterone-system and stimulation of the sympathoadrenal axis to maintain hemodynamic stability and to increase salt and fluid retention [35]. Additionally, a local inflammatory reaction controlling the secretion of cytokines like interleukin 1, 6 and tumour necrosis factor augments the fluid shifts and increases vascular permeability [36]. In our cohort, we detected a marked increase in the capillary leak index due to hypoalbuminaemia and high CRP levels, most probably caused by a systemic inflammatory reaction after surgery [37,38]. Cordemans et al. reported that capillary leak index has a biphasic course with a maximum at day 3 after shock in ventilated critically ill patients [23]. Interestingly, in the present study, the postoperative capillary leak index was a significant individual predictor of change in extracellular volume, besides net perioperative fluid balance and preoperative fluid therapy in multiple regression analysis.

Appropriate perioperative fluid therapy might limit the incidence and severity of systemic inflammation following surgery [9] and might attenuate fluid accumulation with generalized

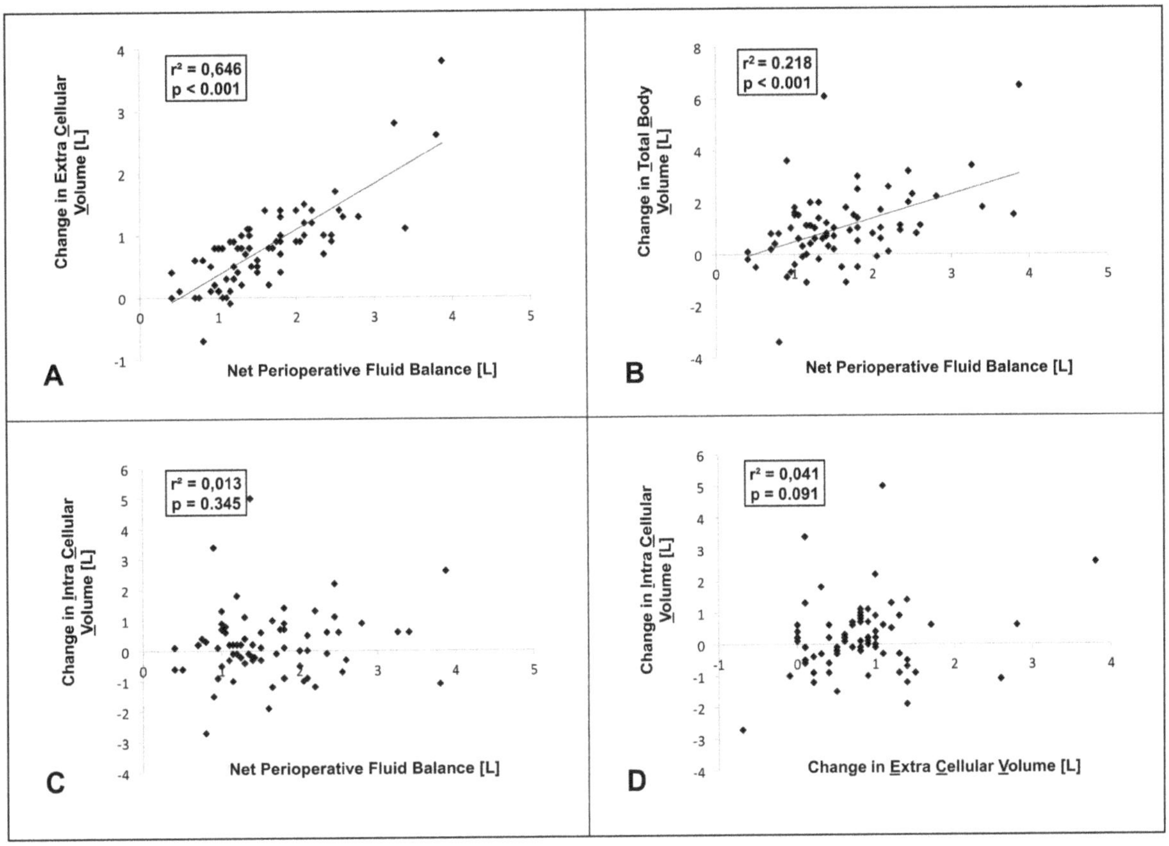


**Figure 1. Associations between pre- to postoperative changes in volume status and net perioperative fluid balance.** Scatter plots. Regression equations are as follows: **A** Change in Extracellular Volume = 0.73 × Net Perioperative Fluid Balance −0.37. **B** Change in Total Body volume = 0.91 × Net Perioperative Fluid Balance −0.43. **C** No linear correlation between Change in Intracellular Volume and Net Perioperative Fluid Balance. **D** No linear correlation between Change in Intracellular Volume and Change in Extracellular Volume. Pearson correlation test. $R^2$ = Coefficient of determination.

oedemas. However, for an acutely ill patient it is not uncommon to receive aggressive fluid therapy, although positive fluid balance, with postoperative fluid-based weight gain more than 10% of body weight is associated with major complications [2,3,5,39–41]. BCM-detected fluid overload in patients with end-stage renal disease has likewise been shown to be associated with greatly increased mortality, the usual cut-off value for "hyper"-hydration and mortality being >15% ECV [16,19,21,22,42]. However, only one patient (1.4%) exceeded this cut-off value for fluid overload after anaesthesia, in this study of relatively healthy, and relatively young patients. High risk surgical patients, and especially those with poor renal function may benefit most from restrictive, intraoperative fluid management, once they have been found to be in a state of fluid overload, measured with BCM.

Our data showed a significant increase of postoperative FO, TBV and ECV, while ICV increased only slightly. It appears surprising to detect this fluid shift at all, because the gynaecological patients had normal renal function, which may leave one wondering why some of the infused volume accumulates in the periphery. Because this fluid status cannot persist indefinitely, the timing of BCM-measurements is important. In future studies, it would be interesting to measure at additional time points postoperatively to observe the return of fluid overload to normal, at least in those patients who are volume overloaded postoperatively.

A net perioperative fluid balance of 1.6±0.7 L led to a measured increase of only 1.0±1.4 L in TBV and to an increase of 0.8±0.7 L in ECV. Thus, roughly 40% of the administered fluid was "missing". One reason for not detecting all of the administered volume in the fluid compartments of the patient may be that respiratory-, cutaneous- and wound fluid losses were not considered. Although the correlation between net perioperative fluid balance and change in extracellular fluid volume was found to be quite strong (r slightly above 0.8, since $r^2 = 0.65$), predicting individual changes in fluid status after iv infusions may remain challenging in patients undergoing surgery, unless it can be clarified that an increase of only 60% is physiologically reasonable. Further methodological issues should be ruled out first.

When applying BIS technology, the bioelectrical properties are measured between the wrist and the ankle under the assumption of a steady fluid distribution. However, if the body can be thought to consist of three segments with different cross-sectional areas and lengths (arm, trunk and leg), the limbs contribute 90%, while the trunk with a large cross sectional area adds only 10% to whole body impedance [24]. After surgery, fluid has been shown to accumulate mostly in the trunk [43]. Because the same amount of fluid leads to different changes in whole-body bioimpedance, depending on whether this fluid is added to or removed from the leg, the arm, or the trunk, whole-body bioimpedance seems to be more sensitive to volume changes in the limbs than in the trunk. Segmental multi-frequency bioelectrical impedance analysis there-

**Table 3.** Association between net perioperative fluid balance and changes in pre- to postoperative extracellular volume, with multiple levels of adjustments.

| | Model 1: net perioperative fluid balance | Model 2: + serum albumin | Model 3: + age | Model 4: + body mass index | Model 5: + serum creatinine | Model 6: + preoperative fluid therapy | Model 7: + preoperative blood pressure | Model 8: + Preoperative capillary leak index | Model 9: + postoperative capillary leak index |
|---|---|---|---|---|---|---|---|---|---|
| Outcome variable: **Delta ECV** | | | | | | | | | |
| $r^2$ | 0.646 | 0.646 | 0.649 | 0.652 | 0.657 | 0.678 | 0.679 | 0.681 | 0.713 |
| **p-value[1]** for each model | **<0.001** | **<0.001** | **<0.001** | **<0.001** | **<0.001** | **<0.001** | **<0.001** | **<0.001** | **<0.001** |
| **p-value[2]** for individual predictors | **<0.001** | 0.845 | 0.479 | 0.435 | 0.330 | **0.046** | 0.639 | 0.540 | **0.011** |
| Beta | **0.804** | 0.014 | −0.056 | 0.060 | −0.077 | **−0.152** | −0.049 | −0.065 | **0.202** |

Multiple regression analysis: After stepwise adjustment the coefficients of determination ($r^2$), the p-value[1] for the combined effect of all predictors for each model, the p-value[2] for the individual effect of a predictor and the correlation coefficient (Beta) represent the association between the outcome and the predictor variables. Boldface indicating statistical significance ($p<0.05$).

fore might be a better approach for determination of ECV changes, because this technique is based on the assumption of a non-uniform fluid distribution within the body [44].

Pneumoperitoneum during laparoscopy increases the intra-abdominal pressure, which affects the cardiovascular system, the respiratory system and renal function [45]. Gülec et al. reported that laparoscopy can constrict the inferior vena cava leading to stasis in the peripheral veins and pooling of blood in the lower limbs [46]. In our cohort, 61% of the patients had laparoscopic surgery, which might influence the efficacy of whole body bioimpedance spectroscopy due the reduced urinary secretion, increased abdominal pressure and venous congestion in the lower limbs.

Additional study limitations: A net perioperative fluid therapy of 1.6 L would increase the body weight, but the postoperative BCM-measurement was performed with the same patient weight, because it was practically impossible to weigh the supine patient in the recovery room after surgery. Entering a patient weight of plus or minus 1.1 kg into the BCM device before performing the measurement has been shown to result in a minimal change of ECV, ICV and FO (0.08 L delta ECV, 0.01 L delta ICV and 0.04 L delta FO, respectively) [47]. Therefore, the perioperative weight difference is expected to interfere only minimally with our results, while a false weight has a higher impact on the BCM-calculated fat mass (1.1 kg higher resulting in 1.04 kg delta Fat) [47].

The present study was an open, non-interventional, observational cohort study, and as such, we were unable to compare our routinely generated BCM results with an additional reference method. Nevertheless, the BCM has been validated against direct estimation methods in more than 500 healthy subjects [14,16,17] and is now widely accepted as a very precise whole body bioimpedance spectroscopy device [48–51]. Future studies, for example using segmental bioimpedance may help clarify whether another bioimpedance method is even better suited to assess the volume status in patients undergoing surgery.

## Conclusion

In conclusion, the results of the present study, obtained with whole body bioimpedance spectroscopy using BCM, show that intraoperative crystalloid fluid administration leads to a significant, and clinically meaningful increase of the extracellular volume compartment, while the intracellular fluid volume increased only slightly. The BCM might serve as a simple and non-invasive device for objective assessment of body fluid distribution in the perioperative setting. Further research is now required to evaluate prospectively, whether BCM-guided fluid administration may improve the postoperative volume status, as well as clinical outcomes in surgical patients.

## Acknowledgments

We thank Paul Chamney and Friedrich K. Port for critically reviewing the manuscript. The corresponding author has had full access to all the data in the study and takes final responsibility for the decision to submit for publication.

## Author Contributions

Conceived and designed the experiments: ME OK PW EF BK MH. Performed the experiments: ME LK BK MH. Analyzed the data: ME LK OK BK PW MH. Contributed reagents/materials/analysis tools: PW KM. Contributed to the writing of the manuscript: ME OK PW MS KM EF BK MH.

## References

1. Doherty M, Buggy DJ (2012) Intraoperative fluids: how much is too much? Br J Anaesth 109: 69–79.
2. Brandstrup B, Tonnesen H, Beier-Holgersen R, Hjortso E, Ording H, et al. (2003) Effects of intravenous fluid restriction on postoperative complications: comparison of two perioperative fluid regimens: a randomized assessor-blinded multicenter trial. Ann Surg 238: 641–648.
3. Lobo DN, Bostock KA, Neal KR, Perkins AC, Rowlands BJ, et al. (2002) Effect of salt and water balance on recovery of gastrointestinal function after elective colonic resection: a randomised controlled trial. Lancet 359: 1812–1818.
4. Lang K, Boldt J, Suttner S, Haisch G (2001) Colloids versus crystalloids and tissue oxygen tension in patients undergoing major abdominal surgery. Anesth Analg 93: 405–409, 403rd contents page.
5. Lowell JA, Schifferdecker C, Driscoll DF, Benotti PN, Bistrian BR (1990) Postoperative fluid overload: not a benign problem. Crit Care Med 18: 728–733.
6. Moller AM, Pedersen T, Svendsen PE, Engquist A (2002) Perioperative risk factors in elective pneumonectomy: the impact of excess fluid balance. Eur J Anaesthesiol 19: 57–62.
7. Holte K, Kehlet H (2006) Fluid therapy and surgical outcomes in elective surgery: a need for reassessment in fast-track surgery. J Am Coll Surg 202: 971–989.
8. Sinclair S, James S, Singer M (1997) Intraoperative intravascular volume optimisation and length of hospital stay after repair of proximal femoral fracture: randomised controlled trial. BMJ 315: 909–912.
9. Frumento RJ B-GE (2003) Newman MF. Perioperative organ protection. Baltimore: Lipincott Williams and Wilkins. 1–27.
10. Lyons FM, Meeran K (1997) The physiology of the endocrine system. Int Anesthesiol Clin 35: 1–21.
11. Miller RD (2010) Intravascular Fluid and Electrolyte Physiology. Miller 's Anesthesia: Elsevier Health Science.
12. Morgan GEM, M.S. (2005) Fluid Management and Transfusion. Clinical Anesthesiology. 4. ed: Lange.
13. Smith TPC (2009) Body Fluids. Fundamentals of Anaesthesia. Third ed: Cambridge University Press.
14. Chamney PW, Wabel P, Moissl UM, Muller MJ, Bosy-Westphal A, et al. (2007) A whole-body model to distinguish excess fluid from the hydration of major body tissues. Am J Clin Nutr 85: 80–89.
15. Hecking M, Karaboyas A, Antlanger M, Saran R, Wizemann V, et al. (2013) Significance of interdialytic weight gain versus chronic volume overload: consensus opinion. Am J Nephrol 38: 78–90.
16. Wabel P, Chamney P, Moissl U, Jirka T (2009) Importance of whole-body bioimpedance spectroscopy for the management of fluid balance. Blood Purif 27: 75–80.
17. Moissl UM, Wabel P, Chamney PW, Bosaeus I, Levin NW, et al. (2006) Body fluid volume determination via body composition spectroscopy in health and disease. Physiol Meas 27: 921–933.
18. Cole KS, Li CL, Bak AF (1969) Electrical analogues for tissues. Exp Neurol 24: 459–473.
19. Chazot C, Wabel P, Chamney P, Moissl U, Wieskotten S, et al. (2012) Importance of normohydration for the long-term survival of haemodialysis patients. Nephrol Dial Transplant 27: 2404–2410.
20. Machek P, Jirka T, Moissl U, Chamney P, Wabel P (2010) Guided optimization of fluid status in haemodialysis patients. Nephrol Dial Transplant 25: 538–544.
21. Van Biesen W, Williams JD, Covic AC, Fan S, Claes K, et al. (2011) Fluid status in peritoneal dialysis patients: the European Body Composition Monitoring (EuroBCM) study cohort. PLoS One 6: e17148.
22. Wizemann V, Wabel P, Chamney P, Zaluska W, Moissl U, et al. (2009) The mortality risk of overhydration in haemodialysis patients. Nephrol Dial Transplant 24: 1574–1579.
23. Cordemans C, De Laet I, Van Regenmortel N, Schoonheydt K, Dits H, et al. (2012) Fluid management in critically ill patients: the role of extravascular lung water, abdominal hypertension, capillary leak, and fluid balance. Ann Intensive Care 2: S1.
24. Kyle UG, Bosaeus I, De Lorenzo AD, Deurenberg P, Elia M, et al. (2004) Bioelectrical impedance analysis-part I: review of principles and methods. Clin Nutr 23: 1226–1243.
25. Kyle UG, Bosaeus I, De Lorenzo AD, Deurenberg P, Elia M, et al. (2004) Bioelectrical impedance analysis-part II: utilization in clinical practice. Clin Nutr 23: 1430–1453.
26. Cagini L, Capozzi R, Tassi V, Savignani C, Quintaliani G, et al. (2011) Fluid and electrolyte balance after major thoracic surgery by bioimpedance and endocrine evaluation. Eur J Cardiothorac Surg 40: e71–76.
27. Itobi E, Stroud M, Elia M (2006) Impact of oedema on recovery after major abdominal surgery and potential value of multifrequency bioimpedance measurements. Br J Surg 93: 354–361.
28. Raimann JG, Zhu F, Wang J, Thijssen S, Kuhlmann MK, et al. (2014) Comparison of fluid volume estimates in chronic hemodialysis patients by bioimpedance, direct isotopic, and dilution methods. Kidney Int 85: 898–908.
29. Piccoli A (2014) Estimation of fluid volumes in hemodialysis patients: comparing bioimpedance with isotopic and dilution methods. Kidney Int 85: 738–741.
30. Forbes GB (1987) Techniques for Estimating Body Composition. Human Body Composition; Growth, Aging, Nutrition, and Activity: Springer- Verlag New York.
31. Wang J, Pierson RN Jr (1976) Disparate hydration of adipose and lean tissue require a new model for body water distribution in man. J Nutr 106: 1687–1693.
32. Ljunggren H (1957) Studies on body composition; with special reference to the composition of obesity tissue and non-obesity tissue. Acta Endocrinol Suppl (Copenh) 25: 1–58.
33. Morse WSJ (1963) The composition of adipose tissue and the non-adipose body of obese and non-obese man. Metab 12: 99–107.
34. Reich DL, Hossain S, Krol M, Baez B, Patel P, et al. (2005) Predictors of hypotension after induction of general anesthesia. Anesth Analg 101: 622–628, table of contents.
35. Desborough JP (2000) The stress response to trauma and surgery. Br J Anaesth 85: 109–117.
36. Sheeran P, Hall GM (1997) Cytokines in anaesthesia. Br J Anaesth 78: 201–219.
37. Pepys MB, Hirschfield GM (2003) C-reactive protein: a critical update. J Clin Invest 111: 1805–1812.
38. Fleck A, Raines G, Hawker F, Trotter J, Wallace PI, et al. (1985) Increased vascular permeability: a major cause of hypoalbuminaemia in disease and injury. Lancet 1: 781–784.
39. Holte K, Jensen P, Kehlet H (2003) Physiologic effects of intravenous fluid administration in healthy volunteers. Anesth Analg 96: 1504–1509, table of contents.
40. Nisanevich V, Felsenstein I, Almogy G, Weissman C, Einav S, et al. (2005) Effect of intraoperative fluid management on outcome after intraabdominal surgery. Anesthesiology 103: 25–32.
41. Rasmussen LA, Rosenberg J, Crawford ME, Kehlet H (1996) [Perioperative fluid therapy. A quality control study]. Ugeskr Laeger 158: 5286–5290.
42. Tsai YC, Tsai JC, Chiu YW, Kuo HT, Chen SC, et al. (2013) Is fluid overload more important than diabetes in renal progression in late chronic kidney disease? PLoS One 8: e82566.
43. Bracco D, Revelly JP, Berger MM, Chiolero RL (1998) Bedside determination of fluid accumulation after cardiac surgery using segmental bioelectrical impedance. Crit Care Med 26: 1065–1070.
44. Tatara T, Tsuzaki K (1998) Segmental bioelectrical impedance analysis improves the prediction for extracellular water volume changes during abdominal surgery. Crit Care Med 26: 470–476.
45. Elliott S, Savill P, Eckersall S (1998) Cardiovascular changes during laparoscopic cholecystectomy: a study using transoesophageal Doppler monitoring. Eur - J Anaesthesiol 15: 50–55.
46. Gulec B, Oner K, Yigitler C, Kocaoglu M, Aydin Y, et al. (2006) Lower extremity venous changes in pneumoperitoneum during laparoscopic surgery. ANZ J Surg 76: 904–906.
47. (2012) BCM - Body Composition Monitor, User Manual: Fresenius Medical Care.
48. Moissl U WP, Chamney PW, Renders L, Bosy-Westphal A, Korth O, Muller MJ (2008) Validation of a bioimpedance spectroscopy method for the assessment of fat free mass. NDT plus 1: ii215.
49. Passauer J, Petrov H, Schleser A, Leicht J, Pucalka K (2010) Evaluation of clinical dry weight assessment in haemodialysis patients using bioimpedance spectroscopy: a cross-sectional study. Nephrol Dial Transplant 25: 545–551.
50. Wabel P RC, Moissl U, Chamney PW, Wizemann V (2007) Accuracy of bioimpedance spectroscopy (BIS) to detect fluid status changes in hemodialysis patients (abstract). Nephrol Dial Transplant 22 (suppl 6).
51. Wizemann V, Rode C, Wabel P (2008) Whole-body spectroscopy (BCM) in the assessment of normovolemia in hemodialysis patients. Contrib Nephrol 161: 115–118.

# 22

# The Impact of Prophylactic Dexamethasone on Nausea and Vomiting after Thyroidectomy

**Zhenhong Zou[1¶], Yuming Jiang[1¶], Mingjia Xiao[2], Ruiyao Zhou[3]***

**1** Department of General Surgery, Nanfang Hospital, Southern Medical University, Guangzhou City, Guangdong Province, China, **2** Department of Hepatobiliary Surgery, Wuxi People's Hospital of Nanjing Medical University, Wuxi, Jiangsu Province, China, **3** Department of General Surgery, The Third Affiliated Hospital of Wenzhou Medical University, Ruian City, Zhejiang Province, China

## Abstract

***Background:*** We carried out a systematic review and meta-analysis to evaluate the impact of prophylactic dexamethasone on post-operative nausea and vomiting (PONV), post-operative pain, and complications in patients undergoing thyroidectomy.

***Methods:*** We searched Pubmed, Embase, and Cochrane Library databases for randomized controlled trials (RCTs) that evaluated the prophylactic effect of dexamethasone versus placebo with or without other antiemetics for PONV in patients undergoing thyroidectomy. Meta-analyses were performed using RevMan 5.0 software.

***Results:*** Thirteen RCTs that considered high quality evidence including 2,180 patients were analyzed. The meta-analysis demonstrated a significant decrease in the incidence of PONV (RR 0.52, 95% CI 0.43 to 0.63, $P<0.00001$), the need for rescue anti-emetics (RR 0.42, 95% CI 0.30 to 0.57, $P<0.00001$), post-operative pain scores (WMD −1.17, 95% CI −1.91 to −0.44, $P=0.002$), and the need for rescue analgesics (RR 0.65, 95% CI 0.50–0.83, $P=0.0008$) in patients receiving dexamethasone compared to placebo, with or without concomitant antiemetics. Dexamethasone 8–10 mg had a significantly greater effect for reducing the incidence of PONV than dexamethasone 1.25–5 mg. Dexamethasone was as effective as other anti-emetics for reducing PONV (RR 1.25, 95% CI 0.86–1.81, $P=0.24$). A significantly higher level of blood glucose during the immediate post-operative period in patients receiving dexamethasone compared to controls was the only adverse event.

***Conclusions:*** Prophylactic dexamethasone 8–10 mg administered intravenously before induction of anesthesia should be recommended as a safe and effective strategy for reducing the incidence of PONV, the need for rescue anti-emetics, post-operative pain, and the need for rescue analgesia in thyroidectomy patients, except those that are pregnant, have diabetes mellitus, hyperglycemia, or contraindications for dexamethasone. More high quality trials are warranted to define the benefits and risks of prophylactic dexamethasone in potential patients with a high risk for PONV.

**Editor:** Richard E. Burney, University of Michigan, United States of America

**Funding:** The authors have no support or funding to report.

**Competing Interests:** The authors have declared that no competing interests exist.

* Email: doctor_zry@126.com

¶ These authors are co-first authors on this work.

## Introduction

Post-operative nausea and vomiting (PONV) is a common and distressing complication associated with surgery. The overall incidence of PONV ranges from 20 to 30% in general surgery and up to 80% in high-risk surgical patients when no prophylactic anti-emetic is given [1,2]. For patients undergoing thyroidectomy, PONV is a risk factor for post-operative bleeding [3,4], and prophylactic anti-emetics may be beneficial.

Previous studies have shown that prophylactic dexamethasone has anti-emetic and analgesic effects. Glucocorticoids are anti-inflammatory and immunosuppressive agents, and dexamethasone may exert its therapeutic actions through central inhibition of prostaglandin synthesis, by decreasing serotonin turnover in the central nervous system, and by influencing the systemic inflammatory response in favor of anti-inflammatory mediators [5–9].

A systematic review demonstrated that prophylactic dexamethasone was safe and effective for reducing the incidence of PONV and post-operative pain in patients undergoing laparoscopic cholecystectomy compared to placebo [10]. In patients undergoing thyroidectomy, a previous meta-analysis demonstrated a significant reduction of PONV in patients treated with a single dose of dexamethasone versus placebo [11]. However, the relatively small sample size included in this review precluded the authors from drawing definitive conclusions, and the optimal dose and timing of dexamethasone administration, and efficacy of combining dexamethasone with other anti-emetics, remains unclear.

The objective of the current study was to confirm, and continue to investigate the impact of prophylactic corticosteroid administration on PONV, post-operative pain, and complications following thyroidectomy.

## Methods

This systematic review and meta-analysis is reported in accordance with the recommendations of the PRISMA statement [12].

### 2.1 Outcome measures

#### 2.1.1 Primary outcome measure

1. Incidence of PONV during the immediate 24 h post-operative period, dichotomized as no nausea versus others; this was evaluated according to a 3-point ordinal scale: no nausea; nausea; retching and/or vomiting

#### 2.1.2 Secondary outcome measures

1. Post-operative pain scores
2. Need for rescue anti-emetic or analgesic agent(s)
3. Incidence of steroid-related complications, including hyperglycemia, wound infection, delayed wound healing, headaches, dizziness, facial flushing, constipation, and abdominal pain

### 2.2 Data collection and analysis

**2.2.1 Searches.** We searched PubMed, Embase, and Cochrane Library databases from their inception to October 1, 2013 using Cochrane Highly Sensitive Search Strategies to identify randomized controlled trials (RCTs) for potential inclusion in our review [13]. We used the following MeSH terms and keywords: thyroid surgery OR thyroidectomy AND corticosteroid, glucocorticoid, steroid, OR dexamethasone. The search strategy is summarized in Table S1. Authors' names were entered as search terms in the PubMed database to check for additional studies. Trials were also identified using the "related articles" function in PubMed. We hand-searched reference lists from articles identified by the electronic search and from previous meta-analyses. This process was performed iteratively until no additional articles could be identified.

**2.2.2 Inclusion and Exclusion Criteria.** We included RCTs that: evaluated the prophylactic effect of dexamethasone versus placebo without other anti-emetics, dexamethasone versus placebo plus concomitant administration of a different anti-emetic, dexamethasone versus a different anti-emetic, and comparisons using different doses of dexamethasone for PONV in patients

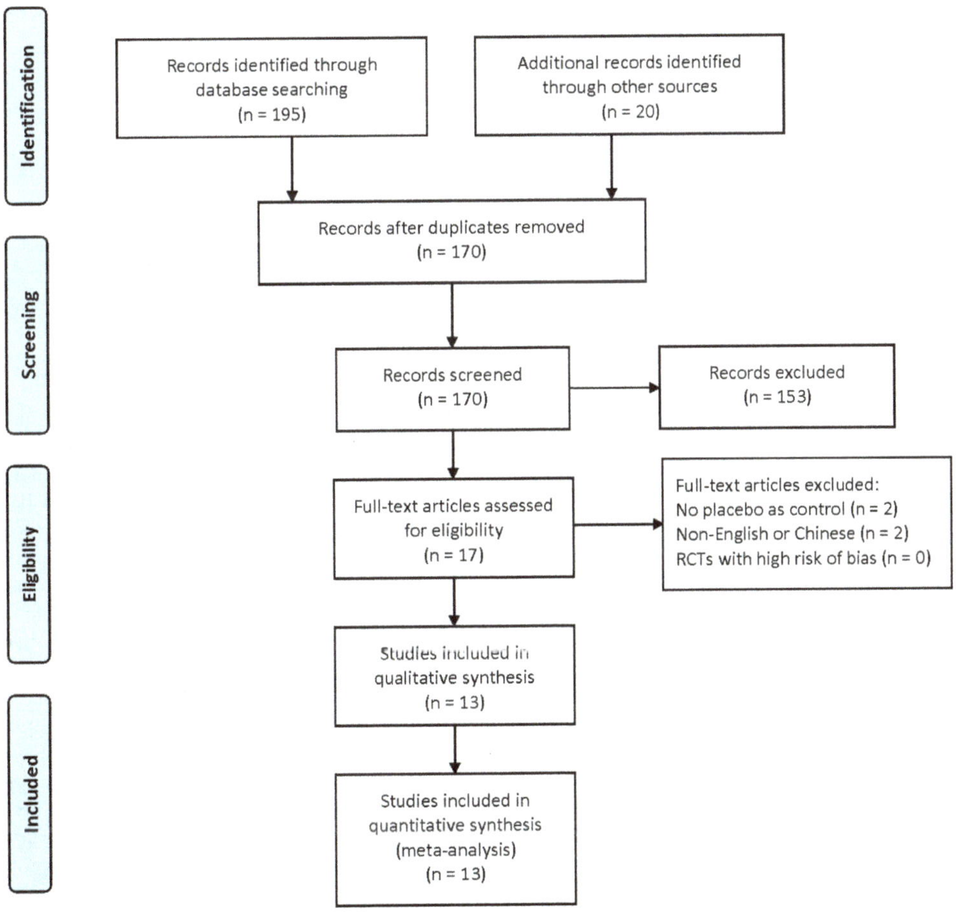


**Figure 1. Flow chart for selecting the trials.** On the basis of the search strategy, 195 articles were identified by the initial search, and 17 required further assessment. Finally, 13 articles were included in this review.

**Table 1.** Characteristics of trials included in the meta-analysis.

| Study | Sample size | Interventions | Studies divided |
|---|---|---|---|
| Wang 1999 [18] | 120 | D 10 mg vs. Droperidol 1.25 mg vs. Placebo, all IV at 1 minute before induction | Wang 1999 D 10: D 10 mg vs. Placebo; Wang 1999: D 10 mg vs. Droperidol 1.25 mg |
| Wang 2000 [19] | 225 | D 10 mg vs. D 5 mg vs. D 2.5 mg vs. D 1.25 mg vs. Placebo, all IV immediately after induction | Wang 2000 D 10: D 10 mg vs. Placebo; Wang 2000 D 5: D 5 mg vs. Placebo; Wang 2000 D 2.5: D 2.5 mg vs. Placebo; Wang 2000 D 1.25: D 1.25 mg vs. Placebo |
| Lee 2001 [20] | 135 | D 8 mg vs. D 5 mg vs. Placebo, all IV before anesthesia | Lee 2001 D 8: D 10 mg vs. Placebo; Lee 2001 D 5: D 5 mg vs. Placebo |
| Fujji 2007 [21] | 75 | D 8 mg vs. D 4 mg vs. Placebo, all IV at the end of surgery | Fujji 2007 D8: D 8 mg vs. Placebo; Fujji 2007 D4: D 4 mg vs. Placebo |
| Worni 2008 [22] | 70 | D 8 mg vs. Placebo, both IV at 45 minutes before anesthesia | Worni 2008 D8: D 8 mg vs. Placebo |
| Feroci 2010 [23] | 102 | D 8 mg vs. Placebo, both IV at 20 minutes before induction | Feroci 2010 D8: D 8 mg vs. Placebo |
| Doksrod 2012 [24] | 120 | D 0.3 mg/kg vs. D 0.15 mg/kg vs. Placebo, all IV within 10 min after induction | Doksrod 2012 D18: D 0.3 mg/kg vs. Placebo; Doksrod 2012 D9: D 0.15 mg/kg vs. Placebo |
| Song 2013 [25] | 123 | D 10 mg vs. Ramosetron 0.3 mg vs. Placebo, both IV immediately after anesthesia | Song 2013 D 10: D10: D 10 mg vs. Placebo; Song 2013: D 10 mg vs. Ramosetron 0.3 mg |
| Barros 2013 [26] | 40 | D 4 mg vs. Placebo, both IV immediately after induction | Barros 2013 D4: D 4 mg vs. Placebo |
| Schietroma 2013 [27] | 328 | D 8 mg vs. Placebo, both IV at 90 minutes before skin incision | Schietroma 2013 D8: D 8 mg vs. Placebo |
| Zhou 2012 [28] | 150 | D 8 mg + T 5 mg vs. D 8 mg vs. T 5 mg, all IV immediately before induction | Zhou 2012 Tropisetron: D 8 mg + T 5 mg vs.T 5 mg; Zhou 2012: D 8 mg vs. T 5 mg |
| Bononi 2010 [29] | 562 | D 4 mg +O 4 mg vs. O 4 mg, D IV at induction and ondansetron IV at 15 minutes before tracheal extubation | Bononi 2010 Ondansetron: D 4 mg +O 4 mg vs. O 4 mg |
| Fujji 2000 [30] | 130 | D 8 mg + G 40 ug/kg vs. G 40 ug/kg, both IV immediately before induction | Fujji 2000 Granisetron: D 8 mg + G 40 ug/kg vs. G 40 ug/kg |

IV: intravenous; ASA, American Society of Anesthesiologists; D: dexamethasone; T: tropisetron; O: ondansetron; G: Granisetron.

undergoing thyroidectomy. The included trials reported at least one of our outcome measures, and clearly reported patient inclusion and exclusion criteria, anesthetic technique, protocols for administration of the experimental drugs, and a definition and evaluation of nausea and vomiting. Studies were excluded if they were not RCTs, included patients who were undergoing other surgical procedures concomitantly, reported insufficient data, or were duplicate studies.

**2.2.3 Selection of studies.** Two reviewers (ZH Zou and YM Jiang) independently examined titles and abstracts to select eligible RCTs. We removed records that were ongoing or unpublished studies, or were published as abstracts or conference proceedings. Where datasets were overlapping or duplicated, only the most recent information was included. We retrieved the full text of potentially relevant studies. Two reviewers (ZH Zou and YM Jiang) independently examined the full text records to determine which studies met the inclusion criteria. We resolved disagreements about selection of studies by discussion and consensus.

**2.2.4 Data extraction and management.** Two reviewers (ZH Zou and YM Jiang) independently extracted data from eligible RCTs including details describing study population, interventions, and outcomes. We resolved disagreements about data extraction by discussion and consensus.

**2.2.5 Assessment of quality of evidence in included studies.** Two reviewers (ZH Zou and YM Jiang) independently assessed RCT quality and risk of bias using tools provided by the Cochrane Collaboration [14]. The reviewers examined six domains including sequence generation, allocation concealment, double-blind evaluation (blinding), complete outcome data, selective outcome reporting, and baseline comparability of groups. The risk of bias was categorized as low, high, or unclear. RCTs with high risk of bias in at least three of six domains were not included in the meta-analysis. Baseline comparability of groups was assessed using seven matching criteria: age, sex, history of motion sickness, previous post-operative emesis, anesthetic technique, operation type (partial or total thyroidectomy), and duration of surgery. Baseline incomparability was defined as non-matching in at least three of the seven criteria. We resolved disagreements about quality of evidence by discussion and consensus.

**2.2.6 Statistical analysis.** Statistical analyses were performed using RevMan (ver. 5.0; The Cochrane Collaboration, Oxford, UK) software and STATA (ver. 11.2; STATA Corpora-

**Table 2.** Details of anesthetic technique, and rescue analgesics and anti-emetics in the included trials.

| Study | Anesthetic technique | Rescue analgesics | Rescue antiemetics |
|---|---|---|---|
| Wang 1999 [18] | Propofol 2.0–2.5 mg/kg, glycopyrrolate 0.2 mg, fentanyl 2.0 ug/kg IV maintained with 1.0%–2.5% isoflurane in oxygen | Diclofenac 75 mg IM q12h | Ondansetron 4 mg IV |
| Wang 2000 [19] | Propofol 2.0–2.5 mg/kg, glycopyrrolate 0.2 mg, fentanyl 2.0 ug/kg IV maintained with 1.0%–2.5% isoflurane in oxygen | Diclofenac 75 mg IM q12h | Ondansetron 4 mg IV |
| Lee 2001 [20] | Glycopyrrolate 0.2 mg, fentanyl 2 ug/kg, thiopental 5 mg/kg IV maintained with desflurane in oxygen | Ketorolac 15 mg IV q6h | Droperidol 1.25 mg IV |
| Fujji 2007 [21] | Propofol 2 mg/kg, fentanyl 2 ug/kg, vecuronium 0.1 mg/kg IV maintained with 1–3% sevoflurane in oxygen | Indomethacin 50 mg rectally | Ranitidine 150 mg orally |
| Worni 2008 [22] | Propofol/thiopental, atracurium, isoflurane, or sevoflurane and fentanyl 5–10 ug/kg | Acetaminophen 4 g/day; second-line metamizole 1g or morphine | Ondansetron 4 mg IV; second-line droperidol 0.625 mg IV |
| Feroci 2010 [23] | Propofol 2 mg/kg, fentanyl 2 ug/kg, vecuronium 0.1 mg/kg IV maintained with sevoflurane in oxygen | Paracetamol 1000 mg IV q8 h; second-line ketorolac 30 mg IV q12h | Metoclopramide 10 mg IV; second-line ondansetron 4 mg IV |
| Doksrod 2012 [24] | Propofol, fentanyl, vecuronium IV maintained with desflurane (4–8%) and itrous oxide (60%) in oxygen | Oxycodone 5 mg orally; second-line metamizole or morphine 2.5 mg IV | Metoclopramide 20 mg IV; second-line ondansetron 4 mg IV |
| Song 2013 [25] | Remifentanil 1 ug/kg, propofol 1–2 mg/kg, rocuroniumin 0.9 mg/kg IV, maintained with desflurane in oxygen–air mixture | Ketorolac 30 mg IV | Metoclopramide 10 mg IV |
| Barros 2013 [26] | Propofol, fentanyl 2.0 ug/kg, cisatracurium 0.15 mg/kg, maintained with sevoflurane in oxygen | Ketorolac 30 mg or parecoxib 40 mg IV | Ondansetron 4 mg IV |
| Schietroma 2013 [27] | Sodium thiopental 5 mg/kg,atracurium besylate 0.5 mg/kg, maintained with oxygen in air, sevoflurane, and remifentanil hydrochloride | Ketorolac tromethamine 30 mg IV q6h | Ondansetron hydrochloride 4 mg IV |
| Zhou 2012 [28] | Propofol 1.5–2.5 mg/kg, midazolam 0.1–0.2 mg/kg, fentanyl 1.0–2.0 ug/kg, maintained with 1.0 3.0% sevoflurane in oxygen | Pethidine 25 mg IV | Metoclopramide 10 mg IV; second-line tropisetron 5 mg IV |
| Bononi 2010 [29] | Not stated[a] | Not stated | Not stated |
| Fujji 2000 [30] | Thiopentone 5 mg/kg, fentanyl 2 ug/kg, vecuronium 0.2 mg/kg maintained with isoflurane (1.0%–3.0%) and nitrous oxide (66%) in oxygen | Indomethacin 50mg rectally for moderae pain and buprenorphiine 0.2 mg IM for severe pain | Domperidone retally |

IV, intravenous; IM, intramuscular; [a]no difference.

**Table 3.** Quality of evidence in included studies.

| Included studies | Country | Sequence generation | Allocation concealment | Double blinding | Complete outcome data | No selective reporting | Baseline comparability | Risk of bias |
|---|---|---|---|---|---|---|---|---|
| Wang 1999 [18] | China | Adequate | Unclear | Yes | Yes | Yes | Yes | Low |
| Wang 2000 [19] | China | Adequate | Unclear | Yes | Yes | Yes | Yes | Low |
| Lee 2001 [20] | China | Adequate | Adequate | Yes | Yes | Yes | Yes | Low |
| Fujii 2007 [21] | Japan | Adequate | Adequate | Yes | Yes | Yes | Yes | Low |
| Worni 2008 [22] | Switzerland | Adequate | Adequate | Yes | Yes | Yes | Yes | Low |
| Feroci 2011 [23] | Italy | Adequate | Adequate | Yes | Yes | Yes | Yes | Low |
| Doksrod 2012 [24] | Norway | Adequate | Adequate | Yes | Yes | Yes | Yes | Low |
| Song 2013 [25] | Korea | Adequate | Adequate | Unclear | Yes | Yes | Yes | Low |
| Barros 2013 [26] | Portugal | Adequate | Adequate | Yes | Yes | Yes | Yes | Low |
| Schietroma 2013 [27] | Italy | Adequate | Adequate | Yes | Yes | Yes | Yes | Low |
| Zhou 2012 [28] | China | Adequate | Adequate | Unclear | Yes | Yes | Yes | Low |
| Bononi 2010 [29] | Italy | Adequate | Adequate | Unclear | Yes | Yes | Yes | Low |
| Fujii 2000 [30] | Japan | Adequate | Adequate | Yes | Yes | Yes | Yes | Low |

tion, College Station, TX, USA) software. Weighted mean differences (WMDs) with 95% confidence intervals (CIs) were calculated for continuous variables, and risk ratios (RRs) with 95% CIs were calculated for dichotomous variables. A random-effects model was used to pool studies with significant heterogeneity, as determined by the chi-squared test ($P \leq 0.10$) and the inconsistency index ($I^2 \geq 50\%$). Potential sources of statistical heterogeneity were explored by carrying out subgroup and sensitivity analyses. Subgroup analyses were performed by stratifying patients according to dose of corticosteroid and timing of dexamethasone administration; sensitivity analyses explored the impact of excluding outlying results. The presence of publication bias was comprehensively assessed using Begg's funnel plot and Begg's rank correlation test of asymmetry. Publication bias was thought to be present when the continuity-corrected $Pr>|z|$ value was $\leq 0.1$ [15]. The GRADE system was used to summarize the overall quality of evidence [16,17].

## Results

### 3.1 Trial identification

The searches identified 195 articles. We screened titles and abstracts, and 17 were identified as potentially eligible for inclusion. We retrieved the full text articles. After analyzing the full text articles, 4 studies were excluded and 13 RCTs [18–30] were found eligible for inclusion according to our criteria for considering studies in this review (Fig. 1).

### 3.2 Characteristics of included studies

The characteristics of the included studies are shown in Table 1. The 13 eligible RCTs included 2,180 patients who underwent general anesthesia for thyroidectomy. The majority of RCTs included patients classified as American Society of Anesthesiologists (ASA) class I or II. Exclusion criteria were: pregnant women, patients with insulin-dependent diabetes mellitus, obesity, and patients with a high risk for PONV. Dexamethasone was administered intravenously in a single or combination dose ranging from 1.25–18 mg. Timing of administration varied from 90 minutes before skin incision to the end of surgery. Controls included placebo, droperidol, granisetron, ondansetron, tropisetron or a combination of these medications. Confounders such as anesthetic technique and rescue analgesics and anti-emetics were standardized within studies (Table 2). Risk of bias was low across all RCTs (Table 3).

### 3.3 Treatment effects

**3.3.1 Primary outcome.** *Incidence of PONV: Dexamethasone versus placebo, with or without concomitant anti-emetics* - Data reporting on the incidence of PONV in thyroidectomy patients treated with dexamethasone versus placebo with or without concomitant anti-emetics are described in 11 RCTs [18–25,28–30]. The meta-analysis demonstrated a significant decrease in the incidence of PONV in patients receiving dexamethasone compared to placebo, with or without concomitant anti-emetics (RR 0.52, 95% CI 0.43 to 0.63, $P<0.00001$; Fig. 2). There was evidence of significant heterogeneity between studies ($P=0.003$, $I^2=56\%$). The dose-response gradient may have caused most of the variation between RCTs (Fig. 3; Fig.S1).

*Incidence of PONV: Dexamethasone versus a different anti-emetic* - Data reporting on the incidence of PONV in thyroidectomy patients treated with dexamethasone versus a different anti-emetic, including droperidol, granisetron, or tropisetron, are described in three RCTs [18,25,28]. The meta-analysis demonstrated no significant difference in the incidence of PONV in

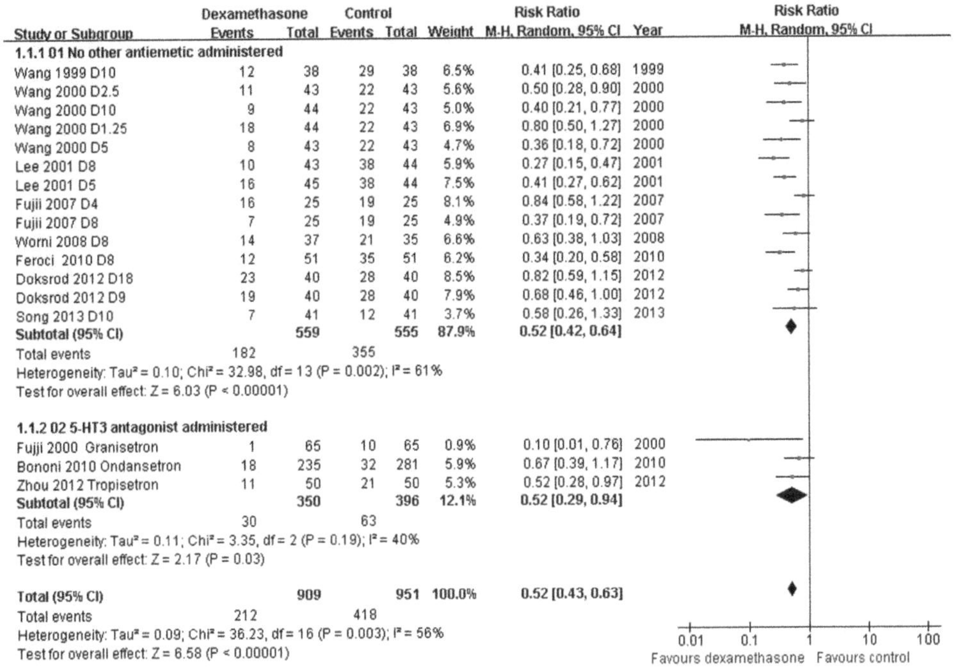


**Figure 2. Incidence of PONV grouped by concomitant anti-emetics.** Eleven studies described the incidence of PONV in thyroidectomy patients treated with dexamethasone versus placebo with or without concomitant anti-emetics (RR 0.52, 95% CI 0.43 to 0.63, $P<0.00001$). There was evidence of significant heterogeneity between studies ($P=0.003$, $I^2=56\%$).

patients receiving dexamethasone compared to these different anti-emetics (RR 1.25, 95% CI 0.86–1.81, $P=0.24$; Fig. 4). There was no evidence of significant heterogeneity between RCTs ($P=0.27$, $I^2=23\%$).

**3.3.2 Secondary outcomes.** *Postoperative pain scores and need for rescue analgesia: Dexamethasone versus placebo with or without concomitant anti-emetics* - Data reporting on post-operative pain scores in thyroidectomy patients treated with dexamethasone versus placebo with or without concomitant anti-emetics are described in six RCTs [18,20,22,23,25,26]. Pain scores were evaluated based on visual analogue scales (VAS) completed by patients 24 h post-operatively. Four RCTs [22,23,25,26] reported data as means ± standard deviations (SDs); two RCTs [18,20] reported data as medians (range) converted to estimated means and SDs [31]. The meta-analysis demonstrated a significantly lower post-operative VAS score in patients receiving dexamethasone compared to placebo, with or without concomitant anti-emetics (WMD −1.17, 95% CI −1.91 to −0.44, $P=0.002$; Fig. 5). There was evidence of significant heterogeneity between RCTs ($P<0.00001$, $I^2=94\%$). The doses of dexamethasone may have caused most of the variation between RCTs. The need for rescue analgesia was significantly less frequent in the patients that received dexamethasone (RR 0.65, 95% CI 0.50–0.83, $P=0.0008$; Fig. 6); there was no evidence of significant heterogeneity between RCTs ($P=0.25$, $I^2=25\%$).

*Need for rescue anti-emetic: Dexamethasone versus placebo with or without concomitant antiemetics* - Data reporting on the need for rescue anti-emetics in thyroidectomy patients treated with dexamethasone versus placebo with or without concomitant anti-emetics are described in six studies [19,25–28,30]. The meta-analysis demonstrated a significant decrease in the need for rescue anti-emetics in patients receiving dexamethasone compared to placebo, with or without concomitant anti-emetics (RR 0.42, 95% CI 0.30 to 0.57, $P<0.00001$; Fig. 7). There was no evidence of significant heterogeneity between RCTs ($P=0.43$, $I^2=0\%$).

*Incidence of adverse events: Dexamethasone versus placebo with or without concomitant anti-emetics* - Data reporting on blood glucose levels in thyroidectomy patients treated with dexamethasone are described in two RCTs. A significantly higher level of blood glucose was observed in patients receiving dexamethasone compared to controls during the first 8 hours post-operatively [23,24]. No statistical differences in symptomatic transient hypocalcemia and asymptomatic transient hypocalcemia were present [23]. One RCT [27] reported that dexamethasone administration prevented recurrent laryngeal nerve palsy; however, this effect was not described elsewhere [23]. There were no significant differences in the incidences of extrapyramidal signs including headache, dizziness, constipation, and muscle pain, and other adverse events such as wound infection and delayed wound healing, in patients receiving dexamethasone compared to controls.

## 3.4 Subgroup analyses

**Incidence of PONV: Dose of dexamethasone.** Subgroup analyses stratified by dose of dexamethasone (range, 1.25 mg to 18 mg) demonstrated that dexamethasone 4–5 mg and 8–10 mg significantly reduced the incidence of PONV compared to controls (1.25–5 mg: RR 0.59, 95% CI 0.44 to 0.79; 8–10 mg: RR 0.45, 95% CI 0.35–0.57), while dexamethasone 18 mg did not (RR 0.82, 95% CI 0.59–1.15) (Fig. 3). Dexamethasone 8–10 mg had a significantly greater effect for reducing the incidence of PONV than dexamethasone 1.25–5 mg (1.25–5 mg RR 0.40, 95% CI 0.28 to 0.55; 8–10 mg: RR 0.23, 95% CI 0.18–0.31; P = 0.02; Fig. S1).

**Incidence of PONV: Timing of dexamethasone administration.** The RCTs included in this review varied with regard to timing of dexamethasone administration. Some patients

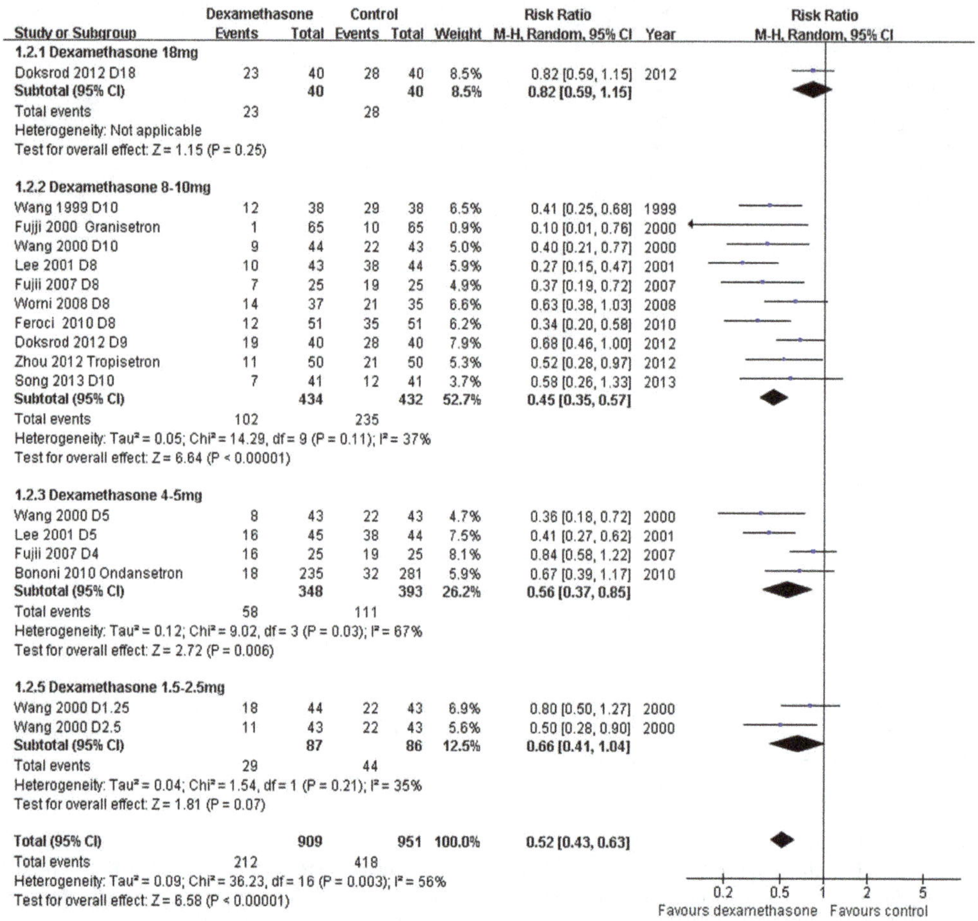


**Figure 3. PONV according to dexamethasone dose.** Higher dexamethasone doses (8–10 mg) were significantly more effective than lower dexamethasone doses (1.25–5 mg) ($P = 0.02$).

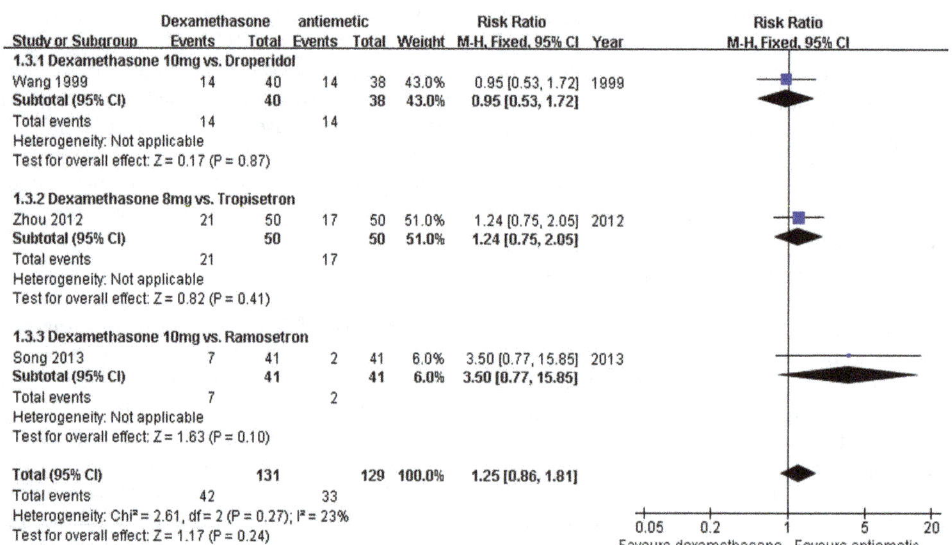


**Figure 4. Comparison of dexamethasone with other anti-emetics.** Three studies described the incidence of PONV in thyroidectomy patients treated with dexamethasone versus other anti-emetics (RR 1.25, 95% CI 0.86–1.81, $P = 0.24$). There was no evidence of significant heterogeneity between RCTs ($P = 0.27$, $I^2 = 23\%$).

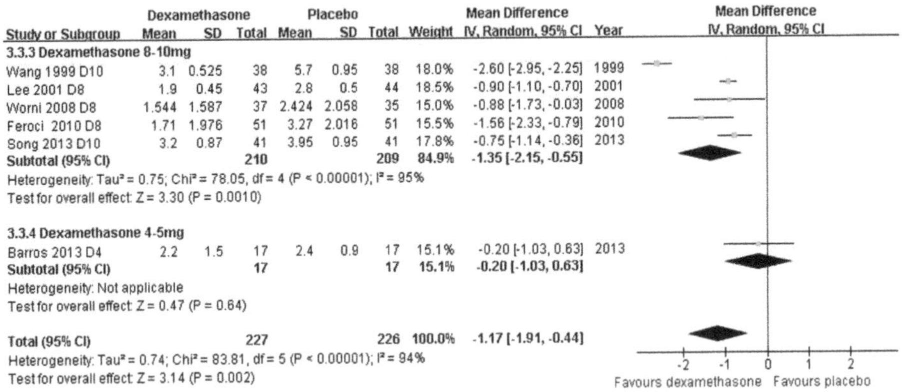


**Figure 5. VAS post-operative pain score grouped by dexamethasone dose.** Six studies described post-operative pain scores in thyroidectomy patients treated with dexamethasone versus placebo with or without concomitant anti-emetics (WMD −1.17, 95% CI −1.91 to −0.44, $P = 0.002$). There was evidence of significant heterogeneity between RCTs ($P < 0.00001$, $I^2 = 94\%$).

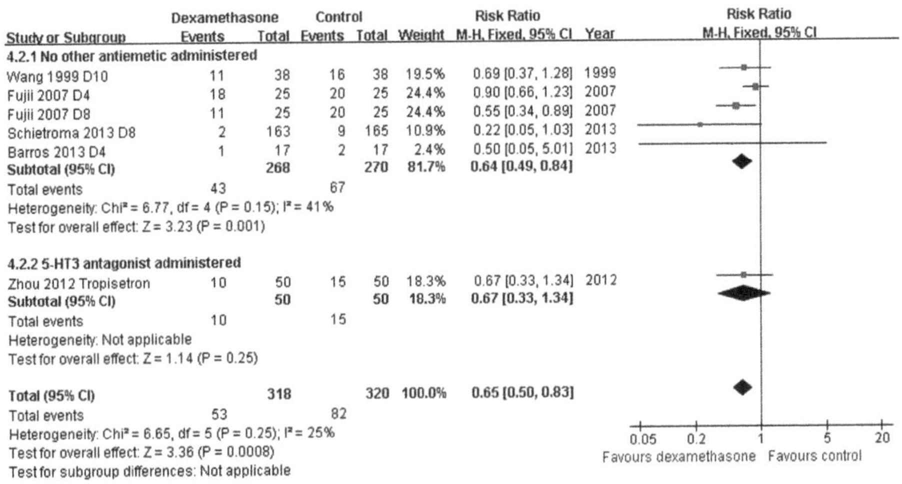


**Figure 6. Need for rescue analgesics grouped by concomitant anti-emetics.** Six studies described the need for rescue analgesics in thyroidectomy patients treated with dexamethasone versus placebo with or without concomitant anti-emetics (RR 0.65, 95% CI 0.50–0.83, $P = 0.0008$). There was no evidence of significant heterogeneity between RCTs ($P = 0.25$, $I^2 = 25\%$).

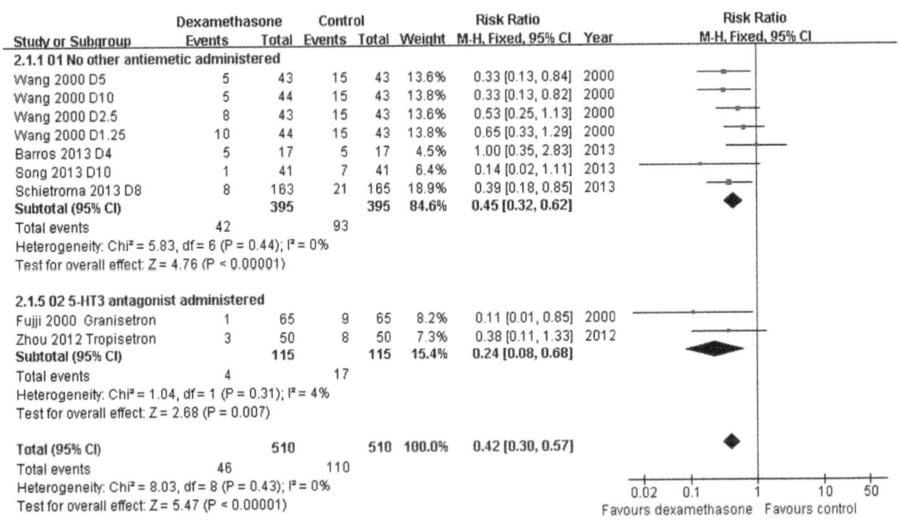


**Figure 7. Need for rescue antiemetics grouped by concomitant antiemetics.** Six studies described the need for rescue antiemetics in thyroidectomy patients treated with dexamethasone versus placebo with or without concomitant antiemetics (RR 0.42, 95% CI 0.30 to 0.57, $P < 0.00001$). There was no evidence of significant heterogeneity between RCTs ($P = 0.43$, $I^2 = 0\%$).

**Table 4.** GRADE evidence.

| Outcomes | Illustrative comparative risks* (95% CI) | | Relative effect (95% CI) | No of Participants (studies) | Quality of the evidence (GRADE) |
|---|---|---|---|---|---|
| | Assumed risk | Corresponding risk | | | |
| | Placebo | Dexamethasone | | | |
| **Dexamethasone versus placebo (in addition to other antiemetics): PONV** | **440 per 1000** | **229 per 1000** (189 to 277) | **RR 0.52** (0.43 to 0.63) | 1860 (17 studies) | ⊕⊕⊕⊕ **high**[1] |
| **Dexamethasone versus placebo (in addition to other antiemetics): rescue antiemetics** | **216 per 1000** | **91 per 1000** (65 to 123) | **RR 0.42** (0.3 to 0.57) | 1020 (9 studies) | ⊕⊕⊕ **high** |
| **Dexamethasone comparison of doses: PONV** | **440 per 1000** | **229 per 1000** (189 to 277) | **RR 0.52** (0.43 to 0.63) | 1860 (17 studies) | ⊕⊕⊕⊕ **high**[2] |
| **Dexamethasone versus placebo: VAS pain score** | | The mean dexamethasone versus placebo: vas pain score in the intervention groups was **1.17 lower** (1.91 to 0.44 lower) | | 453 (6 studies) | ⊕⊕⊕⊖ **moderate**[3] |
| **Dexamethasone versus placebo (in addtion to other antiemetics): resuce analgesic** | **256 per 1000** | **167 per 1000** (128 to 213) | **RR 0.65** (0.5 to 0.83) | 638 (6 studies) | ⊕⊕⊕⊖ **moderate**[4] |
| **Dexamethasone versus a different antiemetic: PONV** | **256 per 1000** | **320 per 1000** (220 to 463) | **RR 1.25** (0.86 to 1.81) | 260 (3 studies) | ⊕⊕⊕⊕ **high** |

*The basis for the **assumed risk** (e.g. the median control group risk across studies) is provided in footnotes. The **corresponding risk** (and its 95% confidence interval) is based on the assumed risk in the comparison group and the **relative effect** of the intervention (and its 95% CI). **CI:** Confidence interval; **RR:** Risk ratio.
GRADE Working Group grades of evidence. **High quality:** Further research is very unlikely to change our confidence in the estimate of effect. **Moderate quality:** Further research is likely to have an important impact on our confidence in the estimate of effect and may change the estimate. **Low quality:** Further research is very likely to have an important impact on our confidence in the estimate of effect and is likely to change the estimate. **Very low quality:** We are very uncertain about the estimate.
[1]Although the PONV results demonstrated significant heterogeneity ($P = 0.003$, $I^2 = 56\%$), it was partly explained by the dose of dexamethasone. [2]Downgraded by not comparing higher dose with lower dose directly, but upgraded by the dose-response gradient. [3]Although there was significant heterogeneity ($P < 0.00001$, $I^2 = 94\%$), it was partly explained by the dose of dexamethasone. [4]Publication bias as $Pr > |z| = 0.06$.
PONV: post-operative nausea and vomiting; VAS: visual analogue scales.
**Patient or population:** patients undergoing thyroidectomy. **Settings:** evidence from China, Japan, Korea, Italy, Switzerland, Norway, Portugal. **Intervention:** dexamethasone. **Comparison:** placebo.

received dexamethasone 90 minutes before skin incision, while others received dexamethasone postoperatively. Wang et al [32] demonstrated that dexamethasone administered before anesthesia was more effective in decreasing early PONV compared to dexamethasone administered after anesthesia. These observations are in accordance with data showing that the onset time of dexamethasone on anti-emesis is approximately 2 hours. In the current study, subgroup analysis stratified by the timing of dexamethasone administration showed that dexamethasone was most effective in preventing PONV when administered before rather than after induction of anesthesia ($P = 0.0002$; Fig. S2).

### 3.5 Sensitivity analysis

To explore the effects of individual RCTs on the pooled OR estimates, we performed a sensitivity analysis omitting one study at a time. No single RCT significantly affected the overall results of the meta-analysis.

### 3.6 Publication bias

Visual inspection of a Funnel plot, Egger's test, and Begg's rank correlation test revealed no significant publication bias (Begg's rank correlation test, continuity-corrected $Pr > |z| > 0.1$), except for RCTs reporting on the need for rescue anti-emetic in patients receiving dexamethasone versus placebo, with or without concomitant antiemetics ($Pr > |z| = 0.06$), (Table S2).

### 3.7 Quality of evidence

Quality of available evidence from RCTs, which was downgraded by inconsistency (heterogeneity between studies), indirectness (variations in study setting), or publication bias, and upgraded by dose-response gradient, varied from moderate to high (Table 4).

## Discussion

PONV is a common and distressing complication for patients undergoing thyroidectomy; therefore, prophylactic anti-emetics may be beneficial. An optimal anti-emetic regimen should be capable of decreasing the incidence of PONV without increasing the risk for adverse events. However, most of the currently used anti-emetics, including anti-histamines, butyrophenones, and dopamine receptor antagonists cause occasional undesirable adverse events, such as excessive sedation, hypotension, dry mouth, dysphoria, hallucinations, and extrapyramidal signs [33]. 5-HT3 antagonists are effective for preventing and treating PONV in patients undergoing various types of surgery [34]. However, the use of prophylactic anti-emetic therapy with 5-HT3 antagonists has been criticized for being too expensive [35].

Our meta-analysis of 13 RCTs demonstrated that prophylactic dexamethasone is effective in reducing the incidence of PONV, post-operative pain scores, and the need for rescue analgesia and anti-emetics compared to placebo administered with or without contaminant anti-emetics in patients undergoing thyroidectomy. In addition, our findings showed that dexamethasone is as effective as other anti-emetics for reducing PONV in this patient population. However, the benefits of administering dexamethasone as a more cost-effective anti-emetic and efficacious analgesic drug[35] should be weighed against the potential side effects. Our study indicated that dexamethasone administration is associated with an increase in blood glucose during the immediate post-operative period, but with no other serious adverse events.

For optimal dose and timing of dexamethasone administration, subgroup analyses showed that higher doses of dexamethasone (8–10 mg) are more effective than lower doses (1.5–5 mg), and dexamethasone is most effective in preventing PONV when administered before rather than after induction of anesthesia.

In terms of populations eligible for treatment, the RCTs in the current study mostly included healthy patients, and excluded pregnant women, patients with insulin-dependent diabetes mellitus, those who were obese, and patients with a high risk for PONV. As such, the impact of prophylactic dexamethasone on outcomes in high-risk patients is not known. A larger sample size and well-performed RCTs including high risk patients are required for further investigations.

This review has several limitations. First, data reporting on the effects of prophylactic dexamethasone on post-operative pain scores and need for rescue analgesics in thyroidectomy patients were limited by substantial heterogeneity and publication bias, respectively. Second, the studies in this systematic review included patients across various age groups receiving dexamethasone according to very different protocols.

## Conclusion

The present meta-analysis shows that prophylactic dexamethasone is safe and effective for reducing the incidence of PONV, post-operative pain, and the need for rescue analgesia and anti-emetics in thyroidectomy patients. Prophylactic dexamethasone 8–10 mg administered before induction of anesthesia should be recommended for patients undergoing thyroidectomy except for those that are pregnant, have diabetes mellitus, hyperglycaemia or contraindications for corticosteroids. More high quality trials are warranted to define the benefits and risks of prophylactic dexamethasone in potential patients with high risk for PONV.

## Supporting Information

**Figure S1 Incidence of PONV stratified according to dexamethasone dose: 8–10 mg and 1.25–5 mg.**

**Figure S2 Incidence of PONV stratified by timing of dexamethasone administration.**

**Table S1 Search strategy from its inception to October 1, 2013.**

**Table S2 Begg's rank correlation test for publication bias.**

**Checklist S1 PRISMA 2009 Checklist.**

## Author Contributions

Conceived and designed the experiments: RZ ZZ MX. Performed the experiments: ZZ YJ. Analyzed the data: ZZ YJ. Contributed reagents/materials/analysis tools: ZZ YJ. Contributed to the writing of the manuscript: RZ MX.

## References


1. Sonner JM, Hynson JM, Clark O, Katz JA (1997) Nausea and vomiting following thyroid and parathyroid surgery. J Clin Anesth 9(5): 398–402.
2. Kranke P, Eberhart LH (2011) Possibilities and limitations in the pharmacological management of postoperative nausea and vomiting. Eur J Anaesthesiol 28: 758–765.
3. Matory YL, Spiro RH (1993) Wound bleeding after head and neck surgery. J Surg Oncol 53(1): 17–19.
4. Schwartz AE, Clark OH, Ituarte P, Lo Gerfo P (1998) Therapeutic controversy: thyroid surgery–the choice. J Clin Endocrinol Metab 83(4): 1097–1105.
5. Fredrikson M, Hursti T, Fürst CJ, Steineck G, Börjeson S, et al. (1992) Nausea in cancer chemotherapy is inversely related to urinary cortisol excretion. Br J Cancer 65: 779–780.
6. Aapro MS, Plezia PM, Alberts DS, Graham V, Jones SE, et al. (1984) Double-blind crossover study of the antiemetic efficacy of high-dose dexamethasone versus high-dose metoclopramide. J Clin Oncol 2: 466–471.
7. Sapolsky RM, Romero LM, Munck AU (2000) How do glucocorticoids influence stress responses? Integrating permissive, suppressive, stimulatory, and preparative actions. Endocr Rev 21: 55–89.
8. Hargreaves KM, Costello A (1990) Glucocorticoids suppress levels of immunoreactive bradykinin in inflamed tissue as evaluated by microdialysis probes. Clin Pharmacol Ther 48: 168–178.
9. Hong D, Byers MR, Oswald RJ (1993) Dexamethasone treatment reduces sensory neuropeptides and nerve sprouting reactions in injured teeth. Pain 55: 171–181.
10. Karanicolas PJ1, Smith SE, Kanbur B, Davies E, Guyatt GH (2008) The Impact of Prophylactic Dexamethasone on Nausea and Vomiting After Laparoscopic Cholecystectomy A Systematic Review and Meta-Analysis. Ann Surg 248(5): 751–762.
11. Chen CC, Siddiqui FJ, Chen TL, Chan ES, Tam KW (2012) Dexamethasone for prevention of postoperative nausea and vomiting in patients undergoing thyroidectomy: meta-analysis of randomized controlled trials. World J Surg 36: 61–68.
12. Moher D, Liberati A, Tetzlaff J, Altman DG, PRISMA Group (2010) Preferred reporting items for systematic reviews and meta-analyses: the PRISMA statement. Int J Surg 8: 336–341.
13. Lefebvre C, Manheimer E, Glanville J (2011) Chapter 6: searching for studies. In: Higgins JPT, Green S (editors). Cochrane Handbook for Systematic Reviews of Interventions Version 5.1.0 [updated March 2011]. The Cochrane Collaboration, 2011. Available: www.cochrane-handbook.org.
14. Higgins JPT, Altman DG, Sterne JAC (2011) Chapter 8: assessing risk of bias in included studies. In: Higgins JPT, Green S (editors). Cochrane Handbook for Systematic Reviews of Interventions Version 5.1.0 [updated March 2011]. The Cochrane Collaboration, 2011. Available: www.cochrane-handbook.org.
15. Begg CB, Mazumdar M (1994) Operating characteristics of a rank correlation test for publication bias. Biometrics 50(4): 1088–1101.
16. Atkins D, Best D, Briss PA, Eccles M, Falck-Ytter Y, et al GRADE Working Group (2004) Grading quality of evidence and strength of recommendations. BMJ 328: 1490–1494.
17. Guyatt G, Gutterman D, Baumann MH, Addrizzo-Harris D, Hylek EM, et al. (2006) Grading strength of recommendations and quality of evidence in clinical guidelines. Chest 129: 174–181.
18. Wang JJ, Ho ST, Lee SC, Liu YC, Liu YH, et al. (1999) The prophylactic effect of dexamethasone on postoperative nausea and vomiting in women undergoing

thyroidectomy: a comparison of droperidol with saline. Anesth Analg 89: 200–203.
19. Wang JJ, Ho ST, Lee SC, Liu YC, Ho CM (2000) The use of dexamethasone for preventing postoperative nausea and vomiting in females undergoing thyroidectomy: a dose-ranging study. Anesth Analg 91: 1404–1407.
20. Lee Y, Lin PC, Lai HY, Huang SJ, Lin YS, et al. (2001) Prevention of PONV with dexamethasone in female patients undergoing desflurane anesthesia for thyroidectomy. Acta Anaesthesiol Sin 39: 151–156.
21. Fujii Y, Nakayama M (2007) Efficacy of dexamethasone for reducing postoperative nausea and vomiting and analgesic requirements after thyroidectomy. Otolaryngol Head Neck Surg 136: 274–277.
22. Worni M, Schudel HH, Seifert E, Inglin R, Hagemann M, et al. (2008) Randomized controlled trial on single dose steroid before thyroidectomy for benign disease to improve postoperative nausea, pain, and vocal function. Ann Surg 248: 1060–1066.
23. Feroci F, Rettori M, Borrelli A, Lenzi E, Ottaviano A, et al. (2011) Dexamethasone prophylaxis before thyroidectomy to reduce postoperative nausea, pain, and vocal dysfunction: a randomized clinical controlled trial. Head Neck 2011; 33: 840–846.
24. Doksrød S, Sagen Ø, Nøstdahl T, Ræder J (2012) Dexamethasone does not reduce pain or analgesic consumption after thyroid surgery; a prospective, randomized trial. Acta Anaesthesiol Scand 56: 513–519.
25. Song YK, Lee C (2013) Effects of ramosetron and dexamethasone on postoperative nausea, vomiting, pain, and shivering in female patients undergoing thyroid surgery. J Anesth 27: 29–34.
26. Barros A, Vale CP, Oliveira FC, Ventura C, Assunção J, et al. (2013) Dexamethasone effect on postoperative pain and tramadol requirement after thyroidectomy. Pharmacology 91: 153–157.
27. Schietroma M, Cecilia EM, Carlei F, Sista F, De Santis G, et al. (2013) Dexamethasone for the prevention of recurrent laryngeal nerve palsy and other complications after thyroid surgery: a randomized double-blind placebo-controlled trial. JAMA Otolaryngol Head Neck Surg 139: 471–478.
28. Zhou H, Xu H, Zhang J, Wang W, Wang Y, et al. (2012) Combination of dexamethasone and tropisetron before thyroidectomy to alleviate postoperative nausea, vomiting, and pain: randomized controlled trial. World J Surg 36: 1217–1224.
29. Bononi M, Amore Bonapasta S, Vari A, Scarpini M, De Cesare A, et al. (2010) Incidence and circumstances of cervical hematoma complicating thyroidectomy and its relationship to postoperative vomiting. Head Neck 32: 1173–1177.
30. Fujii Y, Tanaka H, Kobayashi N (2000) Granisetron/dexamethasone combination for the prevention of postoperative nausea and vomiting after thyroidectomy. Anaesth Intensive Care 28: 266–269.
31. Hozo SP, Djulbegovic B, Hozo I (2005) Estimating the mean and variance from the median, range, and the size of a sample. BMC Med Res Methodol 5: 13.
32. Wang JJ, Ho ST, Tzeng JI, Tang CS (2000) The effect of timing of dexamethasone administration on its efficacy as a prophylactic antiemetic for postoperative nausea and vomiting. Anesth Analg 91(1): 136–9.
33. Watcha MF, White PF (1992) Postoperative nausea and vomiting: its etiology, treatment, and prevention. Anesthesiology 77: 162–84.
34. Kovac AL (2000) Prevention and treatment of postoperative nausea and vomiting. Drugs 59: 213–43.
35. White PF, Watcha MF (1993) Are new drugs cost-effective for patients undergoing ambulatory surgery? Anesthesiology 78(1): 2–5.

23

# Initiation of Bladder Voiding with Epidural Stimulation in Paralyzed, Step Trained Rats

**Parag N. Gad[1], Roland R. Roy[1,4], Hui Zhong[1], Daniel C. Lu[3], Yury P. Gerasimenko[1,5], V. Reggie Edgerton[1,2,3,4]***

**1** Department of Integrative Biology and Physiology, University of California Los Angeles, Los Angeles, California, United States of America, **2** Department of Neurobiology, University of California Los Angeles, Los Angeles, California, United States of America, **3** Department of Neurosurgery, University of California Los Angeles, Los Angeles, California, United States of America, **4** Brain Research Institute, University of California Los Angeles, Los Angeles, California, United States of America, **5** Pavlov Institute of Physiology, St. Petersburg, Russia

## Abstract

The inability to control timely bladder emptying is one of the most serious challenges among the several functional deficits that occur after a complete spinal cord injury. Having demonstrated that electrodes placed epidurally on the dorsum of the spinal cord can be used in animals and humans to recover postural and locomotor function after complete paralysis, we hypothesized that a similar approach could be used to recover bladder function after paralysis. Also knowing that posture and locomotion can be initiated immediately with a specific frequency-dependent stimulation pattern and that with repeated stimulation-training sessions these functions can improve even further, we reasoned that the same two strategies could be used to regain bladder function. Recent evidence suggests that rats with severe paralysis can be rehabilitated with a multisystem neuroprosthetic training regime that counteracts the development of neurogenic bladder dysfunction. No data regarding the acute effects of locomotion on bladder function, however, were reported. In this study we show that enabling of locomotor-related spinal neuronal circuits by epidural stimulation also influences neural networks controlling bladder function and can play a vital role in recovering bladder function after complete paralysis. We have identified specific spinal cord stimulation parameters that initiate bladder emptying within seconds of the initiation of epidural stimulation. The clinical implications of these results are substantial in that this strategy could have a major impact in improving the quality of life and longevity of patients while simultaneously dramatically reducing ongoing health maintenance after a spinal cord injury.

**Editor:** Norbert Weidner, Heidelberg University Hospital, Germany

**Funding:** This research was supported by the National Institute of Biomedical Imaging and Bioengineering (NIBIB) R01EB007615, the National Institute of Health (NIH) R01NS062009, Christopher & Dana Reeve Foundation, the Walkabout Foundation, the Program No.5 and No.7 of the Presidium of RAN; and the Russian Foundation of Basic Research Grants: 13-04-01091 and 13-04-12030-ofi-m. The work is performed according to the Russian Government Program of Competitive Growth of Kazan Federal University. The funding agencies had no role in study design, data collection and analysis, decision to publish, or preparation of the manuscript.

**Competing Interests:** Some of the work described in this submission is the subject of a US patent application(s) filed and owned by the University of California Los Angeles to which some of the authors (VRE, RRR, YPG and DCL) have certain rights (royalty, receipt of intellectual property rights/patent holder); some of the authors (VRE, RRR, YPG and DCL) listed have ownership interest (stock, stock options) in a privately held entity, NeuroRecovery Technologies Inc.

* Email: vre@ucla.edu

## Introduction

The main functions of the lower urinary tract that are compromised after a spinal cord injury (SCI) are the ability to store and to expel urine in a coordinated, controlled manner [1,2]. Two of the major problems after a SCI are an overactive bladder and/or detrusor sphincter dyssynergia (DSD) both of which lead to incomplete bladder voiding due to uncoordinated contractions of the sphincter muscles [1,2]. Maintenance of bladder health and avoiding reflux of urine to the kidneys and other urinary tract infections are of utmost importance after a SCI. In humans, the inability to hold urine and to void when desired (incontinence) is a socially undesirable situation, although not one that is life threatening.

In the normal adult rat, storage of urine is dependent on the inhibition of parasympathetic action on the smooth bladder muscle (detrusor) and on the sympathetic tonic activation of the internal urethral sphincter for outflow resistance. During micturition, efficient voiding is dependent on synchronous activation of the detrusor muscle for contraction, relaxation of the internal urethral sphincter, and bursting activity of the striated external urethral sphincter (EUS) for enhanced urine flow [3,4]. In humans conscious control of the initiation of these largely autonomic functions involves a complex interaction between the cerebral cortex, pontine micturition center, sympathetic and parasympathetic nervous systems, and somatic motoneurons in the lumbar spinal cord. This interaction simultaneously activates stereotypical postural adjustments that are specie as well as gender unique. Although the behavior of the EUS in rats during voiding is different from that of humans, the chronic spinal rat model demonstrates lower urinary tract dysfunction similar to that observed in other species including human subjects [6].

Given the anatomical overlap in the neural networks within the lumbosacral spinal cord that control bladder function [5,6] and locomotor function [7,8,9], interactive effects of bladder function and locomotion are not surprising. For example, de Groat et al. [6] reported that the role of afferents originating in the bladder and EUS projecting to the lumbosacral region of the spinal cord was altered significantly after a mid-thoracic SCI. This overlap in the neural control of somatic and bladder function could represent either two separate neural circuits with some overlap or a single circuit being tuned differentially via varying frequencies of activation. We hypothesize that step training in the presence of electrical enabling motor control (eEmc) [10], a serotoninergic agonist (quipazine) [11] and glycinergic antagonist (strychnine) [12,13] would reinforce the overlapping neural circuitry controlling bladder function and locomotion and that voiding could be tuned by varying the frequencies of eEmc. We further hypothesized that since bladder control is autonomic it should be more amenable to epidural modulation than the less automatic control of locomotion.

The importance of controlling voiding is that the primary danger to the paralyzed individual is bladder overfilling and not partial emptying (incontinence). The spinal rat model does not address all the issues faced by humans after a SCI due to the inability to assess voluntary vs. involuntary responses in rats. This model, however, allowed us to assess the effects of electrical enabling motor control (eEmc) on bladder voiding, since the bladder of spinal rats must be manually expressed post-injury to avoid overfilling [10,12,13]. The main purpose of the present study, therefore, was to assess the acute and chronic effects of varying frequencies of eEmc in the lumbosacral region of the spinal cord on bladder voiding after a complete, mid-thoracic spinal cord transection in adult female rats. In addition, the effects of step training for 6 weeks post-injury on bladder voiding were determined. The results suggest that both eEmc and step training may have positive effects on the recovery of bladder voiding in spinal rats.

## Materials and Methods

### Study design

Data were obtained from 15 (10 trained and 5 untrained) adult female Sprague Dawley rats (270–300 g body weight). Pre- and post-surgical animal care procedures have been described in detail previously [14]. The rats were housed individually with food and water provided *ad libitum*. All survival surgical procedures were conducted under aseptic conditions with the rats deeply anesthetized with isoflurane gas administered via facemask as needed. All procedures described below are in accordance with the National Institute of Health Guide for the Care and Use of Laboratory Animals and were approved by the Animal Research Committee at UCLA. All animals underwent identical surgical procedures including spinal cord transection, intramuscular EMG implantation, and spinal cord epidural electrode implantation. The rats were allowed to recover for 7 days after which step training under the influence of eEmc was initiated. Step training was performed for 6 weeks, 5 days a week for 20 min/day. At 7 weeks post-injury, the rats were tested for their ability to step bipedally on a treadmill with eEmc (40 Hz), motor evoked potentials were generated by spinal cord stimulation (1, 5, and 40 Hz) and recorded in selected hindlimb muscles and the EUS while the rat was suspended in a harness [11,14]. Terminal bladder experiments were performed to determine the most efficient eEmc frequency to enable voiding and to study the activity of the EUS under different bladder conditions, i.e., empty, filled, and voiding. Details of each step are given below.

### Head connector and chronic intramuscular EMG electrode implantation

A small incision was made at the midline of the skull. The muscles and fascia were retracted laterally, small grooves were made in the skull with a scalpel, and the skull was dried thoroughly. Two amphenol head connectors with Teflon-coated stainless steel wires (AS632, Cooner Wire, Chatsworth CA) were securely attached to the skull with screws and dental cement as described previously [11]. Selected hindlimb muscles, i.e., the tibialis anterior (TA) and soleus, were implanted bilaterally with intramuscular EMG recording electrodes as described previously [11]. Skin and fascial incisions were made to expose the belly of each muscle. Two wires extending from the skull-mounted connector were routed subcutaneously to each muscle. The wires were inserted into the muscle belly using a 23-gauge needle and a small notch (~0.5–1.0 mm) was removed from the insulation of each wire to expose the conductor and form the electrodes. The wires were secured in the belly of the muscle via a suture on the wire at its entrance into and exit from the muscle belly. The proper placement of the electrodes was verified during the surgery by stimulating through the head connector and post-mortem via dissection.

### Spinal cord transection, epidural electrode implantation, and post-surgical animal care procedures

A partial laminectomy was performed at the T8–T9 vertebral level to expose the spinal cord. A complete spinal cord transection to include the dura was performed at approximately the T8 spinal level using microscissors. Two surgeons verified the completeness of the transection by lifting the cut ends of the spinal cord and passing a glass probe through the lesion site. Gel foam was inserted into the gap created by the transection as a coagulant and to separate the cut ends of the spinal cord.

For epidural electrode implantation, partial laminectomies were performed to expose the spinal cord at spinal levels L2 and S1. Two Teflon-coated stainless steel wires from the head connector were passed under the spinous processes and above the dura mater of the remaining vertebrae between the partial laminectomy sites. After removing a small portion (~1 mm notch) of the Teflon coating and exposing the conductor on the surface facing the spinal cord, the electrodes were sutured to the dura mater at the midline of the spinal cord above and below the electrode sites using 8.0 Ethilon suture (Ethicon, New Brunswick, NJ). Two common ground (indifferent EMG and stimulation grounds) wires (~1 cm of the Teflon removed distally) were inserted subcutaneously in the mid-back region. All wires (for both EMG and epidural stimulation) were coiled in the back region to provide stress relief.

All incision areas were irrigated liberally with warm, sterile saline. All surgical sites were closed in layers using 5.0 Vicryl (Ethicon, New Brunswick, NJ) for all muscle and connective tissue layers and for the skin incisions in the hindlimbs and 5.0 Ethilon for the back skin incision. All closed incision sites were cleansed thoroughly with saline solution. Analgesia was provided by buprenex (0.5–1.0 mg/kg, s.c. 3 times/day). The analgesics were initiated before completion of the surgery and continued for a minimum of 2 days. The rats were allowed to fully recover from anesthesia in an incubator. The rats were housed individually in

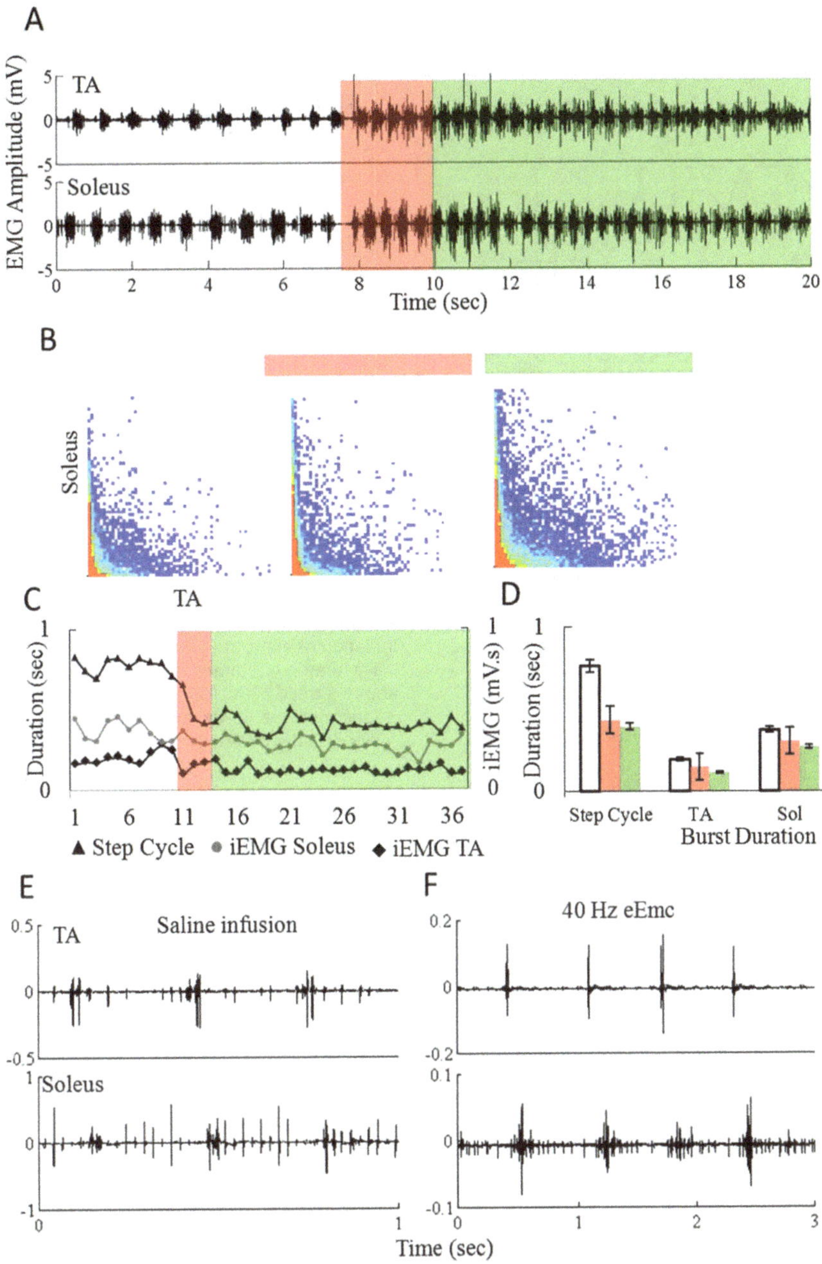


**Figure 1. Interaction between locomotion and bladder circuits.** (A) Representative EMG recordings from the soleus and tibialis anterior (TA) muscles from a spinal rat suspended in a harness and stepping bipedally on a treadmill at 13.5 cm/s under the influence of eEmc (40 Hz between L2 and S1). The rat begins to micturate at the beginning of the green shaded area. Note the shorter step cycle periods and higher EMG amplitudes a few steps prior to (red shaded area) and during (green shaded area) micturition. (B) EMG amplitude distribution plots showing an increase in the amount of co-activation of the soleus and TA muscles during the steps immediately before and during micturition. The red and green bars above the distribution plots correspond to the shaded regions in (A). (C) Step cycle duration and soleus and TA integrated EMG (iEMG) for each step shown in (A). (D) Mean (±SEM) step cycle duration and soleus and TA EMG burst durations for the regions highlighted in (A). Representative EMG recordings from the soleus and TA muscles when the rat hindlimbs were suspended above the treadmill belt (unloaded) during saline infusion (1 cc) into the bladder via a urethral catheter (E) or during 40 Hz eEmc (F).

cages that had ample CareFresh bedding, and the bladders of the spinal rats were expressed manually 3 times daily for the first 2 weeks after surgery and 2 times daily thereafter. During bladder expressions, the urine was collected in a weigh boat and measured using a syringe to quantify the total urine manually expressed each day. The hindlimbs of the spinal rats were moved passively through a full range of motion once per day to maintain joint mobility. These procedures have been described in detail previously [11].

## Step Training

Ten rats were step trained bipedally [11] on a specially designed motor-driven rodent treadmill using a body weight support system [19] under the influence of eEmc between L2 and S1 (40 Hz) and

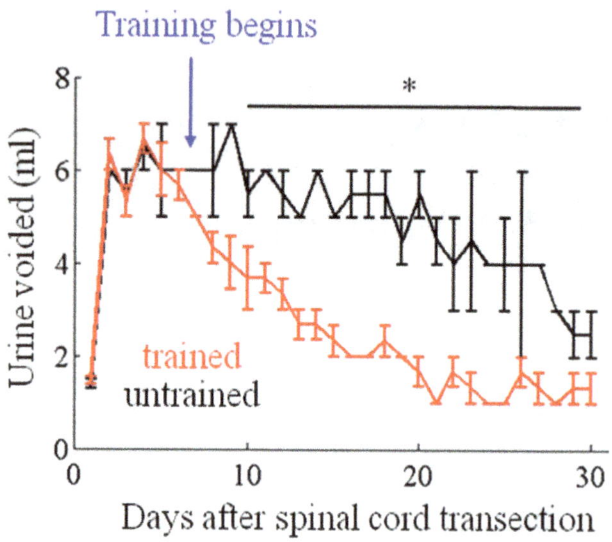


**Figure 2. Total average volume of urine voided manually daily.** Mean (±SEM) total daily volume of urine voided by manual bladder expression in spinal rats trained to step bipedally on a treadmill at 13.5 cm/s beginning 7 days post-surgery or in untrained rats (n = 3 rats/ group). *, significant difference between trained and untrained at $P<0.05$.

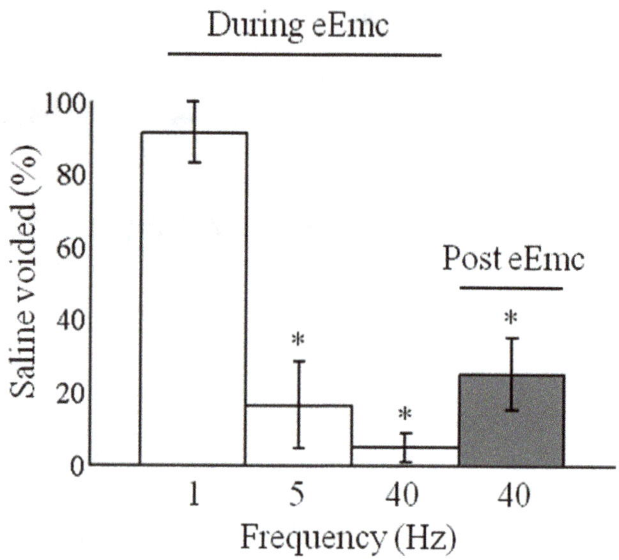


**Figure 3. Voiding efficiency with eEmc.** Mean (±SEM, n = 6 rats, 3 trials each rat) total percent volume voided in the first 90 sec after the initiation of eEmc at different frequencies after infusion of 1cc of saline via a urethral catheter in spinal rats with the hindlimbs suspended above a treadmill belt. In addition, the volume of saline voided within 30 sec after the 40-Hz stimulation was stopped (post-eEmc) is shown. *, significantly different from 1 Hz at $P<0.05$.

quipazine [11] (0.3 mg/kg, i.p.) and strychnine [12,13] (0.5 mg/ kg, i.p.) at a treadmill speed of 13.5 cm/s [13]. The rats were trained for a period of 6 weeks starting one week after the spinal transection surgery. Step training in spinal rats under the influence of pharmacological and/or spinal cord stimulation interventions are routine procedures that have been performed in our lab for several years [11,12,13,14].

## Testing Procedures

All 15 rats (10 trained, 5 untrained) were tested under the following conditions: 1) the rats were tested to step bipedally at a treadmill speed of 13.5 cm/s while in a body weight support system under the influence of eEmc (40 Hz bipolar stimulation between L2 and S1); 2) evoked potentials were recorded from the hindlimb muscles during bipolar epidural stimulation between L2 and S1 (1, 5, and 40 Hz) while the rats were suspended in a harness [11,15,16]; and 3) acute terminal experiments for bladder function were performed 7 weeks post-SCI. Under anesthesia, a PE 50 catheter was inserted via the urethra [17] and secured in place using surgical tape. The EUS muscle was implanted acutely with Teflon coated stainless steel wires (AM systems) as described previously [18]. Once the animal was conscious, they were suspended vertically using the body weight support system with their feet off the treadmill surface (Movie S2). One cc of saline was injected into the bladder via a syringe at a steady pace with no visible leakage of saline. Three trials were conducted at each stimulation frequency (1, 5, and 40 Hz). The saline voided during stimulation at each frequency of stimulation was collected in a large weigh boat positioned below the animal and then the volume measured using a syringe as described above. The bladder was expressed manually between each trial to ensure an empty bladder. No pharmacological agents were administered during the testing procedures.

## Data analysis

EMG recordings from the TA, soleus, and EUS muscles were band-pass filtered (1 Hz to 5 KHz), amplified using an A-M Systems Model 1700 differential AC amplifier (A-M Systems, Carlsborg, WA), and sampled at a frequency of 10 KHz using a custom data acquisition program written in the LabView development environment (National Instruments, Austin, TX) as described previously [11] Custom scripts written in Matlab were used to measure the evoked potentials from the hindlimb and EUS muscles [13]. Step cycle durations and EMG burst durations and amplitudes were determined using a custom program written in the LabView development environment. Burst integrated EMG (iEMG) was calculated as the area under the curve after rectification of the raw EMG signal. EMG amplitude distribution plots were generated using custom scripts written in Matlab: an L-shaped distribution reflects reciprocal activation, whereas a more D-shaped distribution reflects increased co-contraction.

## Statistical analyses

All data are reported as mean ± SEM. Statistically significant differences were determined using a one-way repeated measures analysis of variance (ANOVA) or a paired or unpaired t-test. The criterion level for the determination of a statistical difference was set at $P<0.05$ for all comparisons.

# Results

## Interaction of neural networks controlling locomotion and micturition

Rats with a complete mid-thoracic spinal cord transection can step bipedally on a treadmill when the upper body is supported in a harness [19]. During this body weight supported stepping, spontaneous voiding occurs intermittently with eEmc at 40 Hz between L2 and S1 and there are distinct changes in the locomotor pattern during the transition from no voiding of urine

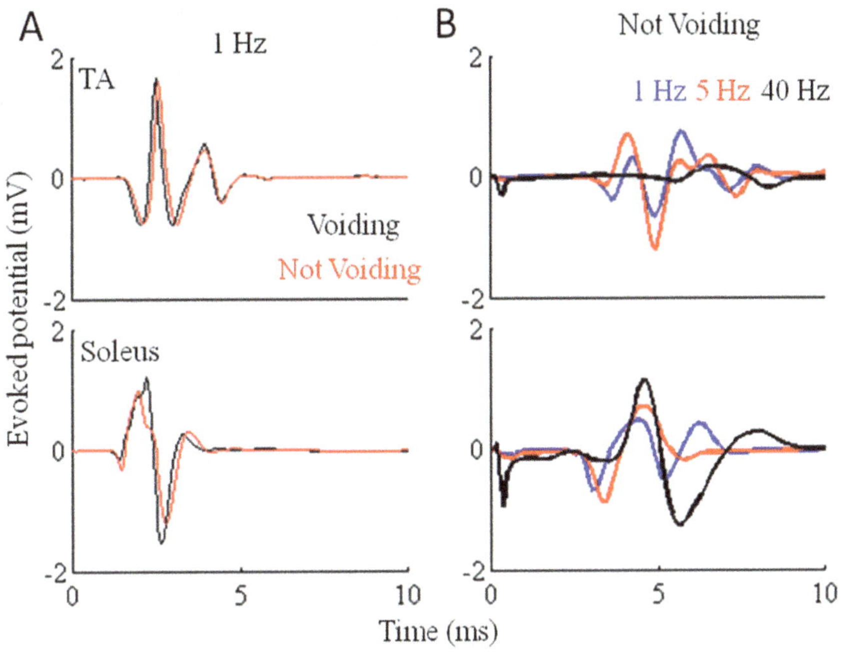


**Figure 4. Hindlimb evoked potentials varying with eEmc and bladder voiding.** (A) Mean evoked potentials (n = 4 rats, 10 potentials for each condition/rat) from the TA and soleus muscles under the influence of eEmc at 1 Hz between L2 and S1 during voiding and not voiding with a filled bladder in a spinal rat with its hindlimbs suspended above a treadmill belt. (B) Mean evoked potentials (n = 7 rats, 10 potentials for each condition/rat) in the soleus and TA induced by eEmc at 1, 5, and 40 Hz. Significant differences ($P<0.05$) in evoked potential amplitudes in the absence of voiding: TA - black < blue < red; Soleus - blue < red < black.

to a state where voiding is initiated (Fig. 1A). Initially consistent stepping with reciprocal activation of the soleus and TA muscles is observed (non-highlighted region). Shortly prior to voiding (~2 sec in this example, red highlighted region) the pattern of stepping changes (Movie S1): there is a shorter step cycle, a higher amount of co-contraction between the TA and soleus, and shorter burst durations and lower iEMG levels in both muscles compared to the prior steps (Fig. 1B–D). During voiding (green highlighted region), the step cycles become even shorter and the amount of co-contraction increases further. The corresponding EMG amplitude distribution plots (Fig. 1B) highlight the differences in the amount of co-contraction between the soleus and TA under each condition. Reciprocal activation of the soleus and TA muscles also is observed when the rat is suspended above the treadmill (no foot contact) and the hindlimbs are air stepping when saline is infused into the bladder via a urethral catheter (Fig. 1E) under the influence of 40 Hz eEmc (Fig. 1F), or when pinching the tail (data not shown). The state of the spinal locomotor circuitry, however, appears to be different under each condition. For example the EMG amplitudes in the flexors and extensors are greater and the cycle periods shorter during saline infusion compared to air stepping (40 Hz) (compare Fig. 1E and F).

## Chronic effects of step training on bladder voiding

Chronic step training under the influence of eEmc (40 Hz between L2 and S1) results in an increase in spontaneous bladder voiding both during routine cage activity as well as during treadmill stepping. The daily average volume of urine voided manually starting after 3 days of training (10 days post-SCI) and continuing for a period of 30 days was lower in step trained vs. untrained rats (Fig. 2), suggesting that the bladder was influenced by the additional sensory input to the spinal circuitry generated by load bearing itself.

## Acute effect of eEmc on bladder voiding after SCI

We determined the effects of different frequencies of stimulation on voiding by infusing controlled quantities of saline into the bladder via a urethral catheter in step trained rats that were suspended in a harness as described above. One cc of saline was infused into the bladder via the urethral catheter at a steady rate since this did not result in any leakage of saline. Any volume higher than 1cc resulted in visible leakage of saline. The most effective voiding was observed with 1-Hz stimulation (pulse width 0.5 ms, ~2.5 V), with almost 90–95% of the volume voided within 90 sec (Fig. 3). Note that the hindlimbs show primarily a flexion motion during voiding (Movie S2). eEmc (40 Hz) resulted in very little voiding of saline (~5%), although a rhythmic alternating bilateral locomotor pattern of the hindlimbs was observed (Fig. 1F). When stimulation at 40 Hz was stopped ~30% of the saline was voided with no movement or evoked potentials observed in the hindlimbs. With 5-Hz stimulation strong oscillatory movements in both hindlimbs were observed but only ~10–20% of the saline was voided.

The responses evoked in a hindlimb extensor (soleus) and flexor (TA) muscle during 1-Hz stimulation were similar when the rats were voiding or not voiding (Fig. 4A). The mean evoked responses in the TA were higher at 1 and 5 Hz vs. 40 Hz, whereas the mean amplitude of the evoked responses was progressively higher with increased stimulation frequencies in the soleus (Fig. 4B). The observations of an increase in the flexor activation at the lower frequencies and of a high voiding efficiency at lower frequencies suggest a facilitating effect of flexion on voiding.

We then investigated the electrophysiological responses to 1-Hz stimulation after infusing saline into the bladder. Infusion of saline initially resulted in a slight increase in the activation of the EUS muscle followed by a period when the EUS was inactive (Fig. 5A). Stimulation at 1 Hz increased EUS activation and bladder voiding

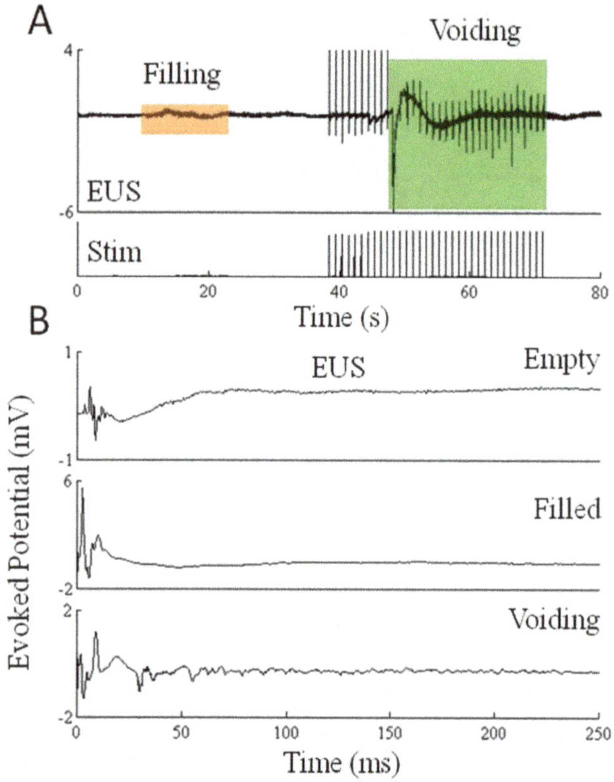


**Figure 5. Changes in EUS activity with and without eEmc.** (A) A representative EMG recording from the EUS muscle during infusion of 1 cc of saline into the bladder (orange highlight) and during voiding under the influence of 1 Hz eEmc (green highlight). (B) Average (20 potentials) evoked potentials recorded from the EUS muscle of a spinal rat at 1-Hz stimulation when the bladder was empty, filled, or voiding.

began after about 10 sec of stimulation. The evoked potentials recorded from the EUS with the bladder empty had a low amplitude with a latency of ~3–5 ms (Fig. 5B). In comparison, these responses with a filled bladder had a higher amplitude and a shorter latency than with an empty bladder. During voiding, the EUS showed two distinct peaks with the first peak having a latency similar to that with a filled bladder but with a lower amplitude and several smaller responses with latencies varying between 20–100 ms.

Stimulation at sub-threshold levels (threshold set at voiding intensity) with a filled bladder resulted in an evoked potential in the EUS (Fig. 6A, black trace). In addition, the amplitude and number of responses increased at voiding threshold and at supra-threshold levels of stimulation (Fig. 6A, blue and red traces, respectively). In comparison, sub-threshold stimulation (same intensity as above) with an empty bladder did not produce an evoked potential (Fig. 6A, black trace). Threshold and supra-threshold levels of stimulation, however, produced an evoked potential in the EUS, although these responses were of lower amplitude compared to those seen with a filled bladder.

## Discussion

It is well known that motor performance can be accompanied by changes of autonomic functions (somatic-visceral interactions) [20,21]. Recent studies of human subjects with motor complete paralysis report improvement in postural control and some voluntary movement in the legs, and the subjects anecdotally have reported improved autonomic function such as bladder, sexual, and thermoregulatory control [23,23]. In this study we show that enabling of locomotor-related spinal neuronal circuits by epidural stimulation also influences neural networks controlling bladder function. Herein we have demonstrated not only the long-term complementary effects of epidural stimulation on locomotor and bladder function, but more importantly we have shown that stimulation at 1 Hz between L2 and S1 can initiate bladder emptying within seconds of the initiation of epidural stimulation. The effect of eEmc on bladder voiding on untrained rats is still not completely understood and will require further investigation.

Given the locations of the neural networks within the spinal cord that control autonomic function, the level and extent of a spinal cord lesion are important factors in the extent of loss of bladder function [24]. A complete mid-thoracic spinal cord transection in rats results in the loss of bladder function initially with some autonomically initiated spontaneous control returning in the following weeks, allowing for occasional but incomplete emptying (Fig. 2). In humans with a thoracic or cervical SCI, descending projections from supraspinal centers often are severed and their axons degenerated. In many such individuals, the reflex pathways mediating continence remain intact, but micturition cannot be initiated in a normal manner [25]. The most common form of this condition is detrusor-sphincter dyssynergia [5,6] in which the detrusor and EUS tend to be activated together rather than reciprocally.

It appears that epidural stimulation raises the net excitability level of spinal neural networks (interneurons and motoneurons) and, when combined with motor training and/or pharmacological interventions, enhances the activation of the sensorimotor pathways that also control bladder function [22]. Data presented herein demonstrate that in addition to the chronic effects, i.e., improved spontaneous bladder emptying associated with epidural stimulation and step training, we have discovered a unique spinal epidural stimulation paradigm which can overcome detrusor-sphincter dyssynergia and induce bladder emptying on demand in unanesthesized rats with a complete mid-thoracic spinal cord transection.

### Spinal cord plasticity mediating locomotor and bladder function after a SCI

Within three days of the initiation of epidural stimulation and step training the rats started voiding spontaneously during cage activity and step training (Fig. 2). After 6 weeks of locomotor training facilitated with eEmc (40 Hz between L2 and S1) plus quipazine and strychnine administration, the spinal rats consistently voided when stimulated at 1 Hz between L2 and S1. Locomotor training [10,12,13] with eEmc chronically engaged the neural networks by lowering the threshold of excitability and apparently when stimulated at 1 Hz the networks were tuned to initiate micturition. An underlying mechanism of the improved spontaneous control of bladder emptying is suggested by the heightened responses of the EUS to the afferent information, i.e., indirectly sensing bladder volume (Fig. 6). More precise measurements to assess bladder function such as urodynamics and loss of fluids during exercise will be required to better understand the interaction between spinal cord stimulation, bladder voiding, and locomotor function. Similar patterns of evoked potentials have been observed in hindlimb muscles in response to eEmc [13,16]. The enhanced spontaneous voiding of the bladder was more efficient in the trained compared to untrained rats (Fig. 2), most likely reflecting the lowered activation threshold due to the chronic engagement of the neural networks in the trained rats. This result is consistent with the observation that after 8 weeks of locomotor

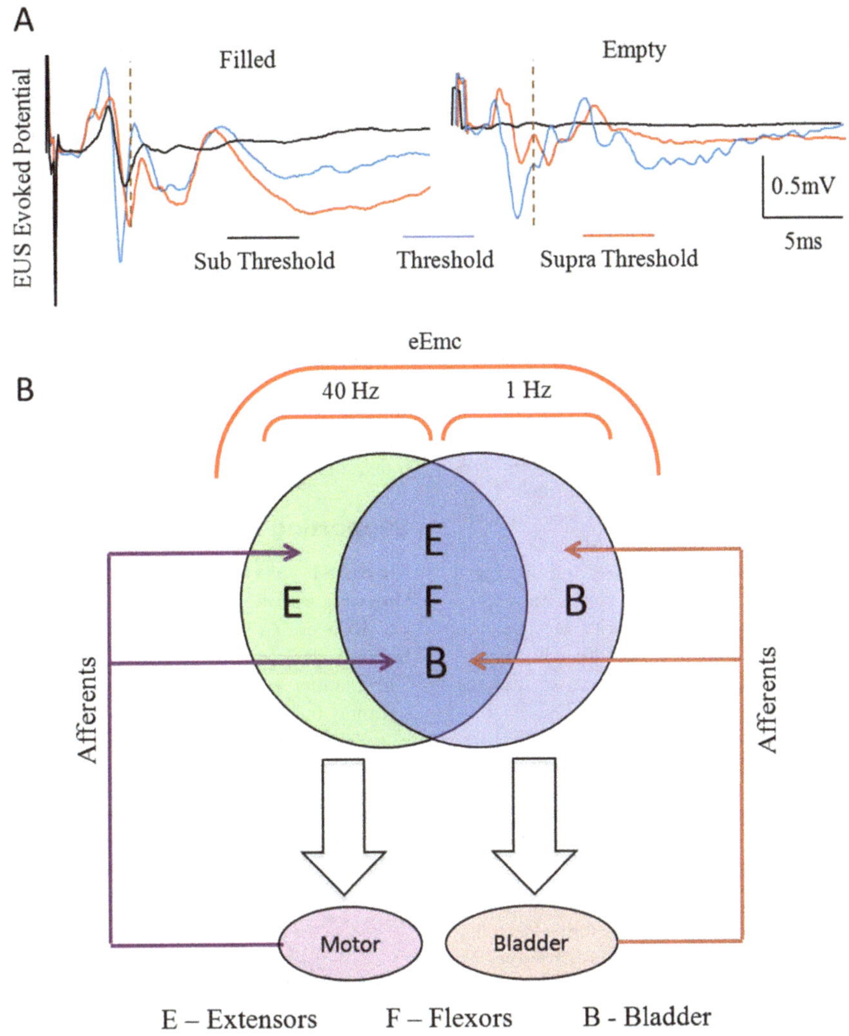


**Figure 6. Changes in EUS evoked potential with varying intensities of eEmc.** (A) Average evoked potentials from the EUS (n = 10 stimulation pulses at 1 Hz) at sub-threshold, threshold, and supra-threshold intensities of stimulation (threshold was determined based on the voltage at which voiding was initiated) with a filled bladder compared to an empty bladder. Note the presence of higher amplitude evoked potentials at a sub-threshold level with a filled bladder compared to an empty bladder and higher amplitude evoked potentials at threshold compared to supra-threshold levels with a filled bladder. Also note the higher amplitudes and longer latencies at threshold and supra-threshold levels in a filled bladder compared to an empty bladder. (B) A schematic representing the overlap of the lumbosacral spinal cord circuitries controlling locomotion and bladder voiding under the influence of eEmc and afferents from the bladder and hindlimbs is shown.

training facilitated by epidural stimulation and pharmacological interventions the contractile responses of the bladder to filling in anesthetized spinal rats were more efficient in trained compared to untrained animals [26]. Direct acute responses to epidural stimulation, however, were not reported.

## Frequency dependent tuning of the automaticity of the spinal cord

The complex functioning of bladder voiding was achieved via an eEmc tonic drive at 1 Hz between L2 and S1 and this was accompanied by increased flexor activity. The conceptual basis of selecting a given eEmc parameter was to activate the neural networks that initiate the automaticity of the coordinated contractions and relaxations of the bladder and EUS that result in bladder voiding. During stimulation at 1 Hz, the bladder contracts tonically. This response occurs in the EUS within a 20 to 100 ms time window (Fig. 5B). These evoked potentials with a long latency may represent the activation of complex interneuronal networks that enable bursting activity of the EUS similar to that observed during voiding in intact rats [18]. Stimulation at higher frequencies (40 Hz) at the same sites on the spinal cord (between L2 and S1) facilitates partial weight-bearing bipedal [10] and quadrupedal [27] stepping of spinal rats on a treadmill belt. A consistent bilateral air stepping pattern also is observed when the rats are suspended in a harness and under the influence of eEmc at 40 Hz and with sufficient levels of current [13] (Fig. 1F). Similar bilateral air stepping-like patterns were observed in the hindlimbs during infusion of saline and tail pinching, suggesting that the afferent information from the bladder and EUS being processed by the neural networks in the lumbosacral region of the spinal cord contribute to these hindlimb responses. These results provide further evidence of an overlap between the networks controlling bladder function and locomotion.

## Neural networks controlling locomotion and micturition

Over the past several decades, multiple techniques have been used to induce micturition after SCI, including stimulation of the bladder wall, the pelvic nerve, and/or the sacral nerve. Directly stimulating the bladder wall induces local contractions, but high currents or a large number of electrodes are needed to induce a more widespread contraction to achieve sufficient bladder emptying. Pelvic nerve stimulation has been shown to contract the bladder wall, but as the pelvic nerve does not innervate the EUS, minimal effect was seen on the EUS resulting in a low voiding efficiency [28]. Voiding was achieved, however, by cutting the pudental nerve. This largely irreversible procedure eliminates sensation from the external genitalia of both sexes and the skin around the anus and perineum, as well as the motor supply to various pelvic muscles, including the EUS and the external anal sphincter. Sacral nerve stimulation seemed to offer the best results, but this requires complicated surgical procedures and a serious risk of permanent damage due to the intradural approach [29]. Recently a closed-loop neuroprosthesis interface was used to measure bladder fullness through implanted afferent dorsal rootlets into microchannel electrodes to measure and interpret sensory activity related to bladder fullness in spinal rats [30]. Voiding was achieved using low frequency anterior sacral nerve stimulation. While promising, the viability of this chronically implanted dorsal root-microchannel electrode system in humans has yet to be established.

Each of the above strategies involves surgically severing nerves, result in permanent loss of some motor and sensory functions, and directly induce contractions in the bladder. Therefore, these strategies completely bypass the automaticity that is intrinsic to the sensorimotor neural circuitries present in the spinal cord. While epidural electrode array implantation also is invasive, similar surgical procedures are followed in routinely performed procedures to alleviate chronic pain. Moreover, no indwelling electrodes in spinal nerves or irreversible surgical denervation of nerves or rootlets are necessary. By preserving the sensorimotor networks that underlie the automaticity of micturition, as occurs with the recovery of stepping and standing after a complete spinal cord transection, bladder function can be largely re-established by enabling the inherent automaticity present within the spinal cord [9,31]. The spinal cord circuitry contains the necessary circuitry to control bladder voiding when provided the appropriate afferent information from the bladder and the EUS. Based on frequency-specific stimulation parameters, the spinal cord can be tuned to enable the appropriate physiological responses (Fig. 6). The clinical implications of this technique are immense and parallel the impact that spinal cord stimulation has had on the recovery of locomotion and postural abilities and some volitional movement after complete paralysis in humans [22,23]. The application of spinal cord stimulation to overcome difficulty in micturition is not likely limited to SCI but could be adapted to other neurological disorders. This protocol could be invaluable in avoiding unnecessary transurethral catheterization, potentially lowering the incidence of urinary tract infections, and reversing the uptake of urine into the kidney.

In summary, the main findings include 1) the demonstration of functional links between the neural control (biomechanical and electrophysiological) of locomotion and micturition in awake unanesthetized rats, 2) the immediate effect of *in vivo* spinal cord stimulation on micturition, and 3) the positive chronic effects of step training under the influence of eEmc and pharmacological interventions on bladder function.

## Supporting Information

**Movie S1 A representative rat with a complete mid-thoracic spinal cord transection stepping on a treadmill at 13.5 cm/s under the influence of eEmc (40 Hz between L2 and S1) spontaneously empties its bladder.** The bladder voiding is accompanied by a change in pattern of stepping and corresponding EMG. Note the pattern change starts ~2 sec prior to the initiation of voiding.

**Movie S2 A representative rat with a complete mid-thoracic spinal cord transection suspended in a harness voids its bladder under the influence of eEmc at 1 Hz between L2 and S1.**

## Acknowledgments

We thank Maynor Herrera for providing excellent animal care and Sharon Zdunowski for technical assistance.

## Author Contributions

Conceived and designed the experiments: VRE RRR PNG. Performed the experiments: RRR PNG. Analyzed the data: PNG. Contributed to the writing of the manuscript: PNG RRR HZ YPG DCL VRE. Performed all of the surgeries: RRR HZ.

## References

1. de Groat W, Araki I, Vizzard M, Yoshiyama M, Yoshimura N, et al (1998) Developmental and Injury Induced Plasticity in the Micturition Reflex Pathway. Behavioral Brain Research 92: 127–140.
2. Shefchyk S (2002) Spinal Cord Neural Organization Controlling the Urinary Bladder and Striated Sphincter. Progress in Brain Research 137: 71–82.
3. Maggi C, Santicioli P, Meli A (1986). The Nonstop Transvesical Cystometrogram in Urethane-Anesthetized Rats: A Simple Procedure for Quantitative Studies on the Various Phases of Urinary Bladder Voiding Cycle. Journal of Pharmacological Methods 15: 157–167.
4. Kruse M, Belton A, de Groat W (1993). Changes in Bladder and External Urethral Sphincter Function after Spinal Cord Injury in the Rat. American Journal of Physiology-Regulatory, Integrative and Comparative Physiology 264: 1157–1163.
5. de Groat W, Kawatani M, Hisamitsu T, Cheng C, Ma C, et al (1990) Mechanisms Underlying the Recovery of Urinary Bladder Function Following Spinal Cord Injury. Journal of the Autonomic Nervous System 30: 71–77.
6. de Groat W, Yoshimura N (2010). Changes in Afferent Activity After Spinal Cord Injury. Neurourology and Urodynamics 29: 63–76.
7. Grillner S, Zangger P (1979). On the Central Generation of Locomotion in the Low Spinal Cat. Experimental Brain Research 34: 241–261.
8. Barbeau H, Rossignol R (1987). Recovery of Locomotion After Chronic Spinalization in the Adult Cat. Brain Research 412: 84–95.
9. Edgerton VR, de Leon R, Harkema S, Hodgson J, London N, et al (2001) Retraining the Injured Spinal Cord. The Journal of Physiology 533: 15–22.
10. Courtine G, Gerasimenko Y, van den Brand R, Yew A, Musienko P, et al (2009) Transformation of Nonfunctional Spinal Circuits Into Functional States After the Loss of Brain Input. Nature Neuroscience 12: 1333–1342.
11. Ichiyama R, Courtine G, Gerasimenko Y, Yang G, van den Brand R, et al (2008) Step Training Reinforces Specific Spinal Locomotor Circuitry in Adult Spinal Rats. The Journal of Neuroscience 28: 7370–7375.
12. Gad P, Choe J, Shah P, Garcia-Alias G, Rath M (2013) Sub-threshold Spinal Cord Stimulation Facilitates Spontaneous Motor Activity in Spinal Rats. Journal of Neuroengineering and Rehabilitation 10: 108.
13. Gad P, Lavrov I, Shah P, Zhong H, Roy R, et al (2013) Neuromodulation of Motor Evoked Potentials During Stepping in Spinal Rats. The Journal of Neurophysiology 110: 1311–1322.
14. Roy R, Hodgson J, Lauretz S, Pierotti D, Gayek R, et al (1992) Chronic Spinal Cord-Injured Cats: Surgical Procedures and management. Laboratory Animal Science 42.

15. Lavrov I, Gerasimenko Y, Ichiyama R, Courtine G, Zhong H, et al (2006) Plasticity of Spinal Cord Reflexes After a Complete Transection in Adult Rats: Relationship to Stepping Ability. Journal of Neurophysiology 96: 1699–1710.
16. Lavrov I, Dy C, Fong A, Gerasimenko Y, Courtine G, et al (2008) Epidural Stimulation Induced Modulation of Spinal Locomotor Networks in Adult Spinal Rats. The Journal of Neuroscience 28: 6022–6029.
17. Rosas-Arellano M, Vergara-Aragón P, Cartas-Heredia L, Guevara-Rojas A (1988). Chronic Bladder Catheterization in the Rat. Physiology & Behavior 43: 127–128.
18. D'Amico S, Collins W (2012). External Urethral Sphincter Motor Unit Recruitment Patterns During Micturition in the Spinally Intact and Transected Adult Rat. Journal of Neurophysiology 108: 2554–2567.
19. de Leon R, Kubasak M, Phelps P, Timoszyk W, Reinkensmeyer D, et al (2002) Using Robotics to Teach the Spinal Cord to Walk. Brain Research Reviews 40: 267–273.
20. Isaev G, Gerasimenko T, Selionov V, Kartashova N (2004). Respiratory Responses to Voluntary and Reflex-induced Stepping Movements in Normal Subjects and Spinal Patients. Journal of Physiology and Pharmacology 55: 77–82.
21. Kunstman K, Orbeli L (1921). Demonstration of a Dog with a Deafferentated Hindlimb, Russian Fiziology 4: 192.
22. Harkema S, Gerasimenko Y, Hodes J, Burdick J, Angeli C, et al (2011) Effect of Epidural Stimulation of the Lumbosacral Spinal Cord on Voluntary Movement, Standing and Assisted Stepping After Motor Complete Paraplegia: a Case Study. Lancet 377: 1938–1947.
23. Angeli C, Edgerton VR, Gerasimenko Y, Harkema S (2014). Alternating Spinal Cord Excitability Enables Voluntary Movements After Chronic Complete Spinal Paralysis in Humans. Brain 137: 1394–1409.
24. Potter P. Disordered Control of the Urinary Bladder After Human Spinal Cord Injury: What are the Problems? Progress in Brain Research 152: 51–57.
25. Barrington F (1941). The Component Reflexes of Micturition in the Cat. Part III. Brain 64: 239–243.
26. Horst M, Heutschi J, van den Brand R, Andersson K, Gobet R, et al (2013) Multisystem Neuroprosthetic Training Improves Bladder Function After Severe Spinal Cord Injury. Journal of Urology 189: 747–753.
27. Gad P, Woodbridge J, Lavrov I, Zhong H, Roy R, et al (2012) Forelimb EMG-Based Trigger to Control an Electronic Spinal Bridge to Enable Hindlimb Stepping After a Complete Spinal Cord Lesion in Rats. Journal of Neuroengineering and Rehabilitation 9: 38.
28. Holmquist B, Tord O (1968). Electromicturition in Female Dogs at Pelvic Nerve Stimulation: An Urethrocystographic Study. Scandinavian journal of urology and nephrology 2: 129–135.
29. Rijkhoff N, Wijkstra H, Van Kerrebroeck P, Debruyne F (1997). Selective Detrusor Activation by Electrical Sacral Nerve Root Stimulation in Spinal Cord Injury. The Journal of Urology 157: 1504–1508.
30. Chew D, Zhu L, Delivopoulos E, Minev I, Musick K, et al (2013) A Microchannel Neuroprosthesis for Bladder Control After Spinal Cord Injury in Rat. Science Translational Medicine 5: 210.
31. Edgerton VR, Tillakaratne N, Bigbee A, de Leon R, Roy R (2004). Plasticity of the Spinal Neural Circuitry After Injury. Annual Review Neuroscience 27: 145–167.

# Adductor Canal Block for Postoperative Pain Treatment after Revision Knee Arthroplasty: A Blinded, Randomized, Placebo-Controlled Study

**Pia Jæger[1]*, Zbigniew J. Koscielniak-Nielsen[1], Henrik M. Schrøder[2], Ole Mathiesen[3], Maria H. Henningsen[1], Jørgen Lund[4], Morten T. Jenstrup[4], Jørgen B. Dahl[1]**

**1** Department of Anaesthesia, Centre of Head and Orthopaedics, Copenhagen University Hospital, Rigshospitalet, Copenhagen, Denmark, **2** Department of Orthopaedic Surgery, Centre of Head and Orthopaedics, Copenhagen University Hospital, Rigshospitalet, Copenhagen, Denmark, **3** Section of Acute Pain Management, Department of Anaesthesia, Centre of Head and Orthopaedics, Copenhagen University Hospital, Rigshospitalet, Copenhagen, Denmark, **4** Department of Anaesthesia, Aleris-Hamlet Hospitals, Copenhagen, Denmark

## Abstract

***Background:*** Revision knee arthroplasty is assumed to be even more painful than primary knee arthroplasty and predominantly performed in chronic pain patients, which challenges postoperative pain treatment. We hypothesized that the adductor canal block, effective for pain relief after primary total knee arthroplasty, may reduce pain during knee flexion (primary endpoint: at 4 h) compared with placebo after revision total knee arthroplasty. Secondary endpoints were pain at rest, morphine consumption and morphine-related side effects.

***Methods:*** We included patients scheduled for revision knee arthroplasty in general anesthesia into this blinded, placebo-controlled, randomized trial. Patients were allocated to an adductor canal block via a catheter with either ropivacaine or placebo; bolus of 0.75% ropivacaine/saline, followed by infusion of 0.2% ropivacaine/saline. Clinicaltrials.gov ID: NCT01191593.

***Results:*** We enrolled 36 patients, of which 30 were analyzed. Mean pain scores during knee flexion at 4 h (primary endpoint) were: 52±22 versus 71±25 mm (mean difference 19, 95% CI: 1 to 37, P = 0.04), ropivacaine and placebo group respectively. When calculated as area under the curve (1–8 h/7 h) pain scores were 55±21 versus 69±21 mm during knee flexion (P = 0.11) and 39±18 versus 45±23 mm at rest (P = 0.43), ropivacaine and placebo group respectively. Groups were similar regarding morphine consumption and morphine-related side effects (P>0.05).

***Conclusions:*** The only statistically significant difference found between groups was in the primary endpoint: pain during knee flexion at 4 h. However, due to a larger than anticipated dropout rate and heterogeneous study population, the study was underpowered.

***Trial Registration:*** Clinicaltrials.gov NCT01191593

**Editor:** Aristidis Veves, Harvard Medical School, United States of America

**Funding:** The authors have no funding or support to report.

**Competing Interests:** The authors have declared that no competing interests exist.

* Email: pia.therese.jaeger@regionh.dk

## Introduction

Revision total knee arthroplasty (TKA) is a challenge, both for surgeons and anesthesiologists. For the surgeon the procedure is technically more difficult, takes longer time, and has a higher rate of complications than primary TKA [1]. For the anesthesiologist the main challenge lies in handling the postoperative pain treatment. Compared with primary TKA, revision TKA is assumed to be even more painful. Many patients suffer from intense preoperative pain [2], often treated with opioids, adding to the complexity of the task. With an increasing volume of primary TKAs being performed, the number of revisions is also inevitably rising; nonetheless, to our knowledge no pain studies have been performed in this subgroup of patients.

The femoral nerve block has been the mainstay for postoperative pain treatment following knee replacement for decades. Current trends however, focus on providing analgesia with minimal motor block. Contrary to the femoral nerve block, the adductor canal block (ACB) is predominantly a sensory nerve block, preserving quadriceps muscle strength and mobilization ability [3–4]. In patients undergoing primary TKA, the ACB reduced postoperative pain and morphine consumption, and enhanced ambulation compared with placebo [5–8].

We hypothesized that the adductor canal block would also reduce postoperative pain following revision TKA. Hence the primary aim of this study was to examine the effect of adductor canal block on pain during knee flexion after revision TKA compared with placebo. Secondary endpoints were pain at rest, morphine consumption and morphine-related side effects.

## Methods

### Ethics statement

This prospective, randomized, blinded, placebo-controlled trial was approved by the local Regional Ethics Committee (H-3-2010-063), the Danish Medicines Agency (2010-021161-71), the Danish Data Protection Agency and registered at clinicaltrials.gov (NCT01191593). After obtaining written informed consent, we recruited patients scheduled for revision TKA from August 2010–March 2013. The study was conducted at the Centre of Head and Orthopaedics, Copenhagen University Hospital, Rigshospitalet, Copenhagen, Denmark and monitored by the Copenhagen University Hospital GCP (Good Clinical Practice) unit. Data are presented in accordance with the CONSORT (Consolidated Standards of Reporting Trials) statement. The protocol for this trial and supporting CONSORT checklist are available as supporting information; see Checklist S1 and Protocol S1.

Eligible patients were Danish speaking adults, scheduled for revision TKA in general anesthesia, aged 40–85 years, with American Society of Anesthesiologists physical status I–III, and body mass index of 18–40 kg/m$^2$. Exclusion criteria were inability to cooperate, allergy to any drug used in the study, alcohol or drug abuse.

### Interventions

Premedication, consisting of 1 g acetaminophen, was given orally one hour before surgery. General anesthesia was induced with propofol, and maintained with propofol (variable rate) and remifentanil 30 μg/kg/h (fixed rate). Thirty minutes prior to the end of surgery, patients were given morphine 0.2 mg/kg intravenously. A femoral tourniquet was applied peri-operatively and intraoperative fluids were administered at the discretion of the anesthetist.

The adductor canal block was performed after the end of surgery, while maintaining general anesthesia until completion of block procedure. A 12L-SC linear ultrasound transducer (GE Medical Systems, Wuxi, China) was placed on the medial part of the thigh, halfway between the superior anterior iliac spine and the patella with the leg slightly externally rotated. The femoral artery was identified in short axis in the adductor canal, underneath the sartorius muscle. After skin disinfection with chlorhexidine gluconate and isopropyl alcohol an 18-gauge, Contiplex Tuohy needle (B.Braun Medical, Melsungen, Germany) was inserted in-plane from the lateral side of the transducer. The needle tip was placed underneath the sartorius muscle, just lateral to the artery and saphenous nerve, using 2–3 ml of saline to ensure correct placement (directional terms are referenced from the US image). A 20-gauge catheter was then advanced 2 cm beyond the tip of the needle, and 30 ml of study medication was slowly injected via the catheter, with repeated aspiration. The position of the catheter tip was adjusted during injection to obtain a semicircular expansion between the sartorius fascia and the artery.

In a double masked fashion patients were allocated to ACB with ropivacaine or placebo (saline) for 24 hours. We administered study medication as an initial bolus of 30 ml 0.75% ropivacaine or saline, followed by another bolus of 15 ml 6 hours later. Immediately after the second bolus, we started infusion of study medication (0.2% ropivacaine or saline) at a rate of 8 ml/h.

Postoperatively, all patients received oral acetaminophen (1 g) and ibuprofen (400 mg) every six hours and a patient-controlled analgesia (PCA) pump with morphine intravenously (bolus 2.5 mg, lock-out time 10 minutes, no background infusion). If analgesia was inadequate patients received an additional bolus of 2.5 mg morphine and/or 0.05 mg fentanyl intravenously until adequate analgesia was obtained (0.1 mg of fentanyl was considered equipotent with 10 mg of morphine). Patients with a daily intake of strong opioids (morphine, oxycodone, methadone, fentanyl, ketobemidone) received their habitual analgesics during the study period. These doses were not included in the cumulative morphine consumption. In case of moderate to severe postoperative nausea or vomiting (PONV), patients received 4 mg of ondansetron intravenously, with supplemental doses of 1 mg, when needed.

### Outcomes

The primary endpoint was pain during 45 degrees flexion of the knee at 4 hours postoperatively.

Secondary endpoints were pain at rest and during flexion of the knee (calculated as area under the curve, 1–8 h and at 24 h), cumulative morphine consumption (0–24 h, 0–8 h and 8–24 h), number of vomiting episodes, ondansetron consumption and degree of nausea and sedation (mean value 1–8 h and 24 h).

### Assessment of outcomes

We assessed all outcomes at 1, 2, 4, 6, 8 and 24 h postoperatively. Pain intensity was assessed on a visual analogue scale (VAS) with 0 mm = no pain, and 100 mm = worst imaginable pain. Patients rated nausea and sedation on a four-point scale (0 = no nausea/sedation, 1 = light, 2 = moderate, 3 = severe), and reported the number of vomiting episodes (volume greater than 10 ml).

To counter the problem of tolerance in patients treated with opioids, we decided that patients with a daily intake of strong opioids should continue with their habitual analgesics during the study period, and that these doses should not be included in the cumulative morphine consumption.

### Randomization and blinding

The pharmacy prepared the study medication in identical pre-packed boxes, consecutively numbered according to a computer generated block randomization list (1:1 ratio, blocks of 10). Subjects were assigned consecutive numbers upon inclusion to the study and received the study medication from the corresponding boxes. A research fellow neither involved in the study nor in the care of the patient administered the study medication in unlabeled syringes for injection and unmarked drug bags for infusion, before handing it over to the investigators. Ropivacaine and saline are identical in appearance.

All investigators, staff and patients were blinded to the treatment groups. The randomization key was first broken after all patients were enrolled, data computed and statistical analyses performed.

### Statistics

We considered a difference of 20 mm in VAS pain scores to be clinically relevant. Assuming a SD of 20, with $\alpha = 0.05$ and power $= 0.80$; 17 patients in each group were required to detect a difference of 20 mm in VAS pain scores. We planned for an inclusion of 36 subjects to compensate for dropouts.

Statistical analyses were conducted using SPSS 19 (SPSS, Chicago, Illinois, USA). Continuous variables are presented as mean ±SD or with medians and 10th–90th percentiles, as appropriate, and ordinal and nominal variables as n (%). The Kolmogorov-Smirnov test was used to assess whether data were normally distributed. If the assumption of normality was met, comparisons between the groups were performed using independent samples t-test; if the assumption of normality was rejected, comparisons were made using Mann-Whitney U test for unpaired data. Nausea and sedation scale scores were compared at 24 h, and by using the mean score from each patient from 1–8 h. We calculated the area under the curve (AUC) for the interval 1–8 h, for VAS pain scores during knee flexion and at rest. Categorical data (ondansetron consumption and vomiting episodes, 0–24 h) were analyzed using the Chi-squared test or by Fischer exact test, as appropriate. The nature of the hypothesis testing was two-tailed, and P<0.05 was considered statistically significant.

### Post hoc analysis

We performed a linear mixed model including pain scores at 1, 2, 4, 6 and 8 hours (originally analyzed as AUC), where we included time as a repeated effect with a first order autoregressive covariance structure (AR(1)). Treatment, time and the interaction treatment*time were set as fixed effects, and preoperative pain scores were included as covariates to compensate for baseline differences. This analysis was performed as an intention to treat analysis.

## Results

We enrolled and randomized 36 patients during a 31-month period, beginning August 2010; 6 patients were excluded prior to receiving any treatment, 2 patients were excluded between 4 and 6 h, and another 4 patients were excluded after completion of the first 8 h of the study protocol. This resulted in 30 patients with data for our primary endpoint (intention to treat analysis): VAS during flexion of the knee at 4 h postoperatively. As for the secondary outcomes all available data were analyzed, although missing data for the final end point in cumulative morphine consumption and pain scores calculated as AUC will in practice render these analyses per protocol analyses. The details of patient flow through the study, including details on patient exclusions, are presented in Figure 1 (CONSORT flow chart). Patients' demographics and perioperative data are presented in Table 1 and 2.

VAS pain scores during flexion of the knee at 4 h postoperatively (primary endpoint) were 52±22 mm in the ropivacaine group and 71±25 mm in the placebo group (mean difference 19, 95% CI: 1 to 37, P = 0.04). At 24 h, pain scores were 50±27 vs. 57±27 mm during knee flexion (mean difference 7, 95% CI: −16 to 30, P = 0.53) and 21±19 vs. 37±24 mm at rest (mean difference 16, 95% CI: −2 to 34, P = 0.09) at rest; ropivacaine and placebo group respectively. When calculated as AUC for the interval 1–8 h/7 h, VAS pain scores during flexion of the knee were 55±21 mm in the ropivacaine group compared with 69±21 mm in the placebo group (mean difference 14, 95% CI: −3 to 31, P = 0.11, Figure 2). At rest, mean pain scores (AUC for the interval 1–8 h/7 h) were 39±18 mm in the ropivacaine group compared with 45±23 mm in the placebo group (mean difference 6, 95% CI: −9 to 22, P = 0.43, figure 3).

Cumulative total morphine consumption was 61±38 versus 74±48 mg from 0–24 h (P = 0.48), 43±34 vs. 44±28 mg at 0–8 h (P = 0.97) and 28±30 vs. 29±18 mg from 8–24 h (P = 0.95), ropivacaine and placebo group respectively (Table 3). There were no differences between the groups regarding morphine-related side effects: nausea (1–8 h: 0.15 vs. 0.24, P = 0.33; 24 h: 0.18 vs. 0.46, P = 0.44), sedation (1–8 h: 1.1 vs. 1.1, P = 0.83; 24 h: 0.64 vs. 0.85, P = 0.50), vomiting episodes (6/16 vs. 6/14 P = 0.77), or in the need of antiemetics (8/16 vs. 7/14, P = 0.46), placebo and ropivacaine group respectively.

All data used for analysis are available in the file: Data S1.

There were no adverse events in the study population.

### Post hoc analysis

Daily intake of strong opioids was omitted from total morphine consumption to counter the problem of tolerance. By chance, more patients in the ropivacaine group had a daily intake of strong opioids (36% vs. 13%, Table 1). If we had included the habitual analgesics from these patients, the cumulative total morphine consumption (0–24 h) would have been 64±39 mg in the ropivacaine group and 81±57 mg in the placebo group (P = 0.43).

Linear mixed models analyses (based on intention to treat) showed a tendency of lower pain scores in the ropivacaine group during knee flexion for the repeated measurements at 1, 2, 4, 6 and 8 hours (estimated difference of 19 mm, P = 0.06) but not for pain at rest (estimated difference 11 mm, P = 0.35).

## Discussion

The ACB reduces pain scores and morphine consumption compared with placebo after primary TKA [5–8]. In this study of ACB for revision TKA, the only statistically significant difference was seen in our primary endpoint: pain during flexion of the knee at 4 h postoperatively. At this time point there was a 19 mm difference in pain scores between the groups. This is very close to what we *a priori* considered to be clinically relevant (20 mm), and what can be expected in a multimodal analgesic setting with patients receiving acetaminophen, ibuprofen and morphine. Pain scores were consistently lower in the ropivacaine group, but mean differences varied between 6–19 mm.

To our knowledge, this is the first postoperative pain study performed exclusively in patients undergoing revision knee arthroplasty. In most studies revision TKA is an exclusion criteria, probably because this group of patients are assumed to have a more complex pathology, and more complex pain problems. As the number of revision TKAs is steadily increasing, we believe it is necessary to perform specific studies in this subgroup of patients.

A major limitation of this study is a larger dropout rate than anticipated, resulting in a reduced study size, especially affecting the secondary outcomes. Six patients were excluded before receiving an ACB. Because allocation assignment was blinded to all investigators and patients, and these six patients neither received an ACB nor any study medication, their exclusion was due to chance and is not likely to have biased our results. Prolonging the study period, although desirable, was not feasible because we stopped performing revision TKAs at our hospital. For our primary endpoint this resulted in a study population four patients short of our *a priori* calculated sample size of n = 17 in each group. Although the exclusion of these first six patients is not likely to have biased our results, additional six patients were excluded after obtaining our primary endpoint at 4 h postoperatively (for further details please see Figure 1), resulting in complete datasets for only 24 subjects for the secondary analysis. This secondary exclusion may have biased the results of our secondary endpoints, as these data points may not be missing at random. Especially the two patients in the placebo group, excluded due to excessive pain and difficulty in self-administration of morphine, may have biased our results. Nevertheless, these

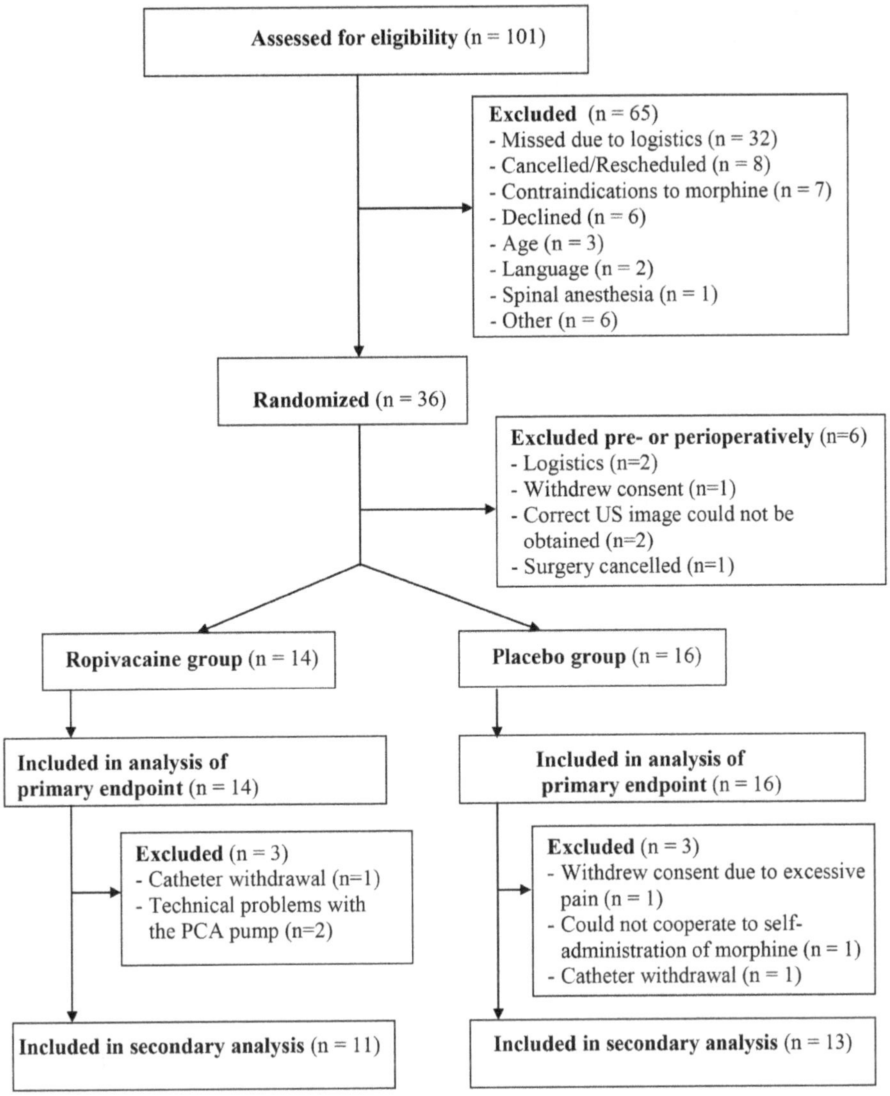


**Figure 1. Flow diagram of patient distribution.** US = ultra sound. PCA = patient-controlled analgesia.

patients were included in the post-hoc analyses using the linear mixed model.

Both total morphine consumption and calculation of AUC requires that the final observation is not missing, because extrapolation of morphine consumption or imputation of data by method of last observation carried forward has been widely criticized [9]. Unfortunately, these limitations will in practice render such analyses per protocol analyses. One of the major advantages of mixed models is that it does not require full data sets, thus allowing an intention to treat analysis. To compensate for the relatively large portion of missing data for our secondary analysis and the large variability in preoperative VAS pain scores, we performed a linear mixed model analysis re-analyzing the repeated VAS pain scores from 1–8 hours (originally compared by calculating the AUC). This revealed a tendency towards lower pain scores during knee flexion in the ropivacaine group (estimated difference 19 mm, $P = 0.06$), but not for pain at rest (estimated difference 11, $P = 0.35$).

Postoperative pain treatment following revision TKA is assumed to be more complex than after primary TKA. The patients suffer more complications, have extended hospital stays, and they are assumed to be in more pain [1]. A previous study, reports of mean preoperative pain scores of 61 mm on a VAS [2] indicating extensively pain issues. In the present study preoperative pain scores were not quite as high, but 16 out of 29 of patients reported moderate-severe pain (VAS≥30 mm) during knee flexion preoperatively (8 in the placebo group, 8 in the ropivacaine group). Preoperative pain and opioid usage are predictors for increased acute postoperative pain and opioid requirements [10], [11].

As the procedure becomes increasingly complicated with each subsequent revision and prior surgery is a predictor for increased pain [11], the demands for optimal postoperative pain treatment accumulate accordingly. Early rehabilitation and avoiding post-operative falls are important aspects of postoperative care in this population. Both of these can be facilitated by the ACB. Our institution is a tertiary referral center which carries out highly specialized functions for all parts of Denmark, and we consider it a strength that all procedures were performed by the same surgeon (HMS). However, half of the patients were 2$^{nd}$, 3$^{rd}$ or 4$^{th}$ time

**Table 1.** Patient characteristics.

| | Ropivacaine group | Placebo group |
|---|---|---|
| **Number of patients** | 14 | 16 |
| **Sex (male/female)** | 8/6 | 8/8 |
| **Age (years)** | 65 (50–78) | 67 (42–83) |
| **Height (cm)** | 170 (162–184) | 170 (150–191) |
| **Weight (kg)** | 94 (69–111) | 88 (58–115) |
| **Preoperative VAS* pain score at rest** | | |
| VAS score in mm | 9 (0–67) | 17 (0–75) |
| *VAS score in proportions:* | | |
| VAS<30 mm | 6/14 (43) | 7/15 (47) |
| VAS 30–59 mm | 4/14 (29) | 5/15 (33) |
| VAS>60 mm | 4/14 (29) | 3/15 (20) |
| **Preoperative VAS* pain score at 45 degrees knee flexion** | | |
| VAS score in mm | 44 (5–76) | 30 (0–78) |
| *VAS score in proportions:* | | |
| VAS<30 mm | 10/14 (71.5) | 11/16 (69) |
| VAS 30–59 mm | 3/14 (21.5) | 3/16 (19) |
| VAS>60 mm | 1/14 (7) | 2/16 (12) |
| **Habitual analgesics:** | | |
| None | 0/14 (0) | 3/16 (19) |
| Paracetamol and/or ibuprofen | 5/14 (36) | 1/16 (6) |
| Weak opioids† | 4/14 (28) | 10/16 (62.5) |
| Daily intake of strong opioids‡ | 5/14 (36) | 2/16 (12.5) |

Values are reported as number of subjects, proportions (percentage) or median (10–90%).
*VAS = visual analogue scale.
†Weak opioids = codeine or tramadol, or a non-daily intake of strong opioids.
‡Strong opioids = morphine, oxycodone, methadone, fentanyl, ketobemidone.

**Table 2.** Perioperative data.

| | Ropivacaine group | Placebo group |
|---|---|---|
| **Number of patients** | 14 | 16 |
| **Operated side (right/left)** | 8/6 | 6/10 |
| **Duration of surgery (min)** | 146 (82–194) | 138 (100–164) |
| **Order of revision performed:** | | |
| 1. Revision | 6/14 (43) | 8/16 (50) |
| 2. Revision | 5/14 (36) | 6/16 (38) |
| 3. Revision | 3/14 (21) | 1/16 (6) |
| 4. Revision | 0/14 (0) | 1/16 (6) |
| **Reason for revision TKA*:** | | |
| Septic loosening | 2/14 (14) | 4/14 (25) |
| Aseptic loosening | 6/14 (43) | 5/14 (31) |
| Component malposition | 3/14 (21.5) | 2/14 (12.5) |
| Instability | 3/14 (21.5) | 3/14 (19) |
| Stiffness | 0/14 (0) | 2/14 (12.5) |
| **Blood loss (ml)** | 150 (0–450) | 200 (0–480) |
| **Isotonic sodium chloride (ml)** | 1250 (650–2625) | 1250 (520–2010) |
| **Hydroxyethyl starch colloids (ml)** | 0 (0–350) | 0 (0–500) |

Values are reported as number of subjects, proportions (percentage) or median (10–90%).
*TKA = total knee arthroplasty.

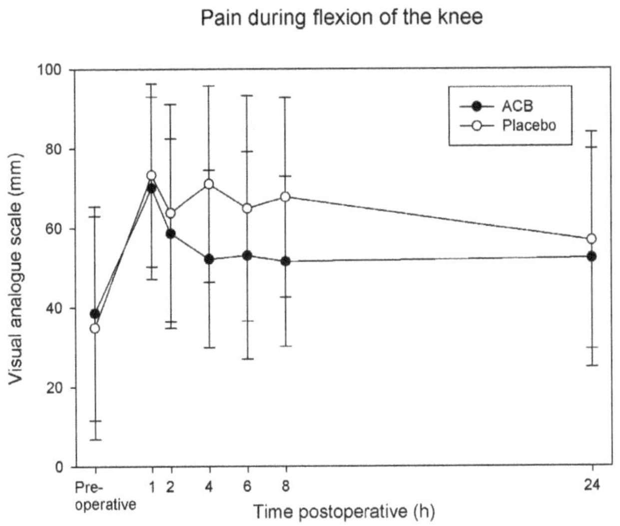


**Figure 2. Effects of the adductor canal block on pain during 45 degrees flexion of the knee.** Pain was assessed with a visual analogue scale (0–100 mm; with 0 equal no pain and 100 being the worst imaginable pain). Pain scores were lower in the ropivacaine group at 4 hours (primary endpoint (P = 0.04), but not when calculated as area under the curve (1–8 h, P = 0.11). Data are expressed as mean ±SD. ACB = adductor canal block.

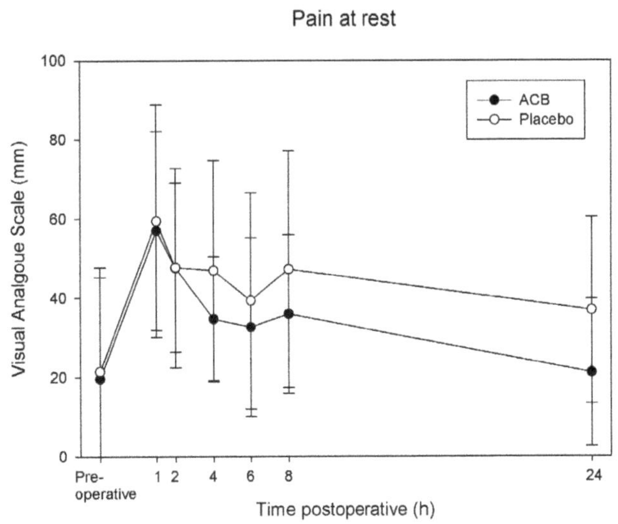


**Figure 3. Effects of the adductor canal block on pain at rest.** Pain was assessed with a visual analogue scale (0–100 mm; with 0 equal no pain and 100 being the worst imaginable pain). Comparisons between the groups were made as area under the curve (AUC) for the interval 1–8 h postoperatively, showing no statistically significant difference between the groups (P = 0.43). Data are expressed as mean ±SD. ACB = adductor canal block.

revisions. Therefore, our study population might not be comparable with the more commonly performed 1st time revisions, and this may reduce generalizability of the study.

To counter the problem of tolerance in patients treated with opioids, we decided that patients with a daily intake of strong opioids should continue with their habitual analgesics during the study period, and that these doses should not be included in the cumulative morphine consumption. By chance, more patients in the ropivacaine group (5/15 (36%) versus 2/16 (12.5%) had a daily intake of strong opioids (Table 1). Including the habitual analgesics from these patients in the cumulative total morphine consumption did not alter the results (P = 0.43). Patients treated with weak opioids may of course develop tolerance too, and as more patients in the placebo group had a daily intake of weak opioids or a non-daily intake of strong opioids, this might have affected our results. However, as there are no differences in morphine consumption between the groups, this would not have affected the conclusion of the study.

As the ACB is a novel technique, we believed it was important to compare the block with a placebo control. If we had compared two active treatments, and had found no significant difference, we would have risked concluding equal efficiency, while on the contrary neither might have been effective [12]. Although the group receiving saline is named "placebo group", the placebo part only refers to the block procedure. Both groups received a standard basic analgesic regimen as recommended by the PROSPECT Working Group [13]. Although the FNB is also recommended by the PROSPECT Working Group, this block is rarely used in Denmark due to the concurrent motor impairment.

Previous reports of the ACB state that intermittent boluses are preferable, in order to ensure spread throughout the aponeurotic canal [5], [14]. However, intermittent boluses might be challenging in every day practice. In the current study, ropivacaine was administered as an initial bolus of 30 ml 0.75% ropivacaine, followed by an additional bolus of 15 ml 0.75% ropivacaine 6 hours later. Because we were not able to ensure proper administration of intermittent boluses thereafter, this was followed by an infusion of 0.2% ropivacaine 8 ml/h. Based upon the results in the current study it is not possible to interpret whether data are a reflection of a single injection block or continuous infusion. The ACB is a relatively new block and further research studies, including dose-ranging studies are required to find the optimal administration of local anesthetic.

Two previous studies reported a success rate of 95 and 98% for the ACB, assessed by temperature discrimination in the saphenous innervation area [5–7]. In contrast, a third study performed an ultrasound control scan in a subgroup of patients, on the second postoperative day, revealing catheter displacement to outside the adductor canal in 5 out of 8 patients [8]. Unfortunately, the authors did not assess for saphenous sensory block in relation to the control scan. In the current study, we did not assess for block failures, but two patients were excluded due to accidental catheter withdrawal.

## Conclusions

Pain scores were consistently lower in the ropivacaine group including clinically relevant differences between groups. However, the mean differences varied and the only statistically significant difference between our groups was seen for pain during knee flexion at 4 hours postoperatively (primary endpoint). Due to a larger than anticipated dropout rate and considerate heterogeneity in the study population (large variability in preoperative pain scores, daily morphine consumption and order of revision being performed), more studies are needed before any recommendations regarding ACB for pain relief after revision TKA can be made. Future studies should include a large enough sample size to balance the distribution of confounders, or alternatively minimize heterogeneity by in- and exclusion criteria.

**Table 3.** Morphine consumption.

| Cumulative total morphine consumption (mg): | Ropivacaine group | Placebo group |
|---|---|---|
| 0–1 h postoperative | 5 (0–40) | 5 (0–39) |
| 0–2 h postoperative | 19 (3–64) | 25 (5–51) |
| 0–4 h postoperative | 28 (5–91) | 34 (5–61) |
| 0–6 h postoperative | 35 (7–105) | 35 (4–73) |
| 0–8 h postoperative | 35 (7–114) | 39 (4–89) |
| 0–24 h postoperative | 55 (8–135) | 60 (6–142) |

Values are presented as medians (10–90 percentiles).

## Supporting Information

**Checklist S1 Supporting CONSORT checklist (Consolidated Standards of Reporting Trials).**

**Protocol S1 The protocol for this trial is available in the supplementary information file.**

**Data S1 All data used for analysis are available in the supplementary information file.**

## Acknowledgments

The authors gratefully acknowledge the invaluable assistance of the entire Operating and Recovery room staff and the nursing staff at the Orthopaedic Ward at Rigshospitalet, Copenhagen University Hospital, Denmark. We also thank the Copenhagen University Hospital GCP Unit, Bispebjerg Hospital, Denmark, for monitoring the study.

**The department and institution to which the work should be attributed:**

Department of Anaesthesia, Centre of Head and Orthopaedics, Copenhagen University Hospital, Rigshospitalet, Copenhagen, Denmark.

## Author Contributions

Wrote the paper: PJ JBD ZJKN HMS OM MHH JL MTJ. Conceived and designed the experiments: PJ JBD ZJKN HMS OM MHH JL MTJ. Performed the experiments: PJ HMS ZJKN MHH. Analyzed the data: PJ JBD.

## References

1. Goldberg VM (2001) Principles of revision total knee arthroplasty: overview. Instr Course Lect 50: 357–358.
2. van Kempen RW, Schimmel JJ, van Hellemondt GG, Vandenneucker H, Wymenga AB (2013) Reason for revision TKA predicts clinical outcome: prospective evaluation of 150 consecutive patients with 2-years followup. Clin Orthop Relat Res 471: 2296–2302. 10.1007/s11999-013-2940-8 [doi].
3. Jaeger P, Nielsen ZJ, Henningsen MH, Hilsted KL, Mathiesen O, et al. (2013) Adductor canal block versus femoral nerve block and quadriceps strength: a randomized, double-blind, placebo-controlled, crossover study in healthy volunteers. Anesthesiology 118: 409–415. 10.1097/ALN.0b013e318279fa0b [doi].
4. Kwofie MK, Shastri UD, Gadsden JC, Sinha SK, Abrams JH, et al. (2013) The effects of ultrasound-guided adductor canal block versus femoral nerve block on quadriceps strength and fall risk: a blinded, randomized trial of volunteers. Reg Anesth Pain Med 38: 321–325. 10.1097/AAP.0b013e318295df80 [doi]; 00115550-201307000-00011 [pii].
5. Jenstrup MT, Jaeger P, Lund J, Fomsgaard JS, Bache S, et al. (2012) Effects of Adductor-Canal-Blockade on pain and ambulation after total knee arthroplasty: a randomized study. Acta Anaesthesiol Scand 56: 357–364.
6. Jaeger P, Zaric D, Fomsgaard JS, Hilsted KL, Bjerregaard J, et al. (2013) Adductor canal block versus femoral nerve block for analgesia after total knee arthroplasty: a randomized, double-blind study. Reg Anesth Pain Med 38: 526–532. 10.1097/AAP.0000000000000015 [doi].
7. Grevstad U, Mathiesen O, Lind T, Dahl JB (2014) Effect of adductor canal block on pain in patients with severe pain after total knee arthroplasty: a randomized study with individual patient analysis. Br J Anaesth. aet441 [pii]; 10.1093/bja/aet441 [doi].
8. Andersen HL, Gyrn J, Moller L, Christensen B, Zaric D (2013) Continuous saphenous nerve block as supplement to single-dose local infiltration analgesia for postoperative pain management after total knee arthroplasty. Reg Anesth Pain Med 38: 106–111.10.1097/AAP.0b013e31827900a9 [doi].
9. White IR, Carpenter J, Horton NJ (2012) Including all individuals is not enough: lessons for intention-to-treat analysis. Clin Trials 9: 396–407. 10.1177/1740774512450098 [doi].
10. Brummett CM, Janda AM, Schueller CM, Tsodikov A, Morris M, et al. (2013) Survey criteria for fibromyalgia independently predict increased postoperative opioid consumption after lower-extremity joint arthroplasty: a prospective, observational cohort study. Anesthesiology 119: 1434–1443. 10.1097/ALN.0b013e3182a8eb1f [doi]; 00000542-201312000-00030 [pii].
11. Liu SS, Buvanendran A, Rathmell JP, Sawhney M, Bae JJ, et al. (2012) Predictors for moderate to severe acute postoperative pain after total hip and knee replacement. Int Orthop 36: 2261–2267. 10.1007/s00264-012-1623-5 [doi].
12. Dahl JB, Rasmussen LS (2012) Comparison of two active analgesic interventions: a suggestion for an 'approximated placebo control'. Acta Anaesthesiol Scand 56: 669–671. 10.1111/j.1399-6576.2012.02680.x [doi].
13. Fischer HB, Simanski CJ, Sharp C, Bonnet F, Camu F, et al. (2008) A procedure-specific systematic review and consensus recommendations for postoperative analgesia following total knee arthroplasty. Anaesthesia 63: 1105–1123.
14. Lund J, Jenstrup MT, Jaeger P, Sorensen AM, Dahl JB (2011) Continuous adductor-canal-blockade for adjuvant post-operative analgesia after major knee surgery: preliminary results. Acta Anaesthesiol Scand 55: 14–19.

# 25

# Electroencephalographic Variation during End Maintenance and Emergence from Surgical Anesthesia

**Divya Chander[1*⁹], Paul S. García[2⁹], Jono N. MacColl[3], Sam Illing[3], Jamie W. Sleigh[3]**

1 Department of Anesthesiology, Perioperative and Pain Medicine, Stanford University School of Medicine, Stanford, California, United States of America, 2 Department of Anesthesiology, Atlanta VA Medical Center/Emory University, Atlanta, Georgia, United States of America, 3 Department of Anaesthesia, Waikato Clinical School, University of Auckland, Hamilton, New Zealand

## Abstract

The re-establishment of conscious awareness after discontinuing general anesthesia has often been assumed to be the inverse of loss of consciousness. This is despite the obvious asymmetry in the initiation and termination of natural sleep. In order to characterize the restoration of consciousness after surgery, we recorded frontal electroencephalograph (EEG) from 100 patients in the operating room during maintenance and emergence from general anesthesia. We have defined, for the first time, 4 steady-state patterns of anesthetic maintenance based on the relative EEG power in the slow-wave (<14 Hz) frequency bands that dominate sleep and anesthesia. Unlike single-drug experiments performed in healthy volunteers, we found that surgical patients exhibited greater electroencephalographic heterogeneity while re-establishing conscious awareness after drug discontinuation. Moreover, these emergence patterns could be broadly grouped according to the duration and rapidity of transitions amongst these slow-wave dominated brain states that precede awakening. Most patients progressed gradually from a pattern characterized by strong peaks of delta (0.5–4 Hz) and alpha/spindle (8–14 Hz) power ('Slow-Wave Anesthesia') to a state marked by low delta-spindle power ('Non Slow-Wave Anesthesia') before awakening. However, 31% of patients transitioned abruptly from Slow-Wave Anesthesia to waking; they were also more likely to express pain in the post-operative period. Our results, based on sleep-staging classification, provide the first systematized nomenclature for tracking brain states under general anesthesia from maintenance to emergence, and suggest that these transitions may correlate with post-operative outcomes such as pain.

**Editor:** Uwe Rudolph, McLean Hospital/Harvard Medical School, United States of America

**Funding:** This work was supported by a collaborative grant from the James S. McDonnell Foundation, and departmental resources of the authors. The funders had no role in study design, data collection and analysis, decision to publish, or preparation of the manuscript.

**Competing Interests:** The authors have declared that no competing interests exist.

* Email: dchander@stanford.edu

⁹ These authors contributed equally to this work.

## Introduction

Both sleep and anesthesia have been tracked in the human electroencephalogram (EEG) since the 1950s [1–3], but a staging nomenclature based on specific EEG features has only been well-developed for natural sleep [4,5]. While there are also stereotyped EEG features, such as a shift in the spectrum toward lower frequencies (<14 Hz), that correlate with anesthesia-induced unresponsiveneses (the historical clinical marker of anesthetic adequacy) [6–11], a standardized nomenclature for anesthetic maintenance and emergence has never been universally accepted by clinicians. Recent focus has been placed on the spatial and temporal distribution of these frequency changes [12–15], and identifies an anteriorization of lower frequency power that correlates with the behavioral transition to loss of consciousness [8,9,16,17]. Studies in which volunteers have been exposed to slowly changing doses of propofol have described spectral power changes upon emergence that appear to be the inverse of induction, i.e. a decrease in power in these low frequency oscillations over the frontal EEG, followed by an increase in higher frequencies as the patient becomes behaviorally responsive to mild stimuli [8,9]. This is in contrast to the termination of natural sleep, which is typically preceded by cyclic transitions into progressively longer episodes of cortical activation [18]. Waking usually occurs from rapid eye movement (REM) sleep (reviewed in Steriade [19]).

Although sleep and anesthesia are not the same, significant overlap in neurotransmitters, circuitry and electrical patterns do exist [20,21], suggesting that anesthetics may achieve part of their hypnotic effect by acting on the normal sleep and arousal systems of the brain [22]. Pharmacologic enhancement of inhibitory signaling, mediated via the gamma aminobutyric acid type A ($GABA_A$) receptor, underlies the mechanisms of most commonly used anesthetic agents [23,24]. Similarly, a physiological GABAergic state also contributes to the thalamocortical oscillations characteristic of non-REM sleep [25], while pharmacologic inhibition of the $GABA_A$ receptor reverses sleepiness in hypersomnic patients [26]. It has been shown that sleep deprivation potentiates the efficacy of anesthetics [27], and these effects can be partially reversed by antagonists to adenosine, an endogenous ligand that accumulates during sleep pressure [28]. Furthermore, activation of subcortical endogenous arousal pathways (e.g. thalamus, basal forebrain, hypothalamus, brain stem) can reverse anesthesia in some animal models [29–36], significantly blurring the distinction between sleep and anesthesia. Perhaps most

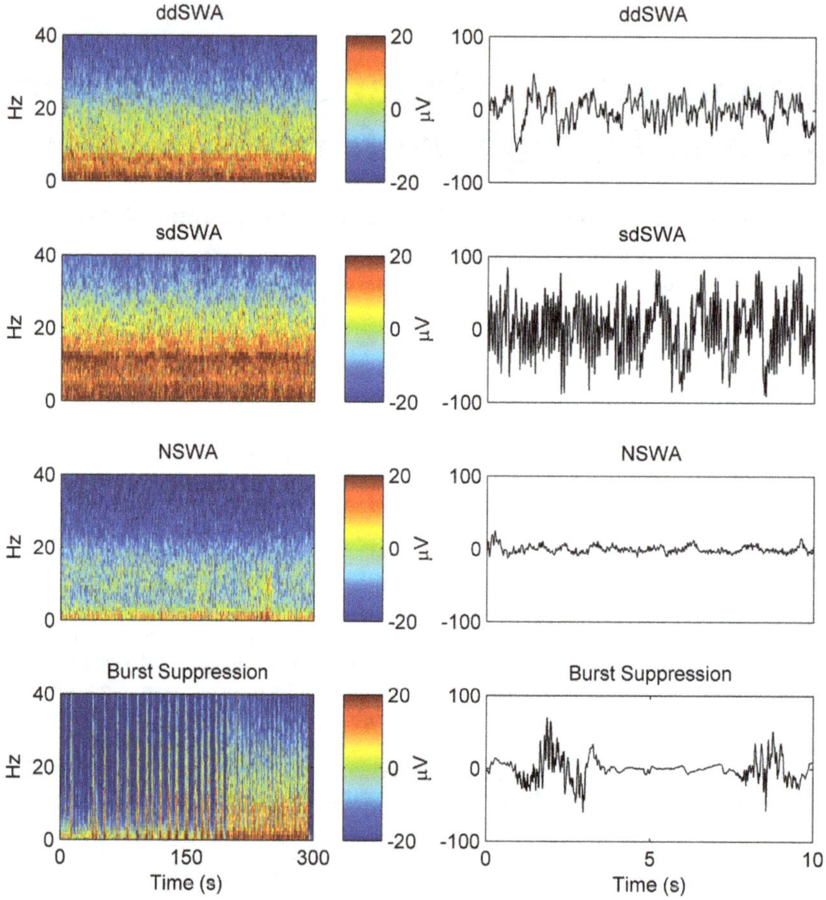


**Figure 1. Spectral patterns at the end of maintenance under sevoflurane general anesthesia comprise 4 basic patterns.** 'Slow-Wave Anesthesia' (SWA) is a spectral pattern in which there is both high delta and spindle power (>7 dB). Panel (A) shows the more common variant, or subclass, of the SWA spectrogram, calculated over 5 minutes prior to turning off the anesthetic, in which delta power is higher than spindle power (point #1 below the diagonal in Figure 2B) termed delta dominant SWA, or ddSWA. An example 10 second raw EEG tracing is take from this period and shown in the right column. Panel (B) is an SWA spectral variant/subclass in which spindle power is higher than delta power, termed spindle-dominant SWA, or sdSWA (point #2 above the diagonal in Figure 2B). Finally, a small subset of patients (5%) showed low amplitude power in both the spindle and delta frequency bands (C). We termed this pattern non Slow-Wave Anesthesia, or NSWA (point #3 in Figure 2B). For completeness, the spectrogram in panel (D) reflects a deeper anesthetic maintenance pattern, burst suppression, transitioning into a ddSWA pattern at approximately 1.5 minutes prior to End Maintenance. The representative 10 second EEG to its right is taken from the burst suppression period.

importantly, both non-REM (NREM) sleep and general anesthesia exhibit similar synchronization and slowing of the EEG [37,38]. Not surprisingly, the same range of lower frequency oscillations that indicate loss of consciousness are also used to separate natural sleep into specific stages [4,5,39,40]. Thalamocortical oscillations in the alpha band (8–14 Hz) are the electroencephalographic hallmark of the loss of perceptual awareness in synchronized sleep [41]. Generated by the reticular nucleus of the thalamus [42], these oscillations consist of waxing and waning of electrical potentials, and are often referred to as sleep spindles [43]. As sleep deepens, spindles are progressively reduced and replaced by slower oscillations (0.5–4 Hz) [44,45]. In contrast, REM sleep is characterized by profound inhibition of motor output, abolition of these low-frequency oscillations, and an EEG resembling the aroused brain [46]. Although the different sleep stages were arbitrarily and heuristically defined, based on EEG patterns described above [5,47], they have been successfully used by clinicians and researchers to relate sleep physiology to functional neuroanatomy [48], consolidation of memory [49–51], and sleep disorders [52,53].

We therefore designed a study with three objectives. The first was to catalogue and define a standardized nomenclature for the EEG during anesthetic maintenance, analogous to that used to describe natural sleep. The second was to characterize the evolution of the human EEG during emergence from general anesthesia during surgery, to determine if there was a single common path, or multiple pathways to re-establishing conscious awareness and interaction with the outside world. Our final goal was to determine if the path by which the patient emerged had any relationship to the quality of a patient's recovery.

We recorded the frontal EEG from 100 human subjects in the operating room, undergoing routine orthopedic surgery with general volatile anesthesia, prior to loss of consciousness, through the maintenance and recovery from anesthesia, until patients were able to be taken safely to the recovery room. Using spectral processing techniques, we propose a nomenclature of four basic EEG patterns, based on the relative dominance of low frequency oscillatory patterns seen during maintenance of general anesthesia (i.e. a degree of hypnosis considered to be commensurate with unconsciousness). We also identified four stereotypical trajectories

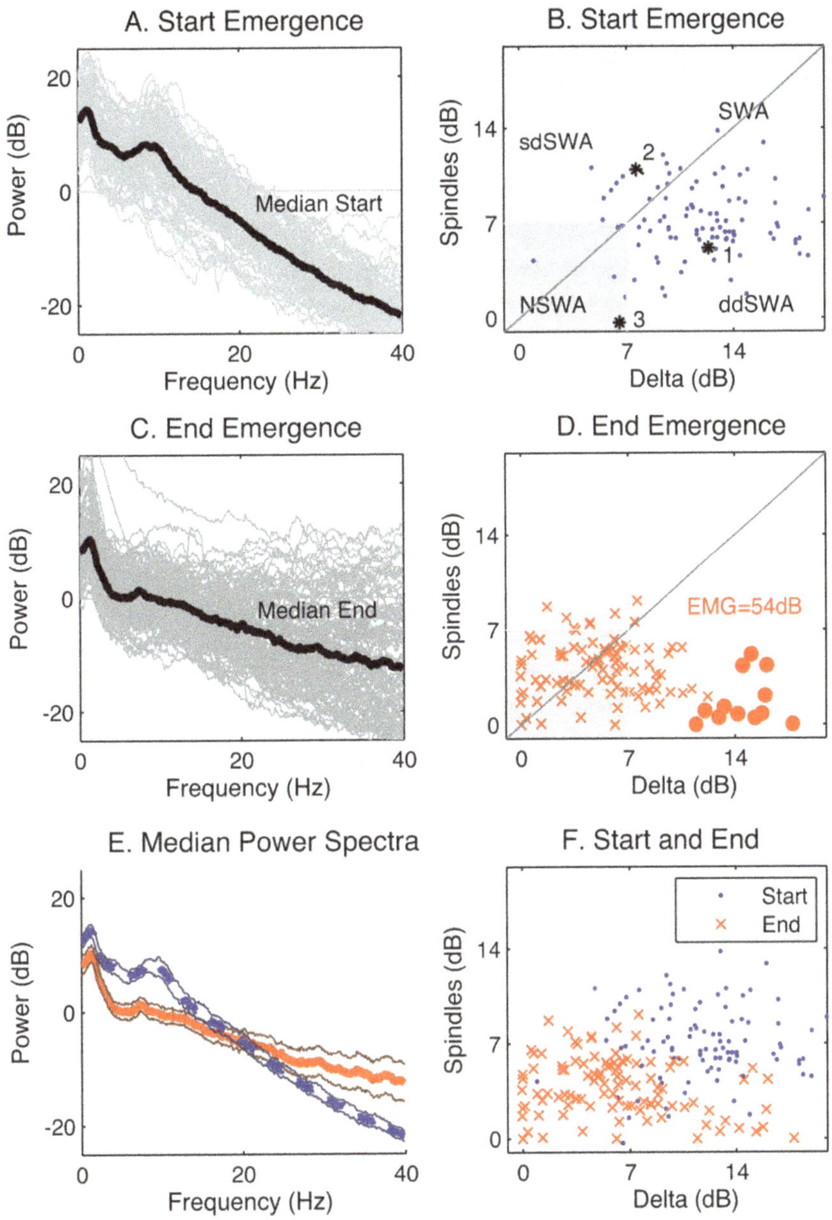


**Figure 2. Emergence from general anesthesia is characterized by a loss in power in the slower spindle and delta frequency bands, and a recovery of power in the higher frequency bands.** Power spectra and scatterplots of delta and spindle power (dB) for all patients, at the start (2A, 2B) and the end (2C, 2D) of emergence. The thick black lines are the median of the power spectra at each frequency for all patients. The median power spectra and 95% confidence intervals of the median, at the start and end, are shown in 2E. Patients were separated into two main spectral classes by thresholding spindle and delta power at 7 dB, whose boundary is marked by the gray box (see also Figure S1). Thus, the most common pattern, seen in 95% patients at Start Emergence, is characterized by high power (>7 dB) in both frequency bands, which we define as '**Slow-Wave Anesthesia (SWA)**'; the alternate pattern, defined as '**Non Slow-Wave Anesthesia (NSWA)**', represents the 5% of patients that fall within the gray box. The fuzzy clusters in 2B are defined in the text: SWA = Slow-Wave Anesthesia, ddSWA = delta-dominant Slow-Wave Anesthesia, sdSWA = spindle-dominant Slow-Wave Anesthesia, NSWA = Non Slow-Wave Anesthesia (gray box). Red circles in 2D are those patients with a high delta power at End Emergence. All except one subject with high delta at End Emergence also had an EMG>40 dB. 2F is the same as 2B and 2D superimposed for ease of visual comparison.

that describe the progression toward conscious awareness during emergence. These emergence patterns do not consistently follow the averaged patterns of volunteers undergoing slow infusions of propofol described in prior studies [8,9], but in some instances do share similarities with sleep stages that precede awakening. Further, we noted that the trajectory taken to re-establish conscious awareness is not correlated to the brain state at the cessation of the anesthetic (End Maintenance), but the path taken to re-establishing awareness does appear to have some correlation with a subject's subsequent level of sedation and post-operative pain. Our work suggests that the central nervous system may not always re-establish connectivity in a canonical sequence after unconsciousness produced by general anesthesia during surgery. We hypothesize that these less typical emergence sequences under

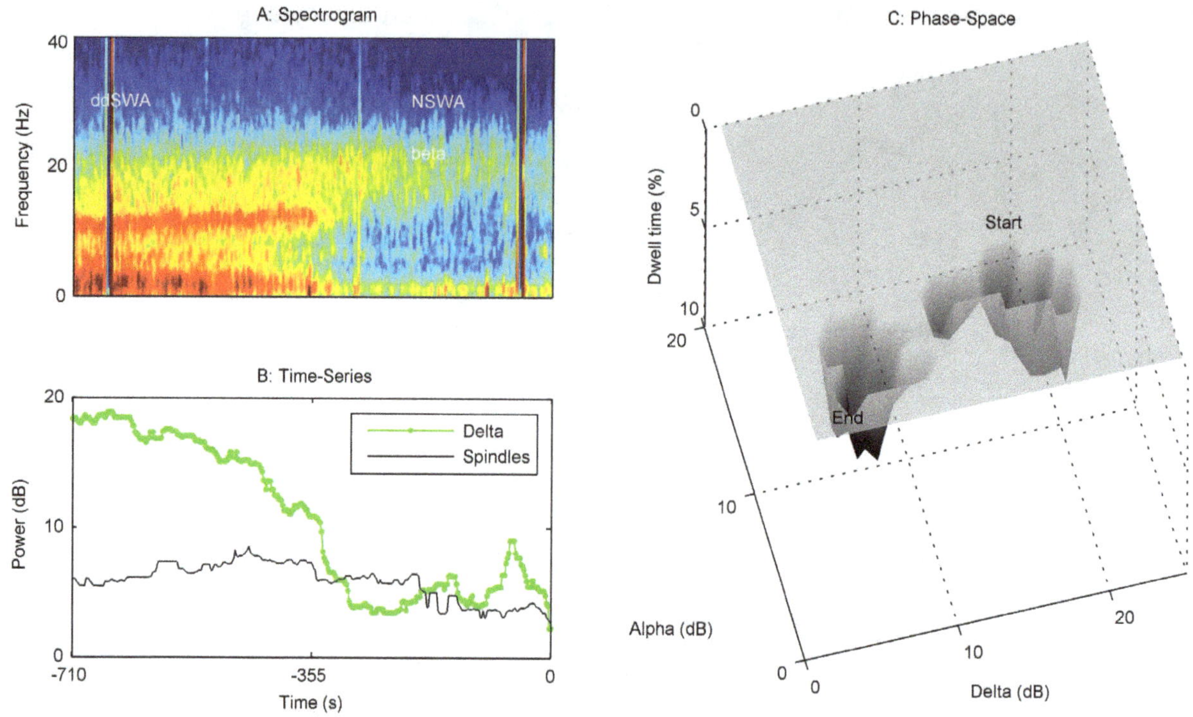


**Figure 3. Emergence Trajectory 1, SWA → NSWA.** The upper left panel (A) is the spectrogram from Start Emergence (measured in negative seconds) to End Emergence (time 0 seconds) for a representative patient (#81); this also corresponds to the time of anesthetic wash-out from the brain. Below it is a time series (B) that quantifies spindle and delta power (dB) over the same emergence period. To the right is a dwell time state-space plot (C). The evolution of spindle and delta power over the emergence trajectory from Start Emergence (upper right) to End Emergence (lower left) is shown where the depth of the contour (y-axis) reflects the time spent in each pixel of the state, as a percentage of the total emergence time. At the start of emergence, this patient remained for a signficant period in a slow-wave state (SWA) characterized by higher delta to spindle power ratio (ddSWA). There was a relatively abrupt transition period of approximately 60 seconds, to a second attractor characterized by lower delta and spindle power (NSWA) prior to waking-up. In our sample, 23% of patients had a similar trajectory.

anesthesia may predispose patients to undesirable wake-ups, in a similar way that parasomnias are exacerbated by disrupted sleep architecture [54].

## Results

### Patterns during maintenance in the human frontal electroencephalograph can be divided into four (4) basic spectral variants

In order to define a nomenclature for anesthetic maintenance, we analyzed the relative contribution amongst major oscillatory features found in the power spectra of the frontal electroencephalogram (EEG) of 100 patients undergoing routine orthopedic surgery under general anesthesia. The time at which the anesthetic was turned off was defined as the 'End Maintenance' or 'Start Emergence' point. A spectrogram of EEG data from a single frontal EEG electrode for 5 minutes prior to End Maintenance was computed for each individual patient. Visual inspection revealed clear peaks in the spectrogram within the delta and alpha bands of some patients, but these peaks showed considerable variation across the population (Figure 1A-D). The power spectra and a scatterplot of delta power against the oscillatory component of alpha power, computed over an 8 second EEG window (see Methods) for all 100 patients at Start Emergence, are shown in Figures 2A and 2B. The oscillatory component of alpha power was quantified by measuring the height of the alpha peak above the underlying broadband activity [55]. This has the advantage that it specifically targets the narrowband oscillatory component of this peak, and is less influenced by the underlying broadband ($1/f$) components of the EEG, making the alpha oscillatory power more orthogonal to the delta power. In this study we have chosen to borrow the term 'spindles' from the sleep literature to describe the specific oscillatory component in the alpha range from the overall composite alpha power [5]. Although the scatterplot in Figure 2B does not readily segregate into discrete clusters, we followed statistical convention and separated the patients into two main spectral classes by thresholding spindle and delta power at 7 dB. Because the bi-variate data appears to follow a unimodal distribution, the 7dB theshold reflects the boundary below which only 5% of the Start Emergence data lay, and the region within which most of the End Emergence data lay (Figure S1). Thus, the most common pattern, seen in 95% patients at Start Emergence, is characterized by high power (>7 dB) in both frequency bands, which we define as '**Slow-Wave Anesthesia (SWA)**;' this includes patients above the 7 dB boundary marked by the gray box. Some patients have a relatively equal distribution of spindle and delta power during SWA, lying on or near the unity diagonal (Figure 2B). However, it was more common in this patient sample for delta power to be greater than spindle power during SWA. This is represented by the preponderance of points lying below the diagonal in Figure 2B. We therefore propose the term '**delta-dominant Slow-Wave Anesthesia**' (**ddSWA**, Figure 1A) to describe this sub-classification. Conversely when spindle power is greater than delta power (i.e. points above the diagonal, Figure 2B), we propose the term '**spindle-dominant Slow-Wave Anesthesia**' (**sdSWA**, Figure 1B). In this sample, we

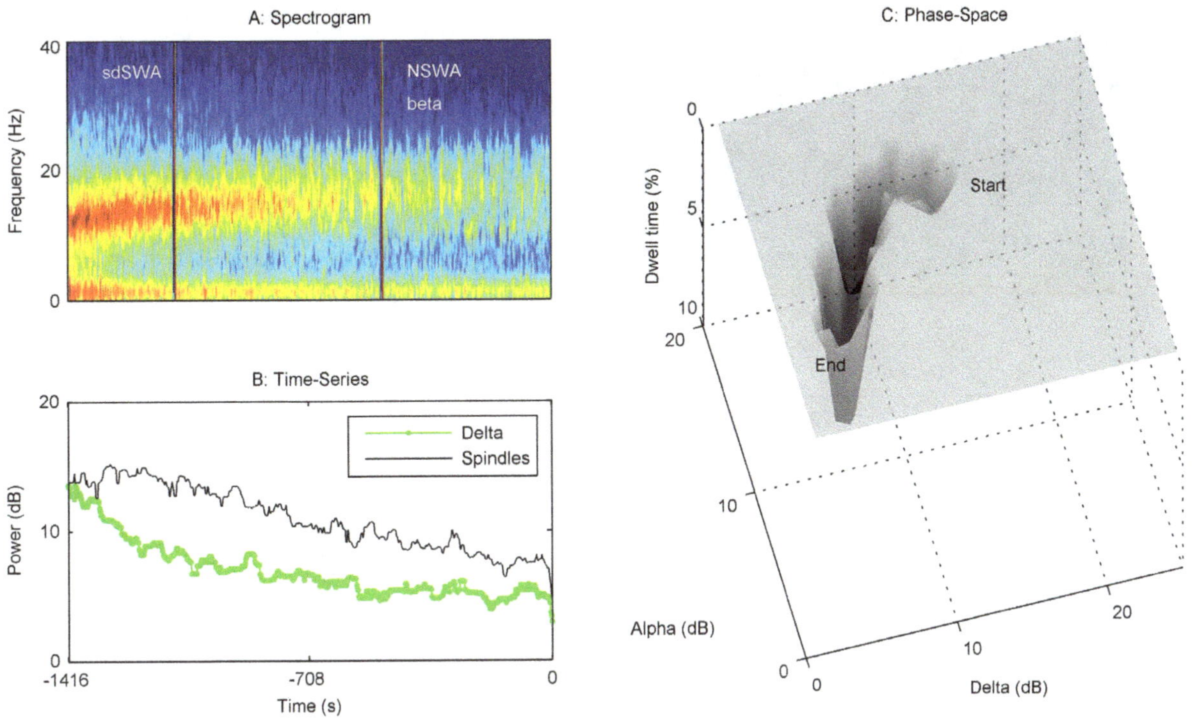


**Figure 4. Emergence Trajectory 2, SWA→NSWA, continuous progression.** The spectrogram (A) and time series (B) from Start Emergence to End Emergence for a representative patient (#36) are shown. To the right is dwell time state-space plot (C). This patient started in a slow-wave state (SWA). Over approximately 1.5 minutes, the patient transitioned into a state characterized by higher spindle power (sdSWA), and then showed a progressive decrease in delta and spindle power towards the NSWA region over about 20 minutes before waking. There was a converse increase in beta power as alpha/spindle power was diminished. No single deep attractor in state-space characterizes this patient's emergence path until reaching NSWA prior to wake-up. In our sample, 20% of patients had a similar trajectory.

noted a continuum of relative spindle and delta power between patients, and even within patients during the course of their anesthetic. Because of this we have purposely left the terms sdSWA and ddSWA somewhat loosely defined – they are convenient labels that indicate a patient (in SWA) has relatively stronger spindle or delta waves. These plots are generated over a short snap-shot in time; thus, a patient in a ddSWA pattern may gradually lose delta power and transition into an sdSWA pattern over the course of an anesthetic. Five percent (5%) of patients had Start Emergence EEGs with a very low spindle and delta power (<7 dB) – we termed these indeterminate patterns "**Non Slow-Wave Anesthesia**" (**NSWA**, Figure 1C). An example of another common maintenance pattern, that of burst suppression (transitioning into SWA) is shown in Figure 1D, for as complete a description as possible of spectral patterns encountered during surgical anesthesia. This pattern is more typically seen post-induction of general anesthesia (i.e. just after loss of consciousness is achieved with a bolus dose of propofol), but may be seen during the entire course of the maintenance phase of anesthesia.

## Emergence from general anesthesia is characterized by a shift from a slow-wave pattern (SWA) to a more uniform distribution of power across all frequency bands

In order to characterize salient features of the EEG at the start (i.e. turning off anesthetic) and end of emergence (i.e. responsiveness to standard verbal stimulation), the power-spectral density (PSD) plots for individual patients were compared in each condition. The plots in the left column of Figure 2 show the power spectra for all patients (gray), derived from the 8 second EEG segments at the start (Figure 2A) and end of emergence (Figure 2C). There is considerable variation in individual patient spectral power, encompassing a 30 dB range (equivalent to an approximately five-fold variation in raw voltage) at both Start and End Emergence, with greater spread in the higher frequency bands (>14 Hz) during End Emergence. The thick black line in both Figures 2A and 2C are the median power spectra for each condition. Distinct peaks are present at Start Emergence/End Maintenance in the delta and spindle frequency bands. At End Emergence, the spindle peak is lost, and the delta peak diminishes in amplitude. The scatterplots in Figures 2B and 2D, in which delta and spindle power are plotted against one another for each patient, clearly show the downward shift in power in both these frequency bands (from 2B to 2D). There is a small subset of patients (12%) at End Emergence that maintains high delta power (red dots in Figure 2D); this subset is also the group that showed high EMG at End Emergence (>40 dB) suggesting that the high delta power is actually broad-band contamination of the EEG with frontalis muscle activity rather than true frontal cortical activity. For ease of comparison, the shifts in median power spectra at Start (blue) and End Emergence (red) are shown in Figure 2E, while the downward shift in spindle-delta power at Start (blue) and End Emergence (red) is summarized in Figure 2F. As a whole, the median power spectra at End Emergence demonstrates a more uniform distribution of power in the 20–40 Hz range, consistent with recent studies in human volunteers receiving propofol infusions [8,9], but with more variability as evidenced by broader confidence intervals.

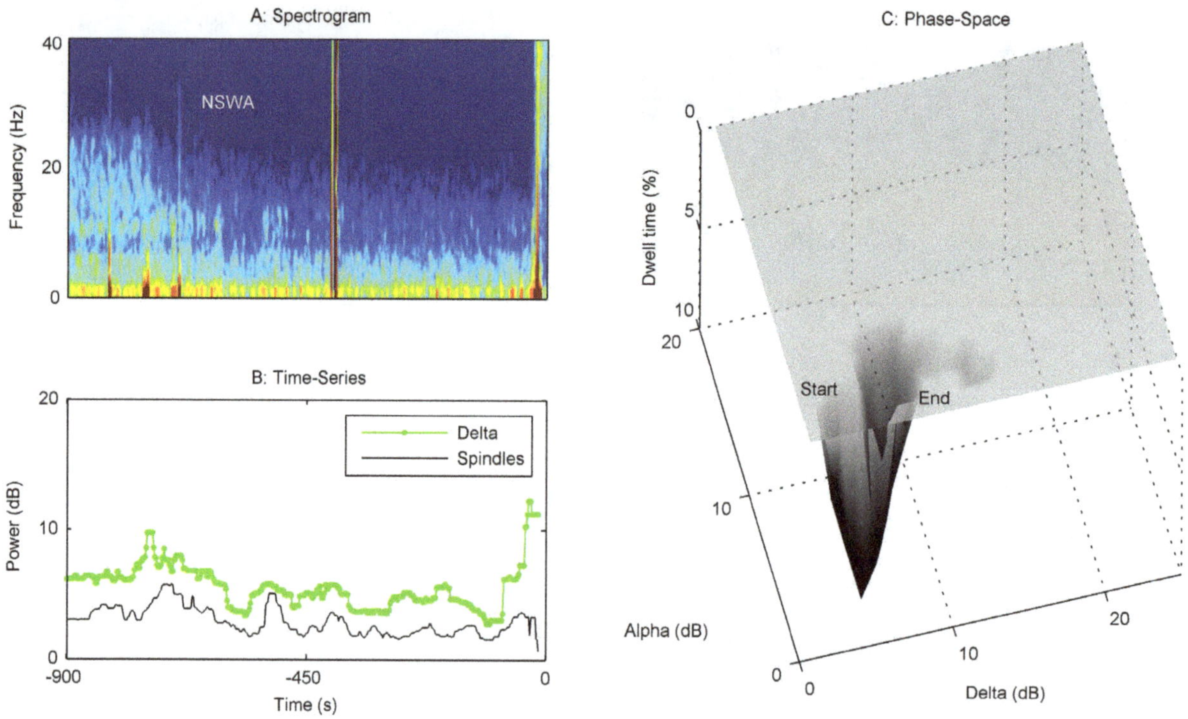


**Figure 5. Emergence Trajectory 3, NSWA→Wakefulness.** The spectrogram (A) and time series (B) from Start Emergence to End Emergence for a representative patient (#19) are shown. To the right is a dwell time state-space plot (C). This patient started and ended in a state characterized by a non slow-wave state (NSWA) attractor prior to waking up. The duration of emergence was long (15 minutes), and the attractor did not move significantly. In our sample, 16% of patients had a similar trajectory.

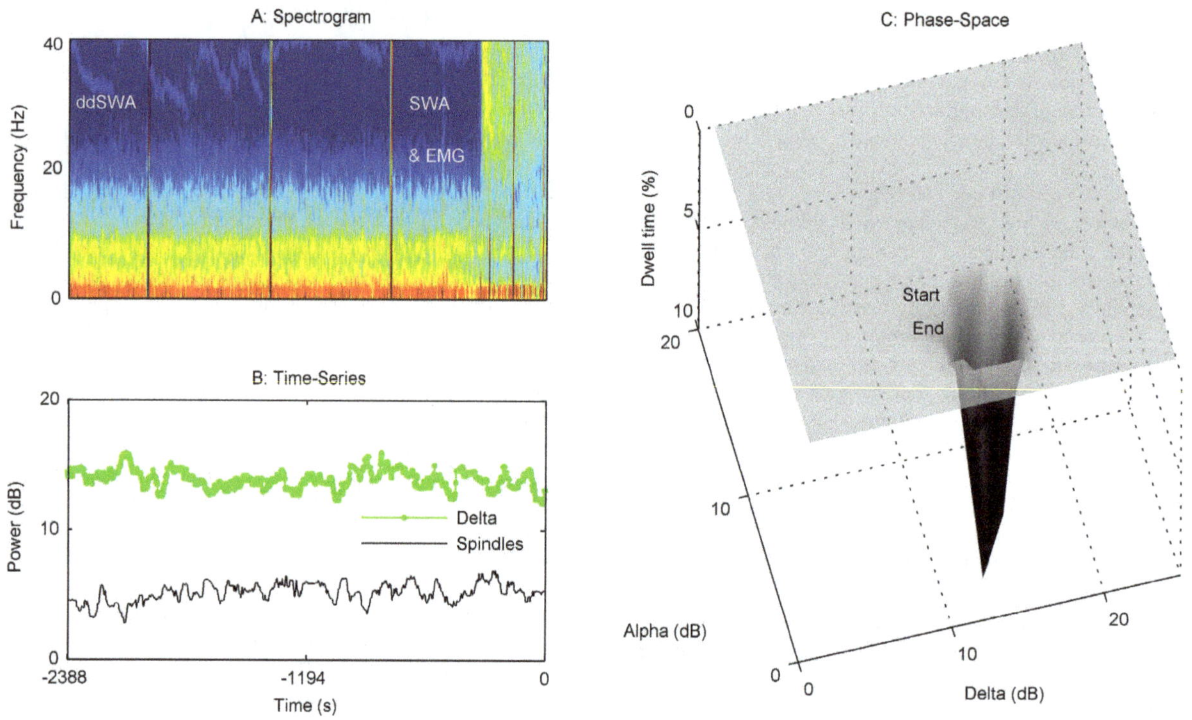


**Figure 6. Emergence Trajectory 4, SWA→Wakefulness.** The spectrogram (A) and time series (B) from Start Emergence to End Emergence for a representative patient (77) are shown. To the right is a dwell time state-space plot (C). This patient started and ended in a state characterized by a slow-wave state (SWA) attractor prior to waking up. Patients who woke up this abruptly from a slow-wave state of anesthesia were more likely to experience high pain in recovery. In our sample, 31% of patients had a similar trajectory.

**Table 1.** Level of Consciousness and Pain.

| | |
|---|---|
| **PACU-Cons Score** | |
| 0 | Confused |
| 1 | Quickly alert (Ramsay score = 2 at 15 minutes) |
| 2 | Somnolent (Ramsay score = 3 or 4 at 15 minutes) |
| **PACU-Pain Score** | |
| 0 | Minimal (NRS = 0–3 and relaxed) |
| 1 | Moderate (NRS = 4–8 and relaxed or going back to sleep) |
| 2 | Severe (NRS = 8–10 or NRS>4 and signs of distress) |

PACU = Post anesthesia care unit, Cons = consciousness, NRS = numerical rating scale

## Evolution of trajectories from Start Emergence to End Emergence vary by patient

Figure 2 captures a static image of the state of the brain at the start and end of emergence. While a shift from one average state to another can be seen in Figure 2E, the variability of individual patient PSDs and spindle-delta power scatterplots suggests that the path from Start to End Emergence may not be identical or stereotyped. Clinically, this is often reflected in the length of time a patient takes to emerge from general anesthesia. We chose not to average patient trajectories, and instead looked for graphical methods to describe changes for individual patients. This involved construction of an 'emergence trajectory' for each patient. A spectrogram from Start to End Emergence was first calculated (Figure 3–6A), and a time series data of spindle and delta power extracted from the power spectrum (Figure 3–6B). Finally, we applied a dynamical systems approach to the data, creating a corresponding 3-D 'dwell time plot' for each patient's emergence trajectory (Figure 3–6C). These graphically depict how the relative spindle and delta power changes for each patient in response to the progressive decline in both anesthetic drug concentrations and the residuum of surgical nociception from the time the anesthetic is turned off until the patient responded to voice. In these 'phase-space' plots, spindle power is reflected on the y-axis, delta power on the x-axis, and the z-axis reflects the time spent in each 'pixel' of state-space as a percentage of the total emergence time ("dwell time"). From these surfaces, we can see that a continuous, progressive decrease in spindle and delta power was **not** the usual pattern of emergence. Instead the majority of patients tended to follow a more "punctated equilibrium" pattern, occupying restricted regions of the state-space for extended periods of time, before relatively rapidly moving to other areas of phase space, or to the waking state. At first approximation, these areas appear to functionally act as point attractors [56]. At Start Emergence, most (95%) of these point attractors can be classified as SWA, or a sub-classification (sdSWA or ddSWA), while at End Emergence, the majority (59%) are classified as NSWA. The path from Start Emergence to End Emergence took variable trajectories. These were roughly classified by the presence of one or two attractors, whether these attractors lay in the SWA or NSWA regions, and whether the transition to a new state was rapid or gradual through the phase-space. Figure 3 demonstrates a common emergence trajectory (23% of patients). It shows an initial attractor in the SWA region, which steps abruptly to a second attractor in NSWA space, followed by arousal. The second trajectory (20%) is similar to the first except it shows a more gradual transition between SWA and NSWA state space (Figure 4). Figure 5 describes a third trajectory (16%), a single attractor in NSWA, which reflects a patient who spends nearly the entire duration of emergence in NSWA before responding to voice. The fourth trajectory (31%) is characterized by a patient who woke up directly from SWA (Figure 6). About 10% of patients fell into indeterminate categories. We would note that during emergence many patients who start emergence in the ddSWA go on to lose their delta power and gained spindle power during their emergence; this resulted in nearly half (49%) of patients spending more than 25% of their time in the sdSWA region. This transition pattern is analogous to that seen in the progression from deep to lighter natural NREM stage 2 sleep. At the other extreme, 27% patients spend no time in the sdSWA region at all, as if NREM stage 2 sleep was skipped during the process of waking.

## Evolution of trajectories from Start Emergence to End Emergence are correlated to nociceptive state and level of consciousness upon waking

We next examined whether there was an association with, the relative time spent in SWA vs. NSWA, and the *quality of emergence*. Two post-anesthesia scores were used to quantify level of consciousness and post-operative pain (Table 1). Because sedation can interfere with reported pain, we measured pain heuristically by combining self-reported pain score with non-reported signs of distress. We found an association between lower pain scores and the relative amount of time spent in NSWA during emergence (Figure 7). Those who spent a long time in a non slow-wave state prior to wake-up were more likely to waken with minimal pain (PACU-Pain = 0) than those who woke directly from a slow-wave state ($p = 0.037$, Chi-squared test; $p = 0.0017$ for delta power distribution, $p = 0.05$ for alpha power distribution; Kolmogorov-Smirnov test). This is reflected in the averaged dwell-time contour map for the low and high pain groups (Figure 8).

## Associations amongst patient variables with delta and spindle power

The delta power at the start of emergence was negatively correlated with age ($r = -0.44$, $p<0.0001$), and positively correlated with the $C_eMAC$ ($r = 0.24$, $p = 0.015$). Combined in a multiple regression model, these two variables explained 21% of the variability in delta power. Addition of anesthetic agent, regional block and gender insignificantly increased this to 24%. Delta power was not correlated with $C_eOpioid$. The spindle power was also negatively correlated with age ($r = -0.34$, $p = 0.0003$) and with duration of operation ($r = -0.29$, $p = 0.002$). When combined with the $C_eMAC$, the model explained 23% of the variation in spindle power. However older patients were also more likely to have longer operations ($r = 0.25$, $p = 0.01$), and receive less volatile anesthetic drug ($r = -0.19$, $p = 0.05$).

## Associations amongst patient variables, emergence time, and post-operative pain

Emergence time was positively correlated with the duration of operation ($r = 0.24$, $p = 0.014$), and weakly influenced by the $C_eMAC$ ($r = 0.18$, $p = 0.07$). Consistent with prior studies [57–60], male patients were slower to emerge ($p = 0.02$) than females. In this study, we found that different volatile drugs had no significant influence on emergence time, but the number of patients receiving desflurane or isoflurane was small. The multivariate model of emergence time is given below (the presence of a regional block is coded as 1, the absence as 0; the difference between the genders was included as a categorical variable [1/0]).

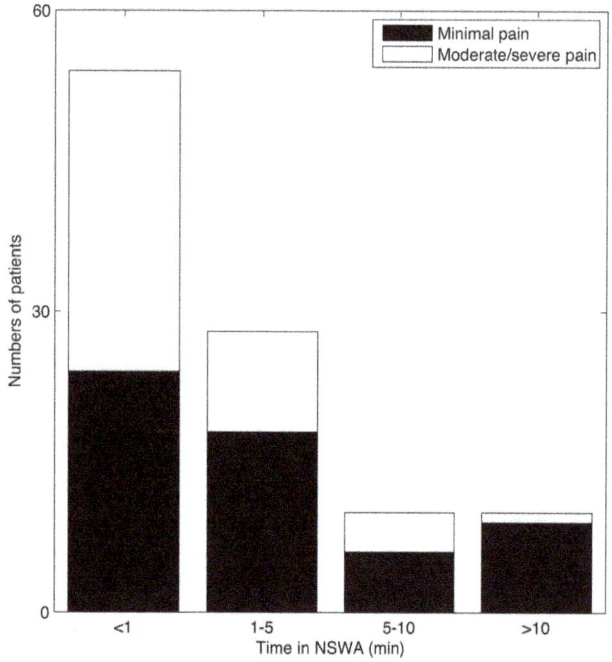


**Figure 7. Increased time spent in a non slow-wave state (NSWA) during emergence is correlated with a lower nociceptive state.** Patients had a variable duration of emergence from the time the anesthetic was turned off, ranging from 2 minutes to more than 10 minutes, as well as a variable dwell-time in the state of NSWA. When divided into 4 groups based on NSWA dwell-time, patients that spent more time in NSWA prior to emerging were more likely to have minimal pain (PACU-pain =0, Table 1). Of the group that spent>10 minutes in NSWA prior to wake-up, 90% had minimal pain. Of the group that spent less than a minute in NSWA prior to wake-up, 44% had minimal pain ($p = 0.037$, Chi-squared test).

$$Log[Emergence\ Time(min)] = 0.75 + 0.004 \times [Riegional\ Block] + 0.20 \times [C_eMAC] + 0.036 \times [Delta\ Power] + 0.05 \times [gender\ Male - Female] + 0.001 \times [Operation\ Duration(min)] \quad (1)$$

Although the model is statistically significant, these explanatory variables are not a very good explanation of the variation in emergence time, as the $r^2$ value was only 0.16.

When combined in the logistic regression model, the effect site concentration of opioid at the start of emergence, expressed in fentanyl equivalents ($C_e$Opioid), duration of NSWA, and male gender were the most significant associations with postoperative pain. A higher opioid concentration was associated with more pain. We attribute this unusual observation to the fact that patients who were expected to have more painful operations would have been given more (but presumably not enough) opioids intraoperatively. This model had a modest predictive capability (area under ROC =0.71), but again the strength of association was quite weak ($r^2 = 0.11$).

$$Probability[Severe\ pain/Mild\ pain] = -0.23 + 1.08 \times [C_e Opioid] - 0.004 \times [NSWA] - 0.61 \times [gender\ Male - Female] \quad (2)$$

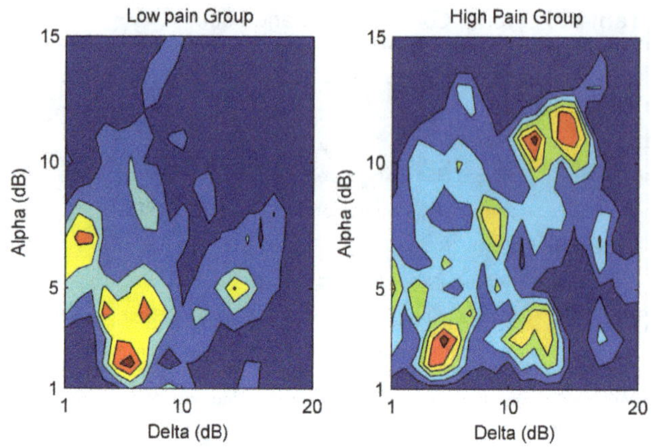


**Figure 8. Patients with low pain scores (0) spend more time in a non slow-wave (NSWA) pattern during emergence while patients with higher pain scores (2) spend more time in a slow-wave pattern (SWA).** This is reflected in the averaged trajectories through the spindle-delta state space for the low (left panel) and high pain (right panel) groups. The heat map from blue to red reflects least to most time.

## Associations amongst patient variables and different EEG patterns of emergence

The heterogeneity in patterns of emergence seem to be largely determined by unknown intrinsic factors, and are not strongly related to the common clinical explanatory variables. We found no significant associations between the EEG emergence pattern group and simple clinical and demographic variables – namely postoperative pain, type of volatile anaesthetic drug, gender, the presence of a regional block, operation duration, or the $C_e$MAC. However those patients that started in SWA, but then spent a period of time in the NSWA attractor before transitioning to wakefulness tended to be younger (mean(SEM) 43(4) years vs. 58(3) years, $p = 0.015$) and have a higher $C_e$Opioid (0.80(0.09) vs. 0.44(0.08) ng/ml fentanyl equivalents, $p = 0.04$), than those who jumped directly from a SWA state to wakefulness. Thus the relationship between $C_e$Opioid, postoperative pain, and EEG emergence pattern, is complex and remains to be fully elucidated in larger studies.

## EMG Activation During Emergence

The BIS EEG monitor attributes the power (dB) in the frequency range 70–110 Hz to the frontalis EMG signal, because it lies above the frequency band at which there is significant scalp EEG power. Typically the EMG power is low during general anaesthesia, and then rather abruptly increases in a stepwise fashion at various points during the emergence period. Often there are no overt clinical signs of an increase in muscle tone, or any gross motor movement. After examination of the EMG records, we chose the point at which the EMG power rose above 40 dB as a time point that reflected the activation of the EMG with reasonable face validity. The most striking feature was that the activation of the EMG often had quite a different time course to the EEG changes. The interval between EMG activation and End Emergence approximately followed an exponential probability distribution. For a quarter of the patients, their EMG became activated coincident with their waking (response to voice). Another one-half of patients woke within 74 seconds of EMG activation. However, a quarter of patients had a prolonged interval of at least 334 seconds between EMG activation and waking. The strongest

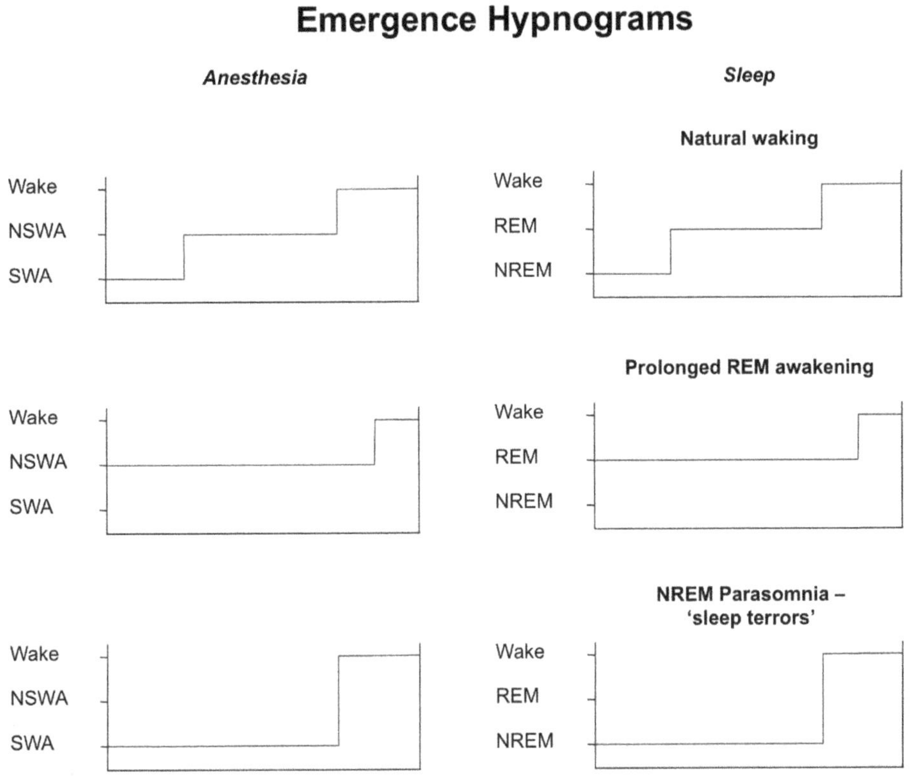


**Figure 9. Hypnograms for emergence from general anesthesia and sleep.** Temporal evolution of stages of arousal during emergence from general anesthesia (GA) are plotted in the left column, and from sleep in the right column. Each GA hypnogram on the left reflects an identified Emergence Trajectory as defined earlier in the text. These trajectories might be loosely correlated with arousal trajectories from various stages of sleep that are placed immediately to the right. SWA = Slow-Wave Anesthesia, NSWA = Non Slow-Wave Anesthesia; NREM = non-REM sleep, REM = REM sleep.

correlations were with duration of operation ($r = 0.23$, $p = 0.02$) and age ($r = 0.21$, $p = 0.03$).

## Discussion

### A Nomenclature for Distinguishing Between Anesthetic Maintenance States

In this study, we present a conceptual framework to discriminate four patterns of anesthetic maintenance comprised of two states, 'Slow-Wave Anesthesia' (SWA) and 'Non Slow-Wave Anesthesia' (NSWA), and two derivative sub-classes of the slow-wave state, 'delta-dominant' (ddSWA) and 'spindle-dominant' (sdSWA). These classes were defined by the relative contribution of delta (0.5–4 Hz) and spindle-alpha (8–14 Hz) power in their spectral signatures (Figure 2B). These sub-14 Hz oscillations that dominate the EEG during both NREM (slow-wave) sleep and general anesthesia have been shown to correspond to diminished responsiveness to mild stimuli in NREM sleep [41,61] and to more aversive stimuli during general anesthesia [9,62,63]. Because these oscillations can also be correlated with specific neural generators in a more generally hyperpolarized reticulothalamocortical circuit, they have been used for decades to classify stages of natural sleep. We were therefore able to capitalize on the methods by which sleep is staged and dynamically tracked over time (Figures 1, 9) to generate a new standardized taxonomy that could be used to describe the maintenace phase of general anesthesia. Although a pattern similar to the spindle-dominant slow-wave pattern (sdSWA) has been previously reported in studies in which volunteers are exposed to slowly changing levels of propofol anesthesia [8,64], the greater diversity of patterns we observed may be due to the lack of spectral averaging in our subjects, the greater diversity of the typical surgical population (e.g. baseline neurological status and co-morbidities, pre-operative medication status, baseline pain sensitivity), and the highly variable surgical environment (e.g. intraoperative medication administration, surgical stimulation, nociception).

### A Description of Emergence Trajectories

We examined the transition from unconsciousness back to conscious awareness (i.e. responsiveness) after general anesthesia was terminated at the conclusion of surgery, from End Maintenance/Start Emergence to End Emergence. We found a general shift from the slow-wave pattern (SWA) to a more uniform distribution of power across frequency bands (NSWA). This trend was immediately visible and highly significant when the grand average of EEG spectra across the entire patient population was performed at the beginning and end of emergence (Figure 2E, $p < 0.05$). However, just as with the maintenance patterns, individual patient emergence trajectories from unconsciousness to waking were more variable than averaged trajectories [8,9] (Figure 2F, Figures 3–6). We speculate that inactivation of endogenous sleep networks, activation of redundant arousal networks, and the nociceptive residuum experienced by the patient, contribute to this variability. In order to minimize non-surgical noxious stimuli, an LMA was used as the airway device, and auditory and tactile stimulation during emergence was limited (see Methods); we

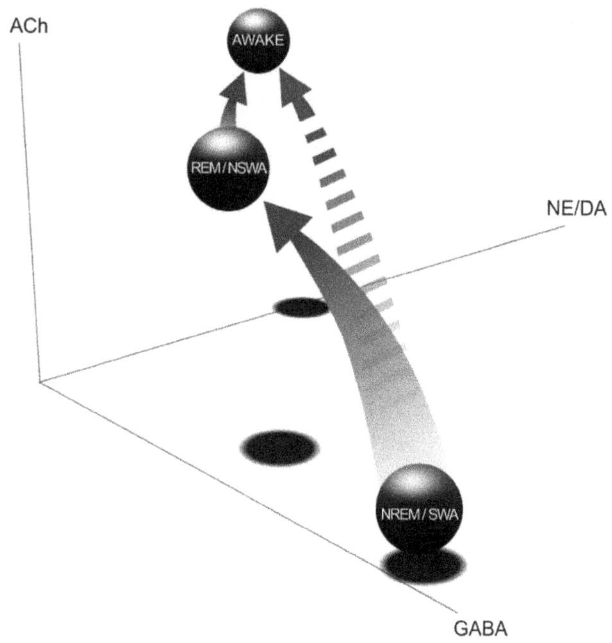


**Figure 10. A putative (shared) 3-D neurotransmitter state space for emergence from sleep and general anesthesia.** Based on spectral power and underlying neural generators, stages of anesthesia and stages of sleep may be analagous, especially on the path from thalamocortical hyperpolarization to waking. During natural NREM sleep, levels of GABA are high, while REM is characterized by high levels of both GABA and acetylcholine (ACh). As the brain passes from REM to waking, levels of GABA diminish, and monoamines such as norepinephrine and dopamine start to increase. The progression on the more typical anesthetic-emergence trajectory from SWA -> NSWA -> waking may reflect a similar shift in neurotransmitter balance as shown in this diagram (solid arrow). The "non-preferred" pathway of emergence that transitions directly from SWA -> waking (somewhat analagous to NREM -> waking) is represented by the broken arrow. NREM = non-REM sleep, REM = rapid eye movement sleep, SWA = Slow-Wave Anesthesia, NSWA = Non Slow-Wave Anesthesia, GABA = GABA-aminobutyric acid, ACh = acetylcholine, NE = norepinephrine, DA = dopamine.

therefore do not attribute this variability to tracheal or general environmental stimulation. More importantly, these diverse emergence patterns suggest that recovery from general anesthesia does not necessarily mirror the induction process, and may reflect a behavioral state barrier, which depends in part on the balance of activation in endogenous sleep and arousal pathways [31,65–67].

Using a dynamical systems approach, we grouped 100 observed emergence trajectories in state-space into categories based on the apparent number of attractors during emergence, the time each subject occupied that stable attractor state, and the time required to transition between attractor states (Figures 3–6). As with any empirical study, the exact dynamical system classification of the attractor topology is provisional. Although the attractors resembled simple point attractors, more detailed studies of the EEG dynamics might reveal some high dimensional chaotic or limit cycle structure within these attractors. With those provisos, almost half (43%) of patients exhibited a canonical sequence: loss of delta, followed by loss of spindles, and then a period of NSWA (characterized by the absence of low frequency oscillatory peaks in the EEG and behavioral unresponsiveness), before waking. In contrast, approximately one-third (31%) of subjects skip the NSWA stage and transition directly from SWA to wakefulness (Trajectory 4), and 16% do not achieve SWA at any stage during end maintenance or emergence (Trajectory 3). We also observed a sharp increase in electromyographic power (EMG) that often precedes the return of consciousness, but is not a necessary prerequisite.

## Connections between Emergence Trajectories and Post-operative Recovery

The time spent in NSWA prior to wake-up (defined on the dwell-time plots from Figures 3–6) was modestly predictive of subsequent pain (Figures 7–8). Patients who spent little of their emergence time in NSWA, were more likely to have high pain, and express a degree of agitation in recovery. (A similarly sudden transition from slow wave sleep directly to wakefulness is associated with some sleep pathologies such as night terrors [53,68], see also FIgure 9). These patients often had more frontal EMG activation during emergence, which in itself was weakly associated with a higher pain score in the PACU. Frontalis muscle activation (EMG) in patients can in itself confound the results. The EMG signature is broad-band and can potentially contaminate, distort or obscure the underlying EEG signal. Conversely EMG activation is a valuable indication of motor system activation as part of the emergence sequence from anesthesia, and we found it to be largely independent of the return of consciousness, as defined by recovery of responsiveness to voice. This observation is in accord with other work suggesting that components of motor systems are relatively resistant to the effects of anesthesia, and that recovery of motor tone is not captured by changing information in the EEG which tends to reflect the hypnotic axis [69]. Different central nervous subsystems may not always reconnect in a well-defined sequence after general anesthesia is discontinued; in some instances, alternate paths or sequences for bringing various brain arousal nuclei or networks on-line preceding the return of consciousness may predispose patients to undesirable wake-ups, in the same way that parasomnias are exacerbated by disrupted sleep architecture [54]. Our measurements also do not assess recovery along the axis of memory, another subsystem affected by anesthetics and sleep.

## The evolution of trajectories from Start to End Emergence can be captured in an emergence hypnogram for general anesthesia

Figure 9 graphically depicts the evolution of each of the emergence trajectory patterns (Figures 3–6) and compares these patterns to arousal from specific stages of sleep. Carrying the analogy between waking from natural sleep and emergence from general anesthesia further, we propose using a hypnogram to capture the emergence trajectories from general anesthesia (left column) seen in Figures 3–6, where the length of the horizontal line at each stages reflects the relative dwell-time in the state-space plot (panel C of Figures 3–6). These can be compared to the sequences of emergence from natural sleep, seen in the right column, in the more classic version of the emergence hypnogram. A transition from SWA to NSWA before waking may correspond most closely to the waking from natural sleep. Waking from very prolonged NSWA may not have a correlate in normal sleep (prolonged REM awakening), but may instead reflect certain hypersomnia subtypes [70]. The emergence trajectory of an abrupt transition from SWA to wakefulness can be compared to arousal during NREM sleep, often associated with parasomnias or sleep disturbances resulting from fragmented sleep [53,54].

**Table 2.** Demographic Data.

| | |
|---|---|
| **Age (yrs)** | 48(19) |
| **Gender (F/M)** | 48/52 |
| **Duration of surgery (min)** | 99(68) |
| **Duration of emergence (min)** | 12.4 [8.4 to 18.9] |
| **Sevo/Des/Isoflurane** | 81/8/11 |
| **$C_eMAC_s$** | 10.79 [0.66 to 0.98] |
| **$C_eMAC_e$** | 0.06 [0.001 to 0.08] |
| **$C_efentanyl_e$ (ng/ml)** | 0.54 [0.31 to 0.78] |
| **PACU-Cons (0/1/2)** | 17/42/41 |
| **PACU-Pain (0/1/2)** | 56/15/29 |

$C_e$ denotes effect site concentration of the drug, and the subscripts 's' and 'e' denote the start and end of emergence. MAC indicates units of age adjusted Minimum Alveolar Concentration, PACU-Cons and PACU-Pain are defined in the text and in Table 1.

## The Neurochemical Relationship Between Sleep Circuitry And General Anesthesia

The degree of thalamocortical hyperpolarization depends on the balance of activity in neurotransmitters systems [71,72]. While there are many regional and nuclear brain differences, NREM sleep tends to be dominated by high GABAergic and low cholinergic and monoaminergic tone, while REM sleep is dominated by both GABAergic and cholinergic tone, and low levels of monoamines [73,74]. We postulate that the presence of spindles and delta oscillations within the stage we define as SWA also reflects overwhelming GABAergic tone and low cholinergic tone, consistent with the mechanism of action of many of our volatile and intravenous anesthetics. The exact sequence of neuromodulator activation during emergence from anaesthesia is unknown, and is probably the main cause for the heterogeneity that we observed in the emergence trajectories. As anesthetic washes out of the brain, the residual GABAergic effects of the drug may be antagonized by depolarizing cholinergic (or aminergic) systems, pushing the brain into the NSWA state. The reason for transition from this point to waking is unclear, but probably involves a switch from high GABAergic tone to high monoaminergic and orexinergic tone, allowing the patient to fully emerge and reconnect with the external world. These pathways may be visualized in a 3-D neurotransmitter diagram for NREM/SWA, REM/NSWA, and waking states (Figure 10). The solid arrow signals a "preferred" wake-up sequence in which a patient moves from SWA to NSWA prior to waking, and experiences a higher degree of conscious awareness and a lower degree of pain and agitation in recovery (i.e. the classic cycle of NREM to REM to waking). The "non-preferred" sequence – in which the brain transitions directly from SWA to waking state – is reflected by the broken arrow, which if compared to sleep, would characterize a parasomnic or less desirable trajectory to re-establishing conscious awareness.

## Underlying Neurobiology of EEG Signatures of Emergence and their Relationship to Sleep

Both sleep and general anesthesia share many similarities, including specific nuclei, circuitry, and neurotransmitter systems. Physiological recordings [75–76] and modeling [64,77] suggest that the oscillatory components of the alpha band (spindles between 8–14 Hz) in the frontal EEG during sleep and anesthesia are generated by hyperpolarizing neurons of the reticular nucleus of the thalamus, in the permissive environment of depressed ascending cholinergic and monoaminergic brainstem activity [75], which switches them to a burst firing mode [78–80]. Spindles predominate in NREM stage 2 sleep, and are more commonly observed during general anesthesia when analgesics are administered to diminish noxious stimulation [63]. NREM stage 3 sleep reflects an even greater degree of thalamocortical hyperpolarization as spindle activity diminishes and slower delta oscillations (0.5–1 Hz) begin to dominate [40]. Because our data demonstrate a positive correlation between anesthetic dose and relative delta power [81] we suggest that NREM stage 3 sleep may be similar to a ddSWA pattern under anesthesia, and NREM stage 2 sleep to an sdSWA pattern. This notion is further supported by the observation that at the midpoint of emergence (with decreasing anesthetic dose) there is an increase in the number of subjects categorized as sdSWA.

A progressive depolarization within the corticothalamic system accompanies the ordered transition to waking from natural sleep. This state is termed REM and is typically the stage of sleep from which most individuals awaken. Similarly, most subjects emerging from general anesthesia appear to move progressively from SWA to NSWA. Can NSWA be likened to REM sleep? Approximately 25% of patients report dream mentation if queried immediately upon waking, and it was more common for the group who reported dreaming to be in NSWA (i.e. have low power in the $<$ 14 Hz range) prior to waking [55]. Thus, SWA and NSWA may directly correspond to different levels of activation in the two distinct networks of conscious awareness (i.e. awareness of environment and awareness of self) described by others [82]. NSWA may reflect an unresponsive state in which some form of internally-directed consciousness has been established (e.g. fronto-parietal connectivity), but there is still insufficient brain function to connect externally. This is consistent with the concept of an unconnected (i.e. with the external world) or covert consciousness, which has been seen using carefully controlled propofol infusions in human volunteers with combined fMRI/EEG [9]. The thalamocortical network is rendered insensate to external inputs, yet activation to stimuli is still observed in cortical areas such as the precuneus. The role of the thalamus is less clear. It plays an important role in sleep, but its contribution to anesthesia has been questioned [83], and thalamic deactivation may not be the cause of unconsciousness but rather a consequence, via a functional thalamic de-afferentation from diminished cortical connectedness [84,85].

One significant limitation to this study is that we only used a frontal EEG electrode strip for our recordings. Our data is therefore constrained to data gathered from accessible frontal leads (corresponding approximatley to FPz, FP1/2 from a traditional 10–20 montage) without simultaneous recording from parietal, temporal or occipital regions. We therefore could not consider other markers of loss and return of consciousness such as global coherence [8,16] or the degree of connectedness and communication between different cortical regions [11,13–15,86]. However, EEG power is largely anteriorized upon loss of consciousness under general anesthesia [11,16,17,87], making the frontal leads reasonable markers for spectral changes that can be observed at the single electrode level. Use of commercially available EEG electrodes that can be easily placed on a patient's forehead intraoperatively as part of the placement of routine monitors also increases the likelihood that our methods for tracking and staging depth of consciousness could be used more routinely by clinicians making real-time decisions in the operating room. Our data indicate that a long period of NSWA before waking is associated with less pain than a direct transition from SWA to waking. Without further prospective randomized clinical studies, it is unclear whether it would actually be clinically useful to specifically titrate anesthetic (or analgesic) drugs to target any particular intraoperative spectral pattern. Apart from the effect of age on spectral power, we found relatively weak correlations between clinical variables and spectral pattern. This would suggest that the spectral pattern for each patient is largely determined by other unknown (possibly inherited) factors. Nevertheless we would hope that this study provides a methodological framework in which these questions could be answered.

## Conclusions

The unconsciousness that accompanies general anesthesia during surgery is marked by several, distinct, oscillatory patterns in the EEG. Because these share features with those observed in natural sleep, it is possible that the underlying neural generators are conserved. Building upon a classification system used to stage sleep, we provide, for the first time, a standardized EEG-based nomenclature by which anesthetic maintenance can be staged and followed intraoperatively. We also applied a dynamical systems approach to characterize the return to consciousness after discontinuation of the anesthetic. We found that recovery of consciousness varies amongst individuals, and that deviations from a canonical sequence of SWA to NSWA occur. Further, the functional path by which the brain re-establishes conscious awareness is correlated with preferred wake-ups (e.g. diminished pain). We have created a descriptive means by which endogenous sleep rhythms and general anesthesia can be compared. Subsequent usage of this nomenclature should further our understanding of the overlapping neural mechanisms of sleep and anesthesia. As the homeostatic, learning and memory benefits of sleep are beginning to be characterized [88], future work may identify targets to improve post-operative cognitive health. The latter is of increasing concern as patients, researchers, and physicians become more apprehensive about the potential for anesthesia to cause or exacerbate adverse neurocognitive sequelae.

## Methods

### Ethics Statement

Studies were approved by the Northern Y Regional Ethics Committee of New Zealand (NTY/11/EXP/077), and written informed consent obtained from each patient. Free and public access to the de-identified data is available from the website: www.accesshq.org.

### Patient Selection

We studied 100 adult patients presenting for routine orthopedic surgery under general anesthesia at Waikato Hospital, New Zealand, from November 2011 to January 2013. Data collection was restricted to patients eligible for laryngeal mask airway (LMA) management, considered less stimulating than an endotracheal tube [89], in order to minimize confounding effects of airway irritation, a strong non-surgical arousal stimulus, on the EEG. We specifically included patients who would be expected to have a wide range of post-surgical pain levels (some augmented with regional nerve blocks). We excluded patients with pre-existing psychiatric illness, chronic substance abuse, chronic pain, or obesity (BMI>35). Patient demographics are represented in Table 2.

### Surgical Procedure and Data Collection

In order to determine the spread of emergence patterns at the conclusion of routine clinical anesthesia, we did not restrict the course of administration of the general anesthetic with the exception of limiting the airway device to an LMA, allowing it proceed according to the clinician's judgment. Patients were induced with a bolus dose of intravenous fentanyl (50–200 μg) followed by propofol (80–200 mg). Patients were maintained on a volatile general anesthetic (VA) of the clinician's choice - sevoflurane, desflurane, or isoflurane - delivered in a mixture of air and oxygen. No neuromuscular blocking drugs were used. Intraoperative analgesia was provided by intravenous morphine (0–25 mg); analgesic adjuncts of paracetamol (1 gm, n = 34), parecoxib (40 mg, n = 39), tramadol (100–200 mg, n = 22) or clonidine (60–120 μg, n = 18) were given as needed. 21 patients received a peripheral nerve block for post-operative analgesia; 14 of these were femoral blocks, done for reduction of postoperative muscle spasm for lower limb joint replacements. Because of the mutineuronal innervation of the knee and hip, most of these nerve blocks achieved incomplete analgesia. Of the others (mainly ankle blocks and brachial plexus blocks), 5 patients had pain scores of 0 on awakening – indicative of a completely successful block.

We used standard American Society of Anesthesiology [90] monitors (pulse oximeter, non-invasive blood pressure cuff, electrocardiogram, capnograph) to measure intraoperative oxygen saturation, hemodynamics, and end-tidal gas concentrations ($O_2$, $CO_2$, VA). In addition to these routine parameters, the times of surgery, tourniquet inflation and release, and drug administration were recorded.

A 2-lead EEG prefrontal electrode strip was placed on the patient's forehead, as per the manufacturer's recommendations (BIS, Covidien Vista). Frontal EEG data (sampling rate 128 Hz) was collected for the duration of the anesthetic, prior to induction through the end of emergence. The frontal EEG waveforms on the BIS sensor strip correlate approximately to the FPz and FP1/2 leads of standard 20 electrode EEG montage. Both electrodes are referenced by an additional electrode over the eyebrow. A separate lead over the temporalis muscle is used as an EMG electrode. Suitable electrode impedance (<5 kOhm) was confirmed using the manufacturer's automatic checking routine. To provide a mechanism to correlate external events with the patient's EEG, the times of surgical incision, cessation of the volatile anesthetic agent, and the exact moment of awakening were marked on the EEG record by tapping the electrodes 4 times in ~1.5 seconds to create a clear stimulus artifact. The patients were allowed to waken without excessive stimulation beyond the usual noise and activity of the operating room and post anesthesia care unit (PACU) environment (e.g. removal and replacement of monitors, background talking). Sustained awakening was confirmed by a positive response to verbal command ("Mrs. X, your operation is over, open your eyes."). 'Emergence' from general anesthesia was specifically defined as the time between the cessation of administration of the maintenance hypnotic drug (VA) and the point at which the patient became responsive to verbal command. Raw EEG and EMG data for each patient were downloaded post-operatively for further analysis.

### Drug Effects

The decreasing effect-site concentrations ($C_e$) of the different volatile anesthetic drugs were estimated as a fraction of age adjusted MAC [91] at Start and End Emergence, and the estimated effect-site concentrations of the intraoperative opioids (fentanyl and morphine) were calculated using standard compartmental pharmacokinetic modeling [92,93]. In order to compare opioid effects across patients, and to take into account the fact that many patients had received both morphine and fentanyl intraoperatively, we expressed the morphine concentrations as fentanyl concentration equivalents ($C_e$ *fentanyl*), assuming a conversion factor of 50. This data is also summarized in Table 2.

## Evaluation of post-emergence level of consciousness and pain

It is common for patients to experience fluctuations in both level of consciousness and pain in the early postoperative period. These changes are hard to capture and analyze [94]. Accordingly we used simple, heuristically derived, descriptions of level of consciousness (PACU-Cons) and pain (PACU-Pain) as described in Table 1. We believe that these classifications have the advantage of capturing the clinically relevant, qualitative aspects of the recovery period. The PACU-Cons score is based on the change in the Ramsay Score over the first 15 minutes in the PACU [95]. The severity of the pain was quantified using a composite of the standard integer numerical verbal rating scale (NRS) – where 0 is no pain and 10 the worst imaginable pain. Because of the questionable validity of the fine gradations in these semi-quantitative scores, the PACU-Pain score bins the numerical rating scale into 'minimal', 'moderate' and 'severe' pain groups [96], which appear to have reasonable clinical validity. However, we also scored the degree of objective distress that the patient manifested, and used this added information to modify these scores as described in Table 1. The first pain score was obtained when the patient had achieved a level of consciousness at which they could maintain a brief conversation. These pain queries were then repeated every 15 minutes. If they were in pain, patients were treated with increments of 1–2 mg IV morphine, 25–50 μg of fentanyl, or 50–100 mg IV tramadol in the PACU, and then discharged to the ward according to institutional criteria based on the Aldrete score [97].

## Spectral Processing, Statistical and Analytical Methods

All data was analyzed using custom scripts written in MATLAB (Mathworks, Natick, Massachusetts). The amplitude and frequency structure of the EEG signal was initially described by the mean power in the traditional frequency bands: delta (0.5–4 Hz), theta (5–7 Hz), alpha (8–14 Hz), and beta (15–25 Hz). The power in each band was then logarithmically transformed so that all spectral power was expressed in units of dB (10× logarithm base 10, referenced to 1 $\mu V^2/Hz$). These band-powers were then smoothed using a 30 second median smoothing filter. In addition we recorded the EMG output (dB) from the Vista monitor. We then extracted EEG features (the delta and alpha bands) that reflected the largest changes in spectral power seen in the prefrontal channels during emergence. Spindle power was specifically derived by measuring the height of the alpha peak above the underlying broadband activity to target the narrowband oscillatory component of this peak [55].

To follow these changes dynamically, we displayed the EEG using typical spectrograms and time series plots of salient features (spindle, delta and EMG power). Spectrograms of the EEG data were made using the 'mtspecgramc.m' function and PSDs using the 'mtspectrumsegc.m' function of the Chronux toolbox (http://chronux.org) [98] on 8 second segments, with 6 second (75%) overlap and tapers of 13 and 8. This segment length was chosen to balance the time required to reliably estimate power in the delta band, while still being short enough to allow for changes in the detection of waveforms within a clinically relevant time frame. 95% confidence intervals for the median PSD for each condition (Start and End Emergence) were calculated using a jackknife estimation method. To create 3-D individualized dwell-time plots for each patient's emergence trajectory (Figures 3–6, panel C), spindle and delta power were plotted against one another in x-y plane, while depth on the z-axis reflected the total amount of time a patient remained in each x-y pixel of the spindle-delta state space as a fraction of total emergence time. This allowed us to capture the changing relationship between oscillations over time, and permitted comparisons across different patients with differing lengths of emergence.

Correlations between pairs of variables were quantified using Pearson's correlation co-efficient (r) if they followed a normal distribution (Kolmogorov-Smirnoff test), otherwise Spearman's rank correlation was used. The multivariate analysis of the interrelationships between all the variables in an observational study is subject to unknown confounding factors. Following conservative statistical practice, we limited the total number of explanatory variables for each model to 5, in order to have 20 data points to estimate the parameter for each variable with reasonable precision. We used multiple linear regression models, with stepwise forward selection, to discover which group of variables were most significantly associated with the continuous outcome variables: namely delta and alpha power at Start Emergence, and emergence time (which was logarithmically transformed to achieve a normal probability distribution). We used similar techniques, but using logistic regression, for binary outcome variables (pain group).

A patient's post-operative nociceptive status was loosely correlated with the emergence trajectory. In order to display those average trajectories, we combined the phase-space data (spindle vs. delta power) for all patients in the low (PACU-Pain = 0) and high (PACU- Pain = 2) groups (Figure 8). More stereotypical patterns were reflected in data points remaining tightly constrained in the 2-D phase space. More variable EEG emergence trajectories were reflected in points spread out over a large area of the 2-D phase space. Cumulative time spent in each area of the phase space was reflected in a color heat map from blue (little time) to red (large amount of time).

## Supporting Information

**Figure S1 This 3-D histogram of spindle and delta power at Start Emergence, calculated on a single 8 second epoch for each patient (z-axis), reveals this data follows a unimodal distribution.** Following statistical convention, patients were separated into two main spectral classes by thresholding spindle and delta power at 7 dB. This theshold reflects the boundary below which only 5% of the Start Emergence data lay, and the region within which most of the End Emergence data lay. Patients who began emergence (i.e. at the termination of general anesthetic delivery) above the 7 dB threshold (above the gray box) were termed to be in Slow-Wave Anesthesia (SWA). Those within the gray box, or below 7 dB, were termed to be in Non Slow-Wave Anesthesia (NSWA).

## Author Contributions

Conceived and designed the experiments: DC PSG JWS. Performed the experiments: JWS JNM SI. Analyzed the data: JWS DC PSG. Contributed reagents/materials/analysis tools: JWS DC. Wrote the paper: DC PSG JWS.

## References


1. Courtin RF, Bickford RG, Faulconer A Jr. (1950) The classification and significance of electro-encephalographic patterns produced by nitrous oxide-ether anesthesia during surgical operations. Proc Staff Meet Mayo Clin 25: 197–206.
2. Kiersey DK, Bickford RG, Faulconer A Jr. (1951) Electro-encephalographic patterns produced by thiopental sodium during surgical operations; description and classification. Br J Anaesth 23: 141–152.
3. Clark DL, Rosner BS (1973) Neurophysiologic effects of general anesthetics. I. The electroencephalogram and sensory evoked responses in man. Anesthesiology 38: 564–582.
4. Dement W, Kleitman N (1957) Cyclic variations in EEG during sleep and their relation to eye movements, body motility, and dreaming. Electroencephalogr Clin Neurophysiol 9: 673–690.
5. Rechtschaffen A, Kales A (1968) A manual of standardized terminology, techniques, and scoring system for sleep stages of human subjects. University of California, Los Angeles: Brain Information Service/Brain Research Institute.
6. Hudson RJ, Stanski DR, Saidman LJ, Meathe E (1983) A model for studying depth of anesthesia and acute tolerance to thiopental. Anesthesiology 59: 301–308.
7. Long CW, Shah NK, Loughlin C, Spydell J, Bedford RF (1989) A comparison of EEG determinants of near-awakening from isoflurane and fentanyl anesthesia. Spectral edge, median power frequency, and delta ratio. Anesth Analg 69: 169–173.
8. Purdon PL, Pierce ET, Mukamel EA, Prerau MJ, Walsh JL, et al. (2013) Electroencephalogram signatures of loss and recovery of consciousness from propofol. Proc Natl Acad Sci U S A 110: E1142–1151.
9. Ni Mhuircheartaigh R, Warnaby C, Rogers R, Jbabdi S, Tracey I (2013) Slow-wave activity saturation and thalamocortical isolation during propofol anesthesia in humans. Sci Transl Med 5: 208ra148.
10. Gugino LD, Chabot RJ, Prichep LS, John ER, Formanek V, et al. (2001) Quantitative EEG changes associated with loss and return of consciousness in healthy adult volunteers anaesthetized with propofol or sevoflurane. Br J Anaesth 87: 421–428.
11. John ER, Prichep LS, Kox W, Valdes-Sosa P, Bosch-Bayard J, et al. (2001) Invariant reversible QEEG effects of anesthetics. Conscious Cogn 10: 165–183.
12. Breshears JD, Roland JL, Sharma M, Gaona CM, Freudenburg ZV, et al. (2010) Stable and dynamic cortical electrophysiology of induction and emergence with propofol anesthesia. Proc Natl Acad Sci U S A 107: 21170–21175.
13. Lee U, Ku S, Noh G, Baek S, Choi B, et al. (2013) Disruption of frontal-parietal communication by ketamine, propofol, and sevoflurane. Anesthesiology 118: 1264–1275.
14. Ku SW, Lee U, Noh GJ, Jun IG, Mashour GA (2011) Preferential inhibition of frontal-to-parietal feedback connectivity is a neurophysiologic correlate of general anesthesia in surgical patients. PLoS One 6: e25155.
15. Boly M, Moran R, Murphy M, Boveroux P, Bruno MA, et al. (2012) Connectivity changes underlying spectral EEG changes during propofol-induced loss of consciousness. J Neurosci 32: 7082–7090.
16. Cimenser A, Purdon PL, Pierce ET, Walsh JL, Salazar-Gomez AF, et al. (2011) Tracking brain states under general anesthesia by using global coherence analysis. Proc Natl Acad Sci U S A 108: 8832–8837.
17. Vijayan S, Ching S, Purdon PL, Brown EN, Kopell NJ (2013) Thalamocortical mechanisms for the anteriorization of alpha rhythms during propofol-induced unconsciousness. J Neurosci 33: 11070–11075.
18. Steriade M, Timofeev I (2003) Neuronal plasticity in thalamocortical networks during sleep and waking oscillations. Neuron 37: 563–576.
19. Steriade M (2004) Acetylcholine systems and rhythmic activities during the waking—sleep cycle. Prog Brain Res 145: 179–196.
20. Zecharia AY, Nelson LE, Gent TC, Schumacher M, Jurd R, et al. (2009) The involvement of hypothalamic sleep pathways in general anesthesia: testing the hypothesis using the GABAA receptor beta3N265M knock-in mouse. J Neurosci 29: 2177–2187.
21. Nelson LE, Guo TZ, Lu J, Saper CB, Franks NP, et al. (2002) The sedative component of anesthesia is mediated by GABA(A) receptors in an endogenous sleep pathway. Nat Neurosci 5: 979–984.
22. Franks NP (2008) General anaesthesia: from molecular targets to neuronal pathways of sleep and arousal. Nat Rev Neurosci 9: 370–386.
23. Bonin RP, Orser BA (2008) GABA(A) receptor subtypes underlying general anesthesia. Pharmacol Biochem Behav 90: 105–112.
24. Garcia PS, Kolesky SE, Jenkins A (2010) General anesthetic actions on GABA(A) receptors. Curr Neuropharmacol 8: 2–9.
25. Huntsman MM, Porcello DM, Homanics GE, DeLorey TM, Huguenard JR (1999) Reciprocal inhibitory connections and network synchrony in the mammalian thalamus. Science 283: 541–543.
26. Rye DB, Bliwise DL, Parker K, Trotti LM, Saini P, et al. (2012) Modulation of Vigilance in the Primary Hypersomnias by Endogenous Enhancement of GABAA Receptors. Sci Transl Med 4: 161ra151.
27. Tung A, Szafran MJ, Bluhm B, Mendelson WB (2002) Sleep deprivation potentiates the onset and duration of loss of righting reflex induced by propofol and isoflurane. Anesthesiology 97: 906–911.
28. Tung A, Herrera S, Szafran MJ, Kasza K, Mendelson WB (2005) Effect of sleep deprivation on righting reflex in the rat is partially reversed by administration of adenosine A1 and A2 receptor antagonists. Anesthesiology 102: 1158–1164.
29. Berridge CW, Bolen SJ, Manley MS, Foote SL (1996) Modulation of forebrain electroencephalographic activity in halothane-anesthetized rat via actions of noradrenergic beta-receptors within the medial septal region. J Neurosci 16: 7010–7020.
30. Alkire MT, McReynolds JR, Hahn EL, Trivedi AN (2007) Thalamic microinjection of nicotine reverses sevoflurane-induced loss of righting reflex in the rat. Anesthesiology 107: 264–272.
31. Kelz MB, Sun Y, Chen J, Cheng Meng Q, Moore JT, et al. (2008) An essential role for orexins in emergence from general anesthesia. Proc Natl Acad Sci U S A 105: 1309–1314.
32. Solt K, Cotten JF, Cimenser A, Wong KF, Chemali JJ, et al. (2011) Methylphenidate actively induces emergence from general anesthesia. Anesthesiology 115: 791–803.
33. Chemali JJ, Van Dort CJ, Brown EN, Solt K (2012) Active emergence from propofol general anesthesia is induced by methylphenidate. Anesthesiology 116: 998–1005.
34. Taylor NE, Chemali JJ, Brown EN, Solt K (2013) Activation of D1 dopamine receptors induces emergence from isoflurane general anesthesia. Anesthesiology 118: 30–39.
35. Vazey EM, Aston-Jones G (2014) Designer receptor manipulations reveal a role of the locus coeruleus noradrenergic system in isoflurane general anesthesia. Proc Natl Acad Sci U S A 111: 3859–3864.
36. Solt K, Van Dort CJ, Chemali JJ, Taylor NE, Kenny JD, et al. (2014) Electrical Stimulation of the Ventral Tegmental Area Induces Reanimation from General Anesthesia. Anesthesiology.
37. Sleigh JW, Andrzejowski J, Steyn-Ross A, Steyn-Ross M (1999) The bispectral index: a measure of depth of sleep? Anesth Analg 88: 659–661.
38. Tung A, Lynch JP, Roizen MF (2002) Use of the BIS monitor to detect onset of naturally occurring sleep. J Clin Monit Comput 17: 37–42.
39. Walters AS, Lavigne G, Hening W, Picchietti DL, Allen RP, et al. (2007) The scoring of movements in sleep. J Clin Sleep Med 3: 155–167.
40. Silber MH, Ancoli-Israel S, Bonnet MH, Chokroverty S, Grigg-Damberger MM, et al. (2007) The visual scoring of sleep in adults. J Clin Sleep Med 3: 121–131.
41. Dang-Vu TT, Bonjean M, Schabus M, Boly M, Darsaud A, et al. (2011) Interplay between spontaneous and induced brain activity during human non-rapid eye movement sleep. Proc Natl Acad Sci U S A 108: 15438–15443.
42. Steriade M, Deschenes M, Domich L, Mulle C (1985) Abolition of spindle oscillations in thalamic neurons disconnected from nucleus reticularis thalami. J Neurophysiol 54: 1473–1497.
43. Steriade M, McCormick DA, Sejnowski TJ (1993) Thalamocortical oscillations in the sleeping and aroused brain. Science 262: 679–685.
44. McCormick DA, Pape HC (1990) Properties of a hyperpolarization-activated cation current and its role in rhythmic oscillation in thalamic relay neurones. J Physiol 431: 291–318.
45. Dossi RC, Nunez A, Steriade M (1992) Electrophysiology of a slow (0.5–4 Hz) intrinsic oscillation of cat thalamocortical neurones in vivo. J Physiol 447: 215–234.
46. Jones BE (1991) Paradoxical sleep and its chemical/structural substrates in the brain. Neuroscience 40: 637–656.
47. Moser D, Anderer P, Gruber G, Parapatics S, Loretz E, et al. (2009) Sleep classification according to AASM and Rechtschaffen & Kales: effects on sleep scoring parameters. Sleep 32: 139–149.
48. Dang-Vu TT, Schabus M, Desseilles M, Sterpenich V, Bonjean M, et al. (2010) Functional neuroimaging insights into the physiology of human sleep. Sleep 33: 1589–1603.
49. Gais S, Molle M, Helms K, Born J (2002) Learning-dependent increases in sleep spindle density. J Neurosci 22: 6830–6834.
50. Rasch B, Buchel C, Gais S, Born J (2007) Odor cues during slow-wave sleep prompt declarative memory consolidation. Science 315: 1426–1429.
51. Molle M, Eschenko O, Gais S, Sara SJ, Born J (2009) The influence of learning on sleep slow oscillations and associated spindles and ripples in humans and rats. Eur J Neurosci 29: 1071–1081.
52. Morgenthaler TI, Kapur VK, Brown T, Swick TJ, Alessi C, et al. (2007) Practice parameters for the treatment of narcolepsy and other hypersomnias of central origin. Sleep 30: 1705–1711.
53. Howell MJ (2012) Parasomnias: an updated review. Neurotherapeutics 9: 753–775.
54. Espa F, Ondze B, Deglise P, Billiard M, Besset A (2000) Sleep architecture, slow wave activity, and sleep spindles in adult patients with sleepwalking and sleep terrors. Clin Neurophysiol 111: 929–939.
55. Leslie K, Sleigh J, Paech MJ, Voss L, Lim CW, et al. (2009) Dreaming and electroencephalographic changes during anesthesia maintained with propofol or desflurane. Anesthesiology 111: 547–555.
56. Hilborn RC (2000) Chaos and nonlinear dynamics: an introduction for scientists and engineers. Oxford; New York: Oxford University Press.

57. Gan TJ, Glass PS, Sigl J, Sebel P, Payne F, et al. (1999) Women emerge from general anesthesia with propofol/alfentanil/nitrous oxide faster than men. Anesthesiology 90: 1283–1287.
58. Myles PS, McLeod AD, Hunt JO, Fletcher H (2001) Sex differences in speed of emergence and quality of recovery after anaesthesia: cohort study. BMJ 322: 710–711.
59. Hoymork SC, Raeder J (2005) Why do women wake up faster than men from propofol anaesthesia? Br J Anaesth 95: 627–633.
60. Bajaj P, Raiger LK, Jain SD, Kumar S (2007) Women emerge from general anesthesia faster than men. Middle East J Anesthesiol 19: 173–183.
61. Steriade M, Contreras D, Curro Dossi R, Nunez A (1993) The slow (<1 Hz) oscillation in reticular thalamic and thalamocortical neurons: scenario of sleep rhythm generation in interacting thalamic and neocortical networks. J Neurosci 13: 3284–3299.
62. Rampil IJ, Matteo RS (1987) Changes in EEG spectral edge frequency correlate with the hemodynamic response to laryngoscopy and intubation. Anesthesiology 67: 139–142.
63. MacKay EC, Sleigh JW, Voss LJ, Barnard JP (2010) Episodic waveforms in the electroencephalogram during general anaesthesia: a study of patterns of response to noxious stimuli. Anaesth Intensive Care 38: 102–112.
64. Ching S, Cimenser A, Purdon PL, Brown EN, Kopell NJ (2010) Thalamocortical model for a propofol-induced alpha-rhythm associated with loss of consciousness. Proc Natl Acad Sci U S A 107: 22665–22670.
65. Steyn-Ross ML, Steyn-Ross DA, Sleigh JW (2004) Modelling general anaesthesia as a first-order phase transition in the cortex. Prog Biophys Mol Biol 85: 369–385.
66. Friedman EB, Sun Y, Moore JT, Hung HT, Meng QC, et al. (2010) A conserved behavioral state barrier impedes transitions between anesthetic-induced unconsciousness and wakefulness: evidence for neural inertia. PLoS One 5: e11903.
67. Joiner WJ, Friedman EB, Hung HT, Koh K, Sowcik M, et al. (2013) Genetic and anatomical basis of the barrier separating wakefulness and anesthetic-induced unresponsiveness. PLoS Genet 9: e1003605.
68. Besset A, Espa F (2001) [Disorders of arousal]. Rev Neurol (Paris) 157: S107–111.
69. Illman H, Antila H, Olkkola KT (2010) Reversal of neuromuscular blockade by sugammadex does not affect EEG derived indices of depth of anesthesia. J Clin Monit Comput 24: 371–376.
70. (2005) International Classification of Sleep Disorders: Diagnostic and Coding Manual (ICSD-2). 2 ed. Westchester NY: American Academy of Sleep Medicine.
71. Basheer R, Sherin JE, Saper CB, Morgan JI, McCarley RW, et al. (1997) Effects of sleep on wake-induced c-fos expression. J Neurosci 17: 9746–9750.
72. Saper CB, Scammell TE, Lu J (2005) Hypothalamic regulation of sleep and circadian rhythms. Nature 437: 1257–1263.
73. Lydic R, Baghdoyan HA (2005) Sleep, anesthesiology, and the neurobiology of arousal state control. Anesthesiology 103: 1268–1295.
74. Van Dort CJ, Baghdoyan HA, Lydic R (2008) Neurochemical modulators of sleep and anesthetic states. Int Anesthesiol Clin 46: 75–104.
75. Keifer JC, Baghdoyan HA, Lydic R (1996) Pontine cholinergic mechanisms modulate the cortical electroencephalographic spindles of halothane anesthesia. Anesthesiology 84: 945–954.
76. Fuentealba P, Timofeev I, Steriade M (2004) Prolonged hyperpolarizing potentials precede spindle oscillations in the thalamic reticular nucleus. Proc Natl Acad Sci U S A 101: 9816–9821.
77. Gottschalk A, Haney P (2003) Computational aspects of anesthetic action in simple neural models. Anesthesiology 98: 548–564.
78. Contreras D, Curro Dossi R, Steriade M (1993) Electrophysiological properties of cat reticular thalamic neurones in vivo. J Physiol 470: 273–294.
79. Ferenets R, Lipping T, Suominen P, Turunen J, Puumala P, et al. (2006) Comparison of the properties of EEG spindles in sleep and propofol anesthesia. Conf Proc IEEE Eng Med Biol Soc 1: 6356–6359.
80. Kroeger D, Amzica F (2007) Hypersensitivity of the anesthesia-induced comatose brain. J Neurosci 27: 10597–10607.
81. Mulholland CV, Somogyi AA, Barratt DT, Coller JK, Hutchinson MK, et al. Association of innate immune single nucleotide polymorphisms with the electroencephalogram during desflurane general anaesthesia. Journal of Molecular Neuroscience: In press.
82. Vanhaudenhuyse A, Demertzi A, Schabus M, Noirhomme Q, Bredart S, et al. (2011) Two distinct neuronal networks mediate the awareness of environment and of self. J Cogn Neurosci 23: 570–578.
83. Alkire MT, Hudetz AG, Tononi G (2008) Consciousness and anesthesia. Science 322: 876–880.
84. Ferrarelli F, Massimini M, Sarasso S, Casali A, Riedner BA, et al. (2010) Breakdown in cortical effective connectivity during midazolam-induced loss of consciousness. Proc Natl Acad Sci U S A 107: 2681–2686.
85. Massimini M, Ferrarelli F, Sarasso S, Tononi G (2012) Cortical mechanisms of loss of consciousness: insight from TMS/EEG studies. Arch Ital Biol 150: 44–55.
86. Imas OA, Ropella KM, Ward BD, Wood JD, Hudetz AG (2005) Volatile anesthetics disrupt frontal-posterior recurrent information transfer at gamma frequencies in rat. Neurosci Lett 387: 145–150.
87. Tinker JH, Sharbrough FW, Michenfelder JD (1977) Anterior shift of the dominant EEG rhytham during anesthesia in the Java monkey: correlation with anesthetic potency. Anesthesiology 46: 252–259.
88. Tononi G, Cirelli C (2014) Sleep and the price of plasticity: from synaptic and cellular homeostasis to memory consolidation and integration. Neuron 81: 12–34.
89. Brimacombe J (1995) The advantages of the LMA over the tracheal tube or facemask: a meta-analysis. Can J Anaesth 42: 1017–1023.
90. (2010) American Society of Anesthesiologists Standards for Basic Anesthetic Monitoring. ASA House of Delegates (Standards and Practice Parameters Committee).
91. Whitlock EL, Villafranca AJ, Lin N, Palanca BJ, Jacobsohn E, et al. (2011) Relationship between bispectral index values and volatile anesthetic concentrations during the maintenance phase of anesthesia in the B-Unaware trial. Anesthesiology 115: 1209–1218.
92. Shafer SL, Varvel JR, Aziz N, Scott JC (1990) Pharmacokinetics of fentanyl administered by computer-controlled infusion pump. Anesthesiology 73: 1091–1102.
93. Villesen HH, Banning AM, Petersen RH, Weinelt S, Poulsen JB, et al. (2007) Pharmacokinetics of morphine and oxycodone following intravenous administration in elderly patients. Ther Clin Risk Manag 3: 961–967.
94. De Jonghe B, Cook D, Appere-De-Vecchi C, Guyatt G, Meade M, et al. (2000) Using and understanding sedation scoring systems: a systematic review. Intensive Care Med 26: 275–285.
95. Haenggi M, Ypparila H, Takala J, Korhonen I, Luginbuhl M, et al. (2004) Measuring depth of sedation with auditory evoked potentials during controlled infusion of propofol and remifentanil in healthy volunteers. Anesth Analg 99: 1728–1736.
96. Mei W, Seeling M, Franck M, Radtke F, Brantner B, et al. (2010) Independent risk factors for postoperative pain in need of intervention early after awakening from general anaesthesia. Eur J Pain 14: 149 e141–147.
97. Aldrete JA (1998) Modifications to the postanesthesia score for use in ambulatory surgery. J Perianesth Nurs 13: 148–155.
98. Mitra P, Bokil B (2008) Observed Brain Dynamics. New York: Oxford University Press.

# Intravenous Remifentanil versus Epidural Ropivacaine with Sufentanil for Labour Analgesia: A Retrospective Study

**Rong Lin**[a], **Yiyi Tao**[a], **Yibing Yu**[a], **Zhendong Xu, Jing Su, Zhiqiang Liu***

Department of Anaesthesiology, Shanghai First Maternity and Infant Hospital, Tongji University School of Medicine, Shanghai, China

## Abstract

Remifentanil with appropriate pharmacological properties seems to be an ideal alternative to epidural analgesia during labour. A retrospective cohort study was undertaken to assess the efficacy and safety of remifentanil intravenous patient-controlled analgesia (IVPCA) compared with epidural analgesia. Medical records of 370 primiparas who received remifentanil IVPCA or epidural analgesia were reviewed. Pain and sedation scores, overall satisfaction, the extent of pain control, maternal side effects and neonatal outcome as primary observational indicators were collected. There was a significant decline of pain scores in both groups. Pain reduction was greater in the epidural group throughout the whole study period (0~180 min) ($P<0.0001$), and pain scores in the remifentanil group showed an increasing trend one hour later. The remifentanil group had a lower $SpO_2$ ($P<0.0001$) and a higher sedation score ($P<0.0001$) within 30 min after treatment. The epidural group had a higher overall satisfaction score ($3.8\pm0.4$ vs. $3.7\pm0.6$, $P=0.007$) and pain relief score ($2.9\pm0.3$ vs. $2.8\pm0.4$, $P<0.0001$) compared with the remifentanil group. There was no significant difference on side effects between the two groups, except that a higher rate of dizziness (1% vs. 21.8%, $P<0.0001$) was observed during remifentanil analgesia. And logistic regression analysis demonstrated that nausea, vomiting were associated with oxytocin usage and instrumental delivery, and dizziness was associated to the type and duration of analgesia. Neonatal outcomes such as Apgar scores and umbilical-cord blood gas analysis were within the normal range, but umbilical pH and base excess of neonatus in the remifentanil group were significantly lower. Remifentanil IVPCA provides poorer efficacy on labor analgesia than epidural analgesia, with more sedation on parturients and a trend of newborn acidosis. Despite these adverse effects, remifentanil IVPCA can still be an alternative option for labor analgesia under the condition of one-to-one bedside care, continuous monitoring, oxygen supply and preparation for neonatal resuscitation.

**Editor:** Sam Eldabe, The James Cook University Hospital, United Kingdom

**Funding:** These authors have no support or funding to report.

**Competing Interests:** The authors have declared that no competing interests exist.

* Email: drliuzhq@hotmail.com

[a] These authors contributed equally to this work.

## Introduction

Epidural analgesia is efficient to relieve labour pain with fewer side effects on parturients and neonatus and regarded as the gold standard for obstetric analgesia [1]. However, some certain clinical conditions restrict its administration, such as maternal rejection or noncooperation, coagulation disorders, infection or tumor close to site of puncture, allergic reaction to local anesthetic, and spinal deformity [2]. It is clear that an effective and safe alternative should be established.

Remifentanil for intravenous patient-controlled analgesia (IVPCA) seems to be a promising option because of its particular pharmacokinetic and pharmacodynamic characteristics. Remifentanil as an ultra short-acting synthetic opioid has a very fast onset time (30~60 s), peak analgesic effect of 2.5 min, a high metabolic rate (context-sensitive half-life about 3~4 min), and no accumulated effect with repeated or long-term use [3–5]. Although it crosses the placental barrier with no difficulty, the drug can be degraded rapidly in the foetus [6].

A lot of studies with respect to the efficacy and complications of remifentanil for labour analgesia have been carried out. A prospective, randomised study from Douma et al. [7] on a group of only 20 patients discovered superior anesthetic effect was provided by epidural analgesia compared with remifentanil IVPCA. Volmanen et al. [8] designed a controlled, double-blinded study (42 parturients were randomly recruited) to observed analgesic efficacy of remifentanil and epidural analgesia just lasting for 60 min during the first stage of labour, and also reached similar conclusions. But they only evaluated fetal heart rate (FHR), umbilical artery pH and 1 min Apgar scores as fetal outcomes. Another randomised, controlled trial of Tveit et al. [9] (EA group 20, RA group 17) reported that remifentanil was more likely to cause sedation and oxygen desaturation, but was safe to neonates. In our recent meta-analysis involving 5 studies, remifentanil IVPCA was not found to afford better pain relief than epidural analgesia, but it did not bring serious adverse outcomes to mother and newborn [10]. Since most of these studies were somewhat limited by small sample sizes, a short observation period or inadequate assessment, it still remains controversial whether we can administrate remifentanil during labour without worry.

Thus we conducted this large sample study to retrospectively investigate maternal and neonatal outcomes of remifentanil IVPCA compared with epidural analgesia.

## Materials and Methods

The study obtained approval from the Research Ethics Committee of Shanghai First Maternity and Infant Hospital. Written consent was obtained from each patient. All electronic medical records of parturients who had accepted intravenous remifentanil or epidural analgesia during labour in our institution from January 2013 to July 2013 were reviewed. Inclusion criteria were as follows: primipara (ASA status I or II), singleton pregnancy with cephalic presentation, gestational age of >36 weeks, spontaneous or induced labour. Records of women with request for caesarean section or stillbirth were excluded. In light of analgesia technique the eligible parturients elected, they were divided into two groups: the remifentanil group and the epidural group (Fig. 1).

### Intravenous remifentanil analgesia regimen

Parturients were directed how to operate the PCA pump (Baxter 6060 Multi-Therapy infusion pump, Baxter Healthcare Corporation, Kista, Sweden) before the start of analgesia. The dosage regimen of remifentanil hydrochloride (Ultiva, GlaxoSmithKline, Oslo, Norway) diluted with saline to a concentration of 20 $\mu g \cdot ml^{-1}$ was set to PCA bolus of 0.4 $\mu g \cdot kg^{-1}$, a continuous background infusion at 0.04~0.05 $\mu g \cdot kg^{-1} \cdot min^{-1}$ and a lockout time of 5 min. PCA doses were calculated according to estimated bodyweight (body height in centimeters -100) [9,11,12].

### Epidural analgesia regimen

An epidural catheter was inserted in the epidural space at L2–3 or L3–4 with the patient in a lateral decubitus position by an anaesthesiologist. Then the same PCA pump was connected to the cannula. Parturients received a 10 ml initial loading dose of 0.068% ropivacaine and 0.3 $\mu g \cdot ml^{-1}$ sufentanil, followed by a maintenance dose at 8 $ml \cdot h^{-1}$ and a PCA bolus dose of 5 ml with a 15-min lockout interval. If necessary, the infusion dose could be adjusted (5–10 $ml \cdot h^{-1}$).

One-to-one nursing service was provided to every parturient entering into the delivery room. The analgesia was applied when the cervix dilated to 3 cm, and terminated before the beginning of the second stage of labor. Before administration of analgesia, intravenous infusion of lactated Ringers solution and oxygen inhalation through nasal tube were given by convention. Routine monitoring, including maternal noninvasive blood pressure (NIBP), heart rate (HR), pulse oxygen saturation ($SpO_2$), uterine activity and FHR by external tocodynamometry were accomplished and measured continuously. Numerical rating scale (NRS) pain score (an 11-point scale, 0 = no pain and 10 = worst pain imaginable) was used to assess the pain level. And the evaluation of sedation referred to the Ramsay sedation score (1 = anxious, agitated, restless; 2 = cooperative, oriented, tranquil; 3 = responds to simple commands only; 4 = brisk response to light glabellar tap or loud auditory stimulation; 5 = sluggish response to light glabellar tap or loud auditory stimulation; 6 = no response to light glabellar tap or loud auditory stimulus). Non-invasive measurements mentioned above as well as pain and sedation scores were recorded before and immediately after treatment, afterwards every 30 min.

The day after delivery, parturients were asked about their overall satisfaction with analgesic therapy on a five-point verbal rating scale (0 = very dissatisfied, 1 = dissatisfied, 2 = neutral [neither satisfied nor dissatisfied], 3 = satisfied, 4 = very satisfied), and to express the degree of pain relief likewise on a 5-point

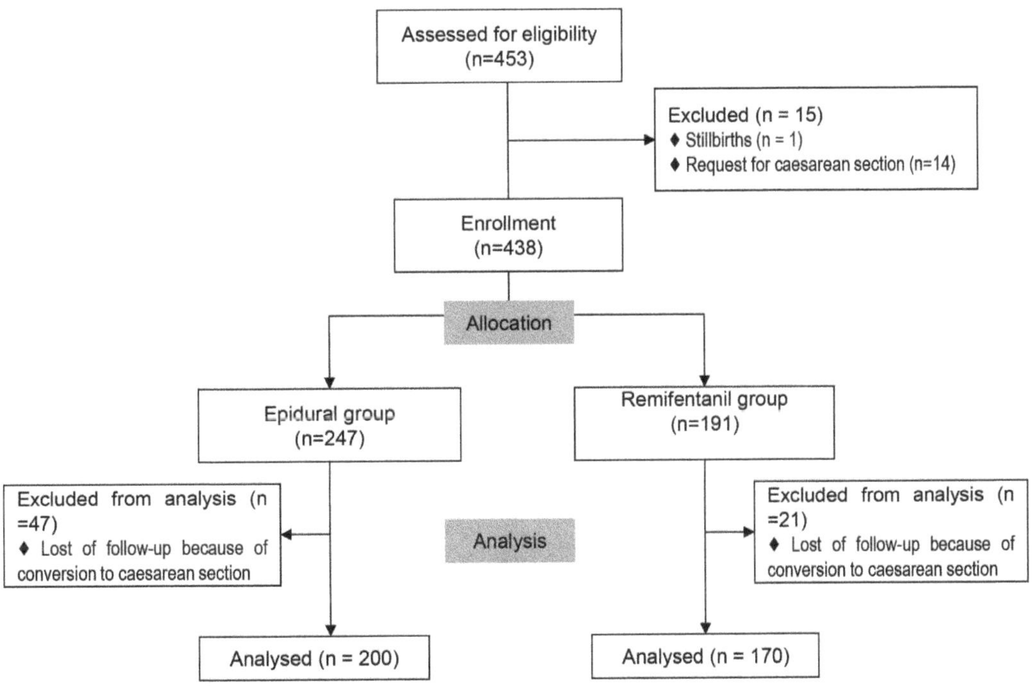


**Figure 1. Flow-process diagram of the retrospective study.**

categorical scale (0 = very poor, 1 = poor, 2 = moderate, 3 = good, 4 = very good) [9].

Excepting above, other data collected included: maternal demographic characteristics (age, gestational weeks, height, weight, BMI), delivery mode, oxytocin treatment, durations of analgesia, maternal adverse reactions (respiratory depression, excessive sedation, nausea and vomiting, skin pruritus), neonatal outcomes (Apgar scores at 1 and 5 min, umbilical-cord blood gas analysis, requirement for resuscitation).

## Statistical analysis

SPSS version 18.0 (SPSS Inc., Chicago, IL, USA) was used for all data analysis. As a general rule, data were expressed as mean ± SD or frequency (percentage). P values less than 0.05 were considered statistically significant. Continuous variables were processed with Student's *t*-test. And Chi-square test was performed for categorical variables. To evaluate the relationship of side effects to other factors, logistic regression analysis was performed.

## Results

Through reviewing the database, we identified 453 medical records that met inclusion criteria. Among them, fifteen subjects were ruled out on account of stillbirth (n = 1) or request for caesarean section (n = 14). Follow-ups of sixty-eight parturients were brought to a close due to their conversion to caesarean section. Finally, the following analysis was on the base of 370 observations (Epidural group 200, Remifentanil group 170) (Fig. 1). The conversive rate of caesarean section in the epidural group is significantly higher than in the remifentanil group (19.0% vs. 11.0%, P = 0.021). But there was no statistically significant difference between the two groups with regard to the indications for cesarean section (Table 1).

Table 1 demonstrated that parturients in the remifentanil group were taller in height and had a shorter duration of analgesia compared to those in the epidural group. Besides that, there was no statistically significant difference between the two groups as regards other demographic characteristics, mode of delivery and oxytocin utilization.

Comparing the two groups, pain scores were similar at baseline. After analgesic therapy, a significant decline in pain scores from baseline was discovered in both groups, and epidural pain scores decreased more at every given point in time (P<0.0001). One-hour treatment later, pain scores in the remifentanil group went steadily up but still inferior to the baseline. By comparison, the ascending tendency was minimal in the epidural group (Fig. 2).

Immediately after remifentanil analgesia, oxygen saturation reduced obviously compared to baseline (P<0.0001). And at that time point and 30 min after analgesia, mean $SpO_2$ of the remifentanil group was lower than that of the epidural group, with significant difference (P<0.0001). Nevertheless, those who suffered from desaturation could recover their original state rapidly by deep breaths and supplementary oxygen. By contrast, oxygen saturation of those receiving epidural analgesia remained stable throughout the whole childbirth (Fig. 3). No respiratory depression (RR<9 breaths/min or $SpO_2$<90%) was discovered in both groups.

The Ramsay sedation scores were significantly higher in the remifentanil group immediately and 30 min after treatment (P< 0.0001 and P<0.001, respectively) (Fig. 4). Six women following remifentanil regimen reached the maximum sedation score of 4.

The epidural group had a higher overall satisfaction score (3.8±0.4 vs. 3.7±0.6, P = 0.007) and pain relief score (2.9±0.3 vs. 2.8±0.4, P<0.0001) compared with the remifentanil group. Although more parturients receiving remifentanil reported nausea, vomiting and pruritus, the incidences of the above adverse reactions were similar between the two regimens. 21.8% of patients in the remifentanil group encountered dizziness, which was far higher than that in the epidural group (Table 2). Furthermore, logistic regression analysis demonstrated that nausea, vomiting were associated with oxytocin usage and

**Table 1.** Maternal demographic characteristics and labour data.

| | Epidural Group (n = 200) | Remifentanil Group (n = 170) | P value |
|---|---|---|---|
| **Age (years)** | 29.3±3.1 | 29.6±3.2 | 0.208 |
| **Gestational age (weeks)** | 39.6±1.1 | 39.6±1.0 | 0.817 |
| **Height (cm)** | 1.60±0.03 | 1.61±0.03 | 0.024 |
| **Weight (kg)** | 71.0±5.3 | 70.1±8.6 | 0.373 |
| **BMI (kg·m$^{-2}$)** | 27.3±1.8 | 27.2±3.0 | 0.837 |
| **Duration of analgesia (min)** | 182.2±96.6 | 171.7±85.8 | 0.033 |
| **Oxytocin** | 88 (44%) | 69 (40.6%) | 0.508 |
| **Mode of delivery, n (%)** | | | 0.925 |
| Spontaneous | 191 (95.5%) | 162 (95.3%) | |
| Instrumental | 9 (4.5%) | 8 (4.7%) | |
| **Conversion to caesarean section, n (%)** | 47/247 (19.0%) | 21/191 (11.0%) | 0.021 |
| **Indications for cesarean delivery, n (%)** | | | |
| Fetal distress | 12/24 (25.5%) | 8/21 (38.1%) | 0.294 |
| Prolonged labor | 14/24 (29.8%) | 7/21 (33.3%) | 0.770 |
| Cephalopelvic disproportion | 13/24 (23.5%) | 3/21 (14.3%) | 0.230 |
| Severe preeclampsia | 3/24 (6.4%) | 1/21 (4.8%) | 0.793 |
| Prenatal fever | 5/24 (10.6%) | 2/21 (9.5%) | 0.889 |

Data are expressed as mean ± standard deviation or n (%). BMI = body mass index.

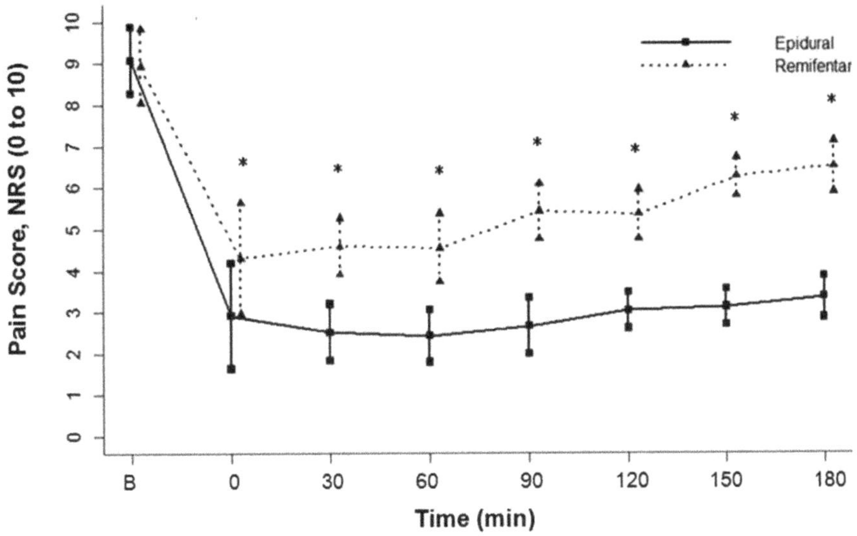


**Figure 2. Comparisons in NRS pain scores between the two groups (Epidural group and Remifentanil group) at each time point.** B represents baseline. NRS = numerical rating scale. *P<0.0001.

instrumental delivery, and dizziness was relative to the type and duration of analgesia (Table 3).

Neonatal data were summarized in Table 4. The analysis showed that there was no difference between the groups in relation to mean birth weight, Apgar scores and the incidence of abnormal FHR. FHR abnormalities included tachycardia, bradycardia, variable decelerations and late decelerations, and all were transient changes. The two groups were also similar with respect to the types of abnormal FHR. But umbilical pH and base excess of neonatus in the remifentanil group were significantly lower. Three newborns had 1 min Apgar scores <7, and all of them were from the epidural group. Two neonates were born after shoulder dystocia with Apgar score 4 and 5 for the 1st minute, and 8 and 7 for the 5th minute, respectively. The other had 1–5 min Apgar scores of 6–9 due to acute fetal distress. In addition, two neonates had an umbilical arterial pH<7.10, they were those who experienced shoulder dystocia in the epidural group. But no umbilical venous pH<7.10 was registered.

## Discussion

This research work shows that epidural analgesia appears to afford more preferable analgesia effect than remifentanil IVPCA. Pain scores reported from the epidural group were significantly lower at each set time-point (0, 30 min, 60 min, 90 min, 120 min, 150 min and 180 min after treatment), and epidural regimen produced more persistent contribution on labor analgesia. In relative terms, administration of remifentanil just had moderate pain reduction with gradual elevation of pain scores as the labor progressed. These findings were consistent with other recent studies [6,8,13–18]. Our previous meta-analysis has also demonstrated that there were higher pain scores at 1 h and 2 h for

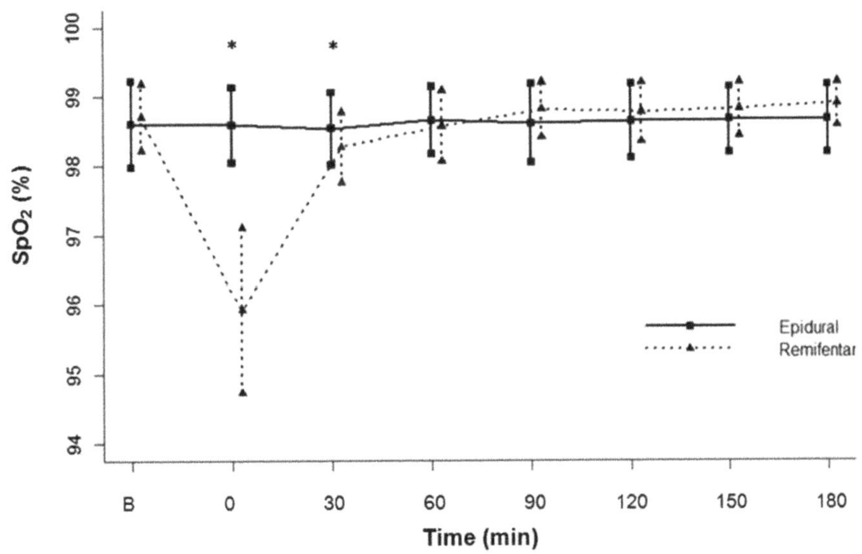


**Figure 3. Comparisons in pulse oxygen saturation ($SpO_2$) between the two groups.**

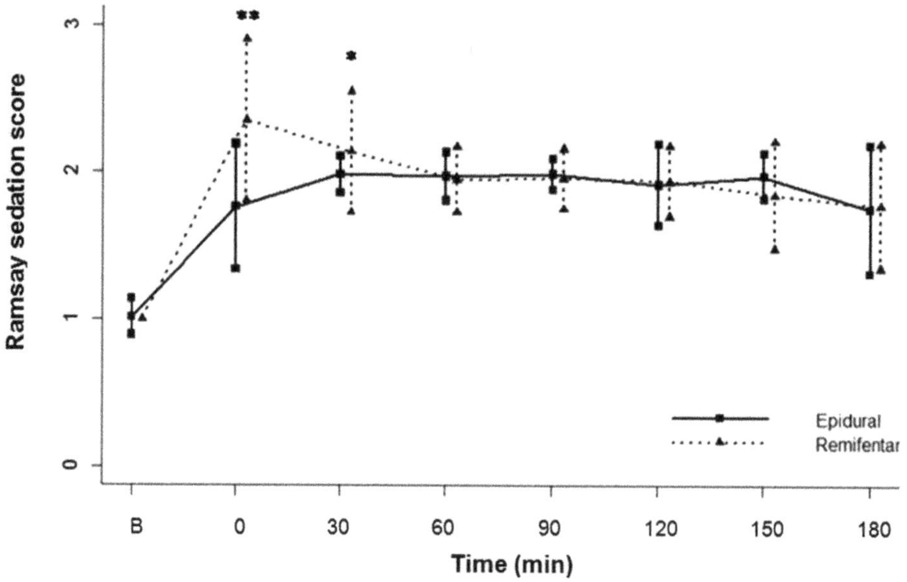


**Figure 4. Comparisons in the Ramsay sedation score between the two groups (Epidural group and Remifentanil group) at each time point.** B represents baseline. **P<0.0001, *P<0.001.

patients with remifentanil IVPCA compared with those receiving epidural analgesia [10]. At the beginning of remifentanil IVPCA, pain relief was still satisfactory because of its rapid onset. Progressive pain of uterus systole with the progress of labor and/or a tolerance to remifentanil after continuous use were probably responsible for the later rising pain scores in the remifentanil group [7,19]. Obviously, local anaesthetic by epidural had more control over the pain stress.

Although 92.4% of parturients with remifentanil IVPCA expressed satisfaction with analgesic effect (very satisfied: 77.1%, satisfied: 15.3%), the overall satisfaction scores and pain relief scores were lower in the remifentanil group, which seemed distinguished from those seen in other researches. Douma et al. [7] found there was no obvious distinction in satisfaction scores after delivery between the remifentanil group and the epidural group. Similarly, in the study of Stourac et al. [20], the level of the parturients' satisfaction with analgesia was similar both in the EA group and in the rPCA group (P = 0.24). One possible explanation for this was that these assessments carried subjective criteria to result in the difference. In addition, interindividual variation in the response to opioid [21,22] and the different administration schedules we adopted were likely to account for the disparity.

**Table 2.** Quality of analgesia and Side effects.

| | Epidural Group (n = 200) | Remifentanil Group (n = 170) | P value |
|---|---|---|---|
| **Overall satisfaction score** | 3.8±0.4 | 3.7±0.6 | 0.007 |
| 4- very satisfied | 167 (83.5%) | 131 (77.1%) | |
| 3- satisfied | 33 (16.5%) | 26 (15.3%) | |
| 2- neutral (neither satisfied nor dissatisfied) | 0 | 13 (7.6%) | |
| 1- dissatisfied | 0 | 0 | |
| 0- very dissatisfied | 0 | 0 | |
| **Pain relief score** | 2.9±0.3 | 2.8±0.4 | <0.0001 |
| 4- very good | 0 | 0 | |
| 3- good | 185 (92.5%) | 132 (77.6%) | |
| 2- moderate | 15 (7.5%) | 38 (22.4%) | |
| 1- poor | 0 | 0 | |
| 0- very poor | 0 | 0 | |
| **Dizziness** | 2 (1%) | 37 (21.8%) | <0.0001 |
| **Nausea** | 11 (5.5%) | 13 (7.6%) | 0.403 |
| **Vomiting** | 9 (4.5%) | 11 (6.5%) | 0.404 |
| **Pruritus** | 3 (1.5%) | 4 (2.4%) | 0.548 |

Data are expressed as mean ± standard deviation or n (%).

**Table 3.** Multiple logistic regression analysis with side effects (nausea, vomiting and dizziness) as the dependent variable.

| | OR | 95% CI | P value |
|---|---|---|---|
| **Nausea** | | | |
| Oxytocin | 0.23 | 0.09–0.59 | 0.0025 |
| Instrumental | 0.21 | 0.06–0.74 | 0.015 |
| **Vomiting** | | | |
| Oxytocin | 0.23 | 0.08–0.66 | 0.0064 |
| Instrumental | 0.17 | 0.05–0.59 | 0.0056 |
| **Dizziness** | | | |
| Type of analgesia | 32.35 | 7.52–139.18 | <0.00015 |
| Duration of analgesia | 1.01 | 1.001–1.009 | 0.02 |

OR = odds ratio; CI = confidence interval.

Up to the present, the most suitable dosage regimen of remifentanil for labour still retains a controversial subject [23]. While the regimen without background infusion has been reported to produce superior effect on obstetric analgesia [14,24–28], recent researches indicated that fixed small PCA boluses with alterable infusion rate could provide effective analgesia with fewer adverse reactions [23]. Our dosage regimen of remifentanil ($0.04\sim0.05$ $\mu g \cdot kg^{-1} \cdot min^{-1}$ infusion and 0.4 $\mu g \cdot kg^{-1}$ PCA bolus) made reference to the previous studies and experiences from our institution. In clinical practice, we found remifentanil presented a delayed peak effect in spite of its quick onset. Thus PCA bolus alone could not act urgently to keep uterine contraction pain under control. Furthermore, a dose-related risk of respiratory depression and excessive sedation exist after remifentanil bolus injection, which has been discovered in healthy volunteers [29]. Some studies have recommended the bolus dose of 0.4 $\mu g \cdot kg^{-1}$ can be used effectively and securely [6,8,18,26,30], the infusion rate more than 0.05 $\mu g \cdot kg^{-1} \cdot min^{-1}$ may be connected with higher incidence of side effects [14].

In this study, a marked drop in maternal $SpO_2$ appeared within 30 min after using remifentanil. It may be related to a transient respiration inhibition at the onset of remifentanil. The oxygen desaturation (defined as $SpO_2<95\%$) episode persisted only for a brief duration, which could be reversed by deep breathing and oxygen inhalation through nasal tube. The incidence of oxygen desaturation we observed was 9.4%, far below other reported rates ($40\%\sim74\%$) [14,16,18,31–33]. Perhaps that had something to do with preventive oxygen supply. And, continuous $SpO_2$ monitoring and bedside-monitor of the anaesthetist or midwife also contributed a great share in preventing desaturation, since hypoxia caused by remifentanil might still occur even in the situation of oxygen supply [8]. Besides, dehydration or exhaustion along with the application of remifentanil also could aggravate respiratory depression [34], so adequate transfusion treatment in advance is recommended.

Despite a higher level of sedation in the remifentanil group, all of patients could be awakened easily by a loud voice or the next uterine contraction pain. 21.8% of patients receiving remifentanil

**Table 4.** Neonatal outcomes.

| | Epidural Group (n = 200) | Remifentanil Group (n = 170) | P value |
|---|---|---|---|
| **Birth weight (g)** | 3399.8±382.9 | 3439.8±371.8 | 0.444 |
| **Apgar score** | | | |
| 1 min | 9.7±0.8 | 9.7±0.6 | 0.984 |
| 5 min | 9.9±0.3 | 9.9±0.3 | 0.712 |
| **Umbilical vein pH** | 7.31±0.07 | 7.29±0.07 | 0.015 |
| **Umbilical artery pH** | 7.28±0.07 | 7.26±0.06 | 0.001 |
| **Umbilical vein base excess ($mol \cdot l^{-1}$)** | −4.50±2.13 | −5.08±2.21 | 0.011 |
| **Umbilical artery base excess ($mol \cdot l^{-1}$)** | −4.96±2.66 | −6.13±2.33 | <0.0001 |
| **Abnormal FHR changes, n (%)** | 27 (13.5%) | 33 (19.4%) | 0.124 |
| During the analgesia period, n (%) | 16/27 (59.3%) | 24/33 (72.7%) | 0.271 |
| - Tachycardia, n (%) | 3/16 (18.8%) | 5/24 (20.8%) | 0.601 |
| - Bradycardia, n (%) | 6/16 (37.5%) | 11/24 (45.8%) | 0.872 |
| - Variable decelerations, n (%) | 5/16 (31.3%) | 7/24 (29.2%) | 0.888 |
| - Late decelerations, n (%) | 2/16 (12.5%) | 1/24 (4.2%) | 0.327 |

Data are expressed as mean ± standard deviation or n (%). FHR = fetal heart rate.

reported dizziness, and we noted that a longer duration of remifentanil analgesia was more likely to cause dizziness. We speculated it might be related to a certain degree of cumulative effect. Yet, nobody complained uncomfortable for it. That being said, one-to-one nursing still needs to be ensured.

The frequencies of nausea, vomiting and pruritus were similar between the two groups, which were consistent with the results from previous studies [6,8,32,35]. Our analyses pointed out that some obstetric factors such as the usage of oxytocin and forceps may be associated with nausea and vomiting which are common during delivery. Studies showed that the occurance of nausea and vomiting is correlated to the degree of hypotension [36]. Higher doses of oxytocin or forceps delivery may lead to sudden haemodynamic change.

The impact of remifentanil on newborns has become a common concern. Neonatal outcomes observed in our study stayed at an acceptable level. Removed from two neonates with shoulder dystocia and one with acute fetal distress, other Apgar scores were normal. Besides, there were no significant differences in the incidence or types of abnormal FHR between the two groups. From the current data, systemic remifentanil seemed have no serious effect on FHR. However the fact that opioids have the capability of producing FHR abnormalities [6] cannot be taken lightly. We guessed close monitoring and routine oxygen supplementation should play a part in this. The mean umbilical cord gases in both groups were kept in normal range as well, whereas umbilical arterial/venous pH and base excess were lower in the remifentanil group. Our findings seemed to be different from previous studies [6,7,9,14,26,35], which found no effect from remifentanil on neonatal outcomes including umbilical pH and base excess. Despite the fact that remifentanil is easy to be metabolized in the neonates [30,37], it still has some influence on neonatal status. Therefore, we recommended neonatal resuscitation should be in train before birth for the neonates whose mothers have received remifentanil. 2010 American Heart Association Guidelines for Neonatal Resuscitation suggested that at least 1 person who must be capable of initiating resuscitation, including administration of positive pressure ventilation and chest compressions, should present at every delivery [38]. 2011 Chinese Neonatal Resuscitation Guidelines also have the same recommendations [39]. In our hospital, every delivery room keeps the necessary equipments and medications for resuscitation available. All practitioners in the delivery rooms including midwives are required to know the whole resuscitation process and have skills to perform the initial steps of resuscitation. The initial steps (about 60 s), which are called "the Golden Minute", will win precious rescue time for skilled personnel's arrival. Coordination between obstetrics and pediatrics, regular training, adequate preparation and prompt initiation of support are a forceful guarantee for successful neonatal resuscitation.

The demographics of two groups were matched except for height and duration of analgesia. The conversive rate and the indications of caesarean section are similar between the two groups. However, we have not been able to determine whether intravenous remifentanil for labour analgesia is helpful with lowering the conversive rate due to limited samples of our present study. As for the conversive rate of caesarean section in our study (15.5% [68/438]), it was really lower than figures reported in other studies. Ismail MT et al. [40] reported that the conversive rate in their study was 24.3%. We guessed it might be related to our inclusion criteria that only healthy primiparas without any obstetrics complications can be included. These patients were less likely to undergo caesarean section. Moreover, one-to-one bedside care, continuous monitoring, timely management and treatment may be also crucial to reduce the conversive rate of caesarean.

As a result of our retrospective study, the probability of missing data and selection bias is unavoidable. It is also the main limitation of our study. For instance, some data relating to blood pressure, heart rate, breathing rate and the quantities of drugs were not recorded completely and missing. A further prospective study will designed to refine the data. However, we believe the omissions and bias may be not big because we adopted a standardized analgesic procedure for labour and a detailed electronic recording system.

In this retrospective study, we confirmed that remifentanil IVPCA produced an observable improvement in pain scores, though not quite as efficacious as epidural analgesia. Furthermore, we also have reached some different conclusions from previous researches. For example, patients' satisfaction scores and neonatal umbilical cord gases in the remifentanil group were lower than those in the epidural group. As a systemic opioid, sedation, dizziness and desaturation were inevitable during using remifentanil. Fortunately, these adverse reactions were temporary and the effects on neonatal outcomes were small. We suggest that remifentanil analgesia can be implemented as an option for pain relief during childbirth under the precondition of ensuring one-to-one bedside care, continuous oxygen saturation monitoring, oxygen supply up front, and immediate availability of neonatal resuscitation.

## Acknowledgments

The authors thank the three anonymous reviewers for their insightful comments and suggestions, which have led to a significantly improved paper.

## Author Contributions

Conceived and designed the experiments: ZL. Performed the experiments: RL YT YY ZX JS. Analyzed the data: RL. Contributed reagents/materials/analysis tools: YT YY. Contributed to the writing of the manuscript: RL ZL.

## References

1. Althaus J, Wax J (2005) Analgesia and anesthesia in labor. Obstet Gynecol Clin North Am 32: 231–244.
2. Miller RD (2010) Miller's anesthesia. Philadelphia, PA: Churchill Livingstone/Elsevier.
3. Babenco HD, Conard PF, Gross JB (2000) The pharmacodynamic effect of a remifentanil bolus on ventilatory control. Anesthesiology 92: 393–398.
4. Egan TD (2000) Pharmacokinetics and pharmacodynamics of remifentanil: an update in the year 2000. Curr Opin Anaesthesiol 13: 449–455.
5. Kapila A, Glass PS, Jacobs JR, Muir KT, Hermann DJ, et al. (1995) Measured context-sensitive half-times of remifentanil and alfentanil. Anesthesiology 83: 968–975.
6. Volikas I, Butwick A, Wilkinson C, Pleming A, Nicholson G (2005) Maternal and neonatal side-effects of remifentanil patient-controlled analgesia in labour. Br J Anaesth 95: 504–509.
7. Douma MR, Middeldorp JM, Verwey RA, Dahan A, Stienstra R (2011) A randomised comparison of intravenous remifentanil patient-controlled analgesia with epidural ropivacaine/sufentanil during labour. Int J Obstet Anesth 20: 118–123.
8. Volmanen P, Sarvela J, Akural EI, Raudaskoski T, Korttila K, et al. (2008) Intravenous remifentanil vs. epidural levobupivacaine with fentanyl for pain relief in early labour: a randomised, controlled, double-blinded study. Acta Anaesthesiol Scand 52: 249–255.
9. Tveit TO, Seiler S, Halvorsen A, Rosland JH (2012) Labour analgesia: a randomised, controlled trial comparing intravenous remifentanil and epidural analgesia with ropivacaine and fentanyl. Eur J Anaesthesiol 29: 129–136.
10. Liu ZQ, Chen XB, Li HB, Qiu MT, Duan T (2014) A comparison of remifentanil parturient-controlled intravenous analgesia with epidural analgesia: a meta-analysis of randomized controlled trials. Anesth Analg 118: 598–603.

11. Egan TD, Huizinga B, Gupta SK, Jaarsma RL, Sperry RJ, et al. (1998) Remifentanil pharmacokinetics in obese versus lean patients. Anesthesiology 89: 562–573.
12. Tveit TO, Halvorsen A, Seiler S, Rosland JH (2013) Efficacy and side effects of intravenous remifentanil patient-controlled analgesia used in a stepwise approach for labour: an observational study. Int J Obstet Anesth 22: 19–25.
13. Balcioglu O, Akin S, Demir S, Aribogan A (2007) Patient-controlled intravenous analgesia with remifentanil in nulliparous subjects in labor. Expert Opin Pharmacother 8: 3089–3096.
14. Balki M, Kasodekar S, Dhumne S, Bernstein P, Carvalho JC (2007) Remifentanil patient-controlled analgesia for labour: optimizing drug delivery regimens. Can J Anaesth 54: 626–633.
15. D'Onofrio P, Novelli AM, Mecacci F, Scarselli G (2009) The efficacy and safety of continuous intravenous administration of remifentanil for birth pain relief: an open study of 205 parturients. Anesth Analg 109: 1922–1924.
16. Douma MR, Verwey RA, Kam-Endtz CE, van der Linden PD, Stienstra R (2010) Obstetric analgesia: a comparison of patient-controlled meperidine, remifentanil, and fentanyl in labour. Br J Anaesth 104: 209–215.
17. Evron S, Ezri T, Protianov M, Muzikant G, Sadan O, et al. (2008) The effects of remifentanil or acetaminophen with epidural ropivacaine on body temperature during labor. J Anesth 22: 105–111.
18. Volmanen P, Akural EI, Raudaskoski T, Alahuhta S (2002) Remifentanil in obstetric analgesia: a dose-finding study. Anesth Analg 94: 913–917, table of contents.
19. Olufolabi AJ, Booth JV, Wakeling HG, Glass PS, Penning DH, et al. (2000) A preliminary investigation of remifentanil as a labor analgesic. Anesth Analg 91: 606–608.
20. Stourac P, Suchomelova H, Stodulkova M, Huser M, Krikava I, et al. (2012) Comparison of parturient - controlled remifentanil with epidural bupivacain and sufentanil for labour analgesia: Randomised controlled trial. Biomed Pap Med Fac Univ Palacky Olomouc Czech Repub.
21. Landau R, Cahana A, Smiley RM, Antonarakis SE, Blouin JL (2004) Genetic variability of mu-opioid receptor in an obstetric population. Anesthesiology 100: 1030–1033.
22. Volmanen P, Alahuhta S (2004) Will remifentanil be a labour analgesic? Int J Obstet Anesth 13: 1–4.
23. Marwah R, Hassan S, Carvalho JC, Balki M (2012) Remifentanil versus fentanyl for intravenous patient-controlled labour analgesia: an observational study. Can J Anaesth 59: 246–254.
24. Blair JM, Dobson GT, Hill DA, McCracken GR, Fee JP (2005) Patient controlled analgesia for labour: a comparison of remifentanil with pethidine. Anaesthesia 60: 22–27.
25. Dhileepan S, Stacey RG (2001) A preliminary investigation of remifentanil as a labor analgesic. Anesth Analg 92: 1358–1359.
26. Evron S, Glezerman M, Sadan O, Boaz M, Ezri T (2005) Remifentanil: a novel systemic analgesic for labor pain. Anesth Analg 100: 233–238.
27. Hill D (2008) Remifentanil in obstetrics. Curr Opin Anaesthesiol 21: 270–274.
28. Volmanen PV, Akural EI, Raudaskoski T, Ranta P, Tekay A, et al. (2011) Timing of intravenous patient-controlled remifentanil bolus during early labour. Acta Anaesthesiol Scand 55: 486–494.
29. Egan TD, Kern SE, Muir KT, White J (2004) Remifentanil by bolus injection: a safety, pharmacokinetic, pharmacodynamic, and age effect investigation in human volunteers. Br J Anaesth 92: 335–343.
30. Kan RE, Hughes SC, Rosen MA, Kessin C, Preston PG, et al. (1998) Intravenous remifentanil: placental transfer, maternal and neonatal effects. Anesthesiology 88: 1467–1474.
31. Shahriari A, Khooshideh M (2007) A randomized controlled trial of intravenous remifentanil compared with intramuscular meperidine for pain relief in labor. J Med Sci 7: 635–639.
32. Thurlow JA, Laxton CH, Dick A, Waterhouse P, Sherman L, et al. (2002) Remifentanil by patient-controlled analgesia compared with intramuscular meperidine for pain relief in labour. Br J Anaesth 88: 374–378.
33. Volmanen P, Akural E, Raudaskoski T, Ohtonen P, Alahuhta S (2005) Comparison of remifentanil and nitrous oxide in labour analgesia. Acta Anaesthesiol Scand 49: 453–458.
34. Bonner JC, McClymont W (2012) Respiratory arrest in an obstetric patient using remifentanil patient-controlled analgesia. Anaesthesia 67: 538–540.
35. Blair JM, Hill DA, Fee JP (2001) Patient-controlled analgesia for labour using remifentanil: a feasibility study. Br J Anaesth 87: 415–420.
36. Ngan Kee WD, Khaw KS, Ng FF (2004) Comparison of phenylephrine infusion regimens for maintaining maternal blood pressure during spinal anaesthesia for Caesarean section. Br J Anaesth 92: 469–474.
37. Ngan Kee WD, Khaw KS, Ma KC, Wong AS, Lee BB, et al. (2006) Maternal and neonatal effects of remifentanil at induction of general anesthesia for cesarean delivery: a randomized, double-blind, controlled trial. Anesthesiology 104: 14–20.
38. Kattwinkel J, Perlman JM, Aziz K, Colby C, Fairchild K, et al. (2010) Neonatal resuscitation: 2010 American Heart Association Guidelines for Cardiopulmonary Resuscitation and Emergency Cardiovascular Care. Pediatrics 126: e1400–1413.
39. (2011) 2011 Neonatal Resuscitation Guidelines. Chin J Perinat Med 14: 415–419.
40. Ismail MT, Hassanin MZ (2012) Neuraxial analgesia versus intravenous remifentanil for pain relief in early labor in nulliparous women. Arch Gynecol Obstet 286: 1375–1381.

# Permissions

All chapters in this book were first published in PLOS ONE, by The Public Library of Science; hereby published with permission under the Creative Commons Attribution License or equivalent. Every chapter published in this book has been scrutinized by our experts. Their significance has been extensively debated. The topics covered herein carry significant findings which will fuel the growth of the discipline. They may even be implemented as practical applications or may be referred to as a beginning point for another development.

The contributors of this book come from diverse backgrounds, making this book a truly international effort. This book will bring forth new frontiers with its revolutionizing research information and detailed analysis of the nascent developments around the world.

We would like to thank all the contributing authors for lending their expertise to make the book truly unique. They have played a crucial role in the development of this book. Without their invaluable contributions this book wouldn't have been possible. They have made vital efforts to compile up to date information on the varied aspects of this subject to make this book a valuable addition to the collection of many professionals and students.

This book was conceptualized with the vision of imparting up-to-date information and advanced data in this field. To ensure the same, a matchless editorial board was set up. Every individual on the board went through rigorous rounds of assessment to prove their worth. After which they invested a large part of their time researching and compiling the most relevant data for our readers.

The editorial board has been involved in producing this book since its inception. They have spent rigorous hours researching and exploring the diverse topics which have resulted in the successful publishing of this book. They have passed on their knowledge of decades through this book. To expedite this challenging task, the publisher supported the team at every step. A small team of assistant editors was also appointed to further simplify the editing procedure and attain best results for the readers.

Apart from the editorial board, the designing team has also invested a significant amount of their time in understanding the subject and creating the most relevant covers. They scrutinized every image to scout for the most suitable representation of the subject and create an appropriate cover for the book.

The publishing team has been an ardent support to the editorial, designing and production team. Their endless efforts to recruit the best for this project, has resulted in the accomplishment of this book. They are a veteran in the field of academics and their pool of knowledge is as vast as their experience in printing. Their expertise and guidance has proved useful at every step. Their uncompromising quality standards have made this book an exceptional effort. Their encouragement from time to time has been an inspiration for everyone.

The publisher and the editorial board hope that this book will prove to be a valuable piece of knowledge for researchers, students, practitioners and scholars across the globe.

# List of Contributors

**Enrico Amico**
Coma Science Group, Cyclotron Research Centre, University of Liège, Liège, Belgium
Faculty of Psychology and Educational Sciences, Department of Data Analysis, Ghent University, Ghent, Belgium

**Francisco Gomez and Damien Lesenfants**
Coma Science Group, Cyclotron Research Centre, University of Liège, Liège, Belgium

**Carol Di Perri**
Department of Neuroradiology, National Neurological Institute C. Mondino, Pavia, Italy

**Audrey Vanhaudenhuyse**
Coma Science Group, Cyclotron Research Centre, University of Liège, Liège, Belgium
Department of Algology and Palliative Care, CHU Sart Tilman Hospital, University of Liège, Liège, Belgium

**Pierre Boveroux**
Coma Science Group, Cyclotron Research Centre, University of Liège, Liège, Belgium
Department of Anesthesia and Intensive Care Medicine, CHU Sart Tilman Hospital, University of Liège, Liège, Belgium

**Vincent Bonhomme**
Coma Science Group, Cyclotron Research Centre, University of Liège, Liège, Belgium
Department of Anesthesia and Intensive Care Medicine, CHU Sart Tilman Hospital, University of Liège, Liège, Belgium
Department of Anesthesia and Intensive Care Medicine, CHR Citadelle, University of Liège, Liège, Belgium

**Jean-François Brichant**
Department of Anesthesia and Intensive Care Medicine, CHU Sart Tilman Hospital, University of Liège, Liège, Belgium

**Daniele Marinazzo**
Faculty of Psychology and Educational Sciences, Department of Data Analysis, Ghent University, Ghent, Belgium

**Steven Laureys**
Coma Science Group, Cyclotron Research Centre, University of Liège, Liège, Belgium
Department of Neurology, University of Liège, Liège, Belgium

**Cihun-Siyong Alex Gong**
Department of Electrical Engineering, School of Electrical and Computer Engineering, College of Engineering, Chang Gung University, Taoyuan, Taiwan
Portable Energy System Group, Green Technology Research Center, College of Engineering, Chang Gung University, Taoyuan, Taiwan

**Shih-Pin Lin, Mei-Yung Tsou and Chien-Kun Ting**
Department of Anesthesiology, Taipei Veterans General Hospital and National Yang-Ming University, Taipei, Taiwan

**M. Susan Mandell**
Department of Anesthesiology, University of Colorado Health Sciences Center, Aurora, Colorado, United States of America

**Yin Chang**
Institute of Biomedical Engineering, National Yang-Ming University, Taipei, Taiwan

**Stéphane Cullati, Patricia Francis and Pierre Chopard**
Quality of care service, University Hospitals of Geneva, Geneva, Switzerland

**Marc-Joseph Licker**
Division of anesthesiology, University Hospitals of Geneva, Geneva, Switzerland

**Adriana Degiorg**
Quality of care unit, Ente Ospedaliero Cantonale, Lugano, Switzerland

**Paula Bezzola**
Patient Safety Foundation Switzerland, Zürich, Switzerland

**Delphine S. Courvoisier**
Division of clinical epidemiology, University Hospitals of Geneva, Geneva, Switzerland

**Seetharamaiah Attili and Simon M. Hughes**
Randall Division of Cell and Molecular Biophysics, Guy's Campus, King's College London, London, United Kingdom

**Juscimar C. Nunes, Jose R. C. Braz, Thais S. Oliveira, Yara M. M. Castiglia and Leandro G. Braz**
Department of Anesthesiology, Botucatu Medical School, UNESP - Univ Estadual Paulista, Botucatu, São Paulo, Brazil

**Lidia R. de Carvalho**
Department of Biostatistics, Institute of Biosciences, UNESP - Univ Estadual Paulista, Botucatu, São Paulo, Brazil

**Tewodros Eyob Woldehaimanot and Tesfahun Chanie Eshetie**
Department of Pharmacy, Jimma University, Jimma, Ethiopia

**Mirkuzie Woldie Kerie**
Department of Health Services Management, Jimma University, Jimma, Ethiopia

**Olav Reikerå**
Institute of Clinical Medicine, Rikshospitalet, Oslo University Hospital, Oslo, Norway

**Pål Borgen**
Martina Hansens Hospital, Oslo, Norway

**Michel Chandon, Yannick Burg, Véronique DesMesnards-Smaja, Christine Foiret, Marc Fischler and Morgan Le Guen**
Department of Anesthesiology, Hôpital Foch, Suresnes, France

**Agnès Bonnet, Carole Barnichon, Brigitte Sitbon and Jamil Rahmani**
Department of Anesthesiology, Institut Hospitalier Franco-Britannique, Levallois-Perret, France

**Jean-François Dreyfus**
Department of Clinical Research and Innovation, Hôpital Foch, Suresnes, France

**Pierre-Antoine Laloë**
Department of Health Education, Bradford Teaching Hospitals, Leeds, United Kingdom

**Carlos M. Acevedo-Arcique, José A. Ibancovichi, Julio R. Chavez, Rafael Moran-Muñoz and Pedro Sanchez-Aparicio**
Department of Anaesthesia and Analgesia, Faculty of Veterinary Medicine, Universidad Autónoma del Estado de México, Toluca, State of Mexico, Mexico

**Eduardo Gutierrez-Blanco**
Department of Animal Health and Preventive Medicine, Faculty of Veterinary Medicine, Universidad Autónoma de Yucatán, Merida, State of Yucatan, Mexico

**José M. Victoria-Mora**
Department of Orthopaedic Surgery and Trauma, Faculty of Veterinary Medicine, Universidad Autónoma del Estado de México, Toluca, State of Mexico, Mexico

**Francisco Tendillo-Cortijo and Martín Santos-González**
Hospital Universitario Clínica Puerta de Hierro, Madrid, España

**Hyungseok Seo, Dong-Min Jang, Jung-Min Yi, Hong-Gi Min and Jai-Hyun Hwang**
Department of Anesthesiology and Pain Medicine, Asan Medical Center, University of Ulsan College of Medicine, Seoul, Republic of Korea

**Carlana Ramlochansingh, Francisco Branoner, Boris P. Chagnaud and Hans Straka**
Department Biology II, Ludwig-Maximilians-University Munich, Planegg, Germany

**Hamed Bahmani and Georgios A. Keliris**
Max Planck Institute for Biological Cybernetics, Tübingen, Germany
Bernstein Center for Computational Neuroscience, Tübingen, Germany

**Yusuke Murayama**
Max Planck Institute for Biological Cybernetics, Tübingen, Germany

**Nikos K. Logothetis**
Max Planck Institute for Biological Cybernetics, Tübingen, Germany
Imaging Science and Biomedical Engineering, University of Manchester, Manchester, United Kingdom

**John V. Roughan, Claire A. Coulter and Paul A. Flecknell**
Comparative Biology Centre, The Medical School, University of Newcastle, Newcastle upon Tyne, United Kingdom

**Huw D. Thomas**
Northern Institute for Cancer Research, The Medical School, University of Newcastle, Newcastle upon Tyne, United Kingdom

**Kenneth J. Sufka**
Research Institute of Pharmaceutical Sciences and Departments of Psychology and Pharmacology, Peabody Building, University of Mississippi, Oxford, Mississippi, United States of America

**Jakub Toczek, Alexis Broisat, Pascale Perret, Marie-Dominique Desruet, Daniel Fagret,Laurent M. Riou and Catherine Ghezzi**
INSERM, UMR 1039, Radiopharmaceutiques Biocliniques; Université Grenoble I, La Tronche, France

**Bradley H. Lee, John Thomas Chan, Obhi Hazarika and Jeffrey W. Sall**
Department of Anesthesia and Perioperative Care, University of California San Francisco, San Francisco, California, Unites States of America

**Laszlo Vutskits**
Department of Anesthesiology, Pharmacology and Intensive Care, University Hospital of Geneva, Geneva, Switzerland

**Herve Delacour and Isabelle Mabboux**
Bégin Military Teaching Hospital, Department of Biology, Unit of Human Genetics, Saint Mandé, France

**Sofya Lushchekina**
Modeling of Biomolecules Lab., N.M. Emanuel Institute of Biochemical Physics, Russian Academy of Sciences, Moscow, Russia

**Aurore Bousquet and Franck Ceppa**
Bégin Military Teaching Hospital, Department of Biology, Unit of Human Genetics, Saint Mandé, France
Val de Grace Military Medical School, Paris, France

**Lawrence M. Schopfer and Oksana Lockridge**
Eppley Institute, University of Nebraska Medical Center, Omaha, Nebraska, United States of America

**Patrick Masson**
Eppley Institute, University of Nebraska Medical Center, Omaha, Nebraska, United States of America
DYNAMOP, Institut de Biologie Structurale, Grenoble, France

**Neil J. Spratt**
School of Biomedical Sciences, University of Newcastle, and Hunter Medical Research Institute, Newcastle, Australia
Hunter New England Local Health District, Newcastle, Australia

**Amelia J. Tomkins, Debbie Pepperall and Damian D. McLeod**
School of Biomedical Sciences, University of Newcastle, and Hunter Medical Research Institute, Newcastle, Australia

**Mike B. Calford**
School of Biomedical Sciences, University of Newcastle, and Hunter Medical Research Institute, Newcastle, Australia
School of Medicine, The University of Tasmania, Hobart, Australia

**Anna R. Gagliardi**
University Health Network, Toronto, Ontario, Canada

**Sharon E. Straus**
St. Michael's Hospital, Toronto, Ontario, Canada

**Kaveh G. Shojania**
Sunnybrook Health Sciences Centre, Toronto, Ontario, Canada

**David R. Urbach**
University Health Network, Toronto, Ontario, Canada

**Stephanie Seah, Abu Bakar Ali Asad and Chih-Liang Chin**
Imaging, Merck & Co. Inc., West Point, Pennsylvania, United States of America
Translational Medicine Research Centre, MSD, Singapore, Singapore

**Richard Baumgartner and Dai Feng**
Biostatistics and Research Decision Sciences, Merck & Co. Inc., Rahway, New Jersey, United States of America

**Donald S. Williams and Jeffrey L. Evelhoch**
Imaging, Merck & Co. Inc., West Point, Pennsylvania, United States of America

**Elaine Manigbas and John D. Beaver**
Imaging, Maccine Pte Ltd, Singapore, Singapore

**Torsten Reese and Brian Henry**
Translational Medicine Research Centre, MSD, Singapore, Singapore

**Luciana M. Camilo, Mariana B. Ávila, Luis Felipe S. Cruz and Walter A. Zin**
Laboratory of Respiration Physiology, Carlos Chagas Filho Institute of Biophysics, Universidade Federal do Rio de Janeiro, Rio de Janeiro, Brazil

**Gabriel C. M. Ribeiro and Antonio Giannella-Neto**
Laboratory of Pulmonary Engineering, Biomedical Engineering Program, Alberto Luis Coimbra Institute of Post-Graduation and Research in Engineering, Universidade Federal do Rio de Janeiro, Rio de Janeiro, Brazil

**Peter M. Spieth**
Pulmonary Engineering Group, Department of Anesthesiology and Intensive Care Medicine, Technische Universität Dresden, Germany

**Andreas A. Reske**
Department of Anesthesiology and Intensive Care Medicine, University of Leipzig, Leipzig, Germany

**Marcelo Amato**
Cardio-Pulmonary Department, Pulmonary Division, Hospital das Clínicas, Universidade de São Paulo, São Paulo, Brazil
Luciana M. Camilo, Mariana B. Ávila, Luis Felipe S. Cruz and Walter A. Zin
Laboratory of Respiration Physiology, Carlos Chagas Filho Institute of Biophysics, Universidade Federal do Rio de Janeiro, Rio de Janeiro, Brazil

**Gabriel C. M. Ribeiro and Antonio Giannella-Neto**
Laboratory of Pulmonary Engineering, Biomedical Engineering Program, Alberto Luis Coimbra Institute of Post-Graduation and Research in Engineering, Universidade Federal do Rio de Janeiro, Rio de Janeiro, Brazil

**Peter M. Spieth**
Pulmonary Engineering Group, Department of Anesthesiology and Intensive Care Medicine, Technische Universität Dresden, Germany

**Andreas A. Reske**
Department of Anesthesiology and Intensive Care Medicine, University of Leipzig, Leipzig, Germany

**Marcelo Amato**
Cardio-Pulmonary Department, Pulmonary Division, Hospital das Clínicas, Universidade de São Paulo, São Paulo, Brazil

**Alysson R. Carvalho**
Laboratory of Respiration Physiology, Carlos Chagas Filho Institute of Biophysics, Universidade Federal do Rio de Janeiro, Rio de Janeiro, Brazil
Laboratory of Pulmonary Engineering, Biomedical Engineering Program, Alberto Luis Coimbra Institute of Post-Graduation and Research in Engineering, Universidade Federal do Rio de Janeiro, Rio de Janeiro, Brazil

**Matthäus Ernstbrunner, Lisa Kostner, Oliver Kimberger, Klaus Markstaller, Edith Fleischmann and Barbara Kabon**
Medical University of Vienna, Department of Anaesthesiology and Critical Care Medicine, Vienna, Austria

**Peter Wabel**
Fresenius Medical Care, Bad Homburg, Germany

**Marcus Säemann**
Medical University of Vienna, Department of Internal Medicine III, Clinical Division of Nephrology & Dialysis, Vienna, Austria

**Manfred Hecking**
Medical University of Vienna, Department of Anaesthesiology and Critical Care Medicine, Vienna, Austria
Medical University of Vienna, Department of Internal Medicine III, Clinical Division of Nephrology & Dialysis, Vienna, Austria

**Zhenhong Zou and Yuming Jiang**
Department of General Surgery, Nanfang Hospital, Southern Medical University, Guangzhou City, Guangdong Province, China

**Mingjia Xiao**
Department of Hepatobiliary Surgery, Wuxi People's Hospital of Nanjing Medical University, Wuxi, Jiangsu Province, China

**Ruiyao Zhou**
Department of General Surgery, The Third Affiliated Hospital of Wenzhou Medical University, Ruian City, Zhejiang Province, China

**Parag N. Gad and Hui Zhong**
Department of Integrative Biology and Physiology, University of California Los Angeles, Los Angeles, California, United States of America

**Roland R. Roy**
Department of Integrative Biology and Physiology, University of California Los Angeles, Los Angeles, California, United States of America
Brain Research Institute, University of California Los Angeles, Los Angeles, California, United States of America

**Daniel C. Lu**
Department of Neurosurgery, University of California Los Angeles, Los Angeles, California, United States of America

**Yury P. Gerasimenko**
Department of Integrative Biology and Physiology, University of California Los Angeles, Los Angeles, California, United States of America
Pavlov Institute of Physiology, St. Petersburg, Russia

**V. Reggie Edgerton**
Department of Integrative Biology and Physiology, University of California Los Angeles, Los Angeles, California, United States of America
Department of Neurobiology, University of California Los Angeles, Los Angeles, California, United States of America
Department of Neurosurgery, University of California Los Angeles, Los Angeles, California, United States of America
Brain Research Institute, University of California Los Angeles, Los Angeles, California, United States of America

**Alysson R. Carvalho**
Laboratory of Respiration Physiology, Carlos Chagas Filho Institute of Biophysics, Universidade Federal do Rio de Janeiro, Rio de Janeiro, Brazil
Laboratory of Pulmonary Engineering, Biomedical Engineering Program, Alberto Luis Coimbra Institute of Post-Graduation and Research in Engineering, Universidade Federal do Rio de Janeiro, Rio de Janeiro, Brazil

**Pia Jæger, Zbigniew J. Koscielniak-Nielsen, Maria H. Henningsen and Jørgen B. Dahl**
Department of Anaesthesia, Centre of Head and Orthopaedics, Copenhagen University Hospital, Rigshospitalet, Copenhagen, Denmark

**Henrik M. Schrøder**
Department of Orthopaedic Surgery, Centre of Head and Orthopaedics, Copenhagen University Hospital, Rigshospitalet, Copenhagen, Denmark

**Ole Mathiesen**
Section of Acute Pain Management, Department of Anaesthesia, Centre of Head and Orthopaedics, Copenhagen University Hospital, Rigshospitalet, Copenhagen, Denmark

**Jørgen Lund and Morten T. Jenstrup**
Department of Anaesthesia, Aleris-Hamlet Hospitals, Copenhagen, Denmark

**Divya Chander**
Department of Anesthesiology, Perioperative and Pain Medicine, Stanford University School of Medicine, Stanford, California, United States of America

**Paul S. García**
Department of Anesthesiology, Atlanta VA Medical Center/Emory University, Atlanta, Georgia, United States of America

**Jono N. MacColl, Sam Illing and Jamie W. Sleigh**
Department of Anaesthesia, Waikato Clinical School, University of Auckland, Hamilton, New Zealand

**Rong Lin, Yiyi Tao, Yibing Yu, Zhendong Xu, Jing Su and Zhiqiang Liu**
Department of Anaesthesiology, Shanghai First Maternity and Infant Hospital, Tongji University School of Medicine, Shanghai, China

# Index

www.ingramcontent.com/pod-product-compliance
Lightning Source LLC
LaVergne TN
LVHW080723210926
848485LV00003B/513
* 9 7 8 1 6 3 2 4 1 5 2 6 4 *